TWELFTH EDITION

LANGE Q&A™

RADIOGRAPHY EXAMINATION

D. A. Saia, MA, RT(R)(M)
Radiography Educator and Consultant
Adjunct Professor, Concordia College
Bronxville, New York

Mc
Graw
Hill
Education

New York   Chicago   San Francisco   Athens   London   Madrid
Mexico City   Milan   New Delhi   Singapore   Sydney   Toronto

Lange Q&A™: Radiography Examination, Twelfth Edition

Previous editions Copyright © 2018, 2016, 2012, 2011, 2008, 2006 by The McGraw Hill Companies, Inc.
Lange Q&A™ is a trademark of McGraw Hill.

7 8 9 10 11 LBC 28 27 26 25

ISBN 978-1-260-46044-5
MHID 1-260-46044-4

Notice

Medicine is an ever-changing science. As new research and clinical experience broaden our knowledge, changes in treatment and drug therapy are required. The authors and the publisher of this work have checked with sources believed to be reliable in their efforts to provide information that is complete and generally in accord with the standards accepted at the time of publication. However, in view of the possibility of human error or changes in medical sciences, neither the authors nor the publisher nor any other party who has been involved in the preparation or publication of this work warrants that the information contained herein is in every respect accurate or complete, and they disclaim all responsibility for any errors or omissions or for the results obtained from use of the information contained in this work. Readers are encouraged to confirm the information contained herein with other sources. For example and in particular, readers are advised to check the product information sheet included in the package of each drug they plan to administer to be certain that the information contained in this work is accurate and that changes have not been made in the recommended dose or in the contraindications for administration. This recommendation is of particular importance in connection with new or infrequently used drugs.

This book was set in Minion Pro by Graphic World, Inc.
The editors were Bob Boehringer and Christie Naglieri.
The production supervisor was Rick Ruzycka.
Project management was provided by Graphic World, Inc.
The cover designer was W2 Design.

Library of Congress Cataloging-in-Publication Data

Names: Saia, D. A. (Dorothy A.), author.
Title: Lange Q & A. Radiography examination / D.A. Saia.
Other titles: Lange Q and A. Radiography examination
Description: Twelfth edition. | New York : McGraw Hill, [2020] | Includes bibliographical references and index. | Summary: "The review resource known as the "yellow Lange book" has become known as the most reliable way to study for the ARRT Radiography exam - our questions set us apart. Includes a total of 1,400 questions, all at a level and in a format that most closely mirror the items found on the actual ARRT exam. All questions include detailed answers, with rationale for both correct And incorrect answers. Content is organized in a way that reflects the content categories of the ARRT exam, while the number of questions in each category parallels the exam as well. NEW! Four color design makes the presentation more visually appealing and increases the utility of the illustrations. NEW! Illustrations will be added in key areas, such as veins, body mechanics, needle positions and body positions. New x-ray images will be added to ensure all images are clear and relevant"—Provided by publisher.
Identifiers: LCCN 2020015001 | ISBN 9781260460445 (paperback) | ISBN 1260460444 (paperback) | ISBN 9781260460452 (ebook)
Subjects: MESH: Radiography | Technology, Radiologic | Examination Questions
Classification: LCC RC78 | NLM WN 18.2 | DDC 616.07/572—dc23
LC record available at https://lccn.loc.gov/2020015001

The following figures were originally published in Saia DA, Radiography PREP: Program Review and Examination Preparation, 9th ed., New York: McGraw Hill, 2018, and are reproduced with permission from McGraw Hill: Figures 2-2, 2-54, 2-55, 2-57, 2-63, 3-6, 3-11, 4-11, 4-24, 5-1, 5-10, 5-13 and 6-24.

McGraw Hill books are available at special quantity discounts to use as premiums and sales promotions, or for use in corporate training programs. To contact a representative please visit the Contact Us page at www.mhprofessional.com.

TWELFTH EDITION

LANGE Q&A™

RADIOGRAPHY
EXAMINATION

Spiritus Sancti gratia,
illuminet sensus et corda nostra.

REVIEWERS

Gloria Albrecht, MS, RT(R)
Program Director
Radiology, CT, MRI
Cleveland Clinic
Cleveland, Ohio

Deanna Butcher, MA, RT(R)
Program Director
School of Diagnostic Imaging
St. Cloud Hospital
St. Cloud, Minnesota

Isaak Miroshenko, MA, RT(R)(CT)
Program Director—Radiography Program
Center for Allied Health Education
Brooklyn, New York

Olive Peart, MS, RT(R)(M)
Radiologic Technology Program Chair
Fortis College
Landover, Maryland

Yana Strochkova, MHS, RT(R)
Instructor—Radiography
Center for Allied Health Education
Brooklyn, New York

CONTENTS

Your feedback on the previous 11 editions of this book has been inspiring and appreciated, and I have enjoyed correspondence with so many of you.

I hope that all who use this book, its companion book *Radiography PREP*, and companion RadReview (at radreviewmhe.com)—educators and students alike—will continue to provide feedback in order that these tools will continue to meet their needs. I invite and encourage you to contact me through McGraw Hill or at dasaia921@yahoo.com with comments, questions, and suggestions for future editions of these learning materials.

The twelfth edition of this *Radiography Q&A* contains new and revised material to reflect changes in the American Registry of Radiologic Technologists (ARRT) Content Specifications published in January 2016 and implemented in January 2017. Exciting new features of this twelfth edition include color illustrations to enhance visualization and improve study effectiveness. New question formats similar to those used by ARRT have been added to improve comprehensive knowledge assessment. The Content Specifications for Examination in Radiography lists the examination's four content categories and provides a detailed list of the topics addressed in each category. *Radiography Q&A* is divided into sections reflecting these four content categories. This edition divides the Safety and Image Production sections into two separate sections, Image Acquisition and Technical Evaluation and Equipment Operation and Quality Assurance, for more focused study. Some very basic introductory CT material is also included—an area becoming increasingly important for the entry-level radiographer. As this field continues to grow, there is increasing need to include its fundamentals in the radiography curriculum. Particularly important is updated and expanded content in digital imaging. Obsolete content has been deleted. SI units are used exclusively, with occasional equivalent traditional unit of measure provided for reference. Thus, study is principally directed and focused on examination-related material.

You have provided us with a very favorable response to the companion online adaptive question bank: *RadReview*. I was very excited about its original implementation and recent updating of this personalized learning tool, and your response has confirmed its usefulness. In addition, *RadReview* has given me the enjoyable opportunity to "meet" so many more of you online.

Robust performance profile of *RadReview* allows users to track their results performance by topic and test scores over time and to compare their scores to others using *RadReview*, including test-takers at the users' specific institutions.

Customization features allow *Students* to:

- Choose the length and subject areas of a test or create a set of randomly selected questions.
- Retake tests composed of questions previously answered incorrectly so they can focus on weak areas.
- Time tests or practice at their own pace.
- Take tests composed of questions that they are seeing for the first time.
- Create a Personal Study Plan which will support their test preparation and allow them to progress according to their customized study plan.

If an institution or program subscribes to *RadReview*, its *Instructors* are able to:

- Access the Instructor Reporting Tool.
- Track individual student's progress.
- Generate reports on class activity or subject area performance.
- Generate assignments for classes or specific students.

RadReview affords students the opportunity to practice CBT prior to taking the computerized ARRT examination. Visit radreviewmhe.com for information about pricing and subscription terms.

I know you realize that review books are not intended to be a "quick fix" preparation for the certification examination administered by the ARRT. It takes at least 2 years of didactic instruction and testing, and hours of clinical practice, to prepare oneself as an entry-level radiographer. During about the last 4 months of radiography education, the actual certification examination becomes a rather scary anticipation. Confident, competent, even cavalier students suddenly become solemn when "the Registry" is mentioned. They begin to question all they ever felt confident about. If you use this book the way it is designed to be used, and perhaps in conjunction with its companion learning tools—RadReview and *Radiography PREP (Program Review and Examination Preparation)*—you should be able to set aside any fears you may have.

I believe that proper use of this text, and its companion tools, will help you overcome your anxieties. First, read the *introductory section* carefully. It presents proven, sensible suggestions to help improve test-taking performance. It elaborates on simple processes to help selection of the correct answer, and several methods and strategies that may be used while taking "the" test. Probably the most important key to reducing apprehension is to reduce the unknowns to the fewest number. You will also find an introduction to CBT with a description of what to expect, and helpful hints to enhance preparation and reduce anxiety. Second, the format and content of the book and the questions on *RadReview* have been specially designed to provide focus and direction for your review, and thus to help you do your very best on your certification examination. Every student and educational program has access to the ARRT online, where they publish regular updates to keep educators and students current on activities and policies. The ARRT publishes its policies and procedures, handbooks, and several other documents that are useful to educators and students in preparation for the certification examination: *Content Specifications for the Examination in Radiography, Standard Terminology for Positioning and Protection, Standard Definitions*—as well as information on accreditation, ethics review pre-application, certification and registration eligibility, advanced placement, brochures, and handbooks. These documents are revised periodically and advise educators and students of terminology, categories, content, and approximate weight of content areas on the ARRT examination. Although the *Content Specifications* by no means serves as a comprehensive radiography curriculum, it does serve as a suitable guide for examination review and preparation. It makes sense to design a review book in which the content, question format, and terminology are similar to that which students can expect to find on their certification examination.

The number of questions found in each chapter here is proportional to the number found in that category on the actual ARRT examination. The questions are designed to test your problem-solving skills and your ability to integrate facts that fit the situation.

Most important and practical are the detailed explanations found at the end of each chapter. *By themselves, many explanations are good reviews of essential material; they provide a "mini-lecture" for each question.* Use them to confirm your correct answers and to better understand your weaker areas. You will see that most explanations will tell you not only why the correct answer is correct but also why the other answer choices (distractors) are incorrect. *Radiography PREP* can be used either *before* this book—as a review of the material this book will test you on—or *with* this book to help you strengthen particular essential areas of study. Similarly, *RadReview* can be used for supplemental study and review.

Once you have finished reviewing the first five chapters, set aside special time for the practice tests in Chapters 6 and 7. Try to simulate the actual examination environment as much as possible. Choose a quiet place free from distractions and interruptions, gather the necessary materials, and arrange to be uninterrupted for up to 3 h.

In summary, use this book as recommended to help ease your precertification examination jitters. *Excessive anxiety can impair clear thinking and lower your score.* Avoiding excessive stress can improve your concentration and information retrieval process. Remember, you have been well prepared by your program director and instructors, and you have studied and worked hard for at least 2 years. So follow the advice found in the Introduction: Prepare yourself sensibly and keep a positive attitude. I totally agree with a remark the famous automaker Henry Ford once made: *"Whether you think you can or whether you think you can't, you're right!"*

I wish you much satisfaction and success in our wonderful profession!

D. A. Saia

ACKNOWLEDGMENTS

Once again, it is a pleasure to recognize and express my sincere appreciation to those who have been so helpful and supportive during the preparation of this twelfth edition.

I am grateful to all the professional staff of McGraw Hill; it is always a pleasure to work with their creative and skilled staff. There would be no twelfth edition without their expert direction and support. Special appreciation is expressed to my editors Rhiannon Wong, Bob Boehringer, and Madison Tucky, who are so generously understanding and supportive. Thank you also to the wonderful project development team of Christie Naglieri and Richard Ruzycka. Jason McAlexander, Biomedical Media Manager at MPS North America LLC developed wonderful color figures for this edition; thank you for your time and patience. Julie Mangoff, Project Manager at Graphic World, Inc., developed a timeline for timely publishing schedule. I had not worked with Julie or Jason before—they have been fantastic to work with; thank you both so very much! An outstanding group of reviewers was recruited for this edition of *Lange Q&A: Radiography Examination*. Gloria Albrecht, Deanna Butcher, Isaak Miroshenko, Olive Peart, and Yana Strochkova are all invaluable resources to the health care and the radiologic imaging communities. They reviewed the manuscript and offered suggestions to improve style and remove ambiguities and inaccuracies. Their participation on this project is deeply appreciated.

A special thank you to Rob Fabrizio and Gregg Cretella of FUJIFILM Medical Systems USA, Inc., for their correspondence, information, and virtual grid images. Several of the new images found in this new edition are contributed by Jayme Shleckler, RT(R), MS of Orthopedic +Fracture Specialists, Portland, OR. Many thanks to Jayme for her support!

Many of the images are reproduced here through the courtesy of Stamford Hospital, Department of Radiology. A number of images found in Image Acquisition and Evaluation have been reproduced through the courtesy of American College of Radiology. A special thank you is also to Conrad P. Ehrlich, MD, for images added to this book and to *Radiography PREP*.

Appreciative and affectionate acknowledgment to all my students—past, present, and those still to come. Their questions, enthusiasm, and desire to learn not only make my job a most pleasant task but also served as the original stimulus for the preparation of this text. Special acknowledgment goes out to the outstanding and supportive faculty of the Concordia College Program in Radiologic Technologies—Dan Sorrentino, MS, RT(R), Program Director; Thai Chan-Grullon, MS, RT(R)(M)(CT), Assistant Professor and Clinical Coordinator; Gregory Torsiello, MS, RT(R)(CT), Assistant Professor and Clinical Instructor. They are wonderful professionals and wonderful friends.

Finally, and most specially, a loving message of appreciation to my husband Tony—the most loving husband in this world. The preparation and revision of two books and a companion website is extraordinarily time-consuming. His love and encouragement (and cooking!) are deeply appreciated throughout the preparation of this, and every edition. I am so proud to be his wife.

D. A. Saia

Completion of the ARRT radiography certification examination is a high point in the career of a radiologic professional. Certification indicates that the individual has acquired a recognized level of knowledge and expertise and is qualified to deliver ionizing radiation in the performance of medical diagnostic testing. On what does success or failure depend?

Relax! It is not as bad as it seems! As the student radiographer nears graduation, there is, understandably, an anxiety that begins to grow. It is a time when you wonder if you are smart enough and if you are skillful enough. Although there will always be room for growth, these concerns arise from the realization that an important landmark has been reached. Formal education will soon be at an end—no more written examinations and no more clinical competencies to complete. You will be on your own, proclaimed competent. How will you perform on the certification examination? How will you perform in the clinical arena? These are indeed sobering thoughts.

Use of the materials presented here is intended to help you overcome your anxieties. You will find several easy and effective suggestions for intelligent preparation and test taking. The suggestions are proven, sensible recommendations to help improve test-taking performance. They elaborate on simple processes to help in selection of the correct answer, and several methods and strategies that may be used while taking your certification examination. Probably the most important key to reducing apprehension is to *reduce the unknowns to the fewest number*.

The format and content of this review book are specially designed to provide focus and direction for your review, thus helping you do your very best on the certification examination. The format and content are based on published ARRT certification examination content, question format, and terminology.

HOW THIS BOOK IS ORGANIZED

There are three primary sections in this book: a topic-by-topic *review* with 1400+ examination-type questions and paragraph-length *explanations*; two 200-question *practice* tests, also with paragraph-length explanations; and this *Introduction*, which includes information necessary to help you get the most out of the book and to do your best on the certification examination.

In addition, its companion *RadReviewEasy.com* has additional questions and answers for further practice in simulated certification conditions; visit the site for pricing and subscription terms.

In summary, this book will provide you, the student, with a review that will better enable you to simulate and prepare for the certification examination by providing an excellent and comprehensive review of radiography.

BEFORE THE EXAMINATION

Pearson VUE testing centers currently administer the ARRT examination. There is no postmarking deadline for ARRT examination applications. Applicants may apply for the examination prior to graduation, but will schedule their examination date within an assigned 90-day window that starts at graduation. Once the ARRT application is processed, and the applicant deemed eligible, the ARRT sends the candidate their CSR—Candidate Status Report. The CSR indicates the candidates' ARRT number and their examination "window" dates. Most educators advise taking the certification examination shortly after completing all didactic and clinical requirements.

It is essential to carefully read the ARRT Radiography Handbook. It describes in detail all the essential testing information required before, during, and after the actual test. Failure to follow the required steps can result in forfeiture of test appointment, application fee, and require reapplication.

ARRT certification examinations are administered at Pearson VUE test centers. To schedule your examination, you will need your ARRT ID from the CSR. Several types of examinations are administered at these test centers. If you believe keyboard sounds might distract you, you are encouraged to request earplugs prior to entering the examination room. They offer a pair of earplugs, upon request, before you enter the room. If you decline the earplugs, you can use a noise-cancelling headset, with clean covers, that is found near your computer.

As noted later in this section, you should plan to arrive at least 15 min early. Many test centers require you to be there 30 min ahead of the scheduled test time. If you are 15 min late, you run the risk of forfeiting your appointment time, and being required to reapply.

Be prepared to show at least two forms of identification, one of which must be government-issued photo ID (e.g., driver's license, state ID card, and passport).

Security requirements upon entry at the examination site include a photograph, digital signature, and palm vein scanning. This process will verify your identity when you check-in, and your identity will be verified a second time before you enter the examination room. You may be asked to pat yourself down and to show both sides of your arms. If you wear glasses, you may be asked to place them on the counter so they can be examined for devices or notes.

Paper, pencils, and so on are not permitted in the examination room—an erasable board and pen are provided. You are not permitted to erase the board during the examination, but are allowed to raise your hand to request another board if you run out of space. A calculator is available on the test computer, or you may request a simple four-function calculator from the test center. Because there are various examinations taking place at the same time, the Testing Center Proctor may not be aware of your needs—be certain to take full responsibility to prepare yourself, otherwise you may not have the necessary supplies. If you have any request/problem during the test, you should raise your hand for assistance (e.g., screen brightness needs adjustment, other problem with computer, or you need earplugs).

ABOUT THE EXAMINATION

The national certification examination for radiography is a standardized test administered by the ARRT and includes 220 multiple-choice questions; 200 questions are scored and 20 questions are unidentified pilot questions. The time allotted for the test is 3½ h; passing score is 75%. Total time, including tutorial and survey, is 4 h.

There is a 20-min tutorial before the start of the examination and a 10-min survey after completion of the examination. Candidates are presented with multiple-choice questions on a computer screen and directed to select an answer using either the keyboard or a mouse. The process allows candidates to review or change any answers to any questions prior to submitting the completed examination for scoring. The tutorial offered at the beginning of the examination allows the candidate to answer several practice questions. This ensures that the candidate is thoroughly familiar with the process.

Multiple-choice questions are presented on the computer screen and the candidate is directed to select the best answer—the mouse or keyboard may be used. There are other types of questions in addition to typical multiple-choice questions. *Select-multiple* questions require you to select all correct options from a list of four to eight possible responses. *Sorted-list* questions require you to place

in order a given list of four to eight options. *Illustration* questions require you to identify numbered labels on an illustration/figure. *Images with "hot spots"* require you to *click on* a particular spot or region. *Videos* require that you view a (silent) video, then answer the question that follows. Videos provide you with a control bar that allows to *play, pause, stop,* and *loop.*

You are able to review any questions you have flagged at the end of the examination before you submit your answers. You may also review any other question by clicking on its number.

STRATEGIES FOR STUDYING AND TEST TAKING

The purpose of a test strategy is to make the most of your knowledge, although no strategy, however elaborate, can help you if you do not know your subject.

A good test strategy can do the following:

1. Prevent you from making mistakes.
2. Help you to use your time efficiently.
3. Improve your odds of getting the right answer.

The single most important trait of a good test strategy is *simplicity*. There are two ways to make and keep a procedure simple—the first way is to design it to be simple; the second is to practice the procedure as it is designed. The second part is up to you. If you use the following test strategies (particularly the elimination strategy) while using this review book, the strategies will become second nature to you, and you can then concentrate all your attention on passing your certification examination.

PREPARING FOR THE EXAMINATION

Designing a Study Schedule

It is important to establish a routine study schedule. This schedule should allow you to study at a time when you are at your optimum. Some students are more alert in the morning for this kind of work, whereas others have better success in the afternoon. It would not be a good plan to try and study late at night after a full day unless this is an optimum time for you.

There are several advantages to designing a schedule. The first is that it forces you to face the reality of your study load. Many students underplay the amount of time it will take to complete a thorough study, and this can adversely affect their performance. If you write out a schedule that includes both your daily responsibilities and the time you need to study, you will have a sense of the pace needed to complete your review. The second advantage to designing a schedule is that it will allow you to increase your concentration because the schedule defines the allotted amount of time for each topic you need to cover. Otherwise, a lot of time can be wasted in determining what to study during each session.

Setting up a Study Plan

After completing the best of radiography programs, even the best of students will have gaps in their knowledge, subjects that were somehow missed or forgotten, or that will not come to mind when needed. These gaps in your knowledge are often small; but one piece of information often builds upon other pieces, so a small gap in your knowledge can sometimes lead to a large drop in your test score. The best way to get around this problem is to use a well-defined study plan. Two alternative plans are listed below for you to consider. The first is *diagnosis and remediation*, and the second is *SQ3R*.

Diagnosis and Remediation

This is a two-step approach: *diagnosis* (finding out what you do not know) and *remediation* (learning the material).

Diagnosis. Many students graduate from their programs without a good idea of what they do or do not know. This book has been designed to make diagnosis simple. By following the steps listed in the following text, you will know what you need to learn before you take the certifying examination.

Step 1. Begin with Chapter 1, Patient Care, or any of the other first five chapters. Go through the questions in one sitting, making the experience as similar to the actual examination as possible. Remember to practice test strategies while answering the questions. This will produce a more valid diagnosis.

While taking the test, you should note or highlight words and phrases from the questions that you do not understand. After you have finished the questions (but before you have graded your work), make a list of the terms you noted and the numbers of the questions that contained them.

Step 2. Analyze your results. Read the answers and make a list of the questions you missed. Compare this list with the subspecialty list at the end of the chapter. This will tell you if you are weak in a particular area. Once you have defined an area of weakness, pay special attention to the explanations provided. If the answer is still unclear, you can research the material in *Radiography PREP* or one of your other texts; you can also follow up with a classmate or one of your professors.

Anytime you go through your work, picking out and correcting your mistakes, you will gain a greater understanding of your strengths and weaknesses. However, by approaching the analysis systematically, the improvement can be dramatic. Concentrate on your areas of weakness, but be sure to read all the explanations at least once. This will allow you to compare your reasoning on right and wrong answers and to check for the possibility that you put down the right answer for the wrong reason.

Step 3. Repeat the process. The purpose of this study plan is to get important information into your long-term memory. The best way to ensure this is to begin your study plan early enough to allow yourself time to repeat your chapter study one more time before the examination. Keep and compare your results from each review and focus on any weaknesses still apparent from the comparison.

Remediation.

Step 1. Read and cross-read. Starting with the subspecialty that you missed most often, make a reading list. For those areas in which you missed three or four questions, a single reference will probably be enough, but if you missed more than four, you should cross-read to cover the same information in more than one text. (You might also want to review these topics in your old class notes.)

When you study from texts, use the index and the table of contents to find the section you need. If you are using more than one text, compare and look for common ideas. Sometimes, writing a summary of your reading helps to clarify the information. This technique has been proven to improve retention and understanding, but it can be time-consuming.

Step 2. Once you have finished your reading, go back to the questions that you missed. If they still are not clear, consult an expert. Most students are reluctant to approach an instructor with a question that does not relate directly to a class. However, most instructors are glad to answer questions that will improve the chances for their students to obtain a high passing score on the certification examination. Instructors appreciate questions that are specific, well thought out, and which show that the student has done some independent work.

SQ3R

This second method for study is best suited for reviewing your textbooks for further study once you have identified a weakness. It is called the SQ3R and is presented by Frances P. Robinson in his book *Effective Study*. It makes reading more efficient and long-term remembering more probable.

SQ3R stands for *Survey, Question, Read, Recite,* and *Review.* The steps are as follows:

Survey. First, skim through an entire chapter.

1. Think about the title of the chapter. What do you already know about the subject? Write ideas in the margins. Read the conclusion. What better way is there to discover the main ideas of a chapter?
2. Read the headings. These are the main topics that have been developed by the author.
3. Read the captions under the diagrams, charts, and graphs.

Allow approximately 10–12 min for the survey step. Surveying will help increase your focus and interest in the material.

Question. Write out two or three questions relating to each heading. These should be questions that you believe will be answered within each section. Use the "who, what, when, where, why, and how" application when generating these questions.

Read. Now, read the first section. Keep in mind the questions you have created and read, with a purpose, as quickly as possible.

Recite. At the end of the section, look away from the book for a few seconds. Recite and think about what you have just learned. It is best to recite aloud because hearing the information will help increase your memorization.

Review. Reviewing is a key step if you want to retain the material you have read. Reviewing as you study results in less time needed for test preparation.

Learning to use the SQ3R method is a skill that takes practice. Often, students feel that it takes too long and is too complicated, but its use results in an increase in comprehension, interest, and memorization. The SQ3R method allows you to study at the same time that you are doing your course reading.

Summary

Everyone does not have the same learning style, and, as a result, effective study techniques are not the same for everyone. It is important to choose the method that is best for you, and this will take some experimentation. For instance, some students become frustrated when they cannot comprehend the textbook material while reading when seated at a desk. Sometimes, just getting up and pacing while memorizing can facilitate the learning process if you are having trouble at your desk. Other students learn faster with audio aids. If these are available to you and you are having trouble with learning just from your books, it may be worth the experiment to see if hearing the material will enhance your learning.

Study Groups

While preparing for an examination, properly organizing or attending a study group can be extremely helpful. However, a study group needs to be very focused with a specific agenda for each session. Otherwise, it can be a time waster. The following are some important points to keep in mind when organizing and conducting a study group:

1. Limit the group size to four or five people.
2. Select classmates who share your academic goals.
3. Meet the first time to discuss the meeting times, meeting place, and group goals.
4. Select a group leader and a timekeeper. The group should meet for 2–3 h for each session to ensure a thorough review.
5. Establish an agenda for each meeting that specifies the topics of discussion. This will save time and lend focus to the group. It ensures that the group reviews all pertinent topics by slotting time for all areas.
6. Establish group norms that define how the group will act. This would include things such as getting there on time, being prepared, and ending on time. It is important to emphasize that all members must do their fair share of the work for the group to gain the maximum benefit.

Study groups are useful to review and compare both lecture and reading notes, to review textbook information together, and to review examination topics. Group sessions are a good time to review the question types used on the certification examination, to discuss test-taking strategies, to help each other design study plans, and to drill or review together all material expected to be on the examination.

Explain the material to a friend! This will help you discover what you know and do not know!

The support of a study group is extremely helpful in building self-confidence and in overall preparation for examinations. They are not intended to replace individual study time, but serve as a *supplement.* If properly utilized, study groups are an enormous asset for test preparation. Finally, when working within a group, many students are more likely to exert their best effort because they are accountable to the other members of the group.

Practice Tests

The practice tests (Chapters 6 and 7) can be used in one of the following two ways: (1) as a way of determining strengths and weaknesses before you go through the review book or (2) as a final preparation for the test after you have done your chapter-by-chapter review.

The practice tests have been designed in an effort to duplicate the experience of taking the certification examination. Test questions are administered in *random order*, questions are not ordered according to topic. Therefore, the practice test questions in this book are in randomized sequence—just as you will find questions presented on the ARRT certification examination. Taking the practice tests will make the process more familiar, so you would not be as nervous when you face the real test. The practice test will help you to determine whether you are answering the questions quickly enough, and whether your score is high enough to pass. In summary, the practice tests simply give you a chance to practice, giving you an opportunity to practice for the *actual* examination.

TEST-TAKING STRATEGIES

Time Management

Keeping track of your time and progress is harder than it might first appear. Most of us have been surprised while taking a test by how little time was left. This experience is even more upsetting in the middle of a certification examination. Knowing when there is a problem and knowing what to do about it are the objectives of time management.

Even with your eye on the clock, calculating the time you have left is not always easy. On the radiography examination, you have 3½ h to complete 220 questions. That gives you about 57 s (0.9 min) per question. In other words, you have to answer approximately 66 questions per hour.

Another way to look at this is by breaking the time into two blocks. If, when you are halfway through the allotted examination time, you have finished a minimum of 110 questions, you are working on time. However, there is one additional complication. Not all questions require equal time to work. It is quite possible to run across a string of difficult questions early in the test and fall behind, and then make up the time with easy questions later in the test. For this reason, being a few questions short at the halfway mark is not a cause for concern. However, if you have finished significantly less than 110 questions after 90 min, you may be starting to fall behind.

If you do fall behind, what can you do to catch up? Sometimes, simply seeing that you are behind and trying to work faster will be enough to motivate you to catch up. If not, you have other options. Try to read through the questions and answers a bit faster. If you have checked only one answer as likely to be right, put that choice down immediately; do not reconsider your answer. Always mark your best choice and move forward.

As a rule of thumb, if a fact question (one requiring you to recall a fact) takes more than a minute or two, select your best answer, "mark" the question (CBT has a "mark" button you can click), and go on. You may not skip a question; you must indicate an answer, but you may mark the question and return to it later for further consideration. For a calculation problem (one requiring you to calculate some quantity), give yourself an extra minute or two. The computer monitor will indicate the question number you are currently answering, compared with the total number of questions (e.g., number 62 of 220). The computer counts down from your allotted time, and the computer screen will indicate the amount of time you have remaining.

Elimination: Finding the Correct Answer

Good test performance is sometimes determined by the ability to recognize the incorrect answers as well as the correct ones. *Eliminating incorrect answers* (termed *distractors*) not just improves your score, it actually makes the test a more accurate measure of your knowledge.

Eliminating a distractor reduces the possible wrong choices. If your knowledge allows you to eliminate two incorrect responses, your odds of a correct response would be increased from one out of four to one out of two. If you can eliminate three distractors, you would have a 100% probability of getting the right answer. Every distractor you eliminate increases your odds of picking the right answer.

Multiple-choice questions usually have one distractor that is obviously wrong, one distractor that is closer to the correct response, and one distractor that is very close to the correct answer. If you know the subject, you can eliminate the distractors that are most incorrect and improve your chances. If you prepare thoroughly, you will be able to eliminate the others. The more you know, the better you will do.

Many books on test taking suggest complicated systems to eliminate bad answers and rank good ones, but to use elimination effectively, you need a procedure that is both quick and simple. For the ARRT CBT examination, you must select an answer in order for the next question to be displayed. If you are unsure of your selection, or just want to come back later to review it, you are able to *mark* the question. All the questions you have marked in this manner will be displayed one by one after you have completed all 220 questions. There is an optional tutorial that you may take prior to starting the examination. Taking the tutorial is a good way to become more familiar with navigating through the examination with greater ease and assurance.

Changing Answers

Everyone has had the experience of trying to remember the answer to a question without success and then *finding that piece of information further along in the test*. A problem that you stare at for an hour without progress might seem simple if you go on to other problems and come back to it later. Very often, another question will jog your memory; this technique can work for you during the CBT examination.

If you are unsure of the correct way to answer a question:

1. If one of the answers seems better than the rest, put it down and mark the question for future reference. Come back and check the question at the end if you have time.
2. If you can eliminate two of the possible answers, make an educated guess between the two remaining possibilities. Then, mark the question for future reference.
3. Ask yourself, "Will more time really help me answer this question?" If your answer is no, do the best you can with what you know, using the process of elimination and making an educated guess. Again, mark the question for future reference so that you can reread it if there is time at the end.

Guessing

You have probably been given a great deal of information and advice about guessing on tests. Most of what you have been told may be confusing or contradictory. It may make the problem easier to think in terms of rolling a die. Imagine a game in which you get a point every time the number 1, for example, comes up. How could you improve your score in this game? One way would be to roll the die as many times as you could. Another way would be to reduce the number of sides on the die so the "right" side would be more likely to come up; this way is called *the process of elimination*, and it plays a good part in test taking when you are unsure of the correct response.

Although we do *not* suggest guessing as an effective method of test taking, we do recognize that there will be times when it can be effective for you. Keep in mind the following things if you need to use this method:

1. The process of elimination will help you significantly in determining the right answer. Use this technique to narrow down the possible choices.
2. *Mark* the question so that, if you have time, you can come back to it. It is possible that the correct response may reveal itself through a question further ahead on the test.
3. Remember that guessing really does not work as an effective strategy by itself. You will need to study hard and use guessing in conjunction with other methods for it to be effective.

PRACTICE TESTS

Taking the Practice Test

To use the practice test to determine how long the test will take you to complete or how high you will score, you must take it under conditions matching, as closely as possible, the actual test conditions. If you try to eat supper while taking the test, take a 5-h break in the middle of the test, or stop after every question to look up the answer, you will not get a clear picture of your current standing or potential to pass the examination. Following are some suggestions on how you can get the most out of the practice test:

1. Keep your schedule completely free. Find a time and a place that will guarantee that you will not be disturbed for the duration of the test. Most libraries work well for this purpose, as do unoccupied classrooms if you can get access to them. If you have to take the test at home, make sure that you would not be bothered by friends or family.
2. Minimize your distractions, do not take phone calls, and do not try to watch TV or concentrate on anything else other than the test.
3. Start at a predetermined time. You may choose to take the practice test at the same time of day your test will be given at the testing center.
4. Bring everything you will need to take the test. The test center will supply you with an erasable board and a simple nonprogrammable calculator. You must remember to *request* a calculator from the testing center personnel during your check-in at the center.
5. Approach the practice tests with the same strategies and attitudes that you plan on using with the actual examination. (Rereading the section on test strategies would be a good idea.)
6. Note time-consuming questions. While taking the test, mark the questions that take longer than 2 or 3 min. Do not spend too much time on any one question.
7. Note how far you get. You should be able to finish the whole practice test in the allotted time, but if you do run out of time, draw a line across the test book to show how far you got and then finish the rest of the test.

Checking Your Results

You should be able to finish all of the questions with enough time left to go back and check your answers on those problems you marked as difficult. Your score should be at least 160 correct answers (80%). If you fail at either of these two goals, you need to go over the test carefully and try to analyze your problem.

Two questions that you can address while analyzing a problem are "Was there a common factor in the questions that gave me trouble?" and "What were the subspecialties of the questions that I missed?" If you keep missing the same type of question, the problem could be easy to fix. Try going back and reworking the section of the book that corresponds to that topic. Upon review of their test, students often report making "silly mistakes" because they did not read carefully enough. When reading in haste, or under stress, we often read what we *expect* to see rather than what is actually written. The importance of careful reading cannot be overstressed.

Review your test-taking techniques. Did you spend too much time on a few questions? Did you spend too much time rereading answers that you had already eliminated as potential answers? Did you misread any questions? If the answer to either of these questions is *yes*, you might want to review the earlier section on test strategies.

TEST STRATEGY CHECKLIST

1. ELIMINATE, CHOOSE, AND MARK
   Eliminate known incorrect answers, *choose* the best of the remaining, *mark* to return to later.
2. DO 50 EVERY 45
   Try to answer at least 50 questions every 45 min.
3. MARK UNCERTAIN ANSWERS
   Mark questions you guessed on so you can come back and double-check them.

OPTIMIZING YOUR RESULTS

When you take the radiography examination, two factors determine your score:

- Your knowledge of the subject
- Your performance on the examination

Of the two, knowledge is the key element needed for success. *Performance is harder to guarantee.* For some people, it seems to come naturally. These people apply test-taking strategies almost unconsciously, concentrating all their attention on the test. For the rest of the population (which includes most people), standardized tests are some of the most stressful and unpleasant experiences that they will ever have to face.

Fortunately, it is possible to significantly improve your performance on tests, even if you have been taking tests all of your life with no apparent improvement. By mastering the following three areas, you can have better results and greatly reduce the trauma of test taking:

1. Know your test strategies.
2. Learn to manage your stress.
3. Avoid surprises on the day of the test.

The important points for each of these areas are explained in detail in the following sections and are summarized in checklists included at the end of each part of the Introduction. These checklists are designed so that you can read them on the day of the test to reassure yourself that you have not forgotten anything.

Test-Taking Strategies

The strategies recommended earlier serve two purposes: (1) to give you a simple, systematic way of eliminating bad choices and improving your odds of getting a correct response and (2) to help you manage your time most efficiently during the test.

Managing Stress

Over the past 30 or so years, educators have become increasingly concerned about the problems of test anxiety and excessive stress that prevent students from doing their best on examinations. In the following sections, you will learn some basics about the nature of stress, the difference between good stress and bad stress, and some management techniques. All of the items listed will be helpful in reducing test anxiety, but the most important point for you to remember is that you are well prepared for the test you are about to take and the odds of your doing well are very good.

Where You Stand

The best way to reduce test anxiety is to address the following points:

1. Know the subject.
2. Master a test-taking routine.
3. Avoid surprises.
4. Understand the role of stress in test taking.
5. Practice relaxation techniques.

The Stress Curve

Recently, stress has received national attention. Magazines discuss it, doctors warn against it, commercials promise to reduce it, and seminars claim to eliminate it. Stress is often treated as a psychological cancer. There is, however, another aspect of stress that receives less attention. In demanding situations requiring optimal performance, moderate stress is not just natural, it is actually helpful. The relationship between stress and performance is called the stress curve; the most important aspect of the curve is the location of the maxima. The maxima is the point of optimal performance, which occurs somewhere between too much stress and no stress at all.

There are plenty of familiar examples of stress improving performance. Athletes often set personal records during pressure situations such as playoff games or international events. Actors give their best performances and musicians play or sing best before an audience. You can probably think of personal examples as well. Most of us have surprised ourselves at one time or another by doing better than we expected under pressure.

How to Recognize Good Stress

If everyone dealt with stress equally well and experienced the same level of stress in the same situation, setting up guidelines for optimal stress levels would be easy. Unfortunately, everyone handles stress differently, and determining what level of stress is best must be judged on an individual basis. Given the importance of the radiography examination and the amount of time you have spent preparing for it, there is little chance of your stress level being too low when you sit for the test.

How do you know if you have too much stress? Feeling nervous does not indicate excessive stress. You are just as likely to feel nervous when you are at your optimal stress level. Stress is excessive when it interferes with the test-taking process. If you have trouble reading the questions, if you lose your place because you are worrying about the test, or if you are too distracted to follow the test strategies you have been practicing, you are experiencing test anxiety.

Relaxation Techniques

Irrespective of whether you anticipate problems with stress, it is a good idea to take a couple of minutes to relax before the test. Stretch your muscles, take deep, slow breaths, and try to think about something unrelated to the test. If, during the test, you have trouble working effectively because of stress, stop, close your eyes, and count to five while taking some deep, slow breaths. Remind yourself that you are extremely well prepared for this test. Many people are now realizing that breathing and anxiety are related, and that taking a minute or two to focus on a deep-breathing relaxation exercise can be extremely helpful in reducing one's level of anxiety.

When you feel anxious, you tend to tighten your chest and shoulder muscles. This results in breathing changes, with movement predominantly in your upper chest rather than your lower abdomen. Breathing this way often leads to undesirable conditions:

1. A reduction of oxygen in your blood, which can affect the way you think and lead to anxiety or fatigue
2. Too much oxygen in your blood, resulting in an uncomfortable condition called *hyperventilation*

It is important, therefore, to learn how to control your breathing, which, in turn, will result in relaxation. When attempting the following breathing exercise, do not try too hard to relax—it can work against you. Instead, try to be as peaceful as possible.

The co-founder of Headspace, Andy Puddicombe, describes one effective breathing relaxation technique as follows. First, take a deep, full breath through your nose and exhale fully and completely through your mouth. Next, inhale again, mentally counting from 1 to 4 while breathing in. Hold this breath in while again counting from 1 to 4. Then, begin fully exhaling through your mouth while slowly counting from 1 to 6. Repeat this sequence 3 times. If you run out of breath before reaching number 6, take deeper breaths and exhale more slowly. If you can learn this technique ahead of time, you can use it while in the examination room without anyone else knowing.

If the stress continues, try to think less about what you are doing. After practicing on 1400 questions, you have developed a kind of "automatic pilot," which will allow you to answer questions almost by reflex. Of course, this is not the best way to take the test, but if you are faced with serious stress problems, it is an option.

Avoiding Surprises

The Week Before the Test

You have spent the past 2–4 years studying radiography, and the past 2–4 months reviewing for this examination. You probably know a great deal more than you think you do. Your top priority now should be getting yourself up to your best testing performance. If you follow these suggestions, you should have a good start.

Take Care of Yourself. When you take the test, you want to be as healthy and well rested as possible. The time it takes to get enough sleep, take a walk, or prepare a balanced meal is better spent than hours of last-minute cramming. Cramming is very stressful!

Make sure you are eating healthy; it will improve your energy, help you study better, and help with relaxation. Caffeine might help to energize you but can interfere with your concentration and make you restless. Excessive fats and carbs make it difficult to focus. Snack on berries, oranges, and nuts for a healthy energy and better relaxation. Be certain to make time for physical activity. Exercise improves your mood and stimulates the memory portions of the brain. Yoga and mindful relaxation can be especially helpful by giving you a break from study, and helping you feel more energized and ready to get back to work.

Reread This Introduction. This may be unnecessary advice, but it is worth mentioning. Pay close attention to the figures and checklists.

Gather Your Supplies. You want to be sure to get everything you need, but, almost as importantly, you want everything organized so that you can avoid extra effort and worry. You might want to bring a sweater or light jacket. This may seem like a strange item, particularly if your test is taken in the summer, but an uncomfortably cold room is extremely distracting, and many public buildings have a wide variation in temperature from room to room. A sweater or windbreaker is a quick, easy solution. Avoid bringing a large purse or other large bundle. Lockers are available for stowing your personal items not allowed in the examination room, but they are often fairly small lockers and will not accommodate a very large purse or other large package.

Scout the Location. It is a *very* good idea to visit the location of the examination if possible. Getting lost on the morning of a test will add unwanted stress. Keep in mind the following questions: (1) What is the best route to the examination? (2) Where is the parking? (3) Where are the doors to the building? If possible, go into the building and look around.

Treat Yourself. Go out and do something special. See a movie. Eat out. Go for a drive. Just let yourself unwind.

The Day of the Test

There are few things more irritating than being told not to worry when you feel like worrying, but not worrying is the best thing to do. To help you avoid worrying, two checklists have been included, one physical checklist (things you need to bring) and one mental checklist (things you need to remember). Check off each item and put it out of your mind. Knowing you are both mentally and physically prepared will help you to relax before the examination.

You should plan to arrive a few minutes early. Many test centers require you to be there 30 min ahead of the scheduled test time.

You will probably want to eat a light meal before taking the test. Digestion tends to slow down when a person is under stress, so a large meal is, in most cases, a bad idea. You will also want to avoid excessive stimulants (and caffeine is definitely considered a stimulant).

This brings up another point. Although you want to be well rested and alert, you should be careful not to disrupt your normal routine any more than necessary. Getting extra rest, eating light, and avoiding stimulants are relative suggestions—relative to your habits and lifestyle. *Do not make drastic changes on the day of the test.* Get an extra half hour or hour of sleep. Eat a lighter meal than you usually would. If you drink coffee, drink a little less than normal.

When you get to the testing center, take a few minutes to relax. Walk around. Stretch your muscles. Remind yourself that you have put a great deal of work into doing well on this test and that work is the main factor for determining success.

PHYSICAL CHECKLIST (What to Bring)

1. Your admission ticket
2. Two current IDs
3. Sweater or windbreaker

MENTAL CHECKLIST

1. Remind yourself that you are well prepared
2. Take the computer tutorial
3. Use your test-taking strategies
4. Focus on the test, not on the surroundings
5. After you have finished, use the same strategies to go over any questions you marked for review

---

REFERENCES

Benson H, Klipper M. *The Relaxation Response.* New York, NY: Avon Books; 1990.

Bosworth S, Brisk M. *Learning Skills for the Science Student.* Clearwater, FL: H&H Publishing Company; 1986.

Coffman S. *How to Survive at College.* Bloomington, IN: College Town Press; 1988.

Hamachek A. *Coping in College: A Guide for Academic Success.* Boston, MA: Allyn and Bacon; 1994.

Krantz H, Kemmelman J. *Keys to Reading and Study Skills.* New York, NY: Holt, Rinehart & Winston; 1985.

Palav S. *Learning Strategies for Allied Health Students.* Philadelphia, PA: WB Saunders; 1995.

Puddicombe A. *Get Some Headspace: 10 Minutes Can Make All the Difference.* London, England: Hodder & Stoughton; 2011.

Robinson F. *Effective Study.* New York, NY: Harper and Row; 1970.

Saia DA. *Radiography Program Review Exam Preparation.* 8th ed. New York, NY: McGraw Hill; 2006.

Vitale B, Nugent P. *Test Success: Test-Taking Techniques for the Health Care Student.* Philadelphia, PA: FA Davis; 2015.

MASTER BIBLIOGRAPHY

Adler AM, Carlton RR. *Introduction to Radiologic and Imaging Sciences and Patient Care.* 7th ed. St Louis, MO: Saunders Elsevier; 2019.

ARRT Standards of Ethics. https://www.arrt.org/docs/default-source/Governing-Documents/arrt-standards-of-ethics.pdf?sfvrsn=10. Accessed March 27, 2017.

ASRT Practice Standards. https://www.asrt.org/docs/default-source/practice-standards-published/ps_rad.pdf?sfvrsn=2. Accessed March 27, 2017.

Bushong SC. *Radiologic Science for Technologists.* 11th ed. St Louis, MO: Mosby; 2017.

Carlton RR, Adler AM, Balas V. *Principles of Radiographic Imaging.* 6th ed. Albany, NY: Delmar; 2020.

Carroll QB. *Radiography in the Digital Age.* 3rd ed. Springfield, IL: Charles C Thomas; 2018.

Carter C, Vealé B. *Digital Radiography and PACS.* 3rd ed. St Louis, MO: Mosby Elsevier; 2019.

Dutton AG, Ryan TA. *Torres' Patient Care in Imaging Technology.* 9th ed. Philadelphia, PA: Lippincott; 2019.

Ehrlich RA, Coakes DM. *Patient Care in Radiography.* 9th ed. St Louis, MO: Mosby; 2017.

Ehrlich RA, Coakes DM. *Patient Care in Radiography.* 10th ed. St Louis, MO: Mosby; 2021.

Fosbinder R, Orth D. *Essentials of Radiologic Science.* Baltimore, MD: Lippincott Williams & Wilkins; 2012.

Fuji Computed Radiography. Minato-Ku, Japan; 2002.

Johnston JN, Fauber TL. *Essentials of Radiographic Physics and Imaging.* 3rd ed. St Louis, MO: Mosby Elsevier; 2020.

Lampignano JP, Kendrick LE. *Bontrager's Textbook of Radiographic Positioning and Related Anatomy.* 9th ed. St Louis, MO: Mosby Elsevier; 2018.

Long BW, Rollins JH, Smith BJ. *Merrill's Atlas of Radiographic Positioning and Procedures.* Vols 1-3. 13th ed. St Louis, MO: Mosby; 2016.

Mills WR. The relation of bodily habitus to visceral form, tonus, and motility. *Am J Roentgenol.* 1917;4:155-169.

NCRP Report No. 99. *Quality Assurance for Diagnostic Imaging.* NCRP; 1990.

NCRP Report No. 102. *Medical X-ray, Electron Beam and Gamma-Ray Protection for Energies up to 50 MeV (Equipment Design, Performance and Use).* NCRP; 1989.

NCRP Report No. 116. *Recommendations on Limits for Exposure to Ionizing Radiation.* NCRP; 1987.

NCRP Report No. 160. *Ionizing Radiation Exposure of the Population of the United States.* NCRP; 2009.

NCRP Report No. 184. *Medical Radiation Exposure of Patients in the United States.* NCRP, 2019

Orth D. *Essentials of Radiologic Science.* 2nd ed. Baltimore, MD: Lippincott Williams & Wilkins; 2017.

Peart O. *Lange Radiographic Positioning Flashcards.* New York, NY: McGraw Hill; 2014.

Saia DA. *Radiography PREP.* 9th ed. New York, NY: McGraw Hill; 2018.

Saladin KS. *Anatomy and Physiology: The Unity of Form and Function.* 7th ed. New York, NY: McGraw Hill; 2015.

Seeram E. *Digital Radiography: An Introduction.* Clifton Park, NY: Delmar Cengage Learning; 2011.

Seeram E, Brennan PC. *Radiation Protection in Diagnostic X-ray Imaging.* Burlington, MA: Jones and Bartlett Learning; 2017.

Shephard CT. *Radiographic Image Production and Manipulation.* New York, NY: McGraw Hill; 2003.

Statkiewicz-Sherer MA, Visconti PJ, Ritenour ER, Haynes KW. *Radiation Protection in Medical Radiography.* 8th ed. St Louis, MO: Mosby; 2018.

Wolbarst AB. *Physics of Radiology.* 2nd ed. Madison, WI: Medical Physics Publishing; 2005.

TWELFTH EDITION

LANGE Q&A™

RADIOGRAPHY EXAMINATION

Patient Care

QUESTIONS

DIRECTIONS: Each of the numbered items or incomplete statements in this section is followed by answers or by completions of the statement. Select the *one* letter answer or completion that is *best* in each case.

1. X-ray verification of central venous catheter (CVC) placement should identify the catheter's distal tip at the
- ❏ A. vena cava near the right atrium
- ❏ B. vena cava near the left atrium
- ❏ C. aorta near the right atrium
- ❏ D. aorta near the left atrium

2. Pathogenic microorganisms that require contact precautions include
1. MRSA
2. *Clostridium difficile (C. difficile)*
3. hepatitis A
- ❏ A. 1 only
- ❏ B. 1 and 2 only
- ❏ C. 2 and 3 only
- ❏ D. 1, 2, and 3

3. From the following, select the four circumstances that violate ARRT Rules of Ethics and can lead to ARRT professional sanction.
1. Soliciting/receiving examination information that uses language similar to that found on the certification examination
2. Providing incorrect/misleading information regarding one's ARRT credentials or qualifications
3. Assisting in billing practices that violate Federal or State laws
4. Inappropriate use of radiographic equipment
5. Failure to respect the patient's privacy
6. Providing false information regarding Continuing Education (CE) compliance
- ❏ A. 1, 2, 3, and 4
- ❏ B. 1, 3, 5, and 6
- ❏ C. 1, 2, 3, and 6
- ❏ D. 2, 4, 5, and 6

4. *Logrolling* is a method of moving patients with suspected
- ❏ A. head injury
- ❏ B. spinal injury
- ❏ C. bowel obstruction
- ❏ D. extremity fracture

5. Fractures of two or more adjacent ribs is termed
- ❏ A. pectus carinatum
- ❏ B. pectus excavatum
- ❏ C. flail chest
- ❏ D. atelectasis

6. An *iatrogenic* infection is the one caused by
- ❏ A. physician intervention
- ❏ B. blood-borne pathogens
- ❏ C. chemotherapy
- ❏ D. infected droplets

7. A radiographer should recognize that gerontologic patients often have undergone physical changes that include loss of
1. muscle mass
2. bone calcium
3. mental alertness
- ❏ A. 1 only
- ❏ B. 1 and 2 only
- ❏ C. 1 and 3 only
- ❏ D. 1, 2, and 3

8. Examples of unintentional misconduct include
1. battery
2. negligence
3. slander
4. malpractice
5. false imprisonment
- ❏ A. 1, 3, and 4
- ❏ B. 2 and 4
- ❏ C. 2, 3, and 5
- ❏ D. 1, 4, and 5

9. X-ray verification of pacemaker leads placement should identify the catheter's tip at the
- ❏ A. apex of the right ventricle
- ❏ B. apex of the left ventricle
- ❏ C. right or left pulmonary artery
- ❏ D. superior or inferior vena cava

10. Examples of a *portal of entry* in the cycle of infection include
1. a break in the skin
2. nasal mucous membrane
3. urinary tract
- ❏ A. 1 only
- ❏ B. 1 and 2 only
- ❏ C. 2 and 3 only
- ❏ D. 1, 2, and 3

11. Administration of a contrast agent for radiographic demonstration of the spinal canal and adjacent structures is performed using which of the following routes?
- ❏ A. Subcutaneous
- ❏ B. Intravenous
- ❏ C. Intramuscular
- ❏ D. Intrathecal

12. Possible side effects of an iodinated contrast medium that is administered intravenously include which of the following?
1. A warm, flushed feeling
2. Altered taste
3. Itching
4. Sneezing
5. Nausea
6. Rash and hives
- ❏ A. 1, 5, and 6
- ❏ B. 1, 2, and 5
- ❏ C. 3, 4, and 5
- ❏ D. 2, 5, and 6

13. If the patient suffers as a result of the radiographer's actions, the radiographer can be charged with professional *negligence*. Many courts will apply *res ipsa loquitur*, "the thing speaks for itself." Select the three circumstances from the following that could subject the radiographer to an accusation of negligence.
1. Failure to explain the x-ray examination to the patient
2. Imaging the wrong patient
3. Cropping/masking an electronic image to make it look collimated
4. Modification of exposure indicator (EI) values
5. Failure to address the patient in a professional manner
- ❏ A. 1, 2, and 3
- ❏ B. 1, 4, and 5
- ❏ C. 2, 3, and 4
- ❏ D. 3, 5, and 6

14. Which of the following statements regarding tracheostomy patients is true?
1. Tracheostomy patients have difficulty in speaking
2. Mobile chest imaging requires any tracheostomy tube to be rotated out of view
3. Audible rattling sounds indicate a need for suction
- ❏ A. 1 only
- ❏ B. 1 and 2 only
- ❏ C. 1 and 3 only
- ❏ D. 1, 2, and 3

15. A small container holding several doses of medication is termed
- ❏ A. an ampoule
- ❏ B. a vial
- ❏ C. a bolus
- ❏ D. a carafe

16. You have encountered a person who is apparently unconscious and unresponsive. There is no rise and fall of the chest, and you can hear no breath sounds. You should first
- ❏ A. begin mouth-to-mouth rescue breathing, giving two full breaths
- ❏ B. proceed with the Heimlich maneuver
- ❏ C. begin with 30 external chest compressions at a rate of 100 compressions/min
- ❏ D. begin with 5 external chest compressions at a rate of 50 compressions/min

17. Examples of biomedical waste include
1. laboratory and pathology waste
2. used bandages and dressings
3. chest tubes
4. bladder catheters
- ❏ A. 1, 3, and 4
- ❏ B. 1, 2, and 3
- ❏ C. 2, 3, and 4
- ❏ D. 1, 2, 3, and 4

18. Types of inflammatory bowel disease include
1. Crohn's disease
2. ulcerative colitis
3. intussusception
- ❏ A. 1 only
- ❏ B. 1 and 2 only
- ❏ C. 2 and 3 only
- ❏ D. 1, 2, and 3

19. Misunderstandings between cultures can happen as a result of
1. looking directly into someone's eyes
2. the use of certain gestures
3. standing too close while speaking to another
- ❏ A. 1 only
- ❏ B. 1 and 2 only
- ❏ C. 2 and 3 only
- ❏ D. 1, 2, and 3

20. From Figure 1-1 select those that illustrate correct body mechanics.
- ❑ A. 1 and 2 are correct
- ❑ B. 1, 2, and 3 are correct
- ❑ C. 2 and 3 are correct
- ❑ D. 3 and 4 are correct

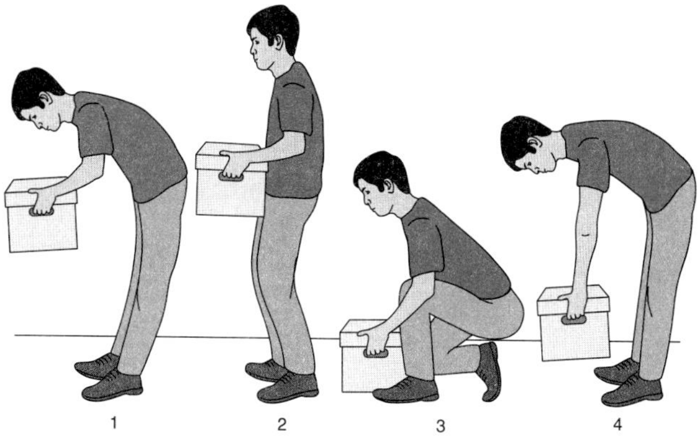

Figure 1-1

21. Some proteins in latex can produce mild-to-severe allergic reactions. Which of the following medical equipment could contain latex?
1. Stethoscopes
2. Enema tips
3. Bed linen
4. Disposable needles
5. Bedpans
6. Syringes
- ❑ A. 1, 2, and 3
- ❑ B. 4, 5, and 6
- ❑ C. 2, 4, and 5
- ❑ D. 1, 2, and 6

22. Which two of the following precautions should be used when microbes are transmitted in air or dust particles?
1. Droplet precautions
2. Airborne precautions
3. Contact precautions
4. Vector precautions
- ❑ A. 1 and 2
- ❑ B. 1 and 4
- ❑ C. 2 and 3
- ❑ D. 3 and 4

23. A large volume of medication introduced intravenously over a longer period of time is termed
- ❑ A. an IV push
- ❑ B. an infusion
- ❑ C. a bolus
- ❑ D. a hypodermic

24. Conditions requiring oxygen therapy include
1. COPD
2. pneumonia
3. sleep apnea
- ❑ A. 1 only
- ❑ B. 1 and 2 only
- ❑ C. 2 and 3 only
- ❑ D. 1, 2, and 3

25. An inanimate object that has been in contact with an infectious microorganism is termed a
- ❑ A. vector
- ❑ B. fomite
- ❑ C. host
- ❑ D. reservoir

26. In which stage of infection do the infective microbes begin to multiply?
- ❑ A. Latent period
- ❑ B. Incubation period
- ❑ C. Disease phase
- ❑ D. Convalescent phase

27. A partially obstructed airway is clinically manifested in which of the following way(s)?
1. Dysphagia
2. Noisy, labored breathing
3. Nail bed and lip cyanosis
- ❑ A. 1 only
- ❑ B. 1 and 2 only
- ❑ C. 2 and 3 only
- ❑ D. 1, 2, and 3

28. All of the following statements regarding hand hygiene and skin care are correct, *except*
- ❑ A. hands should be cleansed before and after every patient examination
- ❑ B. faucets should be opened and closed with paper towels
- ❑ C. hands should be smooth and free from chapping
- ❑ D. any cracks or abrasions should be left uncovered to facilitate healing

29. All of the following are correct concepts of good body mechanics during patient lifting/moving, *except*
- ❑ A. the radiographer should stand with feet approximately 12 inches apart, with one foot slightly forward
- ❑ B. the body's center of gravity should be positioned over its base of support
- ❑ C. the back should be kept straight; avoid twisting
- ❑ D. when carrying a heavy object, hold it away from the body

30. When a patient arrives in the radiology department with a urinary Foley catheter bag, it is important to
- ❏ A. place the drainage bag above the level of the bladder
- ❏ B. place the drainage bag at the same level as the bladder
- ❏ C. place the drainage bag below the level of the bladder
- ❏ D. clamp the Foley catheter

31. While assisting a patient onto an x-ray table, when the patient has one strong side and one weak side, the radiographer should
- ❏ A. start with the weaker side closer to the table
- ❏ B. start with the stronger side closer to the table
- ❏ C. always use a two-person lift
- ❏ D. lift the patient carefully onto the table

32. The radiographer can help to alleviate patient anxiety in which of the following ways?
1. Careful explanation of the procedure
2. Avoiding use of complex medical terms
3. Listening carefully to the patient
- ❏ A. 1 only
- ❏ B. 1 and 2 only
- ❏ C. 2 and 3 only
- ❏ D. 1, 2, and 3

33. What does number 85 represent in the blood pressure reading 145/85 mm Hg?
1. The phase of relaxation of the cardiac muscle tissue
2. The phase of contraction of the cardiac muscle tissue
3. Higher than desirable diastolic pressure
4. Lower than normal diastolic pressure
- ❏ A. 1 and 3
- ❏ B. 1 and 4
- ❏ C. 2 and 3
- ❏ D. 2 and 4

34. Facsimile transmission of health information is
1. not permitted
2. permitted for urgently needed patient care
3. permitted for third-party payer hospitalization certification
- ❏ A. 1 only
- ❏ B. 2 only
- ❏ C. 2 and 3 only
- ❏ D. 1, 2, and 3

35. Forms of intentional misconduct include
1. slander
2. invasion of privacy
3. negligence
- ❏ A. 1 only
- ❏ B. 2 only
- ❏ C. 1 and 2 only
- ❏ D. 1, 2, and 3

36. Which of the following statements is correct with regard to assisting a patient from a wheelchair to an x-ray table?
- ❏ A. The wheelchair should be parallel with the x-ray table
- ❏ B. The wheelchair should be angled 45° to the x-ray table
- ❏ C. The wheelchair should directly face the x-ray table
- ❏ D. The wheelchair footrests should be folded down for foot support during transfer

37. Blood flows into the left ventricle via the
- ❏ A. tricuspid valve during atrial systole
- ❏ B. tricuspid valve during ventricular systole
- ❏ C. bicuspid valve during atrial systole
- ❏ D. bicuspid valve during ventricular systole

38. You and a fellow radiographer have received an unconscious patient from a motor vehicle accident. As you perform the examination, it is important that you
1. refer to the patient by name
2. make only those statements that you would make with a conscious patient
3. reassure the patient about what you are doing
- ❏ A. 1 only
- ❏ B. 1 and 2 only
- ❏ C. 2 and 3 only
- ❏ D. 1, 2, and 3

39. A cathartic is used to
- ❏ A. inhibit coughing
- ❏ B. promote elimination of urine
- ❏ C. stimulate defecation
- ❏ D. induce vomiting

40. The *most* effective method of sterilization is
- ❏ A. dry heat
- ❏ B. moist heat
- ❏ C. pasteurization
- ❏ D. freezing

41. Of the following, which is the most appropriate needle angle for an intravenous injection?
- ❏ A. 90°
- ❏ B. 75°
- ❏ C. 45°
- ❏ D. 15°

42. The belief that one's own cultural ways are superior to any other is termed
- ❏ A. ethnology
- ❏ B. ethnobiology
- ❏ C. ethnocentrism
- ❏ D. ethnography

43. Compliance with HIPAA standards requires which of the following?

1. Protected health care information is accessible to health care workers only
2. A copy of authorization for release of medical information is kept on file
3. Patient information computer files must be encrypted
- ❏ A. 1 only
- ❏ B. 1 and 2 only
- ❏ C. 2 and 3 only
- ❏ D. 1, 2, and 3

44. Which of the following may be used to effectively reduce the viscosity of contrast media?
- ❏ A. Warming
- ❏ B. Refrigeration
- ❏ C. Storage at normal room temperature
- ❏ D. Storage in a cool, dry place

45. The type of shock often associated with pulmonary embolism or myocardial infarction is classified as
- ❏ A. neurogenic
- ❏ B. cardiogenic
- ❏ C. hypovolemic
- ❏ D. septic

46. Symptoms associated with a respiratory reaction to contrast media include

1. sneezing
2. hoarseness
3. wheezing
- ❏ A. 1 and 2 only
- ❏ B. 1 and 3 only
- ❏ C. 2 and 3 only
- ❏ D. 1, 2, and 3

47. What type of precautions is used to prevent the spread of bronchial secretions during coughing?
- ❏ A. Contact precautions
- ❏ B. Airborne precautions
- ❏ C. Protective isolation
- ❏ D. Strict isolation

48. An MRI procedure is contraindicated for a patient who has
- ❏ A. a herniated disk
- ❏ B. cochlear implant
- ❏ C. dental fillings
- ❏ D. subdural bleeding

49. Blood pressure within vessels is highest during
- ❏ A. ventricular diastole
- ❏ B. ventricular systole
- ❏ C. atrial diastole
- ❏ D. atrial systole

50. Each of the following is an example of a fomite, *except*
- ❏ A. a doorknob
- ❏ B. a tick
- ❏ C. a spoon
- ❏ D. an x-ray table

51. Which of the following legal phrases defines a circumstance in which the actions of both the health care provider and the patient are responsible for an injurious outcome?
- ❏ A. Intentional misconduct
- ❏ B. Contributory negligence
- ❏ C. Gross negligence
- ❏ D. None of the above

52. What is the *first* treatment for extravasation of contrast media during an IV injection?
- ❏ A. Apply a hot compress
- ❏ B. Apply a cold compress
- ❏ C. Remove needle and apply pressure to the vein until bleeding stops
- ❏ D. Remove the needle and locate a sturdier vein immediately

53. Which of the following diastolic pressure readings indicates hypertension?
- ❏ A. 40 mm Hg
- ❏ B. 60 mm Hg
- ❏ C. 70 mm Hg
- ❏ D. 90 mm Hg

54. To reduce the back strain that can result from moving heavy objects, the radiographer should
- ❏ A. hold the object away from his or her body when lifting
- ❏ B. bend at the waist and pull
- ❏ C. pull the object
- ❏ D. push the object

55. All the following statements regarding oxygen delivery are true, *except*
- ❏ A. oxygen is classified as a drug and must be prescribed by a physician
- ❏ B. the rate of delivery and mode of delivery must be part of a physician order for oxygen
- ❏ C. oxygen may be ordered continuously or as needed for the patient
- ❏ D. none of the above; all these are true

56. Examples of various diverse cultural groups include which of the following?

1. Generational groups
2. Socioeconomic groups
3. Handicapped groups
- ❏ A. 1 only
- ❏ B. 1 and 2 only
- ❏ C. 2 and 3 only
- ❏ D. 1, 2, and 3

57. Gas-producing powder or crystals usually are ingested preliminary to which of the following examinations?
- ❏ A. Double-contrast barium enema (BE)
- ❏ B. Double-contrast gastrointestinal (GI) series
- ❏ C. Oral cholecystogram
- ❏ D. IV urogram (IVU)

58. According to the CDC, all the following precaution guidelines are true, *except*
- ❏ A. airborne precautions require that the patient wears a mask
- ❏ B. masks are indicated when caring for patients on MRSA precautions
- ❏ C. patients under MRSA precautions require a negative-pressure room
- ❏ D. masks are indicated when caring for a patient on droplet precautions

59. Routes of drug administration include
1. sublingual
2. topical
3. parenteral
- ❏ A. 1 only
- ❏ B. 1 and 2 only
- ❏ C. 2 and 3 only
- ❏ D. 1, 2, and 3

60. You are working in the outpatient department and receive a patient who is complaining of pain in the right hip joint; however, the requisition asks for a left femur examination. What should you do?
- ❏ A. Perform a right hip examination
- ❏ B. Perform a left femur examination
- ❏ C. Perform both a right hip and a left femur examination
- ❏ D. Check with the referring physician

61. If a radiographer performed a lumbar spine examination on a patient who was supposed to have an elbow examination, which of the following charges may be brought against the radiographer?
- ❏ A. Assault
- ❏ B. Battery
- ❏ C. False imprisonment
- ❏ D. Defamation

62. Which of the following diagnostic examinations require(s) restriction of a patient's diet?
1. Barium enema (BE)
2. Pyelogram
3. Metastatic survey
- ❏ A. 1 only
- ❏ B. 1 and 2 only
- ❏ C. 1 and 3 only
- ❏ D. 2 and 3 only

63. Which of the following procedures must be performed by the radiographer before entering a contact isolation room with a mobile x-ray unit?
1. Put on gown and gloves only
2. Put on gown, gloves, mask, and cap
3. Clean the mobile x-ray unit
- ❏ A. 1 only
- ❏ B. 2 only
- ❏ C. 1 and 3 only
- ❏ D. 2 and 3 only

64. Examples of nasogastric (NG) tubes include
1. Swan–Ganz
2. Salem Sump
3. Levin
- ❏ A. 1 and 2 only
- ❏ B. 1 and 3 only
- ❏ C. 2 and 3 only
- ❏ D. 1, 2, and 3

65. All of the following are central venous lines, *except*
- ❏ A. a Port-A-Cath
- ❏ B. a PICC
- ❏ C. a Swan–Ganz
- ❏ D. a Salem Sump

66. Another term used to describe nosocomial infections is
- ❏ A. iatrogenic
- ❏ B. health care–associated infections
- ❏ C. droplet
- ❏ D. airborne

67. The condition in which pulmonary alveoli lose their elasticity and become permanently inflated, causing the patient to consciously exhale, is
- ❏ A. bronchial asthma
- ❏ B. bronchitis
- ❏ C. emphysema
- ❏ D. TB

68. In pediatric imaging, a neonate is usually described as a/an
- ❏ A. preschooler
- ❏ B. toddler
- ❏ C. infant
- ❏ D. newborn

69. A radiologic technologist can be found guilty of a *tort* in which of the following situations?
1. Performing the wrong examination on a patient
2. Imaging the wrong patient
3. Using patient immobilization against his or her will
- ❏ A. 1 only
- ❏ B. 1 and 2 only
- ❏ C. 2 and 3 only
- ❏ D. 1, 2, and 3

70. All of the following statements regarding informed consent are true, *except*
- ❏ A. informed consent is required for research participation
- ❏ B. the physician named on the consent form must perform the procedure
- ❏ C. the consent form cannot be revoked, once signed
- ❏ D. a parent or legal guardian is required to sign for a minor

71. Following pacemaker insertion, care must be taken to
- ❏ A. keep the patient flat for 12 h
- ❏ B. keep the patient Trendelenburg for 12 h
- ❏ C. avoid elevating/abducting the patient's right arm for 24 h
- ❏ D. avoid elevating/abducting the patient's left arm for 24 h

72. On reviewing a patient's blood chemistry, which of the following adult blood urea nitrogen (BUN) ranges is considered normal?
- ❏ A. 0.6–1.5 mg/dL
- ❏ B. 4.5–6 mg/dL
- ❏ C. 7–20 mg/dL
- ❏ D. Up to 50 mg/dL

73. Procedures requiring intravascular iodinated contrast agent for patients being treated with metformin for type 2 diabetes, with no indication of acute kidney disease (AKI) or severe chronic kidney disease, should receive which of the following instructions?
1. Do not discontinue metformin before or after receiving contrast
2. Renal function reassessment not required following the examination
3. Temporarily discontinue metformin at time of (or prior to) the procedure
- ❏ A. 1 only
- ❏ B. 1 and 2 only
- ❏ C. 3 only
- ❏ D. 1, 2, and 3

74. All the following are forms of *mechanical* obstruction seen in neonates or infants, *except*
- ❏ A. paralytic ileus
- ❏ B. meconium ileus
- ❏ C. volvulus
- ❏ D. intussusception

75. The pain experienced by an individual whose coronary arteries are not conveying sufficient blood to the heart is called
- ❏ A. tachycardia
- ❏ B. bradycardia
- ❏ C. angina pectoris
- ❏ D. syncope

76. Which of the following conditions must be met in order for a patient consent to be valid?
1. The patient must sign the consent form before receiving sedation
2. The physician named on the consent form must perform the procedure
3. Blank spaces on the form must be completed by the physician after patient signature
- ❏ A. 1 and 2 only
- ❏ B. 1 and 3 only
- ❏ C. 2 and 3 only
- ❏ D. 1, 2, and 3

77. The advantages of using nonionic, water-soluble contrast media include
1. cost-containment benefits
2. low toxicity
3. fewer adverse reactions
- ❏ A. 1 only
- ❏ B. 1 and 2 only
- ❏ C. 2 and 3 only
- ❏ D. 1, 2, and 3

78. A vasovagal response experienced after injection of a contrast agent is characterized by all of the following symptoms, *except*
- ❏ A. nausea
- ❏ B. syncope
- ❏ C. hypertension
- ❏ D. anxiety

79. Which of the following statements is/are true regarding a two-member team performing mobile radiography on a patient with MRSA precautions?
1. One radiographer remains "clean," that is, he or she has no physical contact with the patient
2. The radiographer who positions the mobile unit also makes the exposure
3. The radiographer who positions the IP also retrieves the IP and removes it from its plastic protective cover
- ❏ A. 1 and 2 only
- ❏ B. 1 and 3 only
- ❏ C. 2 and 3 only
- ❏ D. 1, 2, and 3

80. Which of the following must be included in a patient's medical record or chart?
1. Diagnostic and therapeutic orders
2. Medical history
3. Informed consent
- ❏ A. 1 and 2 only
- ❏ B. 1 and 3 only
- ❏ C. 2 and 3 only
- ❏ D. 1, 2, and 3

81. While in your care for a radiologic procedure, a patient asks to see his medical record/chart. Which of the following is the *appropriate* response?

❑ A. Inform the patient that the records are for health care providers to view, not for the patient

❑ B. Inform the patient that you do not know how to access his records

❑ C. Inform the patient that he has the right to see his records but he should request to view them with his physician so that they are interpreted properly

❑ D. Show the patient his records and leave him alone for a few minutes to review them

82. In which of the following conditions is a double-contrast BE essential for demonstration of the condition?

1. Polyps
2. Colitis
3. Diverticulosis

❑ A. 1 only
❑ B. 1 and 2 only
❑ C. 1 and 3 only
❑ D. 1, 2, and 3

83. Pathologic microorganisms spread by direct or close contact include

1. MRSA
2. conjunctivitis
3. rotavirus

❑ A. 1 only
❑ B. 1 and 2 only
❑ C. 2 and 3 only
❑ D. 1, 2, and 3

84. You receive an ambulatory patient for a GI series. As the patient is being seated on the x-ray table, he tells you he feels faint. You should

1. lay the patient down on the x-ray table
2. elevate the patient's legs or place the table slightly Trendelenburg
3. leave quickly and call for help

❑ A. 1 only
❑ B. 1 and 2 only
❑ C. 1 and 3 only
❑ D. 1, 2, and 3

85. The medical term for *hives* is

❑ A. vertigo
❑ B. epistaxis
❑ C. urticaria
❑ D. aura

86. Blood pressure is measured in units of

❑ A. millimeters of mercury (mm Hg)
❑ B. beats per minute
❑ C. degrees Fahrenheit (°F)
❑ D. liters per minute (L/min)

87. Which ethical principle is related to sincerity and truthfulness?

❑ A. Beneficence
❑ B. Autonomy
❑ C. Veracity
❑ D. Fidelity

88. The medical term for *congenital clubfoot* is

❑ A. coxa plana
❑ B. osteochondritis
❑ C. talipes
❑ D. muscular dystrophy

89. In what order should the following examinations be performed?

1. Upper GI series
2. IVU
3. BE

❑ A. 3, 1, 2
❑ B. 1, 3, 2
❑ C. 2, 1, 3
❑ D. 2, 3, 1

90. Patients are questioned regarding presence of any aneurysm clips, pacemakers, artificial heart valves, or shrapnel during screening for

❑ A. sonography
❑ B. CT
❑ C. MRI
❑ D. fluoroscopy

91. The condition that allows blood to shunt between the right and left ventricles is called

❑ A. patent ductus arteriosus
❑ B. coarctation of the aorta
❑ C. atrial septal defect
❑ D. ventricular septal defect

92. A patient experiencing an episode of syncope should be placed in which of the following positions?

❑ A. Dorsal recumbent with head elevated
❑ B. Dorsal recumbent with feet elevated
❑ C. Lateral recumbent
❑ D. Seated with feet supported

93. The cycle of infection includes which of the following components?

1. Reservoir of infection
2. Susceptible host
3. Mode of transmission

❑ A. 1 only
❑ B. 1 and 2 only
❑ C. 2 and 3 only
❑ D. 1, 2, and 3

94. The act of inspiration will cause elevation of the
1. sternum
2. ribs
3. diaphragm
- ❑ A. 1 only
- ❑ B. 1 and 2 only
- ❑ C. 2 and 3 only
- ❑ D. 1, 2, and 3

95. What venous device can be used for a patient requiring IV injections at frequent or regular intervals?
- ❑ A. Butterfly needle
- ❑ B. Intermittent injection port
- ❑ C. IV infusion
- ❑ D. Hypodermic needle

96. Guidelines for cleaning contaminated objects or surfaces include which of the following?
1. Clean from the least contaminated to the most contaminated areas
2. Clean in a circular motion, starting from the center and working outward
3. Clean from the top down
- ❑ A. 1 only
- ❑ B. 1 and 2 only
- ❑ C. 1 and 3 only
- ❑ D. 1, 2, and 3

97. While performing mobile radiography on a patient, you note that the requisition is for a chest image to check placement of a Swan–Ganz catheter. A Swan–Ganz catheter is a/an
- ❑ A. pacemaker
- ❑ B. chest tube
- ❑ C. IV catheter
- ❑ D. urinary catheter

98. A patient who is warm, flushed, or feverish is said to be
- ❑ A. diaphoretic
- ❑ B. febrile
- ❑ C. cyanotic
- ❑ D. anxious

99. The mechanical device used to correct an ineffectual cardiac rhythm is a
- ❑ A. defibrillator
- ❑ B. cardiac monitor
- ❑ C. crash cart
- ❑ D. resuscitation bag

100. When caring for a patient with an IV line, the radiographer should keep the medication
- ❑ A. 18–24 inches above the level of the vein
- ❑ B. 18–24 inches below the level of the vein
- ❑ C. 28–30 inches above the level of the vein
- ❑ D. 28–30 inches below the level of the vein

101. Diseases that require droplet precautions include
1. rubella
2. mumps
3. influenza
- ❑ A. 1 only
- ❑ B. 1 and 2 only
- ❑ C. 2 and 3 only
- ❑ D. 1, 2, and 3

102. A protective environment or neutropenic precautions (sometimes called *expanded precautions*) as indicated is required in which of the following conditions?
1. TB
2. Burns
3. Leukemia
- ❑ A. 1 only
- ❑ B. 1 and 2 only
- ❑ C. 2 and 3 only
- ❑ D. 1, 2, and 3

103. When a GI series has been requested on a patient with a suspected perforated ulcer, the type of contrast medium that should be used is
- ❑ A. a thin barium sulfate suspension
- ❑ B. a thick barium sulfate suspension
- ❑ C. water-soluble iodinated media
- ❑ D. oil-based iodinated media

104. Nitroglycerin is used
- ❑ A. to relieve pain from angina pectoris
- ❑ B. to prevent a heart attack
- ❑ C. as a vasoconstrictor
- ❑ D. to increase blood pressure

105. For medicolegal reasons, radiographic images are required to include all the following information, *except*
- ❑ A. the patient's name and/or identification number
- ❑ B. the patient's birth date
- ❑ C. a right- or left-side marker
- ❑ D. the date of the examination

106. The diameter of a needle's lumen is called its
- ❑ A. bevel
- ❑ B. gauge
- ❑ C. hub
- ❑ D. length

107. Select the three symptoms/reactions that would be classified as *mild* anaphylactic symptoms.
1. Tingling/itching at injection site
2. Nasal congestion
3. Wheezing
4. Anxious feeling
- ❑ A. 1, 2, and 3
- ❑ B. 2, 3, and 4
- ❑ C. 1, 2, and 4
- ❑ D. 1, 3, and 4

108. A patient in a recumbent position with the feet higher than the head is said to be in which of the following positions?
- ❏ A. Trendelenburg
- ❏ B. Fowler
- ❏ C. Sims
- ❏ D. Caldwell

109. The normal average rate of respiration for a healthy adult patient is
- ❏ A. 5–7 breaths/min
- ❏ B. 8–12 breaths/min
- ❏ C. 12–20 breaths/min
- ❏ D. 20–30 breaths/min

110. Which of the following is a vasopressor and may be used for an anaphylactic reaction or a cardiac arrest?
- ❏ A. Nitroglycerin
- ❏ B. Epinephrine
- ❏ C. Hydrocortisone
- ❏ D. Digitoxin

111. Examples of means by which infectious microorganisms can be transmitted via indirect contact include
1. a fomite
2. soiled equipment
3. nasal or oral secretions
- ❏ A. 1 only
- ❏ B. 1 and 2 only
- ❏ C. 2 and 3 only
- ❏ D. 1, 2, and 3

112. All the following rules regarding proper hand-washing technique are correct, *except*
- ❏ A. keep hands and forearms lower than elbows
- ❏ B. use paper towels to turn water on
- ❏ C. avoid using hand lotions whenever possible
- ❏ D. carefully wash all surfaces and between fingers

113. Which of the following instructions should be given to a patient following a barium sulfate contrast examination?
1. Increase fluid and fiber intake for several days
2. Changes in stool color will occur until all barium has been evacuated
3. Contact a physician if no bowel movement occurs in 24 h
- ❏ A. 1 only
- ❏ B. 2 only
- ❏ C. 1 and 3 only
- ❏ D. 1, 2, and 3

114. Which blood vessels are best suited for determination of pulse rate?
- ❏ A. Superficial arteries
- ❏ B. Deep arteries
- ❏ C. Superficial veins
- ❏ D. Deep veins

115. The medical abbreviation meaning "after meals" is
- ❏ A. gtt
- ❏ B. qid
- ❏ C. qh
- ❏ D. pc

116. Symptoms of inadequate oxygen supply include
1. diaphoresis
2. cyanosis
3. retraction of intercostal spaces
- ❏ A. 1 only
- ❏ B. 1 and 2 only
- ❏ C. 2 and 3 only
- ❏ D. 1, 2, and 3

117. If an emergency trauma patient experiences hemorrhaging from a leg injury, the radiographer should
1. apply pressure to the bleeding site
2. call the emergency department for assistance
3. apply a pressure bandage and complete the examination
- ❏ A. 1 and 2 only
- ❏ B. 1 and 3 only
- ❏ C. 2 and 3 only
- ❏ D. 1, 2, and 3

118. Skin discoloration owing to cyanosis may be observed in the
1. gums
2. earlobes
3. tongue
- ❏ A. 1 only
- ❏ B. 1 and 2 only
- ❏ C. 3 only
- ❏ D. 1, 2, and 3

119. The Controlled Substance Act divides drugs and other controlled substances into five schedules according to
- ❏ A. dosage form
- ❏ B. actions
- ❏ C. potential for abuse
- ❏ D. generic name

120. All of the following are useful resources for non–English-speaking patients, *except*
- ❏ A. automated language lines
- ❏ B. special dual headset phones
- ❏ C. a certified interpreter
- ❏ D. a family member or friend

121. Which of the following is/are symptom(s) of shock?

1. Pallor and weakness
2. Increased pulse
3. Fever
   - ❏ A. 1 only
   - ❏ B. 1 and 2 only
   - ❏ C. 1 and 3 only
   - ❏ D. 1, 2, and 3

122. Increased pain threshold, breakdown of skin, and atrophy of fat pads and sweat glands are all important considerations when working with which of the following groups of patients?

- ❏ A. Infants
- ❏ B. Children
- ❏ C. Adolescents
- ❏ D. Geriatric patients

123. The practice that is used to retard the growth of pathogenic bacteria is termed

- ❏ A. antisepsis
- ❏ B. disinfection
- ❏ C. sterilization
- ❏ D. medical asepsis

124. The usual patient preparation for an upper GI examination is

- ❏ A. nothing by mouth (NPO) 8 h before the examination
- ❏ B. light breakfast only on the morning of the examination
- ❏ C. clear fluids only on the morning of the examination
- ❏ D. 2 ounces of castor oil and enemas until clear

125. Successful, effective communication includes proficiency in which of the following skills?

1. Writing
2. Speech
3. Observation
   - ❏ A. 1 only
   - ❏ B. 1 and 2 only
   - ❏ C. 2 and 3 only
   - ❏ D. 1, 2, and 3

126. When reviewing patient blood chemistry levels, what is considered the normal creatinine range?

- ❏ A. 0.5–1.2 mg/dL
- ❏ B. 4.5–6 mg/dL
- ❏ C. 8–20 mg/dL
- ❏ D. Up to 50 mg/dL

127. Which of the following medical equipment is used to determine blood pressure?

1. Pulse oximeter
2. Stethoscope
3. Sphygmomanometer
   - ❏ A. 1 and 2 only
   - ❏ B. 1 and 3 only
   - ❏ C. 2 and 3 only
   - ❏ D. 1, 2, and 3

128. Diseases whose mode of transmission is through the air include

1. tuberculosis
2. severe acute respiratory syndrome
3. rubeola
   - ❏ A. 1 only
   - ❏ B. 1 and 2 only
   - ❏ C. 1 and 3 only
   - ❏ D. 1, 2, and 3

129. Nosocomial infections are those acquired from

- ❏ A. health care facilities
- ❏ B. physicians
- ❏ C. inanimate objects
- ❏ D. insects

130. Tracheostomy is indicated in cases of tracheal obstruction when the obstruction is located

- ❏ A. below the level of the larynx
- ❏ B. above the level of the larynx
- ❏ C. inferior to the carina
- ❏ D. in the right primary bronchus

131. In her studies on death and dying, Dr Elizabeth Kübler-Ross described the first stage of the grieving process as

- ❏ A. denial
- ❏ B. anger
- ❏ C. bargaining
- ❏ D. depression

132. Disclosing confidential information to an unauthorized individual is termed

- ❏ A. defamation
- ❏ B. slander
- ❏ C. libel
- ❏ D. invasion of privacy

133. The Standard of Ethics is made up of

1. Code of Ethics
2. Rules of Ethics
3. Patient's Bill of Rights
4. Patient Care Partnership
   - ❏ A. 1 and 2
   - ❏ B. 1, 2, and 4
   - ❏ C. 2, 3, and 4
   - ❏ D. 3 and 4

134. Which of the following are enteral routes of drug administration?

1. Intrathecal
2. Rectal
3. Buccal
4. Oral
5. Nasogastric
   - ❏ A. 1 and 3 only
   - ❏ B. 2 and 3 only
   - ❏ C. 1, 3, and 4 only
   - ❏ D. 2, 4, and 5 only

135. Which of the following is the meaning of the legal doctrine *res ipsa loquitur*?

- ❏ A. A matter settled by precedent
- ❏ B. A thing or matter settled by justice
- ❏ C. The thing speaks for itself
- ❏ D. Let the master answer

136. A localized dilatation or bulging in a blood vessel wall is a/an

- ❏ A. cyst
- ❏ B. thrombus
- ❏ C. aneurysm
- ❏ D. angina

137. A creatinine level of 2.2 mg/dL is most likely a/an

- ❏ A. indication for an SB study
- ❏ B. contraindication for an SB study
- ❏ C. indication for an IVU study
- ❏ D. contraindication for an IVU study

138. From the following, select the four functions that are typical of the radiographer's patient assessment prior to starting an x-ray examination.

1. Check admission diagnosis
2. Check/measure body temperature
3. Obtain brief clinical history
4. Note appearance and condition
5. Notice degree of ambulation
6. Check/measure blood pressure
   - ❏ A. 1, 2, 3, and 4
   - ❏ B. 3, 4, 5, and 6
   - ❏ C. 2, 3, 5, and 6
   - ❏ D. 1, 3, 4, and 5

139. Qualities of iodinated contrast agents that are less likely to contribute to side effects and reactions include all of the following, *except*

- ❏ A. low osmolality
- ❏ B. high miscibility
- ❏ C. low toxicity
- ❏ D. high viscosity

140. An abnormal, acquired immune response to a substance that would *not* usually trigger a reaction is called a/an

- ❏ A. allergy
- ❏ B. toxin
- ❏ C. allergen
- ❏ D. antidote

141. A diabetic patient who has taken insulin prior to a fasting radiologic examination is susceptible to

- ❏ A. hypoglycemic reaction
- ❏ B. hyperglycemic reaction
- ❏ C. dyspnea
- ❏ D. dysphagia

142. Positive contrast agents are associated with all of the following, *except*

- ❏ A. high atomic number
- ❏ B. iodine
- ❏ C. carbon dioxide
- ❏ D. radiopaque

143. If the patient is not capable of making decisions regarding his or her health, those rights can be exercised on their behalf by

1. designated proxy
2. designated surrogate
3. parent or spouse
   - ❏ A. 1 only
   - ❏ B. 2 only
   - ❏ C. 1 and 2
   - ❏ D. 2 and 3

144. Examples of nonverbal communication include

1. appearance
2. eye contact
3. touch
   - ❏ A. 1 only
   - ❏ B. 1 and 2 only
   - ❏ C. 2 and 3 only
   - ❏ D. 1, 2, and 3

145. In classifying IV contrast agents, the total number of dissolved particles in solution per kilogram of water defines

- ❏ A. osmolality
- ❏ B. toxicity
- ❏ C. viscosity
- ❏ D. osmolarity

146. The ethical principle that refers to our responsibility to keep our patient from harm and to avoid inflicting harm is

- ❏ A. fidelity
- ❏ B. veracity
- ❏ C. beneficence
- ❏ D. nonmaleficence

147. Which two of the following rules most likely apply when transporting a 3-year-old child from the Pediatric floor to the Imaging department?
1. The child can be carefully carried
2. The child should be transported in a crib
3. The child should be transported on a stretcher
4. If transported via crib, the side rails must be up
5. The child may be transported on a wheelchair
- ❏ A. 1 and 2
- ❏ B. 2 and 4
- ❏ C. 2 and 5
- ❏ D. 3 and 5

148. Which of the following can be transmitted via infected blood?
1. HBV
2. HIV
3. *Mycobacterium tuberculosis*
- ❏ A. 1 only
- ❏ B. 1 and 2 only
- ❏ C. 2 and 3 only
- ❏ D. 1, 2, and 3

149. Organize the Cycle of Infection components listed below.
1. Portal of entry
2. Reservoir of infection
3. Infectious organism
4. Mode of transportation
5. Susceptible host
6. Portal of exit
- ❏ A. 6, 2, 3, 4, 1, 5
- ❏ B. 3, 2, 6, 5, 1, 4
- ❏ C. 3, 6, 2, 4, 5, 1
- ❏ D. 5, 1, 2, 3, 4, 6

150. Methods of sterilization include
1. 5 min in boiling water
2. steam under pressure
3. ethylene oxide
- ❏ A. 1 only
- ❏ B. 1 and 2 only
- ❏ C. 2 and 3 only
- ❏ D. 1, 2, and 3

151. The most frequently used intravenous injection site, which is an anastomosis between other veins, is the
- ❏ A. basilic vein
- ❏ B. cephalic vein
- ❏ C. median cubital vein
- ❏ D. median antecubital vein

152. When a radiographer is obtaining patient history, both subjective and objective data should be obtained. An example of *subjective* data is that
- ❏ A. the patient appears to have a productive cough
- ❏ B. the patient has a blood pressure of 130/95 mm Hg
- ❏ C. the patient states that he or she experiences extreme pain in the upright position
- ❏ D. the patient has a palpable mass in the right upper quadrant of the left breast

153. Therapeutic communication techniques include all of the following, *except*
1. making observation
2. restating the main idea
3. giving advice
4. establishing guidelines
5. defending
- ❏ A. 1 and 3
- ❏ B. 2 and 4
- ❏ C. 2, 4, and 5
- ❏ D. 3 and 5

154. Which of the following is the first step to be taken in the performance of a radiographic examination?
- ❏ A. Obtain clinical history
- ❏ B. Provide appropriate patient assistance
- ❏ C. Verify patient identity
- ❏ D. Use appropriate infection control

155. What document describes the minimally acceptable professional conduct for those certified by the ARRT?
- ❏ A. Code of Ethics
- ❏ B. Rules of Ethics
- ❏ C. Patient's Bill of Rights
- ❏ D. Patient Care Partnership

156. The request for imaging services for hospital patients generally includes which of the following information?
1. Patient name and/or identification number
2. Mode of travel to Imaging department
3. Name of referring physician
- ❏ A. 1 only
- ❏ B. 1 and 2 only
- ❏ C. 2 and 3 only
- ❏ D. 1, 2, and 3

157. The legal document or individual authorized to make an individual's health care decisions, should the individual be unable to make them for himself or herself, is the
1. advance health care directive
2. living will
3. health care proxy
- ❏ A. 1 only
- ❏ B. 1 and 2 only
- ❏ C. 2 and 3 only
- ❏ D. 1, 2, and 3

158. What is the most frequently used device to supplement the oxygen in room air?
- ❏ A. Nasal cannula
- ❏ B. Mechanical ventilator
- ❏ C. Venturi mask
- ❏ D. Partial rebreathing mask

159. Suction may be required when the patient
1. has excessive or very viscous secretions
2. is unconscious
3. experiences ineffective coughing
- ❏ A. 1 only
- ❏ B. 1 and 2 only
- ❏ C. 2 and 3 only
- ❏ D. 1, 2, and 3

160. Instruments required to assess vital signs include
1. a stethoscope
2. a sphygmomanometer
3. a watch with a second hand
- ❏ A. 1 only
- ❏ B. 1 and 2 only
- ❏ C. 1 and 3 only
- ❏ D. 1, 2, and 3

161. Examples of central venous catheters (CVCs) include the
1. Port-A-Cath
2. Swan–Ganz
3. Raaf
4. PICC
5. Hickman
- ❏ A. 1, 2, 3, and 4
- ❏ B. 1, 3, 4, and 5
- ❏ C. 2, 3, 4, and 5
- ❏ D. 1, 2, and 4

162. Pacemakers are most often used to treat
- ❏ A. tachycardia
- ❏ B. bradycardia
- ❏ C. ventricular fibrillation
- ❏ D. PVCs

163. Which of the following drugs is used to treat dysrhythmias?
- ❏ A. Epinephrine
- ❏ B. Lidocaine
- ❏ C. Nitroglycerin
- ❏ D. Verapamil

164. In which of the following situations should a radiographer wear protective eye gear (goggles)?
1. When performing an upper GI radiographic examination
2. When assisting the radiologist during an angiogram
3. When assisting the radiologist in a biopsy/aspiration procedure
- ❏ A. 1 and 2 only
- ❏ B. 1 and 3 only
- ❏ C. 2 and 3 only
- ❏ D. 1, 2, and 3

165. A medication used to reduce fever is called
- ❏ A. emetic
- ❏ B. antihistamine
- ❏ C. antipyretic
- ❏ D. diuretic

ANSWERS AND EXPLANATIONS

1. **(A)** Several specialized tubes/catheters are used to provide regular or continual access to the circulatory system for long-term care requirements such as dialysis, blood transfusion, drug therapy such as chemotherapy, and parenteral nutrition. They can also be used for laboratory blood draws and for monitoring central venous pressure (CVP). These are called *CVCs* (or *central lines*). Examples of these central lines include the Port-A-Cath, the Hickman, the Raaf, and the peripherally inserted central catheter (PICC). For x-ray verification of position placement, there is usually a radiopaque distal tip. The distal tip should be located in the superior or inferior vena cava near the right atrium.

2. **(D)** Any pathogenic microorganism that spreads by direct or close *contact,* such as MRSA and *C. difficile, E. coli,* hepatitis A, and some wounds require *contact precautions.* Contact precaution procedures require the use of gloves and gowns for anyone coming in direct contact with the infected individual or the infected person's environment. Some facilities require health care workers to also wear a mask when caring for a patient with MRSA infection.

3. **(C)** The ARRT Rules of Ethics are mandatory and enforced by the ARRT. Item 1 describes Examination/CQR subversion, items 2, 3, and 6 describe Fraud or Deceptive Practices: fraudulent communication regarding credentials and fraudulent billing practices.

   In addition to rules about subversion of the ARRT certification examination and CE process, the Rules of Ethics provide for ARRT sanctions for parties who are convicted under certain state and federal laws. The ARRT Code of Ethics provides guidelines to the medical imaging professional on ethical behavior; it is aspirational but is not monitored or enforced.

4. **(B)** Patients arriving at the emergency department (ED) with suspected *spinal injury* should not be moved. Anteroposterior (AP) and horizontal lateral projections of the suspected area should be evaluated and a decision should be made about the advisability of further images. For a lateral projection, the patient should be moved along one plane, that is, rolled like a log. It is imperative that twisting motions are avoided.

5. **(C)** Blunt trauma to the chest resulting in fractures of two or more adjacent ribs, causing them to become detached from the rest of the rib cage, is termed *flail chest.* Flail chest is usually associated with additional pulmonary traumatic injury. Rib images should be performed in the erect position, if possible.

Pectus carinatum is a congenital defect in which the sternum protrudes anteriorly, often called "pigeon breast." Pectus excavatum is a congenital defect in which the sternum is depressed posteriorly, often called "sunken" or "funnel" chest. Atelectasis is collapse of all or part of a lung that could be caused by rib fractures.

6. **(A)** The prefix *iatr* comes from the Greek word *iatros,* meaning "physician." An iatrogenic infection is the one caused by physician intervention or by medical or diagnostic treatment/procedures. Examples include infection following surgery and nausea or other illness following prescribed drug use.

7. **(B)** *Gerontology,* or geriatrics, is the study of the elderly. Although bone demineralization and loss of muscle mass occur to a greater or lesser degree in most elderly individuals, the radiographer must not assume that all gerontologic patients are hard of hearing, clumsy, or not mentally alert. Nowadays, many elderly people remain very active, staying mentally and physically agile well into their so-called golden years. The radiographer must keep this in mind as he or she provides age-specific care to the gerontologic patient.

8. **(B)** *Negligence* and *malpractice* are examples of *un*intentional misconduct. Negligence refers to the omission or neglect of reasonable caution/care. Malpractice is professional negligence between a professional and the patient. Failure to correctly identify the patient, with subsequent examination on incorrect patient is an example of negligence. Inadequate patient communication and errors in diagnosis are other examples of professional negligence/malpractice.

False imprisonment, such as unnecessary patient restraint, is intentional misconduct. Slander is a verbal defamation of another and is another type of intentional misconduct. Assault is to threaten harm, battery to carry out the threat; both are examples of intentional misconduct.

9. **(A)** Pacemakers are most often used to treat conduction defects causing bradycardia. They can be positioned under the skin in the upper chest and their wires advanced to the *right side of the heart,* to the *apex of the right ventricle* or to the right atrium *and* right ventricle. Pacemaker insertion is often performed under fluoroscopic control in the imaging catheterization lab. Pacemaker insertion can also be performed in the OR, or in a critical care unit using mobile C-arm fluoroscopy. Care must be taken to avoid elevating or abducting the patient's left arm for 24 h following pacemaker insertion.

10. **(D)** The pathway by which infectious organisms gain entry to the body is termed the *portal of entry*. Potential portals of entry include breaks in the skin, the gastrointestinal tract, mucous membranes of eyes, nose, or mouth, the respiratory tract, and the urinary tract. Entry can be accomplished by ingestion, injection, inhalation, and across mucous membrane; the placenta serves as portal of entry between mother and fetus.

11. **(D)** Myelography is the fluoroscopic and radiographic examination of the spinal canal and adjacent structures to demonstrate herniated disk, spinal cord compression, and related lesions/pathology. Water-soluble nonionic contrast material is used and introduced into the subarachnoid space—this is termed an *intrathecal* injection—in the lumbar area (L2–L3/L3–L4) or at the cisterna magna in the uppermost cervical region. (*Long, Rollins, and Smith, 13th ed, Vol III, p. 6*)

12. **(B)** Nonionic, low-osmolality iodinated contrast agents are associated with far fewer side effects and reactions than ionic, higher osmolality contrast agents. A *side effect* is an effect that is unintended but possibly expected and fundamentally *not harmful*. An *adverse reaction* is a *harmful* unintended effect that can be immediate or delayed. Possible *side effects* of iodinated contrast agents include a warm, flushed feeling, a metallic taste in the mouth, nausea, headache, and pain at the injection site. *Adverse reactions* include itching, anxiety, rash or hives, vomiting, sneezing, dyspnea, and hypotension.

13. **(C)** If the patient's injury results from misperformance of a duty in the routine scope of practice of the radiographer, most courts will apply *res ipsa loquitur*, "the thing speaks for itself." If the patient is obviously injured as a result of the radiographer's/professional's actions, it becomes the professional's burden to *disprove* negligence. Examples include imaging the wrong patient or incorrect limb, surgical removal of a healthy organ or limb, or leaving a sponge or clamp in the patient's body during surgery. Additional examples can include manipulation of, or changes made in, electronic data—for example, cropping or masking an electronic x-ray image of a larger area in an effort to make it look like a collimated smaller area. Potentially useful information can be eliminated via cropping/masking and patient receives unnecessary x-ray exposure. Other examples can include modification of EI values, processing algorithms, and manipulation of brightness and/or contrast values.

14. **(C)** Tracheostomy is the surgical opening of the trachea to provide and secure an open airway. A tracheostomy is often performed in emergency situations when there is *upper* airway obstruction, that is, *above* the level of the larynx. A tracheostomy patient will have difficulty in speaking as a result of redirection of the air past the vocal cords. Gurgling or rattling sounds coming from the trachea indicate an excess accumulation of secretions, requiring suction with sterile catheters. A tracheostomy tube must not be moved because any rotation or movement may cause it to become dislodged, and an obstructed airway may result.

15. **(B)** Injectable medications are available in two different kinds of containers. An *ampoule* is a small container that usually holds a single dose of medication. A *vial* is a somewhat larger container that holds a number of doses of medication. The term *bolus* is used to describe an amount of fluid to be injected. A *carafe* is a narrow-mouthed container; it is not likely to be used for medical purposes.

16. **(C)** The sudden cessation of productive ventilation and circulation is called cardiopulmonary arrest. The radiographer should be trained in basic life support (BLS) for health care providers. The American Heart Association uses the acronym *CAB*—representing *circulation, airway, breathing*—to help individuals remember CPR step sequence. Compressions should be about 100/min, beginning with 30 compressions. After 30 compressions, airway should be established using the head-tilt, chin-lift movement. If the victim is not breathing normally, the professional rescuer should begin mouth-to-mouth breathing. One cycle is considered to be 30 chest compressions followed by two rescue breaths.

17. **(D)** Special precautions must be taken with the disposal of biomedical waste, such as laboratory and pathology waste, used bandages and dressings, discarded gloves, all sharp objects, and liquid waste from suction, bladder catheters, chest tubes, and IV tubes, as well as drainage containers.

Biomedical waste must be packaged in special, easily identifiable, impermeable bags and removed from the premises by an approved biomedical waste hauler.

18. **(B)** The two most common types of chronic inflammation of the intestines are ulcerative colitis and Crohn's disease. The latter can attack any part of the GI tract and it extends through all layers of the intestinal wall (therefore, the possibility of forming fistulous tracks to contiguous structures). Ulcerative colitis attacks only the large bowel and the mucosal layer of the intestinal wall. Curiously, cigarette smoking increases the risk for Crohn's disease and decreases the risk for ulcerative colitis. Intussusception is an obstructive disorder characterized by slippage of a portion of intestine into an adjacent portion ("telescoping") of the intestine.

19. **(D)** Misunderstandings between cultures can occur as a result of the use of gestures that have different meanings in different countries. In the United States and Europe, the "thumbs up" gesture has a positive implication. However, it is considered rude in Australia and obscene in the Middle East. Other examples of potentially misunderstood gestures include the following: if you compliment a Mexican child, you must touch the head, whereas in Asia it is not acceptable to touch the head of a child. In the Philippines, it is rude to beckon with the index finger. Some cultures

such as Asian believe direct eye contact to be rude. Furthermore, in the United States, people are comfortable speaking about 18 inches apart, whereas in the Middle East, people stand much closer together when they talk; in England, people stand further apart.

20. **(C)** Rules of good body mechanics include the following: when carrying a heavy object, hold it *close* to the body; the back should be kept straight; *avoid twisting* when lifting an object; bend the knees and *use leg and abdominal* muscles to lift (rather than using the back muscles); and whenever possible, *push or roll* large heavy objects (rather than lifting or pulling). To transfer the patient with maximum safety, the radiographer must correctly use certain concepts of body mechanics. First, *a broad base of support* lends greater stability; therefore, the radiographer should stand with his or her feet approximately 12 inches apart, with one foot slightly forward. Second, stability is achieved when the body's *center of gravity* (center of the pelvis) is positioned over its base of support. For example, leaning away from the central axis of the body makes the body more vulnerable to losing balance; if the feet are close together, balance is even more difficult to maintain.

21. **(D)** Medical equipment that could contain latex includes disposable gloves, tourniquets, blood pressure cuffs, stethoscopes, IV tubing, oral and nasal airways, enema tips, endotracheal tubes, syringes, electrode pads, catheters, wound drains, and injection ports. It should be noted that when powdered latex gloves are changed, latex protein/powder particles get into the air, where they can be inhaled and come in contact with body membranes. Studies have indicated that when unpowdered gloves are worn, there are extremely low levels of the allergy-producing proteins present.

22. **(A)** Pathogenic microorganisms expelled from the respiratory tract through the mouth or nose can be carried as evaporated *droplets* through the air or as *airborne* dust particles and settle on clothing, utensils, or food. Therefore, patients with respiratory tract infections/diseases who are transported to the radiology department should wear a surgical string mask to prevent such transmission during a cough or sneeze.

23. **(B)** Quantities of medication can be dispensed intravenously over a period of time via an *IV infusion*. A special infusion pump may be used to precisely regulate the quantity received by the patient. An *IV push* refers to a rapid injection; the term *bolus* refers to the quantity of material being injected. The term *hypodermic* refers to administration of medication by any route other than oral.

24. **(D)** Symptoms of inadequate oxygen supply include dyspnea, cyanosis, and distention of the veins of the neck. The radiographer must call for help, assist the patient to a sitting or semi-Fowler position (the recumbent position makes breathing more difficult), and have oxygen and emergency drugs available. Conditions often requiring oxygen therapy are chronic obstructive pulmonary disease (COPD), pneumonia, severe asthma, cystic fibrosis, sleep apnea.

25. **(B)** A *fomite* is an inanimate object that has been in contact with an infectious microorganism. A *reservoir* is a site where an infectious organism can remain alive and from which transmission can occur. Although an inanimate object can be a reservoir for infection, living objects (such as humans) also can be reservoirs. For infection to spread, there must be a *host* environment. Although an inanimate object may serve as a temporary host where microbes can grow, microbes flourish on and in the human host, where there are plenty of body fluids and tissues to nourish and feed the microbes. A *vector* is an animal host of an infectious organism that transmits the infection via bite or sting.

26. **(B)** There are four stages of infection. The infection is introduced and lies dormant in the *latent period*. As soon as the microbes begin to shed, the infection becomes communicable. The microbes reproduce (during the *incubation* period), and during the actual disease period, signs and symptoms of the infection may begin. The infection is most active and communicable at this point. As the patient fights off the infection and the symptoms regress, the *convalescent (recovery) phase* occurs.

27. **(C)** Dyspnea (difficulty breathing) can precede a respiratory arrest event. Dyspnea can be caused by an aspirated foreign object, injury to the chest, tongue obstruction of airway in unresponsive person, drug overdose, and so on. Dyspnea caused by a partially obstructed airway can manifest itself in the patient by wheezing, noisy/labored breathing, cyanosis of the nail beds and lips, distention of the neck veins, and anxiety. The radiographer should not leave the patient alone, should call for assistance, assist the patient to a seated or semi-Fowler position, and prepare to assist with emergency treatment. Dysphagia is the medical term for difficulty in swallowing, usually unrelated to obstructed airway.

28. **(D)** Nowadays, we know that *the most important precaution in the practice of aseptic technique is proper hand hygiene.* The radiographer's hands should be thoroughly washed with soap and warm running water for at least 20 s, or by using an alcohol sanitizer, before and after every patient examination. If the faucet cannot be operated with the knee, it should be opened and closed using paper towels (to avoid contamination of or by the faucet). The radiographer's uniform should not touch the sink. The hands and forearms should always be kept lower than the elbows; care should be taken to wash all surfaces of the hands and between the fingers. Hand lotions should be used to prevent hands from chapping; broken skin permits the entry of microorganisms. Antiseptics, disinfectants, and germicides are substances used to kill pathogenic bacteria, and some of these products are used in hand-washing substances. Cracks or abrasions in the skin should be covered because the broken skin permits the entry of microorganisms. Disinfectants and germicides are often used for hard

surfaces, whereas antiseptics are generally used for tissue. Alcohol-based hand antiseptic sanitizers have been recommended as an alternative to hand washing with soap and water, except when there is visible soiling or after caring for a patient with *Clostridium difficile* (*C. difficile*) infection.

29. **(D)** Rules of good body mechanics include the following: when carrying a heavy object, hold it *close* to the body; the back should be kept straight; *avoid twisting* when lifting an object; bend the knees and *use leg and abdominal* muscles to lift (rather than using the back muscles); and whenever possible, *push or roll* large heavy objects (rather than lifting or pulling). To transfer the patient with maximum safety, the radiographer must correctly use certain concepts of body mechanics. First, *a broad base of support* lends greater stability; therefore, the radiographer should stand with his or her feet approximately 12 inches apart, with one foot slightly forward. Second, stability is achieved when the body's *center of gravity* (center of the pelvis) is positioned over its base of support. For example, leaning away from the central axis of the body makes the body more vulnerable to losing balance; if the feet are close together, balance is even more difficult to maintain.

30. **(C)** When caring for a patient with an indwelling Foley catheter, place the drainage bag and tubing *below the level of the bladder* to maintain the gravity flow of urine. Placement of the tubing or bag above or at the same level with the bladder will allow backflow of urine into the bladder. This reflux of urine can increase the chance of developing a urinary tract infection (UTI).

31. **(B)** While transferring patients, always help the patient transfer toward the *strong* side. That is, begin with the stronger side closer to the x-ray table. Be certain that the wheels of stretchers and wheelchairs are locked during the transfer. A two-person lift is not always necessary; most patients can be transferred with the careful assistance of the radiographer. While assisting a patient in changing, first remove clothing from the unaffected side. If this is done, removing clothing from the affected side will require less movement and effort.

32. **(D)** It is essential that the radiographer takes adequate time for explanation of the procedure to the patient. In addition, there are times when the radiographer must inquire whether proper diet and/or other preparation instructions have been followed prior to the examination. The radiographer requires the cooperation of the patient throughout the course of the examination; therefore, providing a thorough *explanation* will alleviate patient anxieties and permit fuller cooperation. Patient anxiety can also be reduced when the radiographer uses good listening skills, that is, looking at the patient (eye contact) and listening carefully without interruption and answering questions in a simple, clear, and direct manner, avoiding the use of complex medical terminology.

33. **(A)** The normal blood pressure range for adult men and women is a 90–120 mm Hg systolic reading (left/upper number) and a 50–70 mm Hg diastolic reading (right/lower number). Systolic pressure is the contraction phase of the left ventricle, and diastolic pressure is the relaxation phase in the heart cycle. Therefore, in the blood pressure reading 145/85, the systolic pressure of 145 is higher than desirable, and the diastolic pressure of 85 is also higher than desirable. Diastolic pressure 80–89 and systolic pressure 120–139 is usually considered prehypertension. Systolic pressure consistently above 140 and diastolic pressure consistently above 90 is considered hypertension.

34. **(C)** Facsimile transmission of health information is convenient but should be used only to address immediate and urgent patient needs, and every precaution must be taken to ensure its confidentiality. It should be used only with prior patient authorization, when urgently needed for patient care, or when required for third-party payer ongoing hospitalization certification. These recommendations are made by the American Health Information Management Association (AHIMA).

35. **(C)** Verbal defamation of another, or *slander*, is a type of intentional misconduct. *Invasion of privacy* (i.e., public discussion of privileged and confidential information) is intentional misconduct. However, if a radiographer leaves a weak patient standing alone to check images or get supplies and the patient falls and sustains an injury, that would be considered unintentional misconduct, or *negligence*.

36. **(B)** When helping a patient out of a wheelchair, *it must first be locked.* Then, the footrests must be moved up and aside to prevent the patient from tripping over them or tilting the wheelchair forward. The wheelchair should be placed at a 45° angle with the x-ray table or bed, with the patient's *stronger side closest* toward the x-ray table or bed. When returning the patient to the wheelchair, once the patient is seated, the footrests should be lowered into place for the patient's comfort.

37. **(C)** Venous blood is returned to the right atrium via the superior and inferior venae cavae. It also passes from the left atrium through the bicuspid/mitral valve into the left ventricle, and from the right atrium through the tricuspid valve into the right ventricle during atrial systole.

38. **(D)** An unconscious patient frequently is able to hear and understand all that is going on, even though he or she is unable to respond. Therefore, while performing the examination, the radiographer always should refer to the patient by name and take care to continually explain what is being done and reassure the patient.

39. **(C)** *Cathartics* stimulate defecation and are used in preparation for radiologic examinations of the large bowel. *Diuretics* are used to promote urine elimination in individuals whose tissues are retaining excessive fluid. *Emetics* induce vomiting, and *antitussives* are used to inhibit coughing.

40. (B) The most effective method of sterilization is moist heat, using steam under pressure. This is known as *autoclaving*. Sterilization with dry heat requires higher temperatures for longer periods of time than sterilization with moist heat. Chemical sterilization is a low-temperature sterilization. Ethylene oxide is used to sterilize items that cannot tolerate high temperatures or moisture. *Pasteurization* is moderate heating with rapid cooling; it is frequently used in the commercial preparation of milk and alcoholic beverages such as wine and beer. It is not a form of sterilization. *Freezing* also can kill some microbes, but it is not a form of sterilization.

41. (D) Medications can be administered in many ways. *Parenteral* administration refers to drugs administered in a way other than by mouth. Parenteral administration includes intramuscular, subcutaneous, IV, or intrathecal routes. Intramuscular drug injections usually require that the needle form a 90° angle of injection. For subcutaneous injections, the needle should form a 45° angle. *Intravenous* injections generally require that the needle form about a 15°–25° angle with the arm (see Fig. 1-2).

42. (C) *Ethnocentrism* is the belief that one's personal experience and perception of the world is superior to the experiences and perceptions of others, that is, the belief that one's own cultural ways are superior to any other. Ethnocentrism can be found in all cultures and is the most significant barrier to good intercultural communication. *Ethnology* is the comparative study of various cultures. *Ethnobiology* is the study of biological characteristics of various races. *Ethnography* is the study of a single society's culture.

43. (D) Most institutions these days have computerized, paperless systems for patient information transmittal; these systems must ensure confidentiality in compliance with Health Insurance Portability and Accountability Act (HIPAA) of 1996 regulations. *Only health care professionals having been trained in HIPAA compliance may have access* to the computerized system via personal password, thus helping ensure confidentiality of patient information. Computer files containing patient information must be encrypted. If authorization for release of medical information is given, a copy of that authorization must be kept on file. All medical records and other individually identifiable health information, whether electronic, on paper, or oral, are covered by HIPAA legislation and by subsequent Department of Health and Human Services (HHS) rules that took effect in April 2001.

44. (A) Iodinated contrast material can become somewhat *viscous* (i.e., thick and sticky) at normal room temperatures. This makes injection much more difficult. Warming the contrast medium to body temperature serves to reduce viscosity and can be achieved by placing the vial in warm water or putting it into a special warming oven.

45. (B) *Cardiogenic shock* is related to cardiac failure and results from interference with heart function. It can occur in cases of cardiac tamponade, pulmonary embolus, or

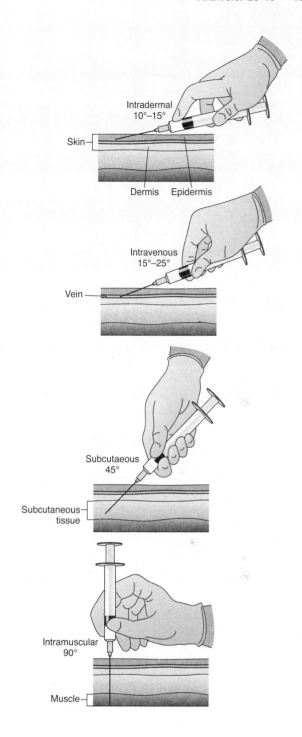

Figure 1-2

myocardial infarction. *Hypovolemic shock* is related to loss of large amounts of blood, either from internal bleeding or from hemorrhage associated with trauma. *Neurogenic shock* occurs in cases of trauma to the central nervous system that results in decreased arterial resistance and pooling of blood in peripheral vessels. *Septic shock,* along with *anaphylactic shock,* generally is classified as *vasogenic shock.*

46. (D) All these symptoms are related to a respiratory reaction. There also may be dyspnea, asthma attack, or cyanosis. The patient who has received contrast media should be watched closely. If any symptoms arise, the radiologist should be notified immediately.

47. (B) Category-specific isolations have been replaced by *transmission-based precautions: airborne, droplet,* and *contact.* Under these guidelines, some conditions or diseases can fall into more than one category. *Airborne precautions* are implemented in patients suspected or known to be infected with *tubercle bacillus (TB), chickenpox (varicella),* or *measles (rubeola).* Airborne precautions *require that the patient wears a string mask* to avoid the spread of bronchial secretions or other pathogens during coughing. If the patient is unable or unwilling to wear a mask, the radiographer must wear one, and for a patient in airborne precautions that would be an N95 particulate respirator mask. The radiographer should wear gloves, but a gown is required only if flagrant contamination is likely. Patients under *airborne precautions* require a *private, specially ventilated (negative-pressure) room.* A private room is also indicated for all patients on *droplet precautions,* that is, with diseases transmitted via *large droplets* expelled from the patient while speaking, sneezing, or coughing. The pathogenic droplets can infect others when they come in contact with mouth or nasal mucosa or conjunctiva. *Rubella* (German measles), *mumps,* and *influenza* are among the diseases spread by droplet contact; a *private room is required* for the patient, and health care practitioners should wear *a string mask* and may also wear *gown and gloves* as needed. Any pathogenic microorganism spread by direct or close *contact,* such as *MRSA, conjunctivitis,* and *hepatitis A,* requires *contact precautions. Contact precautions* require a *private patient room* and the use of *gloves, gown, and sometimes a mask* for anyone coming in direct contact with the infected individual or his or her environment.

48. (B) The presence of surgical clips, cochlear implant, neurostimulator, any implanted metal device, or prosthesis are contraindications for magnetic resonance imaging (MRI). MRI can be performed for a herniated disk and subdural bleeding. Dental fillings do not contraindicate MRI.

49. (B) Blood pressure among individuals varies with age, sex, fatigue, mental or physical stress, disease, and trauma. The blood pressure within vessels is highest during *ventricular systole* (contraction) and lowest during diastole (relaxation). Blood pressure measurements are recorded with the systolic pressure on top and the diastolic pressure on the bottom, as in 100/80.

50. (B) Many microorganisms can remain infectious while awaiting transmission to another host. A contaminated inanimate object such as a food utensil, a doorknob, or an IV pole is called a *fomite.* A *vector* is an insect or animal carrier of infectious organisms, such as a rabid animal, a mosquito that carries malaria, or a mouse/deer tick that carries Lyme disease. These can transmit disease through either direct or indirect contact.

51. (B) A circumstance in which actions of both the health care provider and the patient contribute to an injurious outcome is termed *contributory negligence.* An example would be a patient who fails to follow the physician's orders or fails to show up for follow-up care and then sues the physician when the condition causes permanent damage. Another example would be a patient who deliberately gives false information about the ingestion of drugs, leading to adverse effects from medications administered. Most states do not completely dismiss injury if there has been negligence on the part of the health care institution, even if the patient's actions contributed substantially to the injury. Rather, *comparative negligence* is applied, where the percentage of the injury owing to the patient's actions is compared with the total amount of injury. A jury may decide that a physician was negligent in his or her actions, but because the patient lied about using an illegal street drug that contributed to the injurious outcome, the patient is 80% responsible for his or her condition. The party suing may be awarded $100,000 for injuries but actually would receive only $20,000. *Gross negligence* occurs when there is willful or deliberate neglect of the patient. Assault, battery, invasion of privacy, false imprisonment, and defamation of character all fall under the category of *intentional misconduct.*

52. (C) *Extravasation* of contrast media into surrounding tissue is potentially very painful. If it does occur, the needle should be removed and the extravasation cared for immediately (before looking for another vein). First, *pressure* should be applied to the vein until bleeding stops. Application of *a cold pack* to the affected area helps to relieve pain, and elevate the part. Application of a *warm towel* at the injection site can hasten absorption of any contrast medium.

53. (D) The normal blood pressure range for adult men and women is a 90–120 mm Hg systolic reading (left/upper number) and a 50–70 mm Hg diastolic reading (right number). Systolic pressure is the contraction phase of the left ventricle, and diastolic pressure is the relaxation phase in the heart cycle. Systolic pressure consistently above 140 and diastolic pressure consistently above 90 is considered hypertension.

54. (D) When moving heavy objects, there are several rules that will reduce back strain. When carrying a heavy object, hold it close to your body. Your back should be kept straight; avoid twisting. When lifting an object, bend at the knees and use leg and abdominal muscles to lift (rather than your back muscles). Whenever possible, push or roll heavy objects (i.e., mobile unit), rather than pulling or lifting.

55. (D) None of the statements in the question is false; all are *true.* Oxygen is classified as a drug and must be prescribed by a physician. The rate and mode of delivery of oxygen must be specified in the physician's orders. It can be ordered to be delivered continuously or as needed.

56. (D) Diversity of culture is often thought of as ethnic diversity—a difference in nationality. But cultural groups include religious groups, age groups, racial groups, socioeconomic groups, geographic groups, handicapped groups, generational groups, gender groups, and sexual preference groups. *Ethnocentrism* is the belief that one's own cultural ways are superior to any other way. Ethnocentrism can be found in all cultures and is the most significant barrier to good intercultural communication. It is essential that we have an awareness of our own ethnocentrism.

57. (B) A *double-contrast GI* examination requires the ingestion of gas-producing powder, crystals, pills, or beverage by the patient followed by a small amount of high-density barium. The patient then may be asked to roll in the recumbent position in order to coat the gastric mucosa while the carbon dioxide expands. This procedure provides optimal visualization of the gastric mucosa. Although a *double-contrast BE* uses a negative contrast agent, it is not ingested but rather is delivered rectally. An *oral cholecystogram* (radiographic examination of the gallbladder) can be performed approximately 3 h after ingestion of special ipodate calcium granules. An *IVU* (intravenous/excretory urography, radiographic examination of the excretory/urinary system) requires an IV injection of iodinated contrast medium.

58. (C) Under *transmission-based precautions (airborne, droplet,* and *contact),* some conditions or diseases can fall into more than one category. Airborne precautions are implemented in patients suspected or known to be infected with tubercle bacillus (TB), chickenpox (varicella), or measles (rubeola). *Airborne* precautions require that *the patient wears a string mask* to avoid the spread of bronchial secretions or other pathogens during coughing. If the patient is unable or unwilling to wear a mask, the radiographer must wear a string mask to avoid the spread of bronchial secretions or other pathogens during coughing. The radiographer should wear gloves, but a gown is required only if flagrant contamination is likely. Patients under airborne precautions require a *private, specially ventilated (negative-pressure) room*. A private room is also indicated for all patients on droplet precautions, that is, with diseases transmitted via large droplets expelled from the patient while speaking, sneezing, or coughing. The pathogenic droplets can infect others when they come in contact with mouth or nasal mucosa or conjunctiva. *Rubella* (German measles), *mumps,* and *influenza* are among the diseases spread by droplet contact; a *private room is required* for the patient, and health care practitioners should wear a string mask if within 3 feet of patient. Any disease that spreads by direct or close *contact,* such as methicillin-resistant *Staphylococcus aureus* (MRSA), *conjunctivitis,* and *rotavirus,* requires *contact precautions*. Contact precautions require a *private patient room* and the use of *gloves* and *gowns* for anyone coming in direct contact with the infected individual or his or her environment.

59. (D) Medications can be administered in a number of ways: orally, sublingually, topically, and parenterally. *Oral* denotes delivery by mouth (e.g., analgesics). *Sublingual* refers to medication placed under the tongue and dissolved there for rapid absorption (e.g., nitroglycerine). *Topical* denotes medication that is applied directly onto the skin (e.g., topical anesthetics and transdermal patches). A *parenteral* route of drug administration is one that bypasses the digestive system. The five parenteral routes require different needle placements: under the skin (subcutaneous), through the skin and into the muscle (intramuscular), between the layers of the skin (intradermal), into a vein (intravenous), and into the subarachnoid space (intrathecal).

60. (D) Although it is never the responsibility of the radiographer to diagnose a patient, it is the responsibility of every radiographer to be alert. The patient should not be subjected to unnecessary radiation from an unwanted examination. Rather, it is the radiographer's responsibility to check with the referring physician and report the patient's complaint.

61. (B) A radiographer who performs the wrong examination on a patient may be charged with battery. *Battery* refers to the unlawful laying of hands on a patient. The radiographer also could be charged with battery if a patient is moved about roughly or touched in a manner that is inappropriate or without the patient's consent. *Assault* is the *threat* of touching or laying hands on someone. If a patient feels threatened by a practitioner, either because of the tone or pitch of the practitioner's voice or because the practitioner uses words that are threatening, the practitioner can be accused of assault. *False imprisonment* may be considered if a patient is ignored despite stating that he or she no longer wishes to continue with the procedure or if restraining devices are used improperly or used without a physician's order. The accusation of *defamation* can be upheld when the patient's confidentiality is not respected and, as a result, the patient suffers embarrassment or mockery.

62. (B) A patient who is undergoing a *BE* generally is required to have a low-residue diet for 1 or 2 days, followed by cathartics and cleansing enemas prior to the examination. Any retained fecal material can simulate or obscure pathology. A patient who is scheduled for a *pyelogram* must have the preceding meal withheld to avoid the possibility of aspirating vomitus in case of an allergic reaction. A *metastatic survey* does not require the use of contrast media, and no patient preparation is necessary.

63. (A) When performing bedside radiography in a contact isolation room, the radiographer should wear a gown and gloves. The IRs are prepared for the examination by placing a plastic sleeve over them to protect them from contamination. Whenever possible, one person should manipulate the mobile unit and remain "clean," while the other handles the patient. The mobile unit should be cleaned with a disinfectant on exiting the patient's room, not before entering.

64. (C) The Levin and Salem Sump tubes are NG tubes used for gastric decompression. The *Salem Sump* tube is radiopaque and has a double lumen. One lumen is for gastric air compression, and the other is for removal of fluids. The *Levin* tube is a single-lumen tube that is used to prevent accumulation of intestinal liquids and gas during and following intestinal surgery. The *Swan–Ganz* is a pulmonary artery flow-directed catheter used to measure cardiac output and pressures on the right side of the heart. It is a specific type of IV catheter used to measure the pumping ability of the heart, to obtain pressure readings, and to introduce medications and IV fluids.

65. **(D)** A catheter placed in a large vein is called a *central venous line.* It can be used to deliver frequent medications or nutrition or to monitor cardiac pressures. Catheters can vary in size and number of lumens depending on intended use. The *Port-A-Cath* is a totally implanted access port, and the peripherally inserted central catheter (*PICC*) is inserted through the basilic or subclavian vein and advanced until the tip rests in the superior vena cava—they both permit long-term intravenous treatment. The *Swan–Ganz* catheter is advanced to the pulmonary artery and is used to measure the pumping ability of the heart, to obtain pressure readings, and to introduce medications and IV fluids. The *Levin* and *Salem Sump* tubes are NG tubes used for gastric decompression. The *Salem Sump* tube is radiopaque and has a double lumen, one lumen is for gastric air compression and the other is for removal of fluids.

66. **(B)** *Health care–associated infections* (*HAIs*) are infections acquired by patients while they are in the hospital; these are also termed *nosocomial* infections. Many of these infections are acquired by patients whose resistance has been diminished by their illness and are unrelated to the condition for which the patients were hospitalized. Infection resulting from physician intervention is termed *iatrogenic.* The CDC estimates that 5%–15% of all hospital patients acquire some type of HAI. Hospital personnel can also become infected (occupationally acquired infection).

Individuals weakened by illnesses or diseases are more susceptible to infection than healthy individuals. The most common HAI is the *urinary tract infection* (UTI), often related to the use of urinary catheters, which can allow passage of pathogens into the patient's body. Other types of HAIs include sepsis, wound infection, and respiratory tract infection. These are often attributable to methicillin-resistant *Staphylococcus aureus* (MRSA) and vancomycin-resistant enterococci (VRE).

Droplet and airborne identify types of transmission-based precautions.

67. **(C)** *Emphysema* is a progressive disorder caused by long-term irritation of the bronchial passages, such as by air pollution or cigarette smoking. Emphysema patients are unable to exhale normally because of loss of elasticity of alveolar walls. If emphysema patients receive oxygen, it is usually administered at a very slow flow rate because their respirations are controlled by the level of carbon dioxide in the blood.

68. **(D)** A special population that requires careful consideration in the imaging department is our pediatric patients. Communication and care challenges can be quite different with *children,* depending on their age; they must be provided with a safe environment and never left unattended. A *neonate* is usually described as a child from birth to

28 days (i.e., newborn). Imaging procedures should be explained to the parent/guardian, if they are present. The neonate must be kept warm and staff must constantly be in attendance. *Infant* (up to 1 year of age) care includes minimizing separation anxiety by keeping infant and parent(s) together, keeping a familiar object or two (toy, blanket) with the infant, and limiting the number of staff present in the x-ray room. *Toddlers* (1–2 years of age) should be spoken to at eye level; the radiographer should be cheerful and unhurried. *Preschoolers* (3–5 years of age) benefit from simple explanations. Be honest with *school-age children* (6–12 years of age), explain what you will be doing and let them help whenever possible. *Adolescents* (13–18 years of age) require privacy and modesty. *Young adults* are described as 19–45 years of age.

69. **(D)** A *tort* is an *intentional* or *unintentional* act that involves personal injury or damage to a patient. Allowing a patient to be exposed to unnecessary radiation, either by neglecting to shield the patient or by performing an unwanted examination, would be considered a tort, and the radiographer would be legally accountable. Other examples of negligent/unintentional torts can include imaging the wrong patient or injury to a patient as a result of a fall when left unattended on an x-ray table, in a radiographic room, or on a stretcher without side rails or safety belt. Radiographing the wrong patient or the opposite limb are other examples of *negligence/unintentional tort.* Immobilizing a patient against his or her will is an example of an *intentional* tort.

70. **(C)** Informed consent is required for procedures that involve risk; many imaging procedures require signed consent. Informed consent is also required for procedures that are considered experimental, or for any research in which the patient is participating. The consent form must be complete *before* being signed; there should be no blank spaces on the consent form when the patient signs it. The patient must sign the consent form before receiving sedation. The physician named on the consent form must perform the procedure; no other physician should perform it. In the case of a minor, a parent or guardian is required to sign the form. If a patient is not competent, then the legally appointed guardian must sign the consent form. Remember that obtaining consent is the physician's responsibility, so the *explanation* of the procedural risks should be given by the physician, and not by the radiographer. The informed consent can be revoked by the patient at any time.

71. **(D)** Pacemakers are most often used to treat conduction defects causing bradycardia. They can be positioned under the skin in the upper chest and their wires advanced to the right side of the heart, to the apex of the right ventricle or to the right atrium and right ventricle. Pacemaker insertion is often performed under fluoroscopic control in the imaging catheterization lab. Pacemaker insertion can also be performed in the OR or in a critical care unit using mobile C-arm fluoroscopy. Care must be taken to *avoid elevating or abducting the patient's left arm for 24 h* following pacemaker insertion.

72. (C) The BUN level indicates the quantity of *nitrogen in the blood in the form of urea*. The normal concentration is 7–20 mg/dL. *BUN* and *creatinine* blood chemistry levels should be checked before administering originated contrast agents. An increase in the BUN level often indicates decreased renal function. Increased BUN and/or creatinine levels may forecast an increased possibility of contrast media–induced renal effects and poor visualization of the renal collecting systems. The normal creatinine range is 0.5–1.2 mg/dL.

73. (B) With the use of iodinated contrast agents, there is a potential concern for increased renal damage in patients with AKI and/or in patients with severe chronic kidney disease (as determined by estimated glomerular filtration rate/eGFR). Current (2020) American College of Radiology (ACR) recommendations state that "there have been no reports of lactic acidosis following intravenous iodinated contrast medium administration in patients properly selected for metformin use." The ACR recommends that patients taking metformin (Glucophage) be classified in two categories. Category 1 patients taking metformin are those with no evidence of AKI and with eGFR ≥ 30 mL/min/1.73 m^2; these patients need not discontinue metformin before or after receiving iodinated contrast media, and it is not required that renal function be reassessed following the examination. Category 2 patients taking metformin are those with AKI or severe chronic kidney disease as indicated by eGFR, or those who will be undergoing an arterial catheter study; these patients should temporarily discontinue metformin at the time of (or prior to) the procedure, and withhold metformin for 48 h after the procedure. Metformin should be reinstituted only after renal function studies have been reevaluated and found to be acceptable.(https://www.acr.org/-/media/ACR/Files/Clinical-Resources/Contrast_Media.pdf)

74. (A) *Volvulus* and *intussusception* both involve a mechanical "closure" or obstruction of the intestinal lumen by a change in the continuous pathway of the GI tract—volvulus by a twisting of the bowel on itself causing obstruction and intussusception by "telescoping" of the bowel causing obstruction. *Meconium ileus* is another form of mechanical obstruction where meconium (first feces of a newborn) becomes hardened and impacted, causing obstruction. *Paralytic (or adynamic) ileus,* however, is an obstruction caused by loss of peristaltic movement of the intestine, not considered a mechanical obstruction.

75. (C) An individual whose coronary arteries are not carrying enough blood to the heart muscle (myocardium) as a result of partial or complete blockage of a cardiac vessel experiences crushing pain in the chest, frequently radiating to the left jaw and arm. This is termed *angina pectoris.* It may be relieved by the drug nitroglycerin, which dilates the coronary arteries, thus facilitating circulation. *Tachycardia* refers to rapid heart rate, *bradycardia* refers to slow heart rate, and *syncope* is fainting.

76. (A) Informed consent is required for procedures that involve risk; many imaging procedures require signed consent. Informed consent is also required for procedures that are considered experimental, or for any research in which the patient is participating. The consent form must be complete *before* being signed; there should be no blank spaces on the consent form when the patient signs it. The patient must sign the consent form before receiving sedation. The physician named on the consent form must perform the procedure; no other physician should perform it. In the case of a minor, a parent or guardian is required to sign the form. If a patient is not competent, then the legally appointed guardian must sign the consent form. Remember that obtaining consent is the physician's responsibility, so the *explanation* of the procedural risks should be given by the physician, and not by the radiographer. The informed consent can be revoked by the patient at any time.

77. (C) The relatively low-osmolality and nonionic, water-soluble contrast media available to radiology departments have outstanding advantages, especially for patients with a history of allergic reaction. These were used originally for intrathecal injections (myelography), but were quickly accepted for intravascular injections as well. *Side effects and allergic reactions are less likely and less severe with these media.* One of the very significant disadvantages is their high cost compared with that of ionic contrast media.

78. (C) Reactions to contrast agents are named and categorized according to the body system(s) affected, the nature of the reaction (i.e., allergic vs. nonallergic), and its severity (i.e., mild, moderate, or severe). These reactions are categorized as *mild* (a nonallergic reaction), *anaphylactic* (allergic reaction), and *vasovagal* (life-threatening). *Mild* effects are principally emotional and anxiety based. These are characterized by anxiety, syncope, nausea, lightheadedness, and, sometimes, a few hives. The patient usually requires reassurance and not medical attention. An *anaphylactic* reaction is a true allergic reaction to, for example, iodinated media and can lead to a life-threatening situation. Immediate medical attention is required. Symptoms of anaphylactic reaction include laryngo/bronchospasm, hypotension, moderate-to-severe urticaria, angioedema, and tachycardia. A *vasovagal* reaction is life-threatening and requires a declared emergency (code). Symptoms of a vasovagal reaction include bradycardia, hypotension, and no detectable pulse. The fourth type of reaction, *acute renal failure,* may not manifest for up to 48 h following injection of the contrast agent. Patients should notify their physician if they experience any changes in their urinary habits or any other atypical symptoms. Treatment would include hydration, dispensation of a diuretic (e.g., Lasix), and possibly even renal dialysis.

79. (A) When a two-member team of radiographers is performing mobile radiography on a patient with contact precautions, such as an MRSA patient, one radiographer remains "clean," that is, he or she has no physical contact with the patient. The clean radiographer will position the mobile unit and make the exposure. The other member of the team will position the IP and retrieve the IP. As the two radiographers fold down the IP's protective plastic cover, the "clean" radiographer will remove the IP from the plastic. Both radiographers should be protected with gowns, gloves, and possibly masks if the patient is on contact precautions. In addition, after the examination is completed, the mobile unit should be cleaned with a disinfectant. Conditions requiring the use of contact precautions also include vancomycin-resistant enterococci (VRE) and rotavirus.

80. **(D)** The Joint Commission (formerly the Joint Commission on the Accreditation of Health care Organizations [JCAHO]) is the organization that accredits health care organizations in the United States. The Joint Commission sets forth certain standards for medical records, both written and electronic. In keeping with these standards, all diagnostic and therapeutic orders must appear in the patient's medical record or chart. In addition, patient identification information, medical history, consent forms, and other diagnostic and therapeutic reports, if any, should be part of the patient's permanent record. The patient's chart is a means of communication between various health care providers.

81. **(C)** If a patient in your care asks to see his or her medical records/chart, the appropriate response is to refer the patient to his or her physician. Patients *do* have the right to review their own medical records; however, the patient should do so in the presence of the physician so that the information is not misinterpreted and the physician can address concerns or answer questions. It is not appropriate to provide the patient with his or her records or to deceive him or her into believing that the records are not available for viewing or that the patient has no right to review them.

82. **(B)** Double-contrast studies of the large bowel are particularly useful for demonstration of the *bowel wall* and anything projecting into it, for example, polyps. *Polyps* are projections of the bowel wall mucous membrane into the bowel lumen. *Colitis* is inflammation of the large bowel, often associated with ulcerations of the mucosal wall. A single-contrast study most likely would obliterate these mucosal conditions, but coating of the bowel mucosa with barium and subsequent filling of the bowel with air (double contrast) provide optimal delineation. Single-contrast studies will demonstrate projections/outpouchings from the intestinal wall such as diverticula.

83. **(D)** Category-specific isolations have been replaced by *transmission-based precautions: airborne, droplet,* and *contact.* Under these guidelines, some conditions or diseases can fall into more than one category. Any pathogens spread by direct or close *contact,* such as *MRSA, conjunctivitis,* and *rotavirus,* requires *contact precautions. Contact precautions* require a *private patient room* and the use of *gloves, gown, and possibly a mask* for anyone coming in direct contact with the infected individual or his or her environment. *Airborne precautions* are implemented in patients suspected or known to be infected with *tubercle bacillus*

(TB), chickenpox (varicella), or *measles (rubeola).* Airborne precautions *require that the patient wears a string mask* to avoid the spread of bronchial secretions or other pathogens during coughing. If the patient is unable or unwilling to wear a mask, the radiographer must wear a mask. The radiographer should wear gloves, but a gown is required only if flagrant contamination is likely. Patients under *airborne precautions* require a *private, specially ventilated (negative-pressure) room.* A private room is also indicated for all patients on *droplet precautions,* that is, with diseases transmitted via *large droplets* expelled from the patient while speaking, sneezing, or coughing. The pathogenic droplets can infect others when they come in contact with mouth or nasal mucosa or conjunctiva. *Rubella* (German measles), *mumps,* and *influenza* are among the diseases spread by droplet contact; a *private room is required* for the patient, and health care practitioners should wear a *string mask and possibly gloves and gown* as needed.

84. **(B)** A patient who has been NPO since midnight or who is anxious, frightened, or in pain may suffer an episode of syncope (fainting) on exertion. The patient should be helped to a recumbent position with feet elevated to increase blood flow to the head. A patient who feels like fainting should never be left alone.

85. **(C)** *Urticaria* is a vascular reaction resulting in dilated capillaries and edema and causing the patient to break out in hives. The medical term for *nosebleed* is *epistaxis. Vertigo* refers to a feeling of "whirling" or a sensation that the room is spinning. Some possible causes of vertigo include inner ear infection and acoustic neuroma. An *aura* may be classified as either a feeling or a sensory response (such as flashing lights, tasting metal, or smelling coffee) that precedes an episode such as a seizure or a migraine headache.

86. **(A)** Blood pressure is measured in *millimeters of mercury* (mm Hg). Heart rate, or pulse, is measured in units of *beats per minute.* Temperature is measured in *degrees Fahrenheit* (°F). Oxygen delivery is measured in units of *liters per minute* (L/min). Table 1-1 outlines the normal ranges for vital signs in healthy adults.

Table 1-1. Normal Ranges for Vital Signs in Adults	
Blood pressure	90–120 mm Hg/50–70 mm Hg
Pulse rate	60–100 beats/min
Temperature	97.7°F–99.5°F
Respiration rate	12–20 breaths/min

87. **(C)** *Veracity* (i.e., sincerity) is not only telling the truth but also not practicing deception. *Autonomy* is the ethical principle that is related to the theory that patients have the right to decide what will or will not be done to them. *Beneficence* is related to the idea of doing good and being kind. *Fidelity* is faithfulness and loyalty.

88. **(C)** *Talipes* is the term used to describe congenital clubfoot. There are several types of talipes, generally characterized by

a deformed talus and a shortened Achilles tendon, giving the foot a *clubfoot* appearance. *Osteochondritis* (Osgood–Schlatter disease) is a painful incomplete separation of the tibial tuberosity from the tibial shaft. It is often seen in active adolescent boys. *Coxa plana* (Legg–Calvé–Perthes disease) is ischemic necrosis leading to flattening of the femoral head. *Muscular dystrophy* is a congenital disorder characterized by wasting of skeletal muscles.

89. **(D)** When scheduling patient examinations, it is important to avoid the possibility of residual contrast medium covering areas that will be of interest on later examinations. The IVU (also called *intravenous pyelogram* [IVP]) should be scheduled first because the contrast medium used is excreted rapidly. The BE should be scheduled next. Finally, the upper GI series is scheduled. There should not be enough barium remaining from the previous BE to interfere with the examination of the stomach or duodenum, although a preliminary scout image should be taken in each case.

90. **(C)** MRI uses a very strong magnetic field and all patients are screened regarding cardiac pacemakers, insulin pumps, aneurysm clips, shrapnel, heart valves, eye injuries involving metal, jewelry, metal prostheses, and similar things. Any metallic object will be attracted by the magnet and can cause serious harm to the patient. (*Dutton and Ryan, 9th ed, p. 351*)

91. **(D)** *Ventricular septal defect* is a congenital heart condition characterized by a hole in the interventricular septum that allows oxygenated and unoxygenated blood to mix. Some interventricular septal defects are small and close spontaneously, others require surgery. *Coarctation of the aorta* is a narrowing or constriction of the aorta. *Atrial septal defect* is a small hole (the remnant of the fetal foramen ovale) in the interatrial septum. It usually closes spontaneously in the first few months of life; if it persists or is unusually large, surgical repair is necessary. The ductus arteriosus is a short fetal blood vessel connecting the aorta and pulmonary artery that usually closes within 10–15 h after birth. A *patent ductus arteriosus* is one that persists and requires surgical closure.

92. **(B)** *Syncope*, or fainting, is the result of a drop in blood pressure caused by insufficient blood (oxygen) flow to the brain. The patient should be helped into a dorsal recumbent position with feet elevated to facilitate blood flow to the brain.

93. **(D)** The cycle of infection includes four components: a susceptible host, a reservoir of infection, a pathogenic organism, and a mode of transmission. *Pathogenic organisms* are microscopic and include bacteria, fungi, and viruses. The *reservoir of infection* is the environment in which the microorganism thrives; this can be the human body. A *susceptible host* may have reduced resistance to infection. The *mode of transmission* is either direct (i.e., touch) or indirect (i.e., vector, fomite, or airborne).

94. **(B)** The diaphragm is the major muscle of respiration. On inspiration/inhalation, the diaphragm and abdominal viscera are depressed, enabling filling and expansion of the lungs, accompanied by upward movement of the sternum and ribs. During expiration/exhalation, air leaves the lungs, and these deflate while the diaphragm relaxes and moves to a more superior position along with the abdominal viscera. As the diaphragm relaxes and moves up, the sternum and ribs move inferiorly.

95. **(B)** Other names for an *intermittent injection port* are *saline lock* and *heparin lock*. Intermittent injection ports are used for patients who will require frequent or regular injections. An intravenous catheter is placed in the vein, and an external adapter with a diaphragm allows for repeated injections. This helps to prevent the formation of scarred, sclerotic veins as a result of frequent injections at the same site. Intermittent injection ports provide more freedom than an *IV infusion*, and also allow for repeated access. *Hypodermic needles* usually are used for drawing blood or drawing up fluids, whereas a *butterfly needle* usually is used for venipuncture.

96. **(C)** Hospitals being the refuge of the sick, these can also be the places of disease transmission unless proper infection prevention and control guidelines are followed. When cleaning contaminated objects or surfaces such as the radiographic table, it is important to *clean from the least contaminated to the most contaminated area* and *from the top down*. Soiled gowns and linens should be folded from the outside in and disposed of properly. When the patient's skin is being prepared for surgery, it is often cleaned in circular motion starting from the center and working outward; however, this motion is not used for objects or surfaces.

97. **(C)** A *Swan–Ganz catheter* is a specific type of IV catheter used to measure the pumping ability of the heart, to obtain pressure readings and to introduce medications and IV fluids. A *pacemaker* is a device that is inserted under the patient's skin to regulate heart rate. Pacemakers may be permanent or temporary. *Chest tubes* are used to remove fluid or air from the pleural cavity. Any of these items may be identified on a chest radiograph, provided that the cassette is properly positioned and the correct exposure factors are used. If the physician is interested in assessing the proper placement of a Swan–Ganz catheter, the lungs may have to be slightly overexposed to clearly delineate the proper placement of the tip of the Swan–Ganz catheter, which will overlap the denser cardiac silhouette. A *urinary catheter* will not appear on a chest radiograph.

98. **(B)** When the radiographer initially greets the patient, and as the diagnostic examination progresses, the radiographer should be alert to the patient's appearance and condition, and any subsequent changes in them. These are called *objective* signs. It is important to notice the color, temperature, and moistness of the patient's skin. *Paleness* frequently indicates weakness; the *diaphoretic* patient has

pale, cool skin. The *febrile* patient is usually feverish and exhibits hot, dry skin. "Sweaty" palms may indicate *anxiety.* A patient who becomes *cyanotic* (bluish lips, mucous membranes, or nail beds) needs oxygen and requires immediate medical attention.

99. **(A)** The mechanical device used to correct an ineffectual cardiac ventricular rhythm is a *defibrillator.* The two paddles attached to the unit are placed on a patient's chest and used to introduce an electric current in an effort to correct the dysrhythmia. *Automatic implantable cardioverter defibrillators* (AICDs) are devices that are implanted in the body and deliver a small shock to the heart if a life-threatening dysrhythmia occurs. A *cardiac monitor* is used to display, and sometimes record, electrocardiographic (ECG) readings and some pressure readings. A *crash cart* is a supply cart with various medications and equipment necessary for treating a patient who is suffering from a myocardial infarction or some other serious medical emergency. It is checked and restocked periodically. A *resuscitation bag* is used for ventilation, such as during CPR.

100. **(A)** It is generally recommended that the IV bottle/bag should be kept 18–24 inches above the level of the vein. If the container is too high, the pressure of the IV fluid can cause it to pass through the vein into surrounding tissues, causing a painful and potentially harmful condition. If the IV container is too low, blood may return through the needle into the tubing, form a clot, and obstruct the flow of IV fluid.

101. **(D)** A private room is indicated for all patients on *droplet precaution,* that is, diseases transmitted via large droplets expelled from the patient while speaking, sneezing, or coughing. The pathogenic droplets can infect others when they come in contact with mouth or nasal mucosa or conjunctiva. *Rubella* (German measles), *mumps,* and *influenza* are among the diseases that spread by droplet contact; a *private room is required* for the patient, and health care practitioners must wear a regular (string) *mask* to enter a droplet precautions isolation room.

102. **(C)** A protective environment or neutropenic precautions (sometimes called expanded precautions or reverse isolation) as indicated are used to keep the susceptible patient from becoming infected. Patients who have suffered burns have lost a very important means of protection, their skin, and therefore have increased susceptibility to bacterial invasion. Patients whose immune systems are depressed have lost the ability to combat infection and hence are more susceptible to infection. Active TB requires airborne precautions, not expanded precautions.

103. **(C)** Whenever a perforation of the GI tract is suspected, a water-soluble contrast agent (such as Gastrografin or oral Hypaque) should be used because it is easily absorbed from within the peritoneal cavity. Leakage of barium sulfate into the peritoneal cavity can have serious consequences. Water-soluble contrast agents also may be used in place of barium sulfate when the possibility of barium impaction exists. Oil-based contrast agents are used rarely these days.

104. **(A)** *Angina pectoris* is a crushing chest pain caused by a circulatory disturbance of the coronary arteries. Nitroglycerin is used to dilate blood vessels (vasodilation) and decrease blood pressure in the treatment of pain from angina pectoris. Nitroglycerin usually is given sublingually and thus is absorbed directly into the bloodstream.

105. **(B)** Every radiographic image *must* include (1) the patient's name or ID number; (2) the side marker, right or left; (3) the date of the examination; and (4) the identity of the institution or office. Additional information *may* be included: the patient's birth date or age, name of the attending physician, and the time of day. When multiple examinations (e.g., chest examinations or small bowel images) of a patient are made on the same day, it becomes crucial that the time the radiographs were taken should be included on the image. This allows the physician to track the patient's progress.

106. **(B)** The diameter of a needle is the needle's *gauge.* The higher the gauge number, the smaller is the diameter and the thinner is the needle. For example, a very tiny gauge needle (25 gauge) may be used on a pediatric patient for an IV injection, whereas a large-gauge needle (16 gauge) may be used for donating blood. The *hub* of a needle is the portion of the needle that attaches to a syringe. The *length* of the needle varies depending on its use. A longer needle is needed for intramuscular injections, whereas a shorter needle is used for subcutaneous injection. The *bevel* of the needle is the slanted tip of the needle. For IV injections, the bevel should always face up.

107. **(C)** Adverse reactions to the intravascular administration of iodinated contrast media are not uncommon, and although the risk of a life-threatening reaction is relatively low, the radiographer must be alert to recognize the situation and deal with it effectively should a serious reaction occur. Reactions are typically classified as mild, moderate, and severe. Mild reactions can include the patient feeling nervous or anxious, nasal congestion, tingling/itching at the injection site, a feeling of tightness in the throat. The patient must be closely monitored during examinations that require the use of iodinated contrast media.

108. **(A)** The patient is said to be in the *Trendelenburg* position when the head is positioned lower than the feet (see Fig. 1-3D). This position is helpful in several radiographic procedures, such as for separating redundant bowel loops and demonstration of hiatal hernias. It is also used in treating shock. In the *Fowler* position, the head is *higher* than the feet (Fig. 1-3E). The Fowler position relaxes abdominal muscles and promotes maximum chest expansion with resultant improved lung oxygenation. The *Sims* position (Fig. 1-3F) is the left anterior

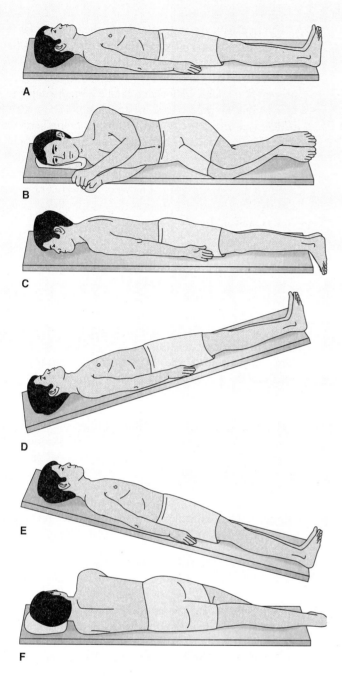

A

B

C

D

E

F

Figure 1-3

vasodilator. *Hydrocortisone* is a steroid that may be used to treat bronchial asthma, allergic reactions, and inflammatory reactions. *Digitoxin* is used to treat cardiac fibrillation.

111. **(B)** Infectious microorganisms can be transmitted from patients to other patients or to health care workers and from health care workers to patients by three routes: *contact, airborne,* and *droplet.* Contact transmission is either via direct contact or indirect contact. *Direct* contact involves *touch. Indirect* contact involves transmission by way of contaminated equipment, supplies, hands. A contaminated object that transmitted infection is called a *fomite.*

Nasal or oral secretions are transmitted via coughs and sneezes; they require *droplet* precautions. *(Dutton and Ryan, 9th ed, pp. 118-120)*

112. **(C)** Frequent and correct hand hygiene is an essential part of medical asepsis; it is the best method for avoiding the spread of microorganisms. Hand hygiene can be accomplished with alcohol-based hand sanitizers if there is no actual soiling on the skin or the patient does not have *Clostridium difficile,* or by washing with soap and water. If the water faucet cannot be operated with the knee or a foot pedal, it should be opened and closed using paper towels. Care should be taken to wash all surfaces of the hand and between the fingers thoroughly. The hands and forearms should always be kept below the elbows. Hand lotions should be used frequently to keep hands from chapping. Unbroken skin prevents the entry of microorganisms; dry, cracked skin breaks down that defense and permits the entry of microorganisms.

113. **(D)** Physicians often prescribe a mild laxative to aid in the elimination of barium sulfate. If a laxative is not given, the patient should be instructed to increase dietary fluid and fiber and to monitor bowel movements (the patient should have at least one within 24 h). Patients should also be aware of the white appearance of their stool that will be present until all the barium is expelled.

114. **(A)** *Superficial arteries* are best suited for determination of pulse rate. The five most easily palpated pulse points are the radial, carotid, temporal, femoral, and popliteal pulses. The radial pulse is used most frequently. The apical pulse, at the apex of the heart, is the most accurate and can be determined with the use of a stethoscope.

115. **(D)** The medical abbreviation *pc* (post cibum) means "after meals." "Three times a day" is indicated by the abbreviation *tid* (ter in die). The abbreviation *qid* (quarter in die) means "four times a day." "Every hour" is represented by *qh* (quaque hora). The medical abbreviation *gtt* (guttae) refers to "drops."

116. **(C)** Oxygen is taken into the body and supplied to the blood to be delivered to all body tissues. Any tissue(s) lacking in or devoid of an adequate blood supply can suffer permanent damage or die. Oxygen may be required in

oblique (LAO) position with the right leg flexed up for insertion of the enema tip. The *Caldwell* position is a radiographic position for imaging the cranium.

109. **(C)** The normal average rate of respiration for a healthy adult patient is between 12 and 20 breaths/min. For children, the rate is higher, averaging between 20 and 30 breaths/min. In addition to monitoring the respiratory rate, it is also important to monitor the depth (shallow or labored) and pattern (regularity) of respiration. A respiratory rate greater than 20 breaths/min in an adult would be considered *tachypnea.*

110. **(B)** *Epinephrine* (adrenalin) is the vasopressor used to treat an anaphylactic reaction or cardiac arrest. *Nitroglycerin* is a

cases of severe anemia, pneumonia, pulmonary edema, and shock. Symptoms of inadequate oxygen supply include *dyspnea, cyanosis, retraction of intercostal spaces, dilated nostrils,* and *distension of the veins of the neck.* The patient who experiences any of these symptoms will be very anxious and must not be left unattended. The radiographer must call for help, assist the patient to a sitting or semi-Fowler position (the recumbent position makes breathing more difficult), and have oxygen and emergency drugs available.

117. (A) It is unlikely that the radiographer will be faced with a wound hemorrhage because bleeding from wounds is controlled before the patient is seen for x-ray examination. However, if a patient does experience hemorrhaging from a wound, you should apply pressure to the bleeding site and call for assistance. Delay can lead to serious blood loss.

118. (B) *Cyanosis* is a condition resulting from a deficiency of oxygen circulating in the blood. It is characterized by bluish discoloration of the gums, nail beds, earlobes, and the area around the mouth. Cyanosis may be accompanied by labored breathing or other types of respiratory distress.

119. (C) The Controlled Substance Act divides drugs and other controlled substances into five schedules according to potential for abuse. Drugs are prescribed to provide safe and optimal patient care; however, some drugs have a high potential for dependence/abuse.

120. (D) Communication difficulties can arise with non–English-speaking patients. Most hospitals and large clinics have a list of resource people, automated systems, language lines, special dual headset phones, or similar accommodations to assist with interpretation when there is a language barrier. A certified interpreter is the most helpful because he or she translates exactly what has been said, rather than a family member or friend who might edit, or try to explain what he or she *thinks* is implied. It is not uncommon for people of any language to experience difficulty in communication during times of trauma, illness, or stress. Volume, speed, and tone of voice may also be determined by culture. Expressions/figures of speech such as "a piece of cake" or "home free" may not be understood by patients/families of all cultures.

121. (B) A patient who is going into shock may exhibit *pallor and weakness,* a significant *drop in blood pressure,* and an *increased pulse.* The patient may also experience *apprehension and restlessness* and may have *cool, clammy skin.* A radiographer recognizing these symptoms should call them to the physician's attention immediately. Fever is generally not associated with shock.

122. (D) Increased pain threshold, breakdown of skin, and atrophy of fat pads and sweat glands are all important considerations when working with *geriatric patients.* Many changes occur as our bodies age. Although muscle

is replaced with fat, the amount of subcutaneous fat is decreased, and the skin atrophies. Therefore, the geriatric patient requires *extra-gentle treatment.* A mattress pad should always be placed on the radiographic table to help prevent *skin injury* or abrasions. If tape is required, paper tape should be used instead of adhesive tape. Geriatric patients are also more sensitive to *hypothermia* because of the breakdown of the sweat glands and always should be kept covered both to preserve modesty and for extra warmth. *Loss of sensation* in the skin increases pain tolerance, so the geriatric patient may not be aware of excessive stress on bony prominences such as the elbow, wrist, coccyx, and ankles.

123. (A) *Antisepsis* is the practice that retards the growth of pathogenic bacteria. The practice of *medical asepsis* reduces the likelihood of transferring pathogenic microorganisms (bacteria) to a vulnerable individual. The *destruction* of pathogens through the use of chemical materials is termed *disinfection.* Examples of disinfectants are hydrogen peroxide, chlorine, iodine, chlorhexidine, and formaldehyde. *Surgical asepsis (sterilization)* refers to the removal of all microorganisms *and* their spores (reproductive cells) and is practiced in the surgical suite. Bacteriostatics reduce microorganism on surfaces. Antiseptics reduce microorganisms on the skin. Bacteriocidals remove all microorganisms. Health care practitioners must practice medical asepsis at all times.

124. (A) To obtain a diagnostic examination of the stomach, it must first be empty. The usual preparation is NPO after midnight (approximately 8 h before the examination). Any material in the stomach can simulate the appearance of disease.

125. (D) Communication can be achieved in many forms; those forms can be verbal or nonverbal. Effective and professional patient communication skills are essential; the interaction between the patient and radiographer generally leaves the patient with a lasting impression of his or her health care experience. The radiographer's communication skills must include a proficiency in *observational* skills, *listening* skills, *speaking* skills, and *writing* skills.

126. (A) *Creatinine* is a normal alkaline constituent of urine and blood, but increased quantities of creatinine are present in advanced stages of renal disease. Creatinine and BUN blood chemistry levels should be checked before beginning an IVU. Increased levels may forecast an increased possibility of contrast media–induced renal effects and poor visualization of the renal collecting systems. The normal creatinine range is 0.5–1.2 mg/dL. The normal BUN range is 7–20 mg/dL.

127. (C) A *stethoscope* and a *sphygmomanometer* are used together to measure blood pressure. The first sound heard is the systolic pressure, and the normal range is 90–120 mm Hg. When the sound is no longer heard, the diastolic pressure is recorded. The normal diastolic range is 50–70 mm Hg. Elevated blood pressure is called *hypertension. Hypotension,* or low blood pressure, is not of concern unless it is caused by injury or disease; in that case, it can result in shock. A *pulse oximeter* is used to measure a patient's pulse rate and oxygen saturation level.

128. **(D)** Transmission-based precautions are used for diseases that are transmitted through the air, requiring *airborne* infection isolation, which include TB, rubeola (measles), varicella (chickenpox), mumps, SARS (severe acute respiratory syndrome), and smallpox. Patients infected with diseases calling for airborne precautions require a private, specially ventilated (negative-pressure) room, and the door must be kept closed. Health care workers must wear an N95 respirator mask. Airborne precautions require the *patient to wear a string mask* when being transported through the hospital.

129. **(A)** *Health care–associated infections (HAIs)* are infections acquired by patients while they are in the hospital or other health care facility; these are also termed *nosocomial* infections. Many of these infections are acquired by patients whose resistance has been diminished by their illness and are unrelated to the condition for which the patients were hospitalized. Infection resulting from physician intervention is termed *iatrogenic.* The CDC estimates that 5%–15% of all hospital patients acquire some type of HAI. Hospital personnel can also become infected (occupationally acquired infection).

Microorganisms can remain infectious while awaiting transmission to another host. A contaminated *inanimate object* such as a food utensil, a doorknob, or an IV pole is called a *fomite.* A *vector* is an *insect or animal carrier* of infectious organisms, such as a rabid animal, a mosquito that carries malaria, or a mouse/deer tick that carries Lyme disease.

130. **(B)** Tracheostomy is the surgical opening of the trachea to provide and secure an open airway. A tracheostomy is often performed in emergency situations when there is *upper* airway obstruction, that is, *above* the level of the larynx. Conditions requiring a tracheostomy include crushing injury of the tracheal rings, inflamed and swollen tracheal mucous membranes, and aspiration of foreign body.

131. **(A)** Dr Elizabeth Kübler-Ross explains that loss requires gradual adjustment and involves several steps. The first is denial or isolation, where the individual often refuses to accept the thought of loss or death. The second step is anger, as the individual attempts to deal with feelings of helplessness. The next is bargaining, in which the patient behaves as though "being good," like a "good patient," will be rewarded by a miraculous cure or return of the loss. Once the individual acknowledges that this is not likely to happen, depression is the next step. This depression precedes acceptance, where the individual begins to deal with fate or loss.

132. **(D) Disclosing** confidential information to unauthorized parties is *invasion of privacy.* If the disclosure is somehow detrimental/harmful to the patient, the radiographer can be accused of *defamation.* Written defamation is *libel;* spoken defamation is *slander.*

133. **(A)** Code of Ethics and Rules of Ethics are the two parts of the Standard of Ethics. The Code of Ethics was adopted by the ASRT and ARRT and describes all aspects of ethical conduct in the radiologic sciences; it is aspirational. The Rules of Ethics are mandatory and enforced by the ARRT. The Rules of Ethics describe the minimally acceptable professional conduct for those certified by ARRT.

134. **(D)** *Enterally* administered drugs are administered into the gastrointestinal track orally, rectally (via suppository or enema), or through a nasogastric (NG) tube.

Parenterally administered drugs are administered by routes other than the GI tract, typically by injection. This avoids GI irritation and produces a more rapid response. Common types of parenteral injections include subcutaneous, intramuscular, intradermal, intra-arterial, intravenous, and intrathecal. Other drug administration sites include sublingual, buccal, and topical.

135. **(C)** The legal doctrine *res ipsa loquitur* relates to a thing or matter that *speaks for itself.* For instance, if the patient went to the hospital to have a kidney stone removed and ended up with an appendectomy, that speaks for itself, and negligence can be proven. *Respondeat superior* is a phrase meaning "let the master answer" or "the one ruling is responsible." If a radiographer were negligent, there may be an attempt to prove that the radiologist was responsible because the radiologist oversees the radiographer. *Res judicata* means of thing or matter settled by justice. *Stare decisis* refers to a matter settled by precedent.

136. **(C)** An *aneurysm* is a localized dilatation/bulging in a weakened blood vessel wall. Aneurysms can occur in the aorta, brain, and other parts of the body. Aneurysms can result in internal bleeding and can be fatal. The location and size of an aneurysm can be identified in medical imaging. A cyst is a fluid-filled sac. A thrombus is a stationary blood clot. Angina is chest pain caused by restricted blood flow to the myocardium.

137. **(D)** Normal creatinine level in the adult is about 0.6–1.5 mg/dL, and a level of 2.0 or more is generally considered to contraindicate the safe administration of iodinated contrast media. *BUN* and *creatinine* values are indicators of renal function. Iodinated contrast medium is contraindicated in cases of elevated BUN and/or creatinine because of potential for renal damage.

138. **(D)** The radiographer assesses a patient's condition before bringing the patient to the radiographic department and continues to be alert to the patient's *appearance and condition* and any changes as the examination proceeds. Assessment begins with a review of the patient's

admission diagnosis, degree of ambulation, preparation for the radiologic procedure (e.g., premedication, effectiveness of cathartic/cleansing enemas), results of laboratory tests (e.g., creatinine, blood urea nitrogen [BUN], GFR), any requirements for collecting the patient's urine, and so on. The radiographer obtains a brief pertinent *clinical history,* and assesses the patient's condition by observing and listening. Facts are gathered to obtain information useful in providing adequate care and accurate diagnosis. To provide safe and effectual care, the radiographer will *assess* the severity of any traumatic injury, degree of motor control, and any need for support equipment or radiographic accessories. Is the patient able to move? Has the patient been NPO? Does the patient have any history of an intolerance to contrast material? Are there any laboratory values or diagnoses that might contraindicate the use of contrast material (e.g., intestinal perforation, diabetes)?

Measurement of body temperature and blood pressure are not typical assessments for radiographic procedures.

139. (D) Qualities of iodinated contrast agents that contribute to discomfort, side effects, and reactions include:

Viscosity: More viscid (thick, sticky) agents are more difficult to inject and produce more heat and vessel irritation; the higher the concentration, the greater is the viscosity; viscosity also increases as room temperature decreases.

Toxicity: Potential toxicity is greater with higher concentration agents and ionic agents.

Miscibility: Contrast agents should be readily miscible (able to mix) with blood.

Osmolality: Low-osmolality agents have fewer particles in a given amount of solution and are less likely to provoke an allergic reaction.

140. (A) An *allergy* is an abnormal, acquired immune response to a substance (i.e., *allergen*) that would not usually trigger a reaction. An initial exposure to the allergen (i.e., *sensitization*) is required. Subsequent contact with the allergen then results in an inflammatory response. Examples of such responses include hay fever, urticaria, allergic rhinitis, eczema, and bronchial asthma. Allergens can be introduced into the body via contact, ingestion (e.g., food), inhalation (e.g., dust, pollen), or injection (e.g., medication, drugs). Allergic reactions of particular importance to the radiographer involve the use of latex products and contrast media. Toxic effects can occur because of sensitivity, overdose, or poor metabolism. An *antidote* is used to treat a toxic effect.

141. (A) The diabetic patient who has taken his or her insulin, and is fasting, is susceptible to a hypoglycemic reaction as a result of low blood sugar. This condition is characterized by restlessness, fatigue, weakness, and irritability. Hypoglycemic reactions can be serious and need to be treated with an immediate dose of sugar in some form (juice, candy).

142. (C) Contrast agents can be described as either positive (*radiopaque*) or negative (radiolucent). Positive contrast agents have a *higher atomic number* than the surrounding soft tissue, resulting in a greater attenuation/absorption of x-ray photons, thereby increasing image contrast. Examples of positive contrast media are *iodinated* agents (both water-based and oil-based) and barium sulfate suspensions. The inert characteristics of barium sulfate render it the least toxic contrast medium. On the contrary, iodinated contrast media have characteristics that increase their likelihood of producing side effects and reactions. Negative, or radiolucent, contrast agents used are air and various gases. Carbon dioxide is absorbed more rapidly by the body than air. Negative contrast is often used *with* positive contrast in examinations termed *double-contrast studies.* The function of the positive agent is usually to *coat* the various parts under study, while the air *fills* the space and permits visualization through the gaseous medium. Examinations that frequently use double-contrast technique are contrast enema (BE), upper GI (UGI), and arthrography.

143. (C) Patient rights can be exercised on the patient's behalf by a *designated surrogate or proxy* decision maker if the patient lacks the decision-making capacity, is legally incompetent, or is a minor. Many people believe that potential legal and ethical issues can be avoided by creating an Advance Health Care Directive or Living Will. Because all individuals have the right to make decisions regarding their own health care, this legal document preserves that right in the event an individual is unable to make those decisions. An Advance Health Care Directive, or Living Will, names the individual authorized to make all health care decisions and can include specifics regarding *DNR* (do not resuscitate), *DNI* (do not intubate), and/or other end-of-life decisions. The parent or spouse could not make decisions for the patient *if* they are identified as a designated surrogate or a proxy.

144. (D) The importance of effective and professional patient *communication* skills cannot be overemphasized; the interaction between the patient and radiographer generally leaves the patient with a lasting impression of his or her health care experience. Of course, communication refers not only to the spoken word (i.e., *verbal* communication) but also to unspoken/*nonverbal* communication. *Facial expression* can convey caring and reassurance or impatience and disapproval. Pursed lips, pointed fingers, frowns, and hands on hips, all indicate disapproval. Similarly, a radiographer's *touch* can convey his or her commitment to considerate care, or it can convey a rough, uncaring, and hurried attitude. Making *eye contact* while speaking is generally considered polite and respectful in the United States, whereas it can be considered just the opposite in other cultures (e.g., Asian, East Indian, and Native American). Our *appearance* gives an impression about how we feel about our work and our patients; it is very much a part of communication and we should strive for a professional appearance/image.

145. (A) In classifying contrast agents, the total number of dissolved particles in solution per kilogram of water defines the *osmolality* of the contrast agent. The term osmolarity refers to the number of particles per liter of solvent. The *toxicity* defines how noxious or harmful a contrast agent is. Contrast agents with low osmolality have been found to cause less tissue toxicity than the ionic IV contrast agents. The *viscosity* defines the thickness or concentration of the contrast agent. The viscosity of a contrast agent can affect its injection rate. A thicker, or more viscous, contrast agent will be more difficult to inject (more pressure is needed to push the contrast agent through the syringe and needle or the angiocatheter). The *miscibility* of a contrast agent refers to its ability to mix with body fluids, such as blood. Miscibility is an important consideration in preventing thrombus formation. It is generally preferable to use a contrast agent with low osmolality and low toxicity because such an agent is safer for the patient and less likely to cause any untoward reaction. When ionic and nonionic contrast agents are compared, a nonionic contrast agent has a lower osmolality. To further understand osmolality, remember that whenever IV contrast media are introduced, there is a notable shift in fluid and ions. This shift is caused by an inflow of water from interstitial regions into the vascular compartment, which increases the blood volume and cardiac output. Consequently, there will be an increase in systemic arterial pressure and peripheral vascular resistance with peripheral *vasodilation.* In addition, the pulmonary pressure and heart rate increase. When the effects of osmolality on the patient are understood, it becomes clear that an elderly patient or one with cardiac disease or impaired circulation would greatly benefit from the use of an agent with lower osmolality.

146. (D) *Nonmaleficence* refers to our responsibility to keep our patient from harm and to avoid inflicting harm on our patients. *Fidelity* refers to keeping promises and fulfilling our commitments. *Veracity* refers to honesty and truthfulness. *Beneficence* refers to our responsibility to do good for our patients.

147. (B) When transporting a young child from Pediatrics to the Imaging department, the safest mode of travel is a crib with the side rails in the up position. Carrying is permissible only when moving from one room to a neighboring room. Stretcher and wheelchair transportation is too risky for a possibly energetic or anxious child.

148. (B) Epidemiologic studies indicate that *HIV* and acquired immunodeficiency syndrome *(AIDS)* can be transmitted only by intimate contact with blood or body fluids of an infected individual. This can occur through the sharing of contaminated needles, through sexual contact, from mother to baby at childbirth, and from transfusion of contaminated blood. *HIV* and *AIDS* cannot be transmitted by inanimate objects. Hepatitis B is an infection that affects the liver and is transmitted via blood, semen, or other body fluid. It is assumed that more than 1 million people in the United States have chronic hepatitis B and, as such, can transmit the disease to others. Acid-fast bacillus (AFB) isolation is implemented in patients suspected or known to be infected with *Mycobacterium tuberculosis (TB).* AFB isolation requires that the patient wears a mask to avoid the spread of AFB (in bronchial secretions) during coughing.

149. (B) The factors involved in the spread of disease begin with the infectious organism (3), or pathogen. Next is the reservoir of infection (2)—a place where the pathogen can thrive, often in/on the bodies of healthy individuals. Other reservoirs of infection include water, food, animals, and soil. The portal of exit (6) refers to the route by which pathogens exit the body; examples include the GI tract, urinary tract, respiratory (sneeze, cough) tract, and bloodstream. The susceptible host (5) might have a compromised immune system. Patients and hospital workers are exposed to a multitude of pathogens. The portal of entry (1) refers to where the pathogen gains access to the susceptible host. The portal of entry can be via mucous membrane of the eyes, nose, mouth, the bloodstream, or GI, urinary, or respiratory system. Modes of transportation (4) include direct contact, airborne transmission, droplet contamination, vectors, vehicles, and fomites.

150. (C) Many spores can resist the heat of boiling water, even for hours, so boiling is not considered a method of sterilization; it is classified as a means of disinfection. Accepted methods of sterilization include the *autoclave (steam under pressure), chemical sterilization,* and *ethylene oxide,* which is used for articles that are unable to tolerate moisture and high temperatures.

151. (C) The cephalic and basilic veins extend proximally from the elbow; the cephalic extends laterally and the basilic extends medially. They anastomose over the cubital fossa to form the *median cubital vein,* which is most frequently used as the site for intravenous injection.

152. (C) Obtaining a complete and accurate history from the patient for the radiologist is an important aspect of a radiographer's job. Both subjective and objective data should be collected. *Objective* data include signs and symptoms that can be observed, such as a cough, a lump, or elevated blood pressure. *Subjective* data relate to what the patient feels and to what extent. A patient may experience pain, but is it mild or severe? Is it localized or general? Does the pain increase or decrease under different circumstances? A radiographer should explore these with the patient and document the information about the requisition for the radiologist.

153. (D) Good communication, both verbal and nonverbal, is essential to good patient care. Therapeutic communication techniques include restating the main idea, reflecting the main idea, establishing guidelines, establishing guidelines, reducing distance, listening, validating, and so on. Defending (a professional whose knowledge/decision the patient is unsure of) is likely to block further patient communication because his or her own opinion has been disregarded/rebuffed. Giving advice is out of our realm of expertise and should always be avoided.

154. (C) Although each of these steps is part of a complete radiologic examination, the all-important first step is careful and accurate patient identification. Patient identification, and correctly matching the patient with the intended examination, is a routine activity in the health care environment. The health care worker has a primary responsibility for checking/verifying the patient's identity. Most facilities require checking *at least two patient identifiers*. Rigorous observance of "timeout" processes prior to procedures can avoid costly events, including those involving patient identification.

155. (B) The Code of Ethics and Rules of Ethics are the two parts are the Standard of Ethics. The Code of Ethics was adopted by the ASRT and ARRT and describes all aspects of ethical conduct in the radiologic sciences; it is aspirational. The Rules of Ethics are mandatory and enforced by the ARRT. The Rules of Ethics describe the minimally acceptable professional conduct for those certified by ARRT.

156. (D) The imaging examination requisition is usually printed with the patient's personal information (name, address, age, referring/admitting physician's name, and the patient's hospital identification number). When examining patients who are admitted to the hospital, the requisition should also include the patient's mode of travel to the radiology department or other imaging facility (e.g., wheelchair vs. stretcher), the type of examination to be performed, pertinent diagnostic information, and any *infection control* or *isolation* information. The radiographer, with access to confidential patient information, must be mindful of compliance with HIPAA regulations.

157. (D) The patient's rights can be exercised on the patient's behalf by a *designated surrogate or proxy* decision maker if the patient lacks decision-making capacity, is legally incompetent, or is a minor. Many people believe that potential legal and ethical issues can be avoided by creating an *advance health care directive* or *living will*. Because all individuals have the right to make decisions regarding their own health care, this legal document preserves that right in the event an individual is unable to make those decisions. An advance health care directive, or living will, names the health care proxy authorized to make all health care decisions and can include specifics regarding DNR (do not resuscitate), DNI (do not intubate), and/or other end-of-life decisions.

158. (A) A patient who experiences symptoms of inadequate oxygen will be very anxious and must not be left unattended. The use of devices to deliver oxygen to patients is determined by the amount of oxygen required by the patient. They are frequently classified as low or high flow. COPD patients require low-flow therapy; high-flow delivery can result in apnea. The *nasal cannula* is the most frequently used device and is used to supplement the oxygen in room air; its short prongs extend approximately 1 cm into the nares. The nasal cannula is a low-flow small-percentage oxygen device. It is convenient and fairly comfortable for the patient. There are various types of oxygen *masks* available for delivery of oxygen. The *Venturi mask* mixes oxygen with room air and can deliver specific (usually, high flow) concentrations of oxygen. The *simple face mask* (low flow) is best suited for short-term oxygen therapy. With extended use, the plastic becomes warm and sticky. Communication is difficult, the mask is easily displaced, and it must be removed at mealtime. The *partial rebreathing mask* (low flow) and *non-rebreathing mask* (low flow) deliver more precise concentrations of oxygen to the patient.

159. (D) The use of a *suction* device is occasionally required to maintain a patient's airway by *aspirating* secretions, blood, or other fluids. Suctioning may be indicated when the patient is unconscious, when secretions have high volume or viscosity, when coughing is ineffective, or when the individual is otherwise unable to clear his or her airway. Suction is available either from a wall outlet, similar to oxygen, or as a mobile apparatus. *(Saia PREP, 9th ed, pp. 32, 33)*

160. (D) The four *vital signs* are *temperature, pulse, respiration,* and *blood pressure*. Because radiographers may be required to take vital signs in an emergency, they should practice these skills. A *thermometer* is required to measure a patient's temperature. A *watch with a second hand* is required to measure a patient's pulse and respiration. To measure blood pressure, a *blood pressure cuff, sphygmomanometer,* and *stethoscope* are required. These are the skills that the radiographer should practice most frequently because these are most likely to be needed in an emergency situation.

161. (B) There are several specialized tubes/catheters used to provide regular or continual access to the circulatory system for long-term care requirements such as dialysis, blood transfusion, drug therapy such as chemotherapy, and parenteral nutrition. They can also be used for laboratory blood draws and for monitoring central venous pressure (CVP). These are called *CVCs* (or *central lines*). Examples of these central lines include the *Port-A-Cath*, the *Hickman*, the *Raaf*, and the *peripherally inserted central catheter* (PICC). For x-ray verification of position placement, they usually have a radiopaque distal tip. The distal tip should be located in the superior or inferior vena cava near the right atrium. A *Swan–Ganz catheter* is a specific type of IV catheter used to measure the pumping ability of the heart, to obtain pressure readings, and to introduce medications and IV fluids

162. (B) Pacemakers are most often used to treat conduction defects causing *bradycardia*. They can be positioned under the skin in the upper chest and their wires advanced to the right side of the heart, to the apex of the right ventricle or to the right atrium and right ventricle. Pacemaker insertion is often performed under fluoroscopic control in the imaging catheterization lab. Pacemaker insertion can also be performed in the OR, or in a critical care unit using mobile C-arm fluoroscopy. Care must be taken to avoid elevating or abducting the patient's left arm for 24 h following pacemaker insertion.

163. **(B)** *Lidocaine* (Xylocaine) is an antiarrhythmic used to prevent or treat cardiac arrhythmias (dysrhythmia). *Epinephrine* (adrenalin) is a bronchodilator. Bronchodilators may be administered in a spray mister, such as for asthma, or by injection to relieve severe bronchospasm.

Nitroglycerin and *verapamil* are vasodilators. Vasodilators permit increased blood flow by relaxing the walls of the blood vessels.

164. **(C)** It is recommended that a radiographer wears protective eye gear (goggles) during any procedure in which there might be splattering of blood or body fluids. This includes both angiography and biopsy/aspiration procedures. This would not be expected during a routine upper GI examination.

165. **(C)** An *antipyretic* is used to reduce fever. An emetic is used to induce vomiting. An antihistamine is used to relieve allergic reactions. A diuretic is used to stimulate the production of urine.

SUBSPECIALTY LIST

Question Number and Subspecialty correspond to subcategories in each of the four ARRT examination specification sections

1. Physical assistance and monitoring
2. Infection control
3. Ethical and legal aspects
4. Physical assistance and monitoring
5. Medical emergencies
6. Infection control
7. Interpersonal communication
8. Ethical and legal aspects
9. Physical assistance and monitoring
10. Infection control
11. Pharmacology
12. Pharmacology
13. Ethical and legal aspects
14. Physical assistance and monitoring
15. Pharmacology
16. Medical emergencies
17. Handling and disposal of toxic or hazardous material
18. Physical assistance and monitoring
19. Interpersonal communication
20. Physical assistance and monitoring
21. Medical emergencies
22. Ethical and legal aspects
23. Pharmacology
24. Physical assistance and monitoring
25. Infection control
26. Infection control
27. Medical emergencies
28. Infection control
29. Physical assistance and monitoring
30. Physical assistance and monitoring
31. Physical assistance and monitoring
32. Interpersonal communication
33. Physical assistance and monitoring
34. Ethical and legal aspects
35. Ethical and legal aspects
36. Physical assistance and monitoring
37. Physical assistance and monitoring
38. Interpersonal communication
39. Pharmacology
40. Infection control
41. Pharmacology
42. Interpersonal communication
43. Ethical and legal aspects
44. Pharmacology
45. Medical emergencies
46. Pharmacology
47. Infection control
48. Ethical and legal aspects
49. Physical assistance and monitoring
50. Infection control
51. Ethical and legal aspects
52. Pharmacology
53. Physical assistance and monitoring
54. Physical assistance and monitoring
55. Physical assistance and monitoring
56. Interpersonal communication
57. Pharmacology
58. Infection control
59. Pharmacology
60. Ethical and legal aspects
61. Ethical and legal aspects
62. Pharmacology
63. Infection control
64. Physical assistance and monitoring
65. Physical assistance and monitoring
66. Infection control
67. Physical assistance and monitoring
68. Ethical and legal aspects
69. Ethical and legal aspects
70. Ethical and legal aspects
71. Physical assistance and monitoring
72. Pharmacology
73. Pharmacology
74. Physical assistance and monitoring
75. Physical assistance and monitoring
76. Ethical and legal aspects
77. Pharmacology
78. Medical emergencies
79. Infection control
80. Ethical and legal aspects
81. Ethical and legal aspects
82. Physical assistance and monitoring
83. Infection control
84. Physical assistance and monitoring
85. Physical assistance and monitoring
86. Physical assistance and monitoring

87. Ethical and legal aspects
88. Physical assistance and monitoring
89. Pharmacology
90. Physical assistance and monitoring
91. Physical assistance and monitoring
92. Physical assistance and monitoring
93. Infection control
94. Physical assistance and monitoring
95. Pharmacology
96. Infection control
97. Physical assistance and monitoring
98. Physical assistance and monitoring
99. Medical emergencies
100. Pharmacology
101. Infection control
102. Infection control
103. Pharmacology
104. Pharmacology
105. Ethical and legal issues
106. Pharmacology
107. Medical emergencies
108. Physical assistance and monitoring
109. Physical assistance and monitoring
110. Medical emergencies
111. Infection control
112. Infection control
113. Pharmacology
114. Physical assistance and monitoring
115. Pharmacology
116. Medical emergencies
117. Medical emergencies
118. Physical assistance and monitoring
119. Pharmacology
120. Interpersonal communication
121. Medical emergencies
122. Physical assistance and monitoring
123. Infection control
124. Pharmacology
125. Interpersonal communication
126. Pharmacology

127. Physical assistance and monitoring
128. Infection control
129. Infection control
130. Ethical and legal issues
131. Ethical and legal issues
132. Ethical and legal issues
133. Ethical and legal issues
134. Pharmacology
135. Ethical and legal issues
136. Physical assistance and monitoring
137. Pharmacology
138. Physical assistance and monitoring
139. From ecology
140. Infection control
141. Medical emergencies
142. Pharmacology
143. Ethical and legal issues
144. Interpersonal communication
145. Pharmacology
146. Ethical and legal issues
147. Physical assistance and monitoring
148. Infection control
149. Infection control
150. Infection control
151. From ecology
152. Interpersonal communication
153. Interpersonal communication
154. Interpersonal communication
155. Ethical and legal issues
156. Ethical and legal issues
157. Ethical and legal issues
158. Physical assistance and monitoring
159. Physical assistance and monitoring
160. Physical assistance and monitoring
161. Physical assistance and monitoring
162. Physical assistance and monitoring
163. Pharmacology
164. Infection control
165. Pharmacology

TARGETED READING

Adler AM, Carlton RR. *Introduction to Radiologic and Imaging Sciences and Patient Care.* 7th ed. St Louis, MO: Saunders Elsevier; 2019.

ARRT Standards of Ethics. https://www.arrt.org/docs/default-source/Governing-Documents/arrt-standards-of-ethics.pdf?sfvrsn=10. Accessed March 27, 2017.

ASRT Practice Standards. https://www.asrt.org/docs/default-source/practice-standards-published/ps_rad.pdf?sfvrsn=2. Accessed March 27, 2017.

Dutton AG, Ryan TA. *Torres' Patient Care in Imaging Technology.* 9th ed. Philadelphia, PA: Lippincott; 2019.

Ehrlich RA, Coakes DM. *Patient Care in Radiography.* 9th ed. St Louis, MO: Mosby; 2017.

Ehrlich RA, Coakes DM. *Patient Care in Radiography.* 10th ed. St Louis, MO: Mosby; 2021.

Saia DA. *Radiography PREP.* 9th ed. New York, NY: McGraw Hill; 2018.

Saladin KS. *Anatomy and Physiology: The Unity of Form and Function.* 7th ed. New York, NY: McGraw Hill; 2015.

Procedures

2

QUESTIONS

DIRECTIONS: Each of the numbered items or incomplete statements in this section is followed by answers or by completions of the statement. Select the *one* letter answer or completion that is *best* in each case.

1. The term *varus* refers to
- ❏ A. turned outward
- ❏ B. turned inward
- ❏ C. rotated medially
- ❏ D. rotated laterally

2. Which elbow fat pad is not visible radiographically in the lateral projection of the normal elbow?
- ❏ A. Anterior
- ❏ B. Posterior
- ❏ C. Supinator
- ❏ D. Pronator

3. What could be done to improve the lateral (mediolateral) projection of the knee seen in Figure 2-1?
1. Angle the x-ray tube 5° cephalad
2. Angle the x-ray tube 5° caudad
3. Rotate the pelvis slightly backward/posteriorly
4. Rotate the pelvis slightly forward/anteriorly
   - ❏ A. 1 and 3
   - ❏ B. 1 and 4
   - ❏ C. 2 and 3
   - ❏ D. 2 and 4

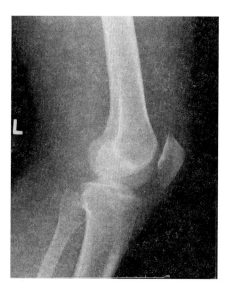

Figure 2-1

4. The proximal radius and ulna are seen free of superimposition in which of the following projections?
- ❏ A. AP elbow
- ❏ B. Lateral elbow
- ❏ C. Medial oblique elbow
- ❏ D. Lateral oblique elbow

5. An RPO position poorly demonstrates the lumbar zygapophyseal articulations and the pedicles are seen on posterior portion of the vertebral body. What does this indicate?
- ❏ A. Excessive rotation
- ❏ B. Insufficient rotation
- ❏ C. Pelvic tilt
- ❏ D. Correct positioning

37

6. Name the structure identified by the number 10 in Figure 2-2.
- ❏ A. Radial head
- ❏ B. Ulnar head
- ❏ C. Lateral epicondyle
- ❏ D. Medial epicondyle

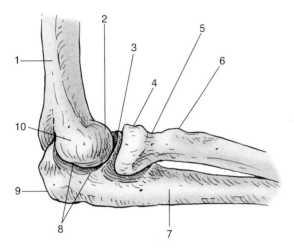

Figure 2-2

7. The term *dorsal* can refer to which three of the following?
1. Anterior surface of body
2. Back of the hand
3. Upper surface of the foot
4. Front of the hand
5. Posterior surface of the body
6. Lower surface of the foot
- ❏ A. 1, 4, and 6
- ❏ B. 2, 1, and 6
- ❏ C. 2, 3, and 5
- ❏ D. 1, 3, and 4
- ❏ E. 3, 4, and 5

8. All of the following statements regarding respiratory structures are true, *except*
- ❏ A. the right lung has two fissures
- ❏ B. the inferior portion of a lung is its base
- ❏ C. each lung is enclosed in pleural membrane
- ❏ D. the main stem bronchi enter the lung fissure

9. All of the following statements regarding a PA projection of the skull are true, *except*
- ❏ A. the OML is perpendicular to the IR
- ❏ B. the petrous pyramids fill the orbits
- ❏ C. the MSP is parallel to the IR
- ❏ D. the CR is perpendicular to the IR and exits the nasion

10. An accurate critique of the PA projection of the chest seen in Figure 2-3 would include which of the following?
1. The pulmonary apices are demonstrated
2. The air-filled trachea and carina are demonstrated
3. Ten posterior ribs are seen above the diaphragm
- ❏ A. 1 only
- ❏ B. 1 and 2 only
- ❏ C. 2 and 3 only
- ❏ D. 1, 2, and 3

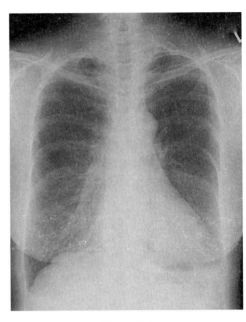

Figure 2-3

11. A congenital defect in which the sternum is depressed posteriorly is termed
- ❏ A. pectus carinatum
- ❏ B. pectus excavatum
- ❏ C. flail chest
- ❏ D. atelectasis

12. Which of the following positions is used to demonstrate vertical patellar fractures and the patellofemoral articulation?
- ❏ A. AP knee
- ❏ B. Lateral knee
- ❏ C. Tangential patella
- ❏ D. Tunnel view

13. Structures located in the right lower quadrant (RLQ) include which of the following?
1. Cecum
2. Vermiform appendix
3. Sigmoid
- ❏ A. 1 only
- ❏ B. 1 and 2 only
- ❏ C. 2 and 3 only
- ❏ D. 1, 2, and 3

14. Which of the following statements are correct regarding Figure 2-4?
1. The image was made in the RPO position
2. The right kidney is more parallel to the IR
3. The procedure is a retrograde pyelogram
4. The right ureter is better visualized
5. The image was made postvoid
6. Kidneys, ureters, and bladder are included
   - ❏ A. 1, 3, and 4
   - ❏ B. 1, 4, and 6
   - ❏ C. 2, 4, and 5
   - ❏ D. 3, 4, and 6

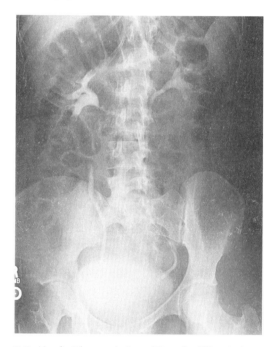

Figure 2-4. Used with permission of Stamford Hospital, Department of Radiology.

15. Structures involved in blowout fractures include the
1. orbital floor
2. inferior rectus muscle
3. zygoma
   - ❏ A. 1 only
   - ❏ B. 1 and 2 only
   - ❏ C. 2 and 3 only
   - ❏ D. 1, 2, and 3

16. Which of the following articulations participate(s) in formation of the ankle mortise?
1. Talotibial
2. Talocalcaneal
3. Talofibular
   - ❏ A. 1 only
   - ❏ B. 1 and 3 only
   - ❏ C. 2 and 3 only
   - ❏ D. 3 only

17. The upper surface of the foot may be described as the
1. plantar surface
2. anterior surface
3. dorsum
   - ❏ A. 1 only
   - ❏ B. 1 and 2 only
   - ❏ C. 2 and 3 only
   - ❏ D. 1, 2, and 3

18. Double-contrast examinations of the stomach or large bowel are performed to better visualize the
   - ❏ A. position of the organ
   - ❏ B. size and shape of the organ
   - ❏ C. diverticula
   - ❏ D. gastric or bowel mucosa

19. Terms used to describe movement include
1. extension
2. eversion
3. erect
   - ❏ A. 1 only
   - ❏ B. 1 and 2 only
   - ❏ C. 1 and 3 only
   - ❏ D. 2 and 3

20. Which of the following is best demonstrated in the AP axial projection (Towne method) of the skull, with the CR directed 30° caudad to the orbitomeatal line (OML) and exiting at the foramen magnum?
   - ❏ A. Occipital bone
   - ❏ B. Frontal bone
   - ❏ C. Facial bones
   - ❏ D. Basal foramina

21. The RPO position (Judet method) of the right acetabulum will demonstrate the
   - ❏ A. anterior rim of the right acetabulum
   - ❏ B. anterior iliopubic column
   - ❏ C. left iliac wing
   - ❏ D. posterior rim of the right acetabulum

22. Select the three correct statements regarding Figure 2-5.
1. The left axillary ribs are well demonstrated
2. The image was obtained in an RPO position
3. Right posterior ribs are well demonstrated
4. The exposure was made on full inspiration
5. The image was made using a 45° oblique
   - ❏ A. 1, 2, and 4
   - ❏ B. 1, 4, and 5
   - ❏ C. 2, 3, and 4
   - ❏ D. 3, 4, and 5

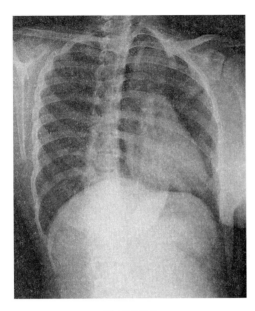

Figure 2-5

23. Which of the following positions/projections is used to demonstrate a nearly frontal view of the sternum?
- ❏ A. AP
- ❏ B. PA
- ❏ C. RAO
- ❏ D. LAO

24. Skeletal muscle is
1. visceral
2. voluntary
3. striated
4. involuntary
- ❏ A. 1 and 3
- ❏ B. 1 and 4
- ❏ C. 2 and 3
- ❏ D. 1, 2, and 3
- ❏ E. 1, 2, and 4

25. Which of the following bones participate(s) in the formation of the knee joint?
1. Femur
2. Tibia
3. Patella
- ❏ A. 1 and 2 only
- ❏ B. 1 and 3 only
- ❏ C. 2 and 3 only
- ❏ D. 1, 2, and 3

26. How should a chest examination to rule out air–fluid levels be obtained on a patient with traumatic injuries?
- ❏ A. Perform the examination in the Trendelenburg position
- ❏ B. Erect inspiration and expiration images should be obtained
- ❏ C. Include a lateral chest examination performed in dorsal decubitus position
- ❏ D. Perform the examination AP supine at 44-inch SID

27. In the axiolateral inferosuperior projection of the hip, the IR should be
- ❏ A. 2 inches medial to the ASIS
- ❏ B. parallel to the central ray
- ❏ C. perpendicular to the femoral neck
- ❏ D. parallel to the femoral neck

28. Which of the following is the recommended method to image the frontal and ethmoidal sinuses seen in Figure 2-6?
- ❏ A. Erect PA, chin extended, OML forming 37° to IR
- ❏ B. Erect PA, OML perpendicular to IR, and CR 15° caudal to IR
- ❏ C. Erect PA, chin extended, OML 15° from horizontal
- ❏ D. Erect PA, chin extended, OML 30° from horizontal

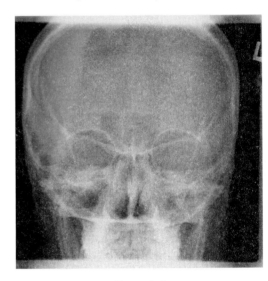

Figure 2-6

29. Which of the following statements is/are true regarding the radiograph in Figure 2-6?
1. The position is used to demonstrate the frontal and ethmoid sinuses
2. The maxillary sinuses are seen near the medial aspect of the orbits
3. The perpendicular plate is visualized in midline of the nasal cavity
- ❏ A. 1 only
- ❏ B. 1 and 2 only
- ❏ C. 1 and 3 only
- ❏ D. 1, 2, and 3

30. To better demonstrate the interphalangeal joints of the hand in the oblique position, the radiographer should
- ❏ A. oblique the hand no more than 45°
- ❏ B. use a support sponge for the phalanges
- ❏ C. clench the fist to bring the carpals closer to the IR
- ❏ D. use ulnar flexion

31. Traumatic rib fractures resulting in their detachment from the rib cage is termed

❏ A. pectus carinatum
❏ B. pectus excavatum
❏ C. flail chest
❏ D. atelectasis

32. The relationship between the fractured ends of long bones is called

❏ A. angulation
❏ B. apposition
❏ C. luxation
❏ D. sprain

33. In the PA axial oblique projection of the cervical spine, the CR should be directed

❏ A. parallel to C4
❏ B. perpendicular to C4
❏ C. 15° cephalad to C4
❏ D. 15° caudad to C4

34. In which of the following positions can small amounts of free air in the peritoneal cavity be demonstrated?

❏ A. Left lateral decubitus
❏ B. Right lateral decubitus
❏ C. AP Trendelenburg
❏ D. AP supine

35. Which of the following anatomic structures is seen most anteriorly in a lateral projection of the chest?

❏ A. Esophagus
❏ B. Trachea
❏ C. Cardiac apex
❏ D. Superimposed scapular borders

36. For an AP projection of the knee in a patient whose measurement from ASIS to tabletop is 17 cm, which CR direction will best demonstrate the knee joint?

❏ A. 3°–5° caudad
❏ B. 10° caudad
❏ C. 3°–5° cephalad
❏ D. 0° (perpendicular)

37. In which of the following projections was the image in Figure 2-7 made?

❏ A. AP
❏ B. Medial oblique
❏ C. Lateral oblique
❏ D. Acute flexion

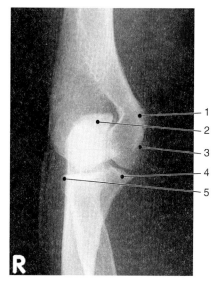

Figure 2-7. Used with permission of Stamford Hospital, Department of Radiology.

38. Which of the following anatomic structures is indicated by the number 1 in Figure 2-7?

❏ A. Medial epicondyle
❏ B. Trochlea
❏ C. Capitulum
❏ D. Radial head

39. Select the correct statement(s) regarding the image shown in Figure 2-8.

1. The femoral neck is parallel to the IR
2. There is insufficient internal rotation
3. The femoral neck is foreshortened

❏ A. 2 only
❏ B. 1 and 2 only
❏ C. 1 and 3 only
❏ D. 2 and 3 only

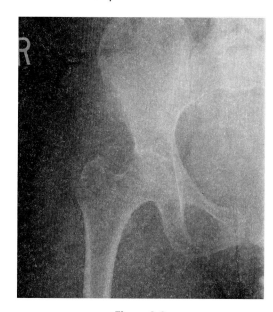

Figure 2-8

40. A patient unable to extend his or her arm is seated at the end of the x-ray table, elbow flexed 90°. The CR is directed 45° medially (toward the shoulder). Which of the following structures will be demonstrated *best*?

1. Radial head
2. Capitulum
3. Coronoid process
   - ❏ A. 1 only
   - ❏ B. 1 and 2 only
   - ❏ C. 2 and 3 only
   - ❏ D. 1, 2, and 3

41. Which of the following projections can be used to supplement the traditional "open-mouth" projection when the upper portion of the odontoid process cannot be well demonstrated?

- ❏ A. AP or PA through the foramen magnum
- ❏ B. AP oblique with right and left head rotation
- ❏ C. Horizontal beam lateral
- ❏ D. AP axial

42. The floor of the cranium includes all of the following bones, *except*

- ❏ A. the temporal bones
- ❏ B. the occipital bone
- ❏ C. the ethmoid bone
- ❏ D. the sphenoid bone

43. Narrowing of the upper airway, as seen in pediatric croup, can be best visualized in the

- ❏ A. AP projection
- ❏ B. lateral projection
- ❏ C. axial projection
- ❏ D. lordotic projection

44. In which of the following positions was the radiograph shown in Figure 2-9 made?

- ❏ A. LAO
- ❏ B. RAO
- ❏ C. AP axial
- ❏ D. Right lateral decubitus

45. The distal ileum is labeled in Figure 2-9 as number

- ❏ A. 3
- ❏ B. 4
- ❏ C. 5
- ❏ D. 6

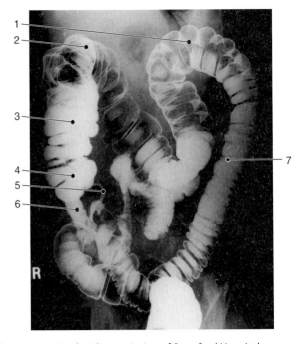

Figure 2-9. Used with permission of Stamford Hospital, Department of Radiology.

46. A kyphotic curve is formed by the

1. sacral vertebrae
2. thoracic vertebrae
3. lumbar vertebrae
4. cervical vertebrae
   - ❏ A. 1, 2, and 4
   - ❏ B. 1 and 2
   - ❏ C. 3 and 4
   - ❏ D. 1, 3, and 4
   - ❏ E. 2 and 4

47. Which of the following projections/positions will best demonstrate a subacromial or subcoracoid dislocation?

- ❏ A. Tangential
- ❏ B. AP axial
- ❏ C. Transthoracic lateral
- ❏ D. PA oblique scapular Y

48. Correct preparation for a patient scheduled for an upper gastrointestinal (GI) series is most likely to be

- ❏ A. iodinated contrast administration evening before examination; water only in the morning
- ❏ B. NPO after midnight
- ❏ C. cathartics and cleansing enemas
- ❏ D. NPO after midnight, cleansing enemas, and empty bladder before scout image

49. Which of the following positions can be used to demonstrate the axillary ribs of the right thorax?

1. LAO
2. LPO
3. RAO
   - ❏ A. 1 only
   - ❏ B. 1 and 2 only
   - ❏ C. 2 and 3 only
   - ❏ D. 1, 2, and 3

50. The interspaces between the first and second cuneiforms are best demonstrated in which of the following projections?
- ❏ A. Lateral oblique foot
- ❏ B. Medial oblique foot
- ❏ C. Lateral foot
- ❏ D. Weight-bearing foot

51. The sternal angle is at approximately the same level as the
- ❏ A. T2–T3 interspace
- ❏ B. T9–T10 interspace
- ❏ C. T5
- ❏ D. costal margin

52. The following are anatomical features of the femur. Rearrange them in order from distal to proximal.
1. Lesser trochanter
2. Medial epicondyle
3. Head
4. Greater trochanter
5. Lateral condyle
6. Body/shaft
- ❏ A. 5, 2, 6, 1, 4, 3
- ❏ B. 2, 5, 4, 1, 6, 3
- ❏ C. 3, 4, 1, 6, 2, 5
- ❏ D. 3, 6, 1, 4, 5, 2

53. Which of the following positions is essential in radiography of the paranasal sinuses?
- ❏ A. Erect
- ❏ B. Recumbent
- ❏ C. Oblique
- ❏ D. Trendelenburg

54. Select the *correct* statement(s) regarding Figure 2-10.
1. The degree of obliquity is correct
2. The middle phalanges are foreshortened
3. The interphalangeal joints are well demonstrated
4. The digits are parallel to the IR
- ❏ **A.** 1, 2, and 4
- ❏ B. 1 and 2
- ❏ C. 3 and 4
- ❏ D. 1, 3, and 4
- ❏ E. 2 and 4

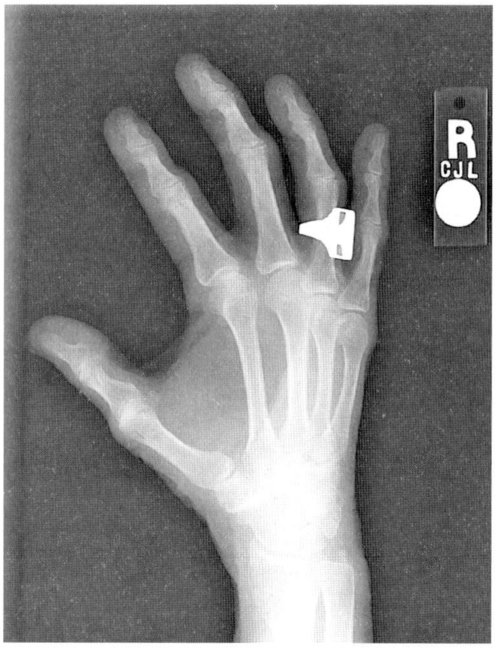

Figure 2-10. Used with permission of Stamford Hospital, Department of Radiology.

55. What is the relationship between the midsagittal and midcoronal planes?
- ❏ A. Parallel
- ❏ B. Perpendicular
- ❏ C. 45°
- ❏ D. 70°

56. All of the following structures are associated with the posterior femur, *except*
- ❏ A. popliteal surface
- ❏ B. intercondyloid fossa
- ❏ C. intertrochanteric line
- ❏ D. linea aspera

57. Which of the following statements is/are correct regarding the Norgaard method, "ball-catcher's position"?
1. Bilateral AP oblique hands are obtained
2. It is used for early detection of rheumatoid arthritis
3. The hands are obliqued about 45°, palm up
- ❏ A. 1 only
- ❏ B. 1 and 2 only
- ❏ C. 2 and 3 only
- ❏ D. 1, 2, and 3

58. What condition(s) is/are demonstrated in Figure 2-11?
1. Emphysema
2. Pneumothorax
3. Pleural effusion
- ❏ A. 1 only
- ❏ B. 1 and 2 only
- ❏ C. 2 and 3 only
- ❏ D. 1, 2, and 3

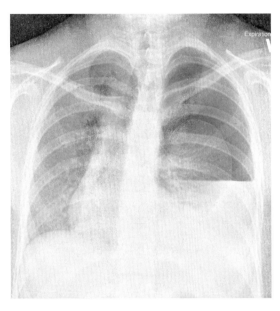

Figure 2-11

59. Which of the following bony landmarks is in the same transverse plane as L2–L3?

❏ A. Inferior costal margin
❏ B. Greater trochanter
❏ C. Iliac crest
❏ D. ASIS

60. To visualize or "open" the right sacroiliac joint, the patient is positioned

❏ A. 30°–40° LPO
❏ B. 30°–40° RPO
❏ C. 25°–30° LPO
❏ D. 25°–30° RPO

61. Which of the following may be used to evaluate the glenohumeral joint?

1. Scapular Y projection
2. Inferosuperior axial
3. Transthoracic lateral
   ❏ A. 1 only
   ❏ B. 1 and 2 only
   ❏ C. 2 and 3 only
   ❏ D. 1, 2, and 3

62. Which of the following is/are distal to the tibial plateau?

1. Intercondyloid fossa
2. Tibial condyles
3. Tibial tuberosity
   ❏ A. 1 only
   ❏ B. 1 and 2 only
   ❏ C. 2 and 3 only
   ❏ D. 1, 2, and 3

63. Evaluation criteria for a lateral projection of the humerus include

1. epicondyles parallel to the IR
2. lesser tubercle in profile
3. superimposed epicondyles
   ❏ A. 1 only
   ❏ B. 1 and 3 only
   ❏ C. 2 and 3 only
   ❏ D. 1, 2, and 3

64. Which of the following are mediastinal structures?

1. Heart
2. Trachea
3. Esophagus
   ❏ A. 1 only
   ❏ B. 1 and 2 only
   ❏ C. 2 and 3 only
   ❏ D. 1, 2, and 3

65. Which of the following statements are correct regarding Figure 2–12?

1. The atlantoaxial articulation is well demonstrated
2. The odontoid process is incompletely visualized
3. More flexion is required to move upper incisors inferiorly
4. More extension is required to move base of skull more inferiorly
   ❏ A. 1 and 2 only
   ❏ B. 1 and 4 only
   ❏ C. 1, 2, and 3 only
   ❏ D. 1, 2, and 4 only

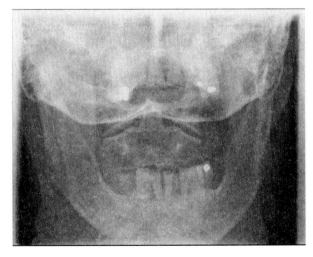

Figure 2-12

66. Which of the following fracture classifications describes a small, bony fragment pulled from a bony process?

❏ A. Avulsion fracture
❏ B. Torus fracture
❏ C. Comminuted fracture
❏ D. Compound fracture

67. That portion of the humerus which articulates with the ulna to help form the elbow joint is the
- ❑ A. semilunar/trochlear notch
- ❑ B. radial head
- ❑ C. capitulum
- ❑ D. trochlea

68. Valid evaluation criteria for a lateral projection of the forearm require that
1. the epicondyles be parallel to the IR
2. the radius and ulna be superimposed distally
3. the radial tuberosity should face anteriorly
- ❑ A. 1 only
- ❑ B. 1 and 2 only
- ❑ C. 2 and 3 only
- ❑ D. 1, 2, and 3

69. In myelography, the contrast medium generally is injected into the
- ❑ A. cisterna magna
- ❑ B. individual intervertebral disks
- ❑ C. subarachnoid space between the first and second lumbar vertebrae
- ❑ D. subarachnoid space between the third and fourth lumbar vertebrae

70. The junction of the sagittal and coronal sutures is the
- ❑ A. diploe
- ❑ B. lambda
- ❑ C. bregma
- ❑ D. pterion

71. Which of the following statements are true regarding the radiograph in Figure 2-13?
1. The image is an oblique projection of the shoulder
2. The glenoid cavity and humeral head are superimposed
3. The acromion process is projected laterally
4. The coracoid process is free of superimposition
5. The coracoid process is projected above the clavicle
- ❑ A. 1 and 2 only
- ❑ B. 1, 2, 3, and 4
- ❑ C. 1, 3, and 4
- ❑ D. 3, 4, and 5 only

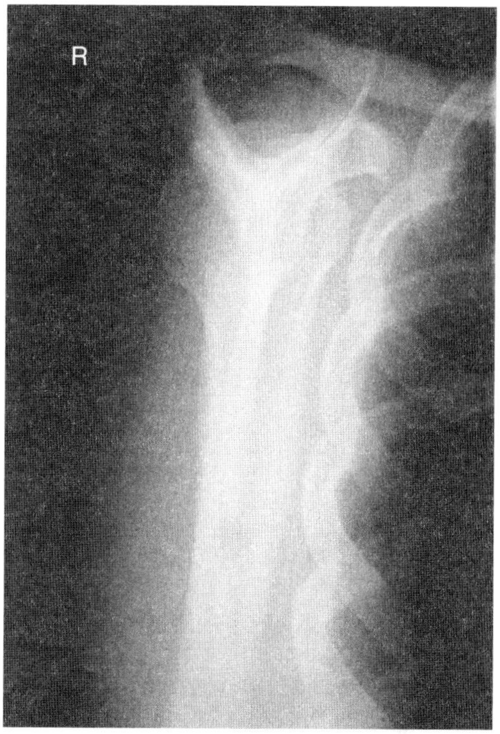

Figure 2-13

72. Which of the following precautions should be observed when radiographing a patient who has sustained a traumatic injury to the hip?
1. When a fracture is suspected, manipulation of the affected extremity should be performed by a physician
2. The AP axiolateral projection should be avoided
3. To evaluate the entire region, the pelvis is typically included in the initial examination
- ❑ A. 1 only
- ❑ B. 1 and 3 only
- ❑ C. 2 and 3 only
- ❑ D. 1, 2, and 3

73. The lumbar vertebral transverse process is represented by which part of the "Scottie dog" seen in a correctly positioned oblique lumbar spine?
- ❑ A. Eye
- ❑ B. Nose
- ❑ C. Body
- ❑ D. Ear

74. Which of the following positions is used to demonstrate the lumbosacral zygapophyseal articulation?
- ❑ A. AP
- ❑ B. Lateral
- ❑ C. 30° RPO
- ❑ D. 45° LPO

75. Which of the following places the anatomical points of the hand's third digit in correct order from proximal to distal?

❏ A. Base of metacarpal, head of middle phalanx, carpometacarpal joint, metacarpophalangeal joint, distal interphalangeal joint, proximal interphalangeal joint, ungual tuft

❏ B. Carpometacarpal joint, base of metacarpal, metacarpophalangeal joint, proximal interphalangeal joint, head of middle phalange, distal interphalangeal joint, ungual tuft

❏ C. Ungual tuft, distal interphalangeal joint, head of middle phalanx, proximal interphalangeal joint, metacarpophalangeal joint, base of metacarpal, carpometacarpal joint

❏ D. Carpometacarpal joint, metacarpophalangeal joint, base of metacarpal, head of middle phalanx, proximal interphalangeal joint, distal interphalangeal joint, ungual tuft

76. Which of the following conditions is limited specifically to the tibial tuberosity?

❏ A. Ewing sarcoma
❏ B. Osgood–Schlatter disease
❏ C. Gout
❏ D. Exostosis

77. Examples of synovial pivot articulations include the

1. atlantoaxial joint
2. radioulnar joint
3. temporomandibular joint

❏ A. 1 only
❏ B. 1 and 2 only
❏ C. 2 and 3 only
❏ D. 1, 2, and 3 only

78. Components of the bony thorax include the

1. scapulae
2. manubrium
3. clavicles
4. ribs
5. thoracic vertebrae

❏ A. 1, 2, and 3 only
❏ B. 2, 3, and 4 only
❏ C. 2, 4, and 5 only
❏ D. 2, 3, 4, and 5 only

79. Aspirated foreign bodies in older children and adults are *most likely* to lodge in the

❏ A. right main stem bronchus
❏ B. left main stem bronchus
❏ C. esophagus
❏ D. proximal stomach

80. The PA chest radiograph shown in Figure 2-14 demonstrates

1. rotation
2. scapulae removed from lung fields
3. adequate inspiration

❏ A. 1 only
❏ B. 1 and 2 only
❏ C. 2 and 3 only
❏ D. 1, 2, and 3

81. The letter B in Figure 2-14 indicates

❏ A. a left anterior rib
❏ B. a right posterior rib
❏ C. a left posterior rib
❏ D. a right anterior rib

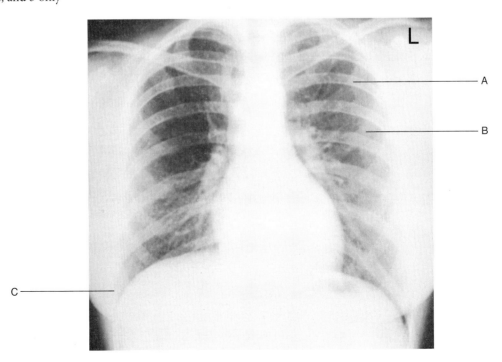

Figure 2-14. Used with permission of Stamford Hospital, Department of Radiology.

82. The laryngeal prominence is formed by the
- ❏ A. thyroid gland
- ❏ B. thyroid cartilage
- ❏ C. vocal cords
- ❏ D. pharynx

83. Types of articulations lacking a joint cavity include
1. fibrous
2. cartilaginous
3. synovial
- ❏ A. 1 only
- ❏ B. 1 and 2 only
- ❏ C. 2 and 3 only
- ❏ D. 1, 2, and 3

84. The thoracic zygapophyseal joints are demonstrated with the
- ❏ A. coronal plane 90° to the IR
- ❏ B. midsagittal plane 90° to the IR
- ❏ C. coronal plane 20° to the IR
- ❏ D. midsagittal plane 20° to the IR

85. The structure located midway between the anterosuperior iliac spine (ASIS) and pubic symphysis is the
- ❏ A. dome of the acetabulum
- ❏ B. femoral neck
- ❏ C. greater trochanter
- ❏ D. iliac crest

86. The structure labeled 4 in Figure 2-15 is the
- ❏ A. maxillary sinus
- ❏ B. sphenoidal sinus
- ❏ C. ethmoidal sinus
- ❏ D. frontal sinus

87. Which of the following would *best* evaluate the structure labeled 3 in Figure 2-15?
- ❏ A. PA axial projection (Caldwell method)
- ❏ B. Parietoacanthial projection (Waters' method)
- ❏ C. Lateral projection
- ❏ D. Submentovertex projection

88. The uppermost portion of the iliac crest is at approximately the same level as the
- ❏ A. costal margin
- ❏ B. umbilicus
- ❏ C. xiphoid tip
- ❏ D. fourth lumbar vertebra

89. The radiograph shown in Figure 2-16 demonstrates the articulation between the
1. talus and the navicular
2. talus and the cuboid
3. talus and the calcaneus
- ❏ A. 1 only
- ❏ B. 1 and 2 only
- ❏ C. 2 and 3 only
- ❏ D. 1, 2, and 3

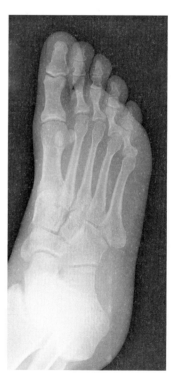

Figure 2-16. Used with permission of Stamford Hospital, Department of Radiology.

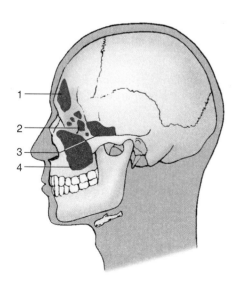

Figure 2-15. Reproduced with permission from DA Saia. *LANGE Radiography Review Flashcards.* New York: McGraw Hill; 2015.

90. The ulnar styloid process seen in Figure 2-17 is indicated by number
- ❑ A. 7
- ❑ B. 8
- ❑ C. 9
- ❑ D. 10

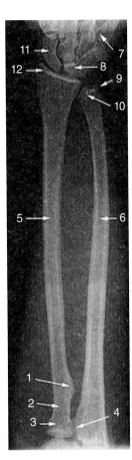

Figure 2-17. Reproduced with permission from DA Saia. *LANGE Radiography Review Flashcards*. New York: McGraw Hill; 2015.

91. The articular facets of L5–S1 are best demonstrated in a/an
- ❑ A. AP projection
- ❑ B. 30° oblique
- ❑ C. 45° oblique
- ❑ D. AP axial projection

92. The patient's chin should be elevated during chest radiography to
- ❑ A. permit the diaphragm to move to its lowest position
- ❑ B. avoid superimposition on the apices
- ❑ C. assist in maintaining an upright position
- ❑ D. keep the MSP parallel

93. That portion of a long bone from which it lengthens/grows is the
- ❑ A. diaphysis
- ❑ B. epiphysis
- ❑ C. metaphysis
- ❑ D. apophysis

94. Posterior displacement of a tibial fracture would be *best* demonstrated in the
- ❑ A. AP projection
- ❑ B. lateral projection
- ❑ C. medial oblique projection
- ❑ D. lateral oblique projection

95. What part of the "Scottie dog," seen in a correctly positioned oblique lumbar spine, represents the vertebral pedicle?
- ❑ A. Eye
- ❑ B. Nose
- ❑ C. Body
- ❑ D. Neck

96. All of the following statements regarding the position shown in Figure 2-18 are true, *except*
- ❑ A. a ventral decubitus position is illustrated
- ❑ B. a right pneumothorax could be demonstrated
- ❑ C. a left pleural effusion could be demonstrated
- ❑ D. the CR is directed horizontally to the level of T7

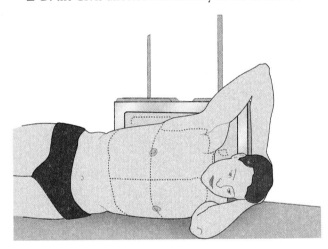

Figure 2-18

97. Which of the following positions *best* demonstrates the proximal tibiofibular articulation?
- ❑ A. AP
- ❑ B. 90° mediolateral
- ❑ C. 45° internal rotation
- ❑ D. 45° external rotation

98. At what level do the carotid arteries bifurcate?
- ❑ A. Foramen magnum
- ❑ B. Trachea
- ❑ C. Pharynx
- ❑ D. C4

99. What is the position of the stomach in a hypersthenic patient?
- ❑ A. High and vertical
- ❑ B. High and horizontal
- ❑ C. Low and vertical
- ❑ D. Low and horizontal

100. Which of the following statements is/are true regarding the shoulder image seen in Figure 2-19?

1. The unaffected arm is adjacent to the IR
2. It provides a lateral view
3. It is useful in trauma situations
   - ❑ A. 1 only
   - ❑ B. 1 and 2 only
   - ❑ C. 2 and 3 only
   - ❑ D. 1, 2, and 3

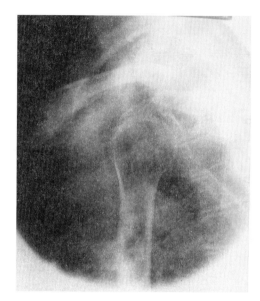

Figure 2-19. Reproduced with permission from DA Saia. *LANGE Radiography Review Flashcards*. New York: McGraw Hill; 2015.

101. Which of the following are characteristics of the hypersthenic body type?

1. Short, wide, transverse heart
2. High and peripheral large bowel
3. Diaphragm positioned low
   - ❑ A. 1 and 2 only
   - ❑ B. 1 and 3 only
   - ❑ C. 2 and 3 only
   - ❑ D. 1, 2, and 3

102. Which of the following conditions is often the result of ureteral obstruction or stricture?

- ❑ A. Pyelonephrosis
- ❑ B. Nephroptosis
- ❑ C. Hydronephrosis
- ❑ D. Cystourethritis

103. Which of the following should be demonstrated in a true AP projection of the clavicle?

1. Clavicular body
2. Acromioclavicular joint
3. Sternocostal joint
   - ❑ A. 1 only
   - ❑ B. 1 and 2 only
   - ❑ C. 2 and 3 only
   - ❑ D. 1, 2, and 3

104. All of the following statements regarding large bowel radiography are true, *except*

- ❑ A. the large bowel must be completely empty prior to examination
- ❑ B. retained fecal material can obscure pathology
- ❑ C. single-contrast studies help to demonstrate intraluminal lesions
- ❑ D. double-contrast studies help to demonstrate mucosal lesions

105. In a lateral projection of the normal knee, the

1. fibular head should be somewhat superimposed on the proximal tibia
2. patellofemoral joint should be visualized
3. femoral condyles should be superimposed
   - ❑ A. 1 only
   - ❑ B. 2 only
   - ❑ C. 1 and 3 only
   - ❑ D. 1, 2, and 3

106. Which of the following conditions is characterized by "flattening" of the hemidiaphragms?

- ❑ A. Pneumothorax
- ❑ B. Pleural effusion
- ❑ C. Emphysema
- ❑ D. Pneumonia

107. The term used to describe the presence of blood in vomit is

- ❑ A. hemoptysis
- ❑ B. hematemesis
- ❑ C. chronic obstructive pulmonary disease (COPD)
- ❑ D. bronchitis

108. The outermost wall of the digestive tract is the

- ❑ A. mucosa
- ❑ B. muscularis
- ❑ C. submucosa
- ❑ D. serosa

109. Which position of the shoulder demonstrates the lesser tubercle in profile medially?

- ❑ A. AP
- ❑ B. External rotation
- ❑ C. Internal rotation
- ❑ D. Neutral position

110. In the PA projection of the hand seen in Figure 2-20, which numeral identifies the proximal interphalangeal joint?

- ❑ A. 4
- ❑ B. 5
- ❑ C. 6
- ❑ D. 7

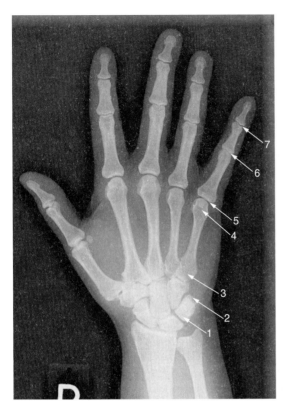

Figure 2-20

111. In which position of the shoulder is the greater tubercle seen superimposed on the humeral head?
- ❏ A. AP
- ❏ B. External rotation
- ❏ C. Internal rotation
- ❏ D. Neutral position

112. With the patient positioned as illustrated in Figure 2-21, which of the following structures is best demonstrated?
- ❏ A. Patella
- ❏ B. Patellofemoral articulation
- ❏ C. Intercondyloid fossa
- ❏ D. Tibial tuberosity

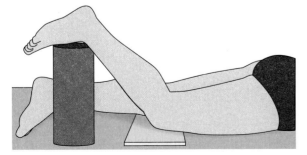

Figure 2-21

113. Which of the following structures is illustrated by the number 2 in Figure 2-22?
- ❏ A. Maxillary sinus
- ❏ B. Coronoid process
- ❏ C. Zygomatic arch
- ❏ D. Coronoid process

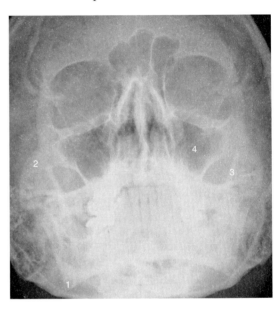

Figure 2-22

114. Which of the following articulations may be described as diarthrotic?
1. Condyloid
2. Sellar
3. Gomphosis
- ❏ A. 1 only
- ❏ B. 3 only
- ❏ C. 1 and 2 only
- ❏ D. 1, 2, and 3

115. Which of the following carpal(s) is/are *best* demonstrated by ulnar flexion/deviation?
1. Medial carpals
2. Lateral carpals
3. Scaphoid
- ❏ A. 1 only
- ❏ B. 1 and 2 only
- ❏ C. 2 and 3 only
- ❏ D. 1, 2, and 3

116. What should be done to better demonstrate the coracoid process shown in Figure 2-23?
- ❏ A. Use a perpendicular CR
- ❏ B. Angle the CR about 30° cephalad
- ❏ C. Angle the CR about 30° caudad
- ❏ D. Angle the MSP 15° toward the affected side

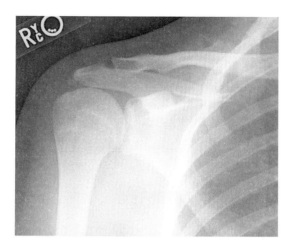

Figure 2-23. Used with permission of Stamford Hospital, Department of Radiology.

117. An LPO fails to clearly demonstrate the lumbar zygapophyseal articulations. The pedicles are seen on the anterior portion of the vertebral body. What does this indicate?
- ❏ A. Excessive rotation
- ❏ B. Insufficient rotation
- ❏ C. Pelvic tilt
- ❏ D. Correct positioning

118. In which type of fracture are the splintered ends of bone forced through the skin?
- ❏ A. Closed
- ❏ B. Compound
- ❏ C. Compression
- ❏ D. Depressed

119. The CR is parallel to the intervertebral foramina in which of the following projections?
1. Lateral cervical spine
2. Lateral thoracic spine
3. Lateral lumbar spine
- ❏ A. 1 only
- ❏ B. 1 and 2 only
- ❏ C. 2 and 3 only
- ❏ D. 1, 2, and 3

120. Which of the following is/are recommended to reduce the amount of scattered radiation reaching the IR in CR/DR imaging of the lumbosacral region?
1. Close collimation
2. Lead mat on table posterior to the patient
3. Decreased SID
- ❏ A. 1 only
- ❏ B. 1 and 2 only
- ❏ C. 2 and 3 only
- ❏ D. 1, 2, and 3

121. Which of the following is/are associated with a Colles fracture?
1. Transverse fracture of the radial head
2. Chip fracture of the ulnar styloid
3. Posterior or backward displacement
- ❏ A. 1 only
- ❏ B. 1 and 3 only
- ❏ C. 2 and 3 only
- ❏ D. 1, 2, and 3

122. Which type of ileus is characterized by cessation of peristalsis?
- ❏ A. Mechanical
- ❏ B. Paralytic
- ❏ C. Asymptomatic
- ❏ D. Sterile

123. The projection/method often used to detect carpal canal defect is the
- ❏ A. PA projection wrist, radial deviation
- ❏ B. PA axial projection wrist, Stecher method
- ❏ C. AP oblique hands/Norgaard method
- ❏ D. tangential projection wrist, Gaynor–Hart method

124. A lateral projection of the hand in extension is often recommended to evaluate
1. a fracture
2. a foreign body
3. soft tissue
- ❏ A. 1 only
- ❏ B. 2 only
- ❏ C. 2 and 3 only
- ❏ D. 1 and 3 only

125. Which of the following statements is/are correct with respect to the images shown in Figure 2-24?
1. Image A was made with cephalad angulation
2. Image B was made with caudal angulation
3. Images A and B were made with CR 15° cephalad
- ❏ A. 1 only
- ❏ B. 1 and 2 only
- ❏ C. 2 and 3 only
- ❏ D. 1, 2, and 3

CHAPTER 2 • PROCEDURES

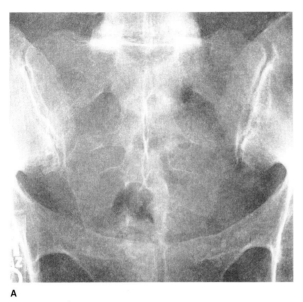
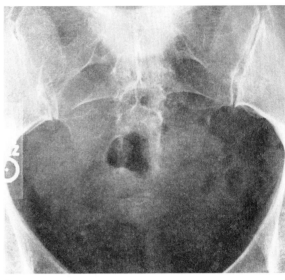

A   B

Figure 2-24. **A** and **B**: Used with permission of Stamford Hospital, Department of Radiology.

126. Which body habitus type is characterized by a long thorax and very low, medial stomach?

❑ A. Asthenic
❑ B. Hyposthenic
❑ C. Sthenic
❑ D. Hypersthenic

127. Which of the following should be performed to rule out subluxation or fracture of the cervical spine?

❑ A. Oblique cervical spine, seated
❑ B. AP cervical spine, recumbent
❑ C. Horizontal beam lateral
❑ D. Laterals in flexion and extension

128. Structures located proximal to the carpal bones include

❑ A. distal interphalangeal joints
❑ B. proximal interphalangeal joints
❑ C. metacarpals
❑ D. radial styloid process

129. Which of the following statements regarding the scapular Y projection of the shoulder is/are true?

1. The midsagittal plane should be about 60° to the IR
2. The scapular borders should be superimposed on the humeral shaft
3. An oblique projection of the shoulder is obtained
    ❑ A. 1 only
    ❑ B. 1 and 2 only
    ❑ C. 2 and 3 only
    ❑ D. 1, 2, and 3

130. An injury to a structure located on the side opposite that of the primary injury is called

❑ A. blowout
❑ B. Le Fort
❑ C. contracture
❑ D. contrecoup

131. The most distal portion of the pharynx is the

❑ A. laryngopharynx
❑ B. nasopharynx
❑ C. epiglottis
❑ D. oropharynx

132. Which part of the mandible will be *best* visualized with the patient's head in a PA position and the CR directed 20° cephalad?

❑ A. Symphysis
❑ B. Rami
❑ C. Body
❑ D. Angle

133. During IV urography, the prone position is generally recommended to demonstrate

1. ureteral filling
2. the renal pelvis
3. superior calyces
    ❑ A. 1 only
    ❑ B. 1 and 2 only
    ❑ C. 1 and 3 only
    ❑ D. 1, 2, and 3

134. The plane passing vertically through the body and dividing it into anterior and posterior halves is the

❑ A. median sagittal plane (MSP)
❑ B. midcoronal plane
❑ C. sagittal plane
❑ D. transverse plane

135. The act of expiration will cause the

1. diaphragm to move inferiorly
2. sternum and ribs to move inferiorly
3. diaphragm to move superiorly
   - ❏ A. 1 only
   - ❏ B. 1 and 2 only
   - ❏ C. 2 and 3 only
   - ❏ D. 1, 2, and 3

136. The number 2 in Figure 2-25 indicates

- ❏ A. body of L2
- ❏ B. spinous process of L1
- ❏ C. spinous process of L3
- ❏ D. transverse process of L3

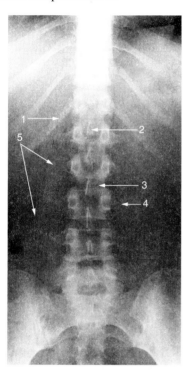

Figure 2-25. Reproduced with permission from DA Saia. *LANGE Radiography Review Flashcards.* New York: McGraw Hill; 2015.

137. The AP axial projection of the cervical spine demonstrates which of the following?

1. C3–C7 cervical bodies
2. Intervertebral foramina
3. Zygapophyseal joints
   - ❏ A. 1 only
   - ❏ B. 1 and 2 only
   - ❏ C. 2 and 3 only
   - ❏ D. 1, 2, and 3

138. Central ray angulation may be required to avoid

1. magnification of anatomic structures
2. foreshortening or self-superimposition
3. superimposition of overlying structures
   - ❏ A. 1 only
   - ❏ B. 1 and 2 only
   - ❏ C. 2 and 3 only
   - ❏ D. 1, 2, and 3

139. Which of the following is recommended to better demonstrate the tarsometatarsal joints in a dorsoplantar projection of the foot?

- ❏ A. Invert the foot
- ❏ B. Evert the foot
- ❏ C. Angle the CR 10° posteriorly
- ❏ D. Angle the CR 10° anteriorly

140. Foot motion caused by turning the ankle outward is termed

- ❏ A. eversion
- ❏ B. inversion
- ❏ C. abduction
- ❏ D. adduction

141. Which of the following positions will provide an AP projection of the L5–S1 interspace?

- ❏ A. Patient supine with CR 30°–35° angle cephalad
- ❏ B. Patient supine with CR 30°–35° angle caudad
- ❏ C. Patient supine with 0° CR angle
- ❏ D. Patient lateral recumbent, CR coned to L5

142. Subject/object unsharpness can result from all of the following, *except* when

- ❏ A. object shape does not coincide with the shape of x-ray beam
- ❏ B. object plane is not parallel with x-ray tube and/or IR
- ❏ C. anatomic object(s) of interest is/are in the path of the CR
- ❏ D. anatomic object(s) of interest is/are at a distance from the IR

143. Patients are instructed to remove all jewelry, hair clips, metal prostheses, coins, and credit cards before entering the room for an examination in

- ❏ A. sonography
- ❏ B. computed tomography (CT)
- ❏ C. magnetic resonance imaging (MRI)
- ❏ D. nuclear medicine

144. The true lateral position of the skull uses which of the following principles?

1. Interpupillary line perpendicular to the IR
2. MSP perpendicular to the IR
3. Infraorbitomeatal line (IOML) parallel to the transverse axis of the IR
   - ❏ A. 1 only
   - ❏ B. 1 and 2 only
   - ❏ C. 1 and 3 only
   - ❏ D. 1, 2, and 3

145. The radiograph shown in Figure 2-26 was most likely made in which of the following positions?

❏ A. Supine recumbent
❏ B. Prone recumbent
❏ C. PA upright
❏ D. Supine Trendelenburg

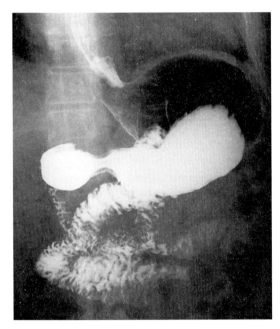

Figure 2-26

146. Persistent connection between the fetal aorta and pulmonary artery is called

❏ A. an atrial septal defect
❏ B. a ventricular septal defect
❏ C. a patent ductus arteriosus
❏ D. coarctation of the aorta

147. To evaluate the interphalangeal joints in the oblique and lateral positions, the fingers

❏ A. rest on the IR for immobilization
❏ B. must be supported parallel to the IR
❏ C. are radiographed in natural flexion
❏ D. are radiographed in palmar flexion

148. The cartilaginous portion of growing bone found at the extremities of long bones is the

❏ A. diaphysis
❏ B. epiphysis
❏ C. metaphysis
❏ D. apophysis

149. How should a mobile chest examination be performed to demonstrate air–fluid levels on a patient seated semi-upright about 70°?

❏ A. With CR directed 20° caudad
❏ B. With CR directed 20° cephalad
❏ C. With CR parallel to the floor
❏ D. With CR perpendicular to coronal plane

150. The ileocecal valve normally is located in which of the following body regions?

❏ A. Right iliac
❏ B. Left iliac
❏ C. Right lumbar
❏ D. Hypogastric

151. Which of the following is/are true regarding radiographic examination of the acromioclavicular joints?

1. The procedure is performed in the erect position
2. Use of weights can improve demonstration of the joints
3. The procedure should be avoided if dislocation or separation is suspected

❏ A. 1 only
❏ B. 1 and 2 only
❏ C. 1 and 3 only
❏ D. 2 and 3 only

152. A type of cancerous bone tumor occurring in children and young adults and arising from bone marrow is

❏ A. Ewing sarcoma
❏ B. multiple myeloma
❏ C. enchondroma
❏ D. osteochondroma

153. With the patient recumbent on the x-ray table with the head lower than the feet, the patient is said to be in the

❏ A. Trendelenburg position
❏ B. Fowler position
❏ C. decubitus position
❏ D. Sims position

154. Which of the following skull positions will demonstrate the cranial base, sphenoidal sinuses, atlas, and odontoid process?

❏ A. AP axial
❏ B. Lateral
❏ C. Parietoacanthial
❏ D. Submentovertical (SMV)

155. Which of the following statements are true with respect to the image seen in Figure 2-27?

1. An oblique cervical spine is shown
2. The zygapophyseal articulations are demonstrated
3. All seven cervical vertebrae are visualized
4. The esophagus is seen filled with air

❏ A. 1 and 2 only
❏ B. 2 and 3 only
❏ C. 1, 3, and 4 only
❏ D. 2, 3, and 4 only

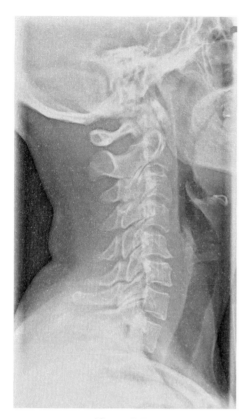

Figure 2-27

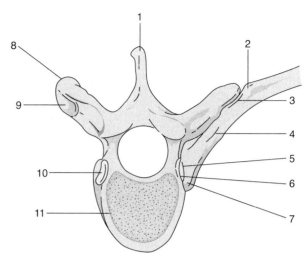

Figure 2-28

156. Which of the following is/are located on the anterior aspect of the femur?

1. Patellar surface
2. Intertrochanteric crest
3. Linea aspera
   ❏ A. 1 only
   ❏ B. 1 and 2 only
   ❏ C. 2 and 3 only
   ❏ D. 1, 2, and 3

157. In which of the following tangential axial projections of the patella is complete relaxation of the quadriceps femoris required for an accurate diagnosis?

1. Supine flexion 45° (Merchant)
2. Prone flexion 90° (Settegast)
3. Prone flexion 55° (Hughston)
   ❏ A. 1 only
   ❏ B. 1 and 2 only
   ❏ C. 2 and 3 only
   ❏ D. 1, 2, and 3 only

158. In Figure 2-28, the structure indicated as number 2 is which of the following?

❏ A. Facet for rib articulation
❏ B. Spinous process
❏ C. Tubercle of the rib
❏ D. Head of rib

159. Which of the following statements is/are correct with respect to evaluation criteria for a PA projection of the chest for lungs?

1. Sternal extremities of clavicles are equidistant from vertebral borders
2. Ten posterior ribs are demonstrated above the diaphragm
3. The esophagus is visible in the midline
   ❏ A. 1 only
   ❏ B. 1 and 2 only
   ❏ C. 2 and 3 only
   ❏ D. 1, 2, and 3

160. In which of the following positions/projections will the talocalcaneal joint be visualized?

❏ A. Dorsoplantar projection of the foot
❏ B. Plantodorsal projection of the os calcis
❏ C. Medial oblique position of the foot
❏ D. Lateral foot

161. In the lateral projection of the ankle, the

1. talotibial joint is visualized
2. talofibular joint is visualized
3. tibia and fibula are superimposed
   ❏ A. 1 only
   ❏ B. 1 and 2 only
   ❏ C. 1 and 3 only
   ❏ D. 1, 2, and 3

162. The position illustrated in the radiograph in Figure 2-29 may be obtained with the patient

1. supine and the CR angled 30° caudad
2. supine and the CR angled 30° cephalad
3. prone and the CR angled 30° cephalad
   ❏ A. 1 only
   ❏ B. 2 only
   ❏ C. 1 and 3 only
   ❏ D. 2 and 3 only

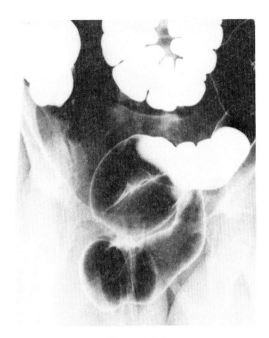

Figure 2-29

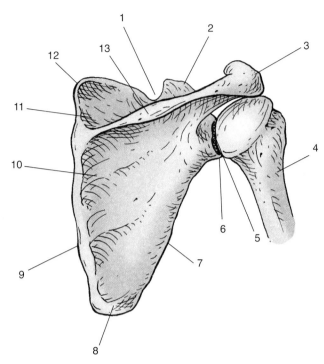

Figure 2-30

163. All of the following positions are likely to be used for both single- and double-contrast examinations of the large bowel, *except*
- ❏ A. lateral rectum
- ❏ B. AP axial rectosigmoid
- ❏ C. right and left lateral decubitus abdomen
- ❏ D. RAO and LAO abdomen

164. Which of the following projections best demonstrates the ankle mortise?
- ❏ A. Medial oblique 15°–20°
- ❏ B. Lateral oblique 15°–20°
- ❏ C. Medial oblique 45°
- ❏ D..Lateral oblique 45°

165. Which type of pediatric fracture specifically involves the bony growth plate?
- ❏ A. Hip dysplasia
- ❏ B. Salter–Harris
- ❏ C. Talipes
- ❏ D. Osgood–Schlatter

166. Which aspect(s) of the scapula is/are demonstrated in Figure 2-30?
1. Its posterior aspect
2. Its costal surface
3. Its sternal articular surface
    - ❏ A. 1 only
    - ❏ B. 1 and 2 only
    - ❏ C. 1 and 3 only
    - ❏ D. 1, 2, and 3

167. Which of the following is represented by the number 3 in Figure 2-30?
- ❏ A. Acromion process
- ❏ B. Superior angle
- ❏ C. Coracoid process
- ❏ D. Apex

168. Which of the following is represented by the number 8 in Figure 2-30?
- ❏ A. Superior angle
- ❏ B. Spine
- ❏ C. Lateral angle
- ❏ D. Apex

169. With the patient in the PA position and the OML and CR perpendicular to the IR, the resulting image will demonstrate the petrous pyramids
- ❏ A. below the orbits
- ❏ B. in the lower third of the orbits
- ❏ C. completely within the orbits
- ❏ D. above the orbits

170. When evaluating a PA axial projection of the skull with a 15° caudal angle, which of the following should be demonstrated?
1. Petrous pyramids in the lower third of the orbits
2. Equal distance from the lateral border of the skull to the lateral rim of the orbit bilaterally
3. Symmetrical petrous pyramids
    - ❏ A. 1 and 2 only
    - ❏ B. 1 and 3 only
    - ❏ C. 2 and 3 only
    - ❏ D. 1, 2, and 3

171. Which of the following barium-filled anatomic structures is *best* demonstrated in the LPO position?

❏ A. Hepatic/right colic flexure
❏ B. Splenic/left colic flexure
❏ C. Sigmoid colon
❏ D. Ileocecal valve

172. Hysterosalpingography may be performed for demonstration of

1. uterine tubal patency
2. mass lesions in the uterine cavity
3. uterine position
   ❏ A. 1 and 2 only
   ❏ B. 1 and 3 only
   ❏ C. 2 and 3 only
   ❏ D. 1, 2, and 3

173. During a double-contrast BE, which of the following positions would afford the *best* double-contrast visualization of the lateral wall of the descending colon and the medial wall of the ascending colon?

❏ A. AP or PA erect
❏ B. Right lateral decubitus
❏ C. Left lateral decubitus
❏ D. Ventral decubitus

174. In the PA axial oblique position of the cervical spine, the structures best seen are the

❏ A. intervertebral foramina nearest the IR
❏ B. intervertebral foramina furthest from the IR
❏ C. interarticular joints
❏ D. intervertebral joints

175. During chest radiography, the act of inspiration

1. elevates the diaphragm
2. raises the ribs
3. depresses the abdominal viscera
   ❏ A. 1 only
   ❏ B. 1 and 2 only
   ❏ C. 2 and 3 only
   ❏ D. 1, 2, and 3

176. All of the following are palpable bony landmarks that can be used in radiography of the pelvis, *except*

❏ A. the femoral neck
❏ B. the pubic symphysis
❏ C. the greater trochanter
❏ D. the iliac crest

177. Which of the following statements is/are true regarding Figure 2-31?

1. It demonstrates RAO sternum
2. Exposure was made during shallow respiration
3. Sternum is projected in the left thorax
   ❏ A. 1 only
   ❏ B. 2 only
   ❏ C. 2 and 3 only
   ❏ D. 1, 2, and 3

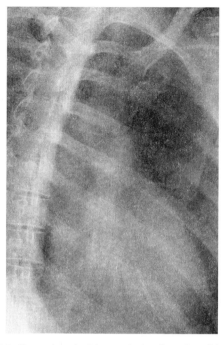

Figure 2-31. Reproduced with permission from David Sack, B.S., R.T. (R), CRA, FAHRA.

178. To better visualize the knee-joint space in the radiograph in Figure 2-32, the radiographer should

❏ A. flex the knee more acutely
❏ B. flex the knee less acutely
❏ C. direct the CR 5°–7° cephalad
❏ D. direct the CR 5°–7° caudad

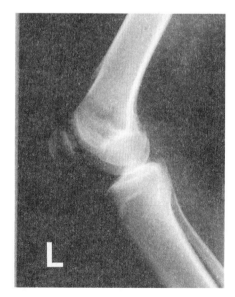

Figure 2-32

179. During an air-contrast BE, in what part of the colon is air most likely to be visualized in the AP recumbent position?

❏ A. Transverse colon
❏ B. Descending colon
❏ C. Ascending colon
❏ D. Left and right colic flexures

180. With which of the following does the trapezium articulate?
- ❏ A. Fifth metacarpal
- ❏ B. First metacarpal
- ❏ C. Distal radius
- ❏ D. Distal ulna

181. Which of the following statements is/are true regarding a PA projection of the paranasal sinuses?
1. The OML is elevated 15° from the horizontal
2. The petrous pyramids completely fill the orbits
3. The frontal and ethmoidal sinuses are visualized
- ❏ A. 1 only
- ❏ B. 1 and 2 only
- ❏ C. 1 and 3 only
- ❏ D. 1, 2, and 3

182. With a patient in the PA position and the OML perpendicular to the table, a 15°–20° caudal angulation would place the petrous ridges in the lower third of the orbit. To achieve the same result in an infant or a small child, it is necessary for the radiographer to modify the angulation to
- ❏ A. 10°–15° caudal
- ❏ B. 25°–30° caudal
- ❏ C. 15°–20° cephalic
- ❏ D. 3°–5° caudal

183. During GI radiography, the position of the stomach may vary depending on
1. the respiratory phase
2. body habitus
3. patient position
- ❏ A. 1 and 2 only
- ❏ B. 1 and 3 only
- ❏ C. 2 and 3 only
- ❏ D. 1, 2, and 3

184. For which of the following conditions is operative cholangiography a useful tool?
1. Patency of the biliary ducts
2. Biliary tract calculi
3. Duodenal calculi
- ❏ A. 1 only
- ❏ B. 1 and 2 only
- ❏ C. 2 and 3 only
- ❏ D. 1, 2, and 3

185. For the average patient, the CR for a lateral projection of a barium-filled stomach should enter
- ❏ A. midway between the midcoronal line and the anterior abdominal surface
- ❏ B. midway between the vertebral column and the lateral border of the abdomen
- ❏ C. at the midcoronal line at the level of the iliac crest
- ❏ D. perpendicular to the level of L2

186. In the lateral projection of the foot, the
1. plantar surface should be perpendicular to the IR
2. metatarsals are superimposed
3. talofibular joint should be visualized
- ❏ A. 1 only
- ❏ B. 1 and 2 only
- ❏ C. 2 and 3 only
- ❏ D. 1, 2, and 3

187. Which of the following is/are appropriate technique(s) for imaging a patient with a possible traumatic spine injury?
1. Instruct the patient to turn slowly and stop if anything hurts
2. Maneuver the x-ray tube instead of moving the patient
3. Call for help and use the log rolling method to turn the patient
- ❏ A. 1 and 2 only
- ❏ B. 1 and 3 only
- ❏ C. 2 and 3 only
- ❏ D. 1, 2, and 3

188. All elbow fat pads are best demonstrated in which position?
- ❏ A. AP
- ❏ B. Lateral
- ❏ C. Acute flexion
- ❏ D. AP partial flexion

189. The structure labeled 4 in Figure 2-33 is the
- ❏ A. anterior arch of C1
- ❏ B. body of C1
- ❏ C. body of C2
- ❏ D. odontoid process

190. In Figure 2-33, the posterior arch of the atlas is indicated by the number
- ❏ A. 3
- ❏ B. 4
- ❏ C. 5
- ❏ D. 6

191. Which of the following examinations is used to demonstrate vesicoureteral reflux?
- ❏ A. Retrograde urogram
- ❏ B. Intravenous urogram (IVU)
- ❏ C. Voiding cystourethrogram
- ❏ D. Retrograde cystogram

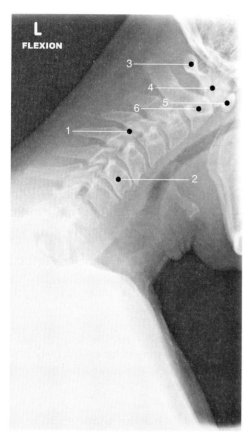

Figure 2-33. Used with permission of Stamford Hospital, Department of Radiology.

192. Important considerations for radiographic examinations of traumatic injuries to the upper extremity include

1. the joint closest to the injured site should be supported during movement of the limb
2. both joints must be included in long bone studies
3. two views, at 90° to each other, are required
   - ❏ A. 1 only
   - ❏ B. 1 and 2 only
   - ❏ C. 2 and 3 only
   - ❏ D. 1, 2, and 3

193. In which of the following projections is the talofibular joint *best* demonstrated?

- ❏ A. AP
- ❏ B. Lateral oblique
- ❏ C. Medial oblique
- ❏ D. Lateral

194. In the AP projection of the ankle, the

1. plantar surface of the foot is vertical
2. fibula projects more distally than the tibia
3. calcaneus is well visualized
   - ❏ A. 1 only
   - ❏ B. 1 and 2 only
   - ❏ C. 2 and 3 only
   - ❏ D. 1, 2, and 3

195. Which of the following sequences correctly describes the path of blood flow as it leaves the left ventricle?

- ❏ A. Arteries, arterioles, capillaries, venules, veins
- ❏ B. Arterioles, arteries, capillaries, veins, venules
- ❏ C. Veins, venules, capillaries, arteries, arterioles
- ❏ D. Venules, veins, capillaries, arterioles, arteries

196. Which of the following is demonstrated in a 25° RPO position with the CR entering 1 inch medial to the elevated ASIS?

- ❏ A. Left sacroiliac joint
- ❏ B. Right sacroiliac joint
- ❏ C. Left ilium
- ❏ D. Right ilium

197. An acromioclavicular (AC) separation will be best demonstrated in which of the following projections?

- ❏ A. AP recumbent, affected shoulder
- ❏ B. AP recumbent, both shoulders
- ❏ C. AP erect, affected shoulder
- ❏ D. AP erect, both shoulders

198. Causes of death in 70% of people older than 65 years include

1. stroke
2. heart disease
3. digestive disorders
   - ❏ A. 1 only
   - ❏ B. 1 and 2 only
   - ❏ C. 1 and 3 only
   - ❏ D. 1, 2, and 3

199. In the axiolateral projection of the hip, the CR should be

- ❏ A. 2 inches medial to the ASIS
- ❏ B. parallel to the IR
- ❏ C. perpendicular to the femoral neck
- ❏ D. parallel to the femoral neck

200. Select the statements that correctly describe the image seen in Figure 2-34.

1. An axial projection of the calcaneus is seen
2. The talocalcaneal joint is visualized
3. The sinus tarsi is visualized
4. The tibiotalar joint is visualized
5. The ankle is dorsiflexed
6. The sustentaculum tali is visualized
   - ❏ A. 1, 3, 4, and 5
   - ❏ B. 2, 4, 5, and 6
   - ❏ C. 1, 2, 5, and 6
   - ❏ D. 2, 3, 5, and 6

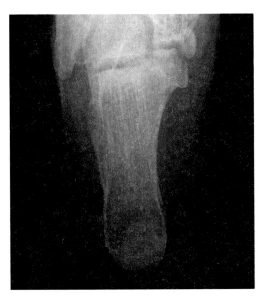

Figure 2-34. Used with permission of Orthopedic + Fracture Specialists, Portland, OR.

201. The inhalation of liquid or solid particles into the nose, throat, or lungs is called
- ❏ A. asphyxia
- ❏ B. aspiration
- ❏ C. atelectasis
- ❏ D. asystole

202. Endoscopic retrograde cholangiopancreatography (ERCP) usually involves
1. cannulation of the hepatopancreatic ampulla
2. introduction of contrast medium into the common bile duct
3. introduction of barium directly into the duodenum
- ❏ A. 1 only
- ❏ B. 1 and 2 only
- ❏ C. 1 and 3 only
- ❏ D. 1, 2, and 3

203. The long, flat structures that project posteromedially from the pedicles are the
- ❏ A. transverse processes
- ❏ B. vertebral arches
- ❏ C. laminae
- ❏ D. pedicles

204. The axiolateral, or horizontal beam, projection of the hip requires the IR to be placed
1. parallel to the central ray (CR)
2. parallel to the long axis of the femoral neck
3. in contact with the lateral surface of the body
- ❏ A. 1 only
- ❏ B. 1 and 2 only
- ❏ C. 2 and 3 only
- ❏ D. 1, 2, and 3

205. Appropriate radiation protection strategies for the pediatric patient include which of the following?
1. Use appropriate gonadal shielding
2. Shield torso when examining upper extremities
3. Examine thorax and skull in AP position rather than PA
- ❏ A. 1 only
- ❏ B. 1 and 2 only
- ❏ C. 2 and 3 only
- ❏ D. 1, 2, and 3

206. Which of the following interventional procedures can be used to increase the diameter of a stenosed vessel?
1. Percutaneous transluminal angioplasty (PTA)
2. Stent placement
3. Peripherally inserted central catheter (PICC line)
- ❏ A. 1 only
- ❏ B. 1 and 2 only
- ❏ C. 1 and 3 only
- ❏ D. 1, 2, and 3

207. Which of the following examinations involves the introduction of a radiopaque contrast medium through a uterine cannula?
- ❏ A. Retrograde pyelogram
- ❏ B. Voiding cystourethrogram
- ❏ C. Hysterosalpingogram
- ❏ D. Myelogram

208. Arteries and veins enter and exit the medial aspect of each lung at the
- ❏ A. root
- ❏ B. hilus
- ❏ C. carina
- ❏ D. epiglottis

209. The contraction and expansion of arterial walls in accordance with forceful contraction and relaxation of the heart are called
- ❏ A. hypertension
- ❏ B. elasticity
- ❏ C. pulse
- ❏ D. pressure

210. Which of the following structures should be visualized through the foramen magnum in an AP axial projection (Towne method) of the skull for occipital bone?
1. Posterior clinoid processes
2. Dorsum sella
3. Posterior arch of C1
- ❏ A. 1 only
- ❏ B. 2 only
- ❏ C. 1 and 2 only
- ❏ D. 2 and 3 only

211. Which of the following projections/positions would be the *best* choice for a right shoulder examination to rule out fracture?

❏ A. Internal and external rotation
❏ B. AP and tangential
❏ C. AP and AP axial
❏ D. AP and scapular Y

212. Which of the following projections will best demonstrate the tarsal navicular with minimal superimposition?

❏ A. AP oblique, medial rotation
❏ B. AP oblique, lateral rotation
❏ C. Mediolateral
❏ D. Lateral weight-bearing

213. Which of the following bones participate(s) in the formation of the obturator foramen?

1. Ilium
2. Ischium
3. Pubis

❏ A. 1 and 2 only
❏ B. 1 and 3 only
❏ C. 2 and 3 only
❏ D. 1, 2, and 3

214. All of the following are associated with the knee joint, *except*

❏ A. labrum
❏ B. fat pad
❏ C. menisci
❏ D. collateral ligament

215. The AP projection of the sacrum requires that the CR should be directed

1. 15° cephalad
2. two inches superior to the pubic symphysis
3. 10° caudad

❏ A. 1 only
❏ B. 2 only
❏ C. 1 and 2 only
❏ D. 1 and 3 only

216. Which of the following positions/projections would *best* demonstrate cartilage degeneration in the knees?

❏ A. AP recumbent
❏ B. Lateral recumbent
❏ C. AP erect
❏ D. Medial oblique

217. Elements of correct positioning for PA projection of the chest include

1. weight evenly distributed on feet
2. elevation of the chin
3. shoulders elevated and rolled forward

❏ A. 1 only
❏ B. 1 and 2 only
❏ C. 2 and 3 only
❏ D. 1, 2, and 3

218. Which of the following statements is/are true regarding the images shown in Figure 2-35?

1. Image A demonstrates internal rotation
2. Image B demonstrates internal rotation
3. The greater tubercle is better demonstrated in image A

❏ A. 1 only
❏ B. 2 only
❏ C. 1 and 3 only
❏ D. 2 and 3 only

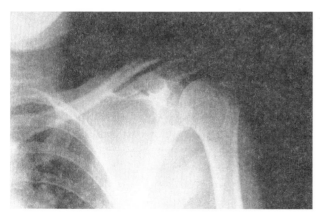 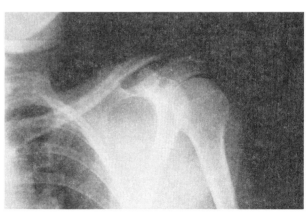

A

B

Figure 2-35. A and **B**. Used with permission of Stamford Hospital, Department of Radiology.

219. Which of the following will best demonstrate the size and shape of the liver and kidneys?
- ❏ A. Lateral abdomen
- ❏ B. AP abdomen
- ❏ C. Dorsal decubitus abdomen
- ❏ D. Ventral decubitus abdomen

220. The adult cranial bones contain a layer of cancellous tissue between their inner and outer layers called
- ❏ A. canaliculi
- ❏ B. Haversian layer
- ❏ C. diploe
- ❏ D. suture

221. In the AP axial projection, or bilateral "frog-leg" position, which of the following is most likely to place the long axes of the femoral necks parallel with the plane of the IR?
- ❏ A. Adducted 25° from the horizontal
- ❏ B. Abducted 25° from the vertical
- ❏ C. Adducted 40° from the horizontal
- ❏ D. Abducted 40° from the vertical

222. AP stress studies of the ankle may be performed
1. to demonstrate fractures of the distal tibia and fibula
2. following inversion or eversion injuries
3. to demonstrate a ligament tear
- ❏ A. 1 only
- ❏ B. 1 and 2 only
- ❏ C. 2 and 3 only
- ❏ D. 1, 2, and 3

223. Which of the following projections require(s) that the humeral epicondyles be perpendicular to the IR?
1. AP humerus
2. Lateral forearm
3. Internal rotation shoulder
- ❏ A. 1 only
- ❏ B. 1 and 2 only
- ❏ C. 2 and 3 only
- ❏ D. 1, 2, and 3

224. Image identification markers should include
1. patient's name and/or ID number
2. date
3. a right or left marker
- ❏ A. 1 only
- ❏ B. 1 and 2 only
- ❏ C. 1 and 3 only
- ❏ D. 1, 2, and 3

225. To demonstrate the entire circumference of the radial head, exposure(s) must be made with the
1. epicondyles perpendicular to the IR
2. hand pronated and supinated as much as possible
3. hand lateral and in internal rotation
- ❏ A. 1 only
- ❏ B. 1 and 2 only
- ❏ C. 1 and 3 only
- ❏ D. 1, 2, and 3

226. The image shown in Figure 2-36 was made in what position?
- ❏ A. AP or PA erect
- ❏ B. Dorsal decubitus
- ❏ C. Left lateral decubitus
- ❏ D. Right lateral decubitus

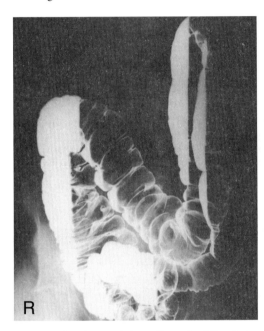

Figure 2-36. Used with permission of Stamford Hospital, Department of Radiology.

227. Which of the following equipment is required when preparing the examining room for myelography?
1. Footboard for fluoroscopy table
2. Shoulder support for fluoroscopy table
3. Surgical masks
4. Oil-based nonionic contrast
5. Water-soluble nonionic contrast
6. Image intensifier in unlocked position
- ❏ A. 1, 2, and 4
- ❏ B. 1, 2, and 6
- ❏ C. 1, 2, 3, and 5
- ❏ D. 1, 3, and 4
- ❏ E. 2, 4, 5, and 6

228. Which of the following positions is most likely to place the right kidney parallel to the IR?
- ❏ A. AP
- ❏ B. PA
- ❏ C. RPO
- ❏ D. LPO

229. Which of the following is/are effective in reducing exposure to sensitive tissues for frontal views during scoliosis examinations?
1. Use of PA projection
2. Use of breast shields
3. Use of compensating filtration
- ❏ A. 1 only
- ❏ B. 1 and 2 only
- ❏ C. 2 and 3 only
- ❏ D. 1, 2, and 3

230. Which type of articulation is evaluated in arthrography?
- ❏ A. Synarthrodial
- ❏ B. Diarthrodial
- ❏ C. Amphiarthrodial
- ❏ D. Cartilaginous

231. With the patient seated at the end of the x-ray table, elbow resting on table and flexed 80°, and the CR directed 45° laterally *from the shoulder to the elbow joint,* which of the following structures will be demonstrated best?
- ❏ A. Radial head
- ❏ B. Ulnar head
- ❏ C. Coronoid process
- ❏ D. Olecranon process

232. Free air in the abdominal cavity is *best* demonstrated in which of the following?
- ❏ A. AP projection, left lateral decubitus position
- ❏ B. AP projection, right lateral decubitus position
- ❏ C. PA recumbent position
- ❏ D. AP recumbent position

233. Which of the following examinations most likely would be performed to diagnose Wilms' tumor?
- ❏ A. BE
- ❏ B. Upper GI
- ❏ C. IVU
- ❏ D. Bone survey

234. A radiolucent sponge can be placed under the patient's waist for a lateral projection of the lumbosacral spine to
1. make the vertebral column parallel with the IR
2. place the intervertebral disk spaces perpendicular to the IR
3. decrease the amount of SR reaching the IR
- ❏ A. 1 only
- ❏ B. 1 and 2 only
- ❏ C. 2 and 3 only
- ❏ D. 1, 2, and 3

235. Which of the following sinus groups is best demonstrated with the patient positioned as for a parietoacanthial projection (Waters' method) with the CR directed through the patient's open mouth?
- ❏ A. Frontal
- ❏ B. Ethmoidal
- ❏ C. Maxillary
- ❏ D. Sphenoidal

236. Which of the following women is likely to have the most homogenous glandular breast tissue?
- ❏ A. A postpubertal adolescent
- ❏ B. A 20-year-old with one previous pregnancy
- ❏ C. A menopausal woman
- ❏ D. A 65-year-old postmenopausal woman

237. Standard radiographic protocols may be reduced to include two views, at right angles to each other, in which of the following situations?
- ❏ A. Barium examinations
- ❏ B. Spine radiography
- ❏ C. Skull radiography
- ❏ D. Emergency and trauma radiography

238. Which of the following structures is/are located in the right upper quadrant (RUQ)?
1. Spleen
2. Gallbladder
3. Hepatic flexure
- ❏ A. 1 only
- ❏ B. 1 and 2 only
- ❏ C. 2 and 3 only
- ❏ D. 1, 2, and 3

239. The facial bones include the
1. palatine
2. sphenoid
3. maxilla
4. ethmoid
5. vomer
6. mandible
- ❏ A. 1, 2, 3, 5, and 6
- ❏ B. 1, 3, 5, and 6
- ❏ C. 2, 3, 4, and 6
- ❏ D. 2, 3, 4, and 5

240. Which of the following projections is *most likely* to demonstrate the carpal pisiform free of superimposition?
- ❏ A. Radial flexion/deviation
- ❏ B. Ulnar flexion/deviation
- ❏ C. AP (medial) oblique
- ❏ D. AP (lateral) oblique

CHAPTER 2 • PROCEDURES

241. Myelography is a diagnostic examination used to demonstrate

1. internal disk lesions
2. posttraumatic swelling of the spinal cord
3. posterior disk herniation
   ❑ A. 1 only
   ❑ B. 2 only
   ❑ C. 2 and 3 only
   ❑ D. 1, 2, and 3

242. Which of the following blood chemistry levels must the radiographer check prior to excretory urography?

1. Creatinine
2. Blood urea nitrogen (BUN)
3. Red blood cells (RBCs)
   ❑ A. 1 only
   ❑ B. 1 and 2 only
   ❑ C. 2 and 3 only
   ❑ D. 1, 2, and 3

243. Which of the following are components of a trimalleolar fracture?

1. Fractured lateral malleolus
2. Fractured medial malleolus
3. Fractured anterior tibia
   ❑ A. 1 only
   ❑ B. 1 and 2 only
   ❑ C. 2 and 3 only
   ❑ D. 1, 2, and 3

244. Which of the following descriptive terms could be associated with an AP recumbent position?

1. Supine
2. Dorsal decubitus
3. Ventral decubitus
   ❑ A. 1 only
   ❑ B. 1 and 2 only
   ❑ C. 1 and 3 only
   ❑ D. 1, 2, and 3

245. The four major arteries supplying the brain include the

1. brachiocephalic artery
2. common carotid arteries
3. vertebral arteries
   ❑ A. 1 and 2 only
   ❑ B. 1 and 3 only
   ❑ C. 2 and 3 only
   ❑ D. 1, 2, and 3

246. Ingestion of barium sulfate is contraindicated in which of the following situations?

1. Suspected perforation of a hollow viscus
2. Suspected large-bowel obstruction
3. Preoperative patients
   ❑ A. 1 only
   ❑ B. 1 and 3 only
   ❑ C. 2 and 3 only
   ❑ D. 1, 2, and 3

247. The term that refers to parts away from the source or beginning is

❑ A. cephalad
❑ B. proximal
❑ C. distal
❑ D. lateral

248. Which of the following is/are well demonstrated in the lumbar spine shown in Figure 2-37?

1. Zygapophyseal articulations
2. Intervertebral foramina
3. Inferior articular processes
   ❑ A. 1 only
   ❑ B. 1 and 2 only
   ❑ C. 1 and 3 only
   ❑ D. 1, 2, and 3

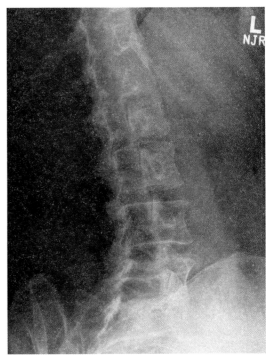

Figure 2-37. Used with permission of Orthopedic + Fracture Specialists, Portland, OR.

249. Which of the following statements is/are correct, with respect to a left lateral projection of the chest?

1. The MSP must be perfectly vertical and parallel to the IR
2. The right posterior ribs will be projected slightly posterior to the left posterior ribs
3. Arms must be raised high to prevent upper-arm soft-tissue superimposition on lung field
   ❑ A. 1 only
   ❑ B. 1 and 2 only
   ❑ C. 1 and 3 only
   ❑ D. 1, 2, and 3

250. Which of the following is well demonstrated just posterior to the lumbar vertebra in Figure 2-38?
- ❏ A. Inferior vena cava
- ❏ B. Aorta
- ❏ C. Gallbladder
- ❏ D. Psoas muscle

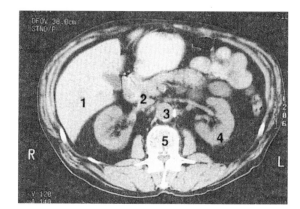

Figure 2-38. Used with permission of Stamford Hospital, Department of Radiology.

251. Which of the following can be used to demonstrate the intercondyloid fossa?
1. Prone, knee flexed 40°, CR directed caudad 40° to the popliteal fossa
2. Supine, IR under flexed knee, CR directed cephalad to knee, perpendicular to tibia
3. Prone, patella parallel to IR, heel rotated 5°–10° lateral, CR perpendicular to knee joint
- ❏ A. 1 only
- ❏ B. 1 and 2 only
- ❏ C. 2 and 3 only
- ❏ D. 1, 2, and 3

252. In the lateral projection of the scapula, the
1. vertebral and axillary borders are superimposed
2. acromion and coracoid processes are superimposed
3. inferior angle is superimposed on the ribs
- ❏ A. 1 only
- ❏ B. 1 and 2 only
- ❏ C. 1 and 3 only
- ❏ D. 1, 2, and 3

253. Lateral deviation of the nasal septum may be *best* demonstrated in the
- ❏ A. lateral projection
- ❏ B. PA axial (Caldwell method) projection
- ❏ C. parietoacanthial (Waters' method) projection
- ❏ D. AP axial (Towne method) projection

254. The AP Trendelenburg position is often used during an upper GI examination to demonstrate
- ❏ A. the duodenal loop
- ❏ B. filling of the duodenal bulb
- ❏ C. hiatal hernia
- ❏ D. hypertrophic pyloric stenosis

255. What is the structure labeled number 2 in Figure 2-39?
- ❏ A. Trapezium
- ❏ B. Scaphoid
- ❏ C. Lunate
- ❏ D. Pisiform

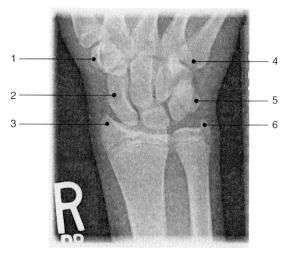

Figure 2-39. Used with permission of Stamford Hospital, Department of Radiology.

256. What is the structure labeled number 3 in Figure 2-39?
- ❏ A. Trapezium
- ❏ B. Scaphoid
- ❏ C. Ulnar styloid
- ❏ D. Radial styloid

257. Which of the following positions of the abdomen is obtained with the patient lying supine on the radiographic table and the CR directed horizontally to the iliac crest?
- ❏ A. AP abdomen
- ❏ B. PA abdomen
- ❏ C. Ventral decubitus position
- ❏ D. Dorsal decubitus position

258. Which of the following is a functional study used to demonstrate the degree of AP motion present in the cervical spine?
- ❏ A. Open-mouth projection
- ❏ B. Moving-mandible AP
- ❏ C. Flexion and extension laterals
- ❏ D. Right and left bending AP

259. If a patient's zygomatic arch has been traumatically depressed or the patient has flat cheekbones, the arch may be demonstrated by modifying the SMV projection and rotating the patient's head
- ❏ A. 15° toward the side being examined
- ❏ B. 15° away from the side being examined
- ❏ C. 30° toward the side being examined
- ❏ D. 30° away from the side being examined

260. A traumatic injury involving the bases of the first and second metatarsals and cuneiforms is termed

❏ A. Osgood–Schlatter fracture
❏ B. Lisfranc injury
❏ C. Jones fracture
❏ D. Pott fracture

261. What is the degree of difference between the baselines numbered 1 and 3 in Figure 2-40 and used for various projections of the skull?

❏ A. 7°
❏ B. 9°
❏ C. 15°
❏ D. 23°

262. Referring to Figure 2 -40, which of the following positions of the skull requires that baseline number 3 be parallel to the IR?

❏ A. Parietoacanthial
❏ B. PA axial (Caldwell)
❏ C. AP axial (Towne)
❏ D. Lateral

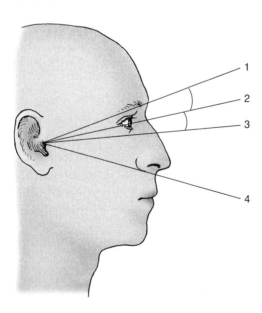

Figure 2-40

263. Radiographic measurement of long bones of an upper or lower extremity requires which of the following?

1. Special ruler/Bell–Thompson scale
2. Precise collimation
3. Cannula

❏ A. 1 only
❏ B. 1 and 2 only
❏ C. 1 and 3 only
❏ D. 1, 2, and 3

264. Which of the following is/are demonstrated in a lateral projection of the cervical spine?

1. Intervertebral foramina
2. Zygapophyseal joints
3. Intervertebral joints

❏ A. 1 only
❏ B. 1 and 2 only
❏ C. 2 and 3 only
❏ D. 1, 2, and 3

265. In a lateral projection of the nasal bones, the CR is directed

❏ A. half inch posterior to the anterior nasal spine
❏ B. half inch posterior to the glabella
❏ C. half inch distal to the nasion
❏ D. half inch anterior to the EAM

266. The tissue that occupies the central cavity of the adult long bone body/shaft is

❏ A. red marrow
❏ B. yellow marrow
❏ C. endosteum
❏ D. cancellous tissue

267. Which of the following statements are true regarding knee x-ray arthrography?

1. Ligament tears can be demonstrated
2. Sterile technique is observed
3. MRI can follow x-ray

❏ A. 1 and 2 only
❏ B. 1 and 3 only
❏ C. 2 and 3 only
❏ D. 1, 2, and 3

268. During an upper GI examination of a stomach of average size and shape, a barium-filled fundus and double contrast of the pylorus and duodenal bulb are demonstrated. The position used is most likely

❏ A. AP erect
❏ B. PA
❏ C. RAO
❏ D. LPO

269. Inspiration and expiration projections of the chest are performed to demonstrate

1. partial or complete collapse of pulmonary lobe(s)
2. air in the pleural cavity
3. foreign body

❏ A. 1 only
❏ B. 1 and 2 only
❏ C. 1 and 3 only
❏ D. 1, 2, and 3

270. Shoulder arthrography is performed to
1. evaluate humeral luxation
2. demonstrate complete or partial rotator cuff tear
3. evaluate the glenoid labrum
   - ❏ A. 1 only
   - ❏ B. 1 and 2 only
   - ❏ C. 2 and 3 only
   - ❏ D. 1, 2, and 3

271. Which of the following positions will separate the radial head, neck, and tuberosity from superimposition on the ulna?
- ❏ A. AP
- ❏ B. Lateral
- ❏ C. Medial oblique
- ❏ D. Lateral oblique

272. Select the terms associated with trabeculae.
1. Haversian system
2. Cancellous
3. Spongy
4. Red bone marrow
   - ❏ A. 1 and 2
   - ❏ B. 1, 2, and 3
   - ❏ C. 1, 3, and 4
   - ❏ D. 2, 3, and 4

273. Which of the following structures is located at the level of the interspace between the second and third thoracic vertebrae?
- ❏ A. Manubrium
- ❏ B. Jugular notch
- ❏ C. Sternal angle
- ❏ D. Xiphoid process

274. For the AP projection of the scapula, the
1. patient's arm is abducted at right angles to the body
2. patient's elbow is flexed with the hand supinated
3. exposure is made during quiet breathing
   - ❏ A. 1 and 2 only
   - ❏ B. 1 and 3 only
   - ❏ C. 3 only
   - ❏ D. 1, 2, and 3

275. The innominate bone is located in the
- ❏ A. middle cranial fossa
- ❏ B. posterior cranial fossa
- ❏ C. foot
- ❏ D. pelvis

276. Which type of fracture involves the distal end of the fourth or fifth metacarpal?
- ❏ A. Colles fracture
- ❏ B. Boxer fracture
- ❏ C. Pott fracture
- ❏ D. Bennett fracture

277. Deoxygenated blood from the head and thorax is returned to the heart by the
- ❏ A. pulmonary artery
- ❏ B. pulmonary veins
- ❏ C. superior vena cava
- ❏ D. thoracic aorta

278. Below diaphragm, ribs are better demonstrated when
1. the patient is in the AP erect position
2. respiration is suspended at the end of full exhalation
3. the patient is in the recumbent position
   - ❏ A. 1 only
   - ❏ B. 1 and 2 only
   - ❏ C. 2 and 3 only
   - ❏ D. 1, 2, and 3

279. To demonstrate esophageal varices, the patient must be examined in
- ❏ A. the recumbent position
- ❏ B. the erect position
- ❏ C. the anatomic position
- ❏ D. the Fowler position

280. What projection of the calcaneus is obtained with the leg extended, the plantar surface of the foot vertical and perpendicular to the IR, and the CR directed 40° cephalad?
- ❏ A. Axial plantodorsal projection
- ❏ B. Axial dorsoplantar projection
- ❏ C. Lateral projection
- ❏ D. Weight-bearing lateral projection

281. To demonstrate the first two cervical vertebrae in the AP projection, the patient is positioned so that
- ❏ A. the glabellomeatal line is vertical
- ❏ B. the acanthiomeatal line is vertical
- ❏ C. a line between the mentum and the mastoid tip is vertical
- ❏ D. a line between the maxillary occlusal plane and the mastoid tip is vertical

282. Tracheotomy is an effective technique used to restore breathing when there is
- ❏ A. respiratory pathway obstruction above the larynx
- ❏ B. crushed tracheal rings owing to trauma
- ❏ C. respiratory pathway closure owing to inflammation and swelling
- ❏ D. respiratory pathway obstruction below the larynx

283. The structure labeled number 7 in Figure 2-41 is the
- ❏ A. right subclavian artery
- ❏ B. brachiocephalic artery
- ❏ C. right common carotid artery
- ❏ D. left vertebral artery

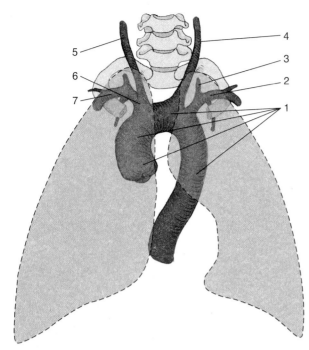

Figure 2-41. Reproduced with permission from Doherty GM, ed. *Current Surgical Diagnosis & Treatment*, 12th ed. New York: McGraw Hill; 2006:824.

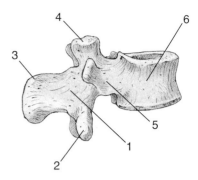

Figure 2-42

284. The structure labeled number 4 in Figure 2-41 is the
- ❑ A. right subclavian artery
- ❑ B. brachiocephalic artery
- ❑ C. left common carotid artery
- ❑ D. left vertebral artery

285. How should an AP projection be obtained when examining a patient whose elbow is in partial flexion?
1. With humerus parallel to IR, CR perpendicular
2. With forearm parallel to IR, CR perpendicular
3. Through the partially flexed elbow, resting on the olecranon process, CR perpendicular
- ❑ A. 1 only
- ❑ B. 1 and 2 only
- ❑ C. 2 and 3 only
- ❑ D. 1, 2, and 3

286. Which of the following positions demonstrates the sphenoid sinuses?
1. Modified Waters' (mouth open)
2. Lateral
3. PA axial
- ❑ A. 1 only
- ❑ B. 1 and 2 only
- ❑ C. 2 and 3 only
- ❑ D. 1, 2, and 3

287. The number 5 in Figure 2-42 represents which of the following structures?
- ❑ A. Body
- ❑ B. Pedicle
- ❑ C. Inferior articular process
- ❑ D. Superior articular process

288. To demonstrate the mandibular body in the PA projection, the
- ❑ A. CR is directed perpendicular to the IR
- ❑ B. CR is directed cephalad to the IR
- ❑ C. skull is obliqued away from the affected side
- ❑ D. skull is obliqued toward the affected side

289. Which of the following equipment is necessary for ERCP?
1. A fluoroscopic unit with imaging device and tilt-table capabilities
2. A fiberoptic endoscope
3. Polyethylene catheters
- ❑ A. 1 and 2 only
- ❑ B. 1 and 3 only
- ❑ C. 2 and 3 only
- ❑ D. 1, 2, and 3

290. Types of mechanical obstruction found in pediatric patients include
1. volvulus
2. intussusception
3. paralytic ileus
- ❑ A. 1 only
- ❑ B. 1 and 2 only
- ❑ C. 2 and 3 only
- ❑ D. 1, 2, and 3

291. To demonstrate a profile view of the glenoid fossa, the patient is AP recumbent and obliqued 45°
- ❑ A. toward the affected side
- ❑ B. away from the affected side
- ❑ C. with the arm at the side in the anatomic position
- ❑ D. with the arm in external rotation

292. An intrathecal injection is associated with which of the following examinations?
- ❑ A. Intravenous urogram
- ❑ B. Retrograde pyelogram
- ❑ C. Myelogram
- ❑ D. Cystogram

293. The vertebral/neural arch is formed by the
1. articular processes
2. pedicles
3. laminae
4. transverse processes
5. vertebral body
- ❑ A. 2 and 3 only
- ❑ B. 1, 2, and 3
- ❑ C. 2, 3, and 5
- ❑ D. 2, 3, and 4

294. Which of the following positions will *best* demonstrate the right zygapophyseal articulations of the lumbar vertebrae?
- ❑ A. PA
- ❑ B. Left lateral
- ❑ C. RPO
- ❑ D. LPO

295. What projection was used to obtain the image seen in Figure 2-43?
- ❑ A. AP, internal rotation
- ❑ B. AP, external rotation
- ❑ C. AP, neutral position
- ❑ D. AP axial

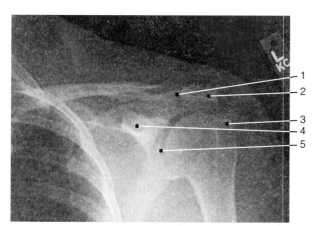

Figure 2-43. Used with permission of Conrad P. Ehrlich, MD.

296. The structure labeled number 4 in Figure 2-43 is the
- ❑ A. acromion process
- ❑ B. coracoid process
- ❑ C. greater tubercle
- ❑ D. lesser tubercle

297. The structure labeled number 1 in Figure 2-43 is the
- ❑ A. sternoclavicular joint
- ❑ B. acromioclavicular joint
- ❑ C. glenohumeral joint
- ❑ D. acromiohumeral joint

298. Which projection of the elbow will demonstrate the coronoid process free of superimposition?
- ❑ A. AP
- ❑ B. Lateral
- ❑ C. Medial oblique
- ❑ D. Lateral oblique

299. Which of the following is/are required for a lateral projection of the skull?
1. The IOML is parallel to the IR
2. The MSP is parallel to the IR
3. The CR enters ¾ inch superior and anterior to the EAM
- ❑ A. 1 only
- ❑ B. 1 and 2 only
- ❑ C. 2 and 3 only
- ❑ D. 1, 2, and 3

300. Which of the following projections require(s) that the humeral epicondyles be superimposed?
1. Lateral thumb
2. Lateral wrist
3. Lateral humerus
- ❑ A. 1 only
- ❑ B. 1 and 2 only
- ❑ C. 2 and 3 only
- ❑ D. 1, 2, and 3

301. What is the name of the condition that results in the forward slipping of one vertebra upon the vertebra below it?
- ❑ A. Spondylitis
- ❑ B. Spondylolysis
- ❑ C. Spondylolisthesis
- ❑ D. Spondylosis

302. What is that portion of bone labeled **C** in the pediatric PA hand image seen in Figure 2-44?
- ❑ A. Diaphysis
- ❑ B. Epiphysis
- ❑ C. Metaphysis
- ❑ D. Apophysis

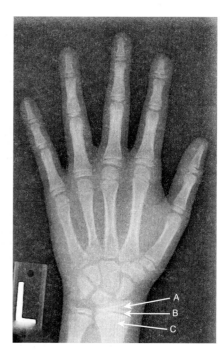

Figure 2-44

303. The female bony pelvis differs from the male bony pelvis in which of the following ways?
1. The male greater/false pelvis is deep
2. The male acetabulum faces more laterally
3. The female coccyx is more vertical
   - ❏ A. 1 only
   - ❏ B. 1 and 2 only
   - ❏ C. 2 and 3 only
   - ❏ D. 1, 2, and 3

304. The structures visualized when positioned as in Figure 2-45 could also be seen when performed with the patient in which of the following positions?
1. Lateral recumbent
2. Seated
3. Erect AP
   - ❏ A. 1 only
   - ❏ B. 1 and 2 only
   - ❏ C. 2 and 3 only
   - ❏ D. 1, 2, and 3

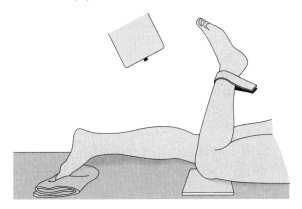

Figure 2-45

305. Which of the following conditions is demonstrated in Figure 2-46?
   - ❏ A. Right upper lobe atelectasis
   - ❏ B. Left upper lobe atelectasis
   - ❏ C. Pneumothorax
   - ❏ D. Dextrocardia

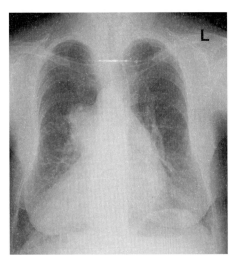

Figure 2-46

306. Which of the following is/are well demonstrated in the lumbar spine seen in Figure 2-47?
1. Pedicles
2. Vertebral foramina
3. Zygapophyseal articulations
   - ❏ A. 1 only
   - ❏ B. 1 and 2 only
   - ❏ C. 2 and 3 only
   - ❏ D. 1, 2, and 3

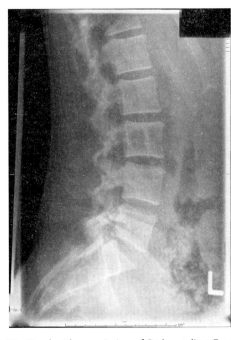

Figure 2-47. Used with permission of Orthopedic + Fracture Specialists, Portland, OR.

307. With the patient in the PA position, which of the following tube angle and direction combinations is correct for an axial projection of the clavicle?
   - ❏ A. 5°–15° caudad
   - ❏ B. 5°–15° cephalad
   - ❏ C. 15°–30° cephalad
   - ❏ D. 15°–30° caudad

308. Correct preparation for a patient scheduled for a lower GI series is *most likely* to be
   - ❏ A. iodinated contrast administration evening before examination; water only in the morning
   - ❏ B. NPO after midnight
   - ❏ C. cathartics and cleansing enemas
   - ❏ D. NPO after midnight, cleansing enemas, and empty bladder before scout image

309. Mineral homeostasis, protection, and triglyceride storage are functions of which body system?
   - ❏ A. Endocrine
   - ❏ B. Integumentary
   - ❏ C. Skeletal
   - ❏ D. Muscular

310. Which of the following is a major cause of bowel obstruction in children?

❑ A. Appendicitis
❑ B. Intussusception
❑ C. Regional enteritis
❑ D. Ulcerative colitis

311. The most significant risk factor for breast cancer is

❑ A. age
❑ B. gender
❑ C. family history
❑ D. personal history

312. With the patient in a 40° RPO position, affected side down, hip joint centered to IR, and CR directed perpendicularly to the IR at the level of the ASIS, the structure best demonstrated is the

❑ A. right SI joint
❑ B. left SI joint
❑ C. right ilium
❑ D. left ilium

313. Which of the following techniques would provide a posteroanterior (PA) projection of the gastroduodenal surfaces of a barium-filled high and transverse stomach?

❑ A. Place the patient in a 35°–40° right anterior oblique (RAO) position
❑ B. Place the patient in a lateral position
❑ C. Angle the CR 35°–45° cephalad
❑ D. Angle the CR 35°–45° caudad

314. With the patient PA, the MSP centered to the IR, the OML forming a 37° angle with the IR, and the CR perpendicular and exiting the acanthion, which of the following is *best* demonstrated?

❑ A. Occipital bone
❑ B. Frontal bone
❑ C. Facial bones
❑ D. Basal foramina

315. Which of the following articulate(s) with the bases of the metatarsals?

1. The heads of the first row of phalanges
2. The cuboid
3. The cuneiforms
   ❑ A. 1 only
   ❑ B. 1 and 2 only
   ❑ C. 2 and 3 only
   ❑ D. 1, 2, and 3

316. Features of the first cervical vertebra include

1. lateral masses
2. transverse foramina
3. odontoid process
4. body
5. posterior arch
   ❑ A. 1, 3, and 4
   ❑ B. 1, 2, and 5
   ❑ C. 2, 3, and 4
   ❑ D. 2, 4, and 5

317. Patients can experience involuntary motion as a result of

1. tremor
2. chill
3. age
4. peristalsis
5. breathing
   ❑ A. 1, 2, and 3
   ❑ B. 1, 2, and 4
   ❑ C. 3, 4, and 5
   ❑ D. 2, 3, and 4

318. The inferior costal margin is an external landmark that can be used to identify which level?

❑ A. T9–T10
❑ B. T12–L1
❑ C. L2–L3
❑ D. L4–L5

319. Articulations without a joint cavity include

1. cartilaginous joints
2. fibrous joints
3. synovial joints
   ❑ A. 1 only
   ❑ B. 3 only
   ❑ C. 1 and 2 only
   ❑ D. 1 and 3 only

320. Correctly order the following parts of the humerus from distal to proximal.

1. Anatomical neck
2. Body/shaft
3. Trochlea
4. Head
5. Lesser tubercle
6. Surgical neck
7. Medial epicondyle
   ❑ A. 7, 3, 6, 2, 1, 5, 4
   ❑ B. 4, 1, 5, 6, 2, 7, 3
   ❑ C. 3, 7, 2, 6, 5, 1, 4
   ❑ D. 1, 4, 6, 5, 7, 2, 3

ANSWERS AND EXPLANATIONS

1. **(B)** The term *varus* refers to bent or turned *inward*. In genu varum, the tibia or femur turns inward causing bow-legged deformity; in talipes varus, the foot turns inward (clubfoot deformity). The term *valgus* refers to a part turned/deformed *outward*—as in hallux valgus and talipes valgus. Hallux valgus is angulation of the great toe away from the midline; talipes valgus is a foot deformity with the heel turned outward—a component of clubfoot.

2. **(B)** There are three important fat pads associated with the elbow, best demonstrated in the *true* lateral projection. They are not demonstrated in the AP projection because of their superimposition on bony structures. The *anterior* fat pad is located just anterior to the distal humerus. The *posterior* fat pad is located within the olecranon fossa at the distal posterior humerus. The *supinator* fat pad/stripe is located at the proximal radius just anterior to the head, neck, and tuberosity. The *posterior* fat pad *is not visible* radiographically in the *normal* elbow. The posterior fat pad is visible in cases of trauma or other pathology and when the elbow is insufficiently flexed, that is, extended somewhat beyond the 90° flexion.

3. **(A)** Figure 2-1 shows a lateral (mediolateral) projection of the knee. The femoral condyles are not superimposed posteriorly and too much of the fibular head is visualized, indicating incorrect degree of forward/anterior or backward/posterior rotation. The magnified medial femoral condyle is obscuring the patellofemoral articulation, so it indicates excessive anterior rotation and the need to rotate the pelvis backward/posteriorly. In addition, the magnified medial femoral condyle is obscuring the femorotibial joint space, the CR should be directed 5° cephalad to superimpose the condyles and open the joint space.

4. **(D)** The *lateral oblique* elbow projection demonstrates the proximal radius and ulna free of superimposition. The coronoid process is located on the proximal anterior ulna. The *medial oblique* projection of the elbow demonstrates the coronoid process in profile, as well as the ulnar olecranon process within the humeral olecranon fossa. There is some superimposition of the radius and ulna in both the AP and lateral projections.

5. **(A)** The posterior oblique positions (LPO and RPO) are used to demonstrate the zygapophyseal articulations of L1–L4. When correctly positioned, the classic "Scottie dog" should be visualized. If the zygapophyseal articulations are not clearly visualized, and the pedicle is seen on the *posterior* aspect of the vertebral body, patient rotation should be decreased. If the zygapophyseal articulations are not clearly visualized and the pedicle is seen on the *anterior* aspect of the vertebral body, patient rotation should be increased. Pelvic tilt is indicated when iliac crests are not opposite one another.

6. **(C)** Figure 2-2 shows a lateral elbow formed by the humerus, radius, and ulna. Number 1 is the humerus and number 10 is its lateral epicondyle. Just distal to the lateral epicondyle is the capitulum (number 2), which articulates with the radial head (number 4). The radial neck (number 5) and tuberosity (number 6) are seen just distal to the radial head. Number 9 is the olecranon process, number 8 is the semilunar/trochlear notch, and number 3 is the coronoid process.

7. **(C)** The term *dorsal* refers to the *posterior* aspect of a structure/part. The "back" of the hand (dorsum manus), the posterior surface of the body, and the upper surface of the foot (dorsum pedis) are all dorsal aspects of these parts.

8. **(D)** The trachea bifurcates into left and right *main stem bronchi,* each entering its respective lung hilum. The *left* bronchus divides into *two* portions, one for each lobe of the left lung. The left lung has one fissure: the oblique. The *right* bronchus divides into *three* portions, one for each lobe of the right lung (Fig. 2-48). The right lung has two fissures: the horizontal and the oblique. The lungs are conical in shape, consisting of upper pointed portions, termed the *apices* (plural of apex) and broad lower portions (or *bases*). The lungs are enclosed in a double-walled serous membrane called the *pleura.*

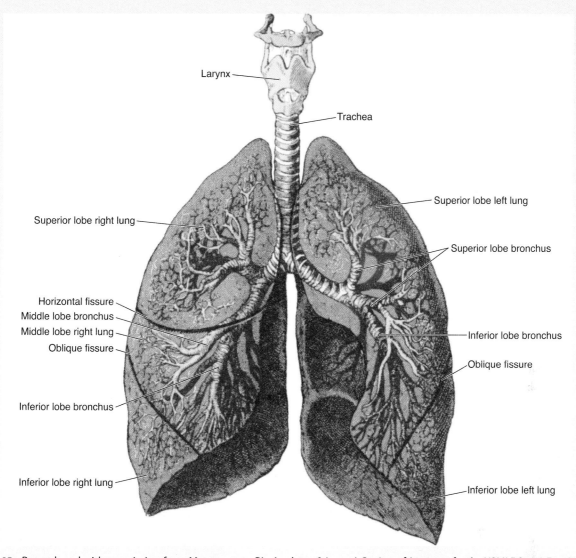

Larynx

Trachea

Superior lobe left lung

Superior lobe right lung

Superior lobe bronchus

Horizontal fissure
Middle lobe bronchus
Middle lobe right lung
Oblique fissure

Inferior lobe bronchus

Oblique fissure

Inferior lobe bronchus

Inferior lobe right lung

Inferior lobe left lung

Figure 2-48. Reproduced with permission from Montgomery RL. *Appleton & Lange's Review of Anatomy for the USMLE Step I*. East Norwalk, CT: Appleton & Lange; 1995:27.

9. **(C)** In the exact PA projection of the skull, the perpendicular CR exits the nasion and the petrous pyramids should be demonstrated *filling* the orbits (Fig. 2-49). As the CR is angled caudally, the petrous ridges/pyramids are projected lower in the orbits. At about 25°–30° caudad, they are projected *below* the orbits. The OML must be *perpendicular* to the IR for the petrous pyramids to be projected into the expected location, that is, within the orbital cavities. The MSP must be *perpendicular* to the IR, or the skull will be rotated and left/right symmetry will be lost.

10. **(D)** Figure 2-3 illustrates a PA projection of the chest. This projection demonstrates the air-filled trachea, the carina at the bifurcation of the trachea, the lungs from apices to costophrenic angles, both hemidiaphragms, the heart, and aortic arch. The shoulders have been rolled forward to effectively remove the scapulae from the lung fields. Adequate inspiration is demonstrated by visualization of 10 posterior ribs above the diaphragm (see numbered ribs in Fig. 2-50).

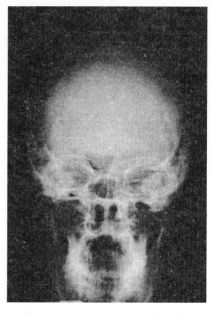

Figure 2-49. Used with permission of Stamford Hospital, Department of Radiology.

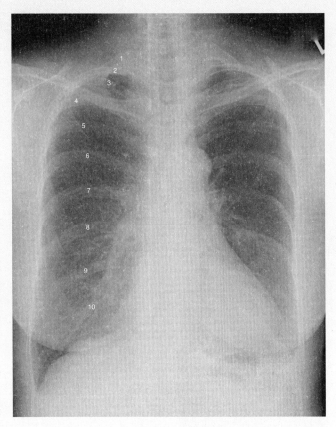

Figure 2-50

11. (B) *Pectus excavatum* is a congenital defect in which the sternum is depressed posteriorly, often called "sunken" or "funnel" chest and can be associated with pulmonary or cardiac difficulties. *Pectus carinatum* is a congenital defect in which the sternum protrudes anteriorly, often called "pigeon breast." Blunt trauma to the chest resulting in fractures of two or more adjacent ribs, causing them to become detached from the rest of the rib cage, is termed *flail chest.* Atelectasis is collapse of all or part of a lung.

12. (C) In the tangential (sunrise) projection of the patella, the CR is directed parallel to the longitudinal plane of the patella, thereby demonstrating a vertical fracture and providing the best view of the patellofemoral articulation. The AP knee projection could demonstrate a vertical fracture through the superimposed femur, but it does not demonstrate the patellofemoral articulation. The tunnel view of the knee is used to demonstrate the intercondyloid fossa.

13. (B) The cecum is a blind pouch located at the most proximal (first) portion of the large intestine. Extending from the lower end of the cecum is the wormlike vermiform appendix. The cecum and the vermiform appendix are both located in the RLQ. The sigmoid colon is located in the *left* lower quadrant (LLQ).

14. (B) The image shown in Figure 2-4 is one of a series of IVU images taken 15 min after injection of the contrast medium. The urinary collecting system is well demonstrated. An RPO position is illustrated, with the right marker indicating the right side; also, the right ilium is more "open" (i.e., parallel to the IR) than the left. The RPO position places the *left kidney* and *right ureter* parallel to the IR. The urinary bladder contains considerable contrast, indicating that it is most likely a *prevoid image.* A retrograde pyelogram is not performed intravenously; a retrograde study would demonstrate catheters instilled through urethra into ureters.

15. (B) *Blowout fractures* of the orbital floor are caused by a direct blow to the eye. The orbital floor is caused to collapse; this carries the *inferior rectus muscle* through the fracture site and into the *maxillary sinus.* Diplopia (double vision) often results. Blowout fractures are well demonstrated with the Waters' method (parietoacanthial projection) and CT studies. A parietoacanthial projection with the OML perpendicular and the CR angled 30° caudad also will demonstrate the orbital floor in profile. The *zygoma* usually is not involved with a blowout fracture but rather with a *tripod* fracture.

16. (B) The ankle mortise, or ankle joint, is formed by the articulation of the tibia, fibula, and talus (Fig. 2-51). Two articulations form the ankle mortise: the talotibial and talofibular articulations. The calcaneus is not associated with formation of the ankle mortise.

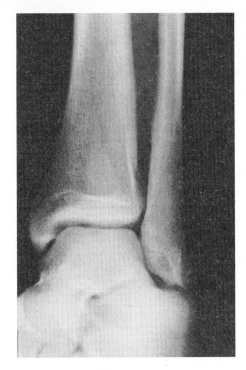

Figure 2-51

17. **(C)** The foot has anterior, posterior, medial, and lateral surfaces. The upper surface is the *anterior* or *dorsum*/dorsal surface. The lower surface is the plantar surface. Hence, the AP projection of the foot is also called the dorsoplantar projection of the foot (describing the path of the CR traversing from dorsum to plantar surface).

18. **(D)** Double-contrast studies of the stomach or large intestine involve coating the organ with a thin layer of barium sulfate and then introducing air. This allows visualization of the interior of the organ, its *mucosal* lining, and the structures behind the organ. A barium-filled stomach or large bowel demonstrates the position, size, and shape of the organ and any lesion that projects *out* from its walls, such as diverticula. Polypoid lesions, which project *inward* from the wall of an organ, may go unnoticed unless a double-contrast examination is performed.

19. **(B)** *Extension* increases the angle as a body part moves from a flexed position to a straightened position, for example, the elbow or knee. The term *eversion* refers to an outward stress movement of the foot and ankle as the plantar surface is moved away from the median plane. The term *erect* is a positioning term describing a general physical position of the body in the upright position.

20. **(A)** The AP axial projects the anterior structures (frontal and facial bones) downward, thus permitting visualization of the *occipital bone* without superimposition (Towne method). The dorsum sella and posterior clinoid processes of the sphenoid bone should be visualized within the foramen magnum. This projection may also be obtained by angling the CR 37° caudad to the IOML. The CR passes through the level of the EAM and exits at the foramen magnum (Fig. 2-52). The *frontal bone* is best shown with the patient PA and with a perpendicular CR. The parietoacanthial projection is the single best position for *facial bones*. *Basal foramina* are well demonstrated in the submentovertical projection.

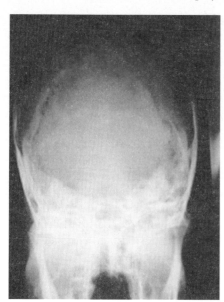

Figure 2-52. Used with permission of Stamford Hospital, Department of Radiology.

21. **(A)** The posterior oblique positions (AP oblique projections) of the acetabulum (Judet method) require a 45° obliquity of the entire MSP. With the *internal* oblique position, affected side *up,* the anterior iliopubic column and/or posterior rim of the acetabulum are best demonstrated. With the *external* oblique position, affected side *down,* the posterior ilioischial column and/or anterior rim of the acetabulum are best demonstrated. In the RPO position, the *down* side (the *right* side in this case) will demonstrate the *anterior rim of the right acetabulum,* the *right posterior ilioischial column,* and the *right iliac wing*. When centered to the *up* side (*left* in this case), the structures demonstrated are the posterior rim of the left acetabulum, left anterior iliopubic column, and the left obturator foramen.

22. **(B)** Figure 2-5 demonstrates an LPO position, used to demonstrate left axillary and posterior portions of ribs. The RPO position is used to demonstrate right axillary and posterior ribs. Exposure was made on full inspiration and adequately demonstrates the first nine ribs. The part was positioned correctly at a 45° oblique, demonstrating about twice the distance between the vertebrae and lateral border of the affected ribs, compared with that seen on the unaffected side.

23. **(C)** Because the sternum and vertebrae would be superimposed in a direct PA or AP projection, a slight oblique (just enough to separate the sternum from superimposition on the vertebrae) is used instead of a direct frontal projection. In the RAO position, the heart superimposes a homogenous tissue density over the sternum, thereby providing more clear radiographic visualization of its bony structure. If the *LAO* position were used to project the sternum to the *right* of the thoracic vertebrae, the posterior ribs and pulmonary markings would cast confusing shadows over the sternum because of their differing densities.

24. **(C)** *Skeletal* muscle attaches to bones. It is *striated,* having long threadlike-shaped cells/fibers. Skeletal muscle is called *voluntary* because we have conscious control over these muscles.

Visceral muscle forms walls of hollow organs. It is involuntary, smooth, and nonstriated. The stomach, intestine, urinary bladder, blood vessels, and other structures are associated with smooth, involuntary muscle. In the stomach and intestines, smooth/involuntary muscle cells contract in wavelength sequence as impulse travels from one cell to another (peristalsis).

Cardiac muscle is found in the wall of the heart (myocardium). It is striated in appearance, but involuntary. Cardiac muscle has little or no regeneration of fibers after injury. Healing is accomplished by scar formation.

25. **(A)** The knee (tibiofemoral joint) is the largest joint of the body, formed by the articulation of the femur and tibia. The "knee" actually consists of three articulations: the patellofemoral joint, the lateral tibiofemoral joint (lateral femoral

condyle with tibial plateau), and the medial tibiofemoral joint (medial femoral condyle with tibial plateau). Although the knee is classified as a synovial (diarthrotic), hinge-type joint, the patellofemoral joint actually is a gliding joint, and the medial and lateral tibiofemoral joints are hinge type.

26. (C) One of the most important principles in chest radiography is that it should be performed, whenever possible, in the erect position. It is in this position that the diaphragm can descend to its lowest position during inspiration, and any air–fluid levels can be detected. However, patients with traumatic injuries frequently must be examined in the supine position. An AP supine chest is performed first. If the examination is also being performed to rule out air–fluid levels, this can be determined by performing the *lateral projection in the dorsal decubitus position*. The patient is lying supine, and a *horizontal* (cross-table) x-ray beam is used.

27. (D) The femoral head articulates with the acetabulum to form the hip joint. The femoral neck angles upward approximately 120° and forward (anteversion) approximately 15°. The *axiolateral inferosuperior projection* of the hip (also commonly called a cross-table lateral, horizontal beam lateral, or Danelius–Miller method) is often used to evaluate suspected femoral neck fracture.

The patient is supine with *un*affected leg elevated. If possible, the pelvis is elevated 1–2 inches from the stretcher/x-ray table and the affected leg rotated internally 15° to avoid anteversion; *however, rotation must never be attempted when femoral neck fracture or destructive disease is suspected.*

The top of the IR is placed just above the crest and adjusted to be parallel to the femoral neck and perpendicular to the CR.

The femoral neck is located 1–2 inches (3–5 cm) medial and 3–4 inches (8–10 cm) distal to the ASIS. The femoral neck is seen radiographically in the same transverse plane as the pubic symphysis and greater trochanters.

28. (C) The radiograph shown in Figure 2-6 is a PA projection (Caldwell method) of the frontal and anterior ethmoidal sinuses. The frontal sinuses are seen centrally in the vertical plate of the frontal bone behind the glabella and extending laterally over the superciliary arches. The ethmoidal sinuses are seen adjacent and inferior to the medial aspect of the orbits. The patient is positioned PA erect with the chin extended so that the OML is 15° from the horizontal. This will project the petrous ridges in the lower third of the orbits; CR angulation is not used when examining the paranasal sinuses because it could distort/obliterate any fluid levels. With the OML perpendicular to the IR, the petrous pyramids would fill the orbits (true PA).

In the PA position with chin extended (choice A) and OML 37° to the IR (parietoacanthial projection, Waters' method), the petrous pyramids are projected below the maxillary sinuses.

29. (C) The radiograph shown in Figure 2-6 is a PA projection (Caldwell method) of the *frontal and anterior ethmoid sinuses.* The frontal sinuses are seen centrally in the vertical plate of the frontal bone behind the glabella and extending laterally over the superciliary arches. The *ethmoid* sinuses are seen adjacent and inferior to the medial aspect of the orbits. The nasal cavity is seen, with the perpendicular plate and vomer, in the midline. The patient is positioned PA erect with the chin extended so that the OML is 15° from the horizontal.

30. (B) The oblique projection of the hand should demonstrate minimal overlap of the third, fourth, and fifth metacarpals. Excessive overlap of these metacarpals is caused by obliquing the hand *more than 45°*. The use of a 45° foam wedge ensures that the fingers will be extended and parallel to the IR, thus permitting visualization of the interphalangeal joints and avoiding foreshortening of the phalanges. Clenching of the fist and ulnar flexion are maneuvers used to better demonstrate the carpal scaphoid.

31. (C) Blunt trauma to the chest resulting in fractures of two or more adjacent ribs, causing them to become detached from the rest of the rib cage, is termed *flail chest*. Atelectasis is collapse of all or part of a lung. *Pectus excavatum* is a congenital defect in which the sternum is depressed posteriorly, sometimes called "sunken" or "funnel" chest and can be associated with pulmonary or cardiac difficulties. *Pectus carinatum* is a congenital defect in which the sternum protrudes anteriorly, sometimes called "pigeon breast."

32. (B) Various terms are used to describe the position of fractured ends of long bones. The term *apposition* is used to describe the *alignment,* or *misalignment,* between the ends of fractured long bones. The term *angulation* describes the *direction* of misalignment. The term *luxation* refers to a dislocation. A *sprain* refers to a wrenched articulation with ligament injury.

33. (D) The *PA axial oblique* projections (LAO and RAO positions) of the cervical spine require a 15° caudal angulation and demonstrate the intervertebral foramina *closest* to the IR. The *AP axial oblique* projections (LPO and RPO positions) require that the CR be directed 15° cephalad to C4. PA axial oblique projections (LAO and RAO) demonstrate the intervertebral foramina *closer to* the IR.

34. (A) Air or fluid levels will be clearly delineated only if the CR is directed parallel to them. Therefore, to demonstrate air or fluid levels, the erect or decubitus position should be used. Small amounts of *fluid* are best demonstrated in the lateral decubitus position, *affected side down*. Small amounts of air are best demonstrated in the lateral decubitus position, *affected side up*. The left lateral decubitus abdomen best visualizes free air within the peritoneal cavity against the liver and away from air in the stomach.

35. (C) The relationship of these three structures is easily appreciated in a lateral projection of the chest. The *heart* is seen in the anterior half of the thoracic cavity, with its apex extending inferior and anterior. The air-filled *trachea* can be seen in about the center of the chest, and the air-filled *esophagus* is seen just posterior to the trachea (Fig. 2-53). The superimposed vertebral and axillary borders of the scapulae would be seen most posteriorly.

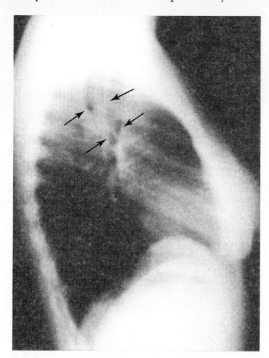

Figure 2-53. From the American College of Radiology Learning File. Used with permission of the ACR.

36. (A) The knee structures are formed by the proximal tibia, the patella, and the distal femur, which articulate to form the *femorotibial* and *femoropatellar* joints. The knee joint is the femorotibial joint. Body habitus can considerably change the knee joint and tabletop/IR relationship. The CR should be directed to ½ inch below patellar apex (knee joint). The direction of CR depends on the distance between the ASIS and tabletop/IR. When this distance is up to 19 cm (thin pelvis), the CR is directed 3°–5° caudad; when the distance is between 19 and 24 cm, the CR is directed vertically/perpendicular (0°); when the distance is greater than 24 cm (thick pelvis), the CR is directed 3°–5° cephalad.

37. (B) Figure 2-7 illustrates a *medial oblique (internal rotation)* projection of the elbow with epicondyles 45° to the IR. An oblique view of the proximal radius and ulna and the distal humerus is obtained. This projection is particularly useful to demonstrate the *coronoid process* in profile, the *trochlea*, and the *medial epicondyle*. The external oblique (lateral rotation) projection demonstrates the radial head free of superimposition as well as the radial neck and the humeral capitulum. The acute flexion projection (Jones method) of the elbow is a two-projection method demonstrating the elbow anatomy when the part cannot be extended for an AP projection.

38. (A) Figure 2-7 illustrates a *medial oblique (internal rotation)* projection of the elbow with epicondyles 45° to the IR. An oblique view of the proximal radius and ulna and the distal humerus is obtained. This projection is particularly useful to demonstrate the *coronoid process* in profile (number 4), the *trochlea* (number 3), and the *medial epicondyle* (number 1). The olecranon process (number 2) fits into the olecranon fossa during extension of the elbow. A small portion of the radial head (number 5) not superimposed on the ulna can be seen. The external oblique (lateral rotation) projection demonstrates the entire radial head free of superimposition as well as the radial neck and the humeral capitulum.

39. (D) The AP projection of the hip requires sufficient internal leg rotation to place the femoral neck parallel to the IR. Insufficient internal rotation is demonstrated here by foreshortening (i.e., not parallel with the IR) of the femoral neck and visualization of the lesser trochanter beyond the medial border of the femur (there should be no, or very little, visualization of the lesser trochanter).

40. (B) The axial trauma lateral (Coyle) position is described. If routine elbow projections in extension are not possible because of limited part movement, this position can be used to demonstrate the coronoid process and/or radial head. With the elbow flexed *90°* and the CR directed to the elbow joint at an angle of 45° medially (i.e., toward the shoulder), the joint space between the *radial head* and capitulum should be revealed. With the elbow flexed *80°* and the CR directed to the elbow joint at an angle of 45° laterally (i.e., from the shoulder toward the elbow), the elongated *coronoid process* will be visualized.

41. (A) A diagnostic image of C1–C2 depends on adjusting the flexion of the neck *so that the maxillary occlusal plane and the base of the skull are superimposed.* Accurate adjustment of these structures will usually allow good visualization of the odontoid process and the atlantoaxial articulation. Should the patient anatomy occasionally prevent the usual visualization, the odontoid process can be visualized through the foramen magnum, either AP or PA. In the AP position (Fuchs method) or the PA position (Judd method), the patient's chin is extended to be in line vertically with the mastoid tip (similar to a Waters' or reverse Waters' position). The CR is directed to the midline and perpendicularly at the level of the mastoid tip. The resulting image demonstrates the odontoid process through the foramen magnum. These positions should not be attempted if the patient has a suspected, new, or healing fracture or destructive disease.

42. (B) The skull is divided into two parts: the cranial bones and the facial bones. There are eight cranial bones. Four of them comprise the *calvarium:* the frontal, the two parietals, and the occipital. The bones that comprise the *floor* of the cranium are the *two temporals,* the *ethmoid,* and the *sphenoid.*

43. (A) Croup is a viral infection generally seen in children 1–3 years of age. It is characterized by a dry cough, sometimes accompanied by fever. Soft-tissue projections of the neck are frequently used to evaluate the upper airway. Narrowing of the upper airway is best demonstrated in the AP projection.

44–45. (44, A; 45, D) The radiograph shown in Figure 2-9 is an oblique position of a double-contrast study of the large bowel, illustrating an "open" view of the splenic/left colic flexure (number 1) and descending colon, with the hepatic/right colic flexure (number 2) somewhat superimposed on the transverse and ascending (number 3) colon. Therefore, the radiograph must have been made in either an *RPO* (if the patient was supine) or an *LAO* (if the patient was prone) position. The LPO and RAO positions are used to demonstrate the hepatic flexure and ascending colon free of self-superimposition. The distal ileum is well visualized (number 6), as well as the commencement of the large bowel—the cecum (number 4)—and its vermiform appendix (number 5). The descending colon is labeled number 7. The AP or PA axial position is generally used to visualize the rectosigmoid colon.

46. (B) The thoracic and sacral vertebrae exhibit *primary kyphotic* curves, those that are present at birth. The *lordotic* curves are *secondary* curves, that is, they develop sometime after birth. The cervical and lumbar vertebrae form lordotic curves.

47. (D) The *scapular Y* refers to the characteristic Y formed by the humerus, acromion, and coracoid processes. The patient is placed in a PA oblique position—an RAO or LAO position depending on which is the affected side. The midcoronal plane is adjusted approximately 60° to the IR, and the affected arm remains relaxed at the patient's side. The scapular Y position is used *to demonstrate anterior (subcoracoid) or posterior (subacromial) humeral dislocation.* The humerus is normally superimposed on the scapula in this position; any deviation from this may indicate dislocation.

48. (B) Diagnostic x-ray examinations that require contrast agents include upper GI series, lower GI series (BE), and intravenous urogram (IVU). Patient preparation is somewhat different for each of these examinations. The patient scheduled for an *upper* GI series must be NPO (nothing by mouth) after midnight. A *lower* GI series (BE) requires that the large bowel be very clean prior to the administration of barium; this requires the administration of *cathartics* (laxatives) and cleansing enemas. Preparation for an IVU requires that the patient be NPO after midnight; some institutions also require that the large bowel be cleansed of gas and fecal material. Aftercare for barium examinations is very important. Patients typically are instructed to take Milk of Magnesia, increase their intake of fiber, drink plenty of water, and expect changes in stool color until all barium is evacuated and to call their physician if they do not have a bowel movement within 24 h. Because water is removed from the barium sulfate suspension in the large bowel, it is essential to make patients understand the importance of these instructions to avoid barium impaction in the large bowel. The use of barium sulfate suspensions is contraindicated when ruling out *visceral perforation.*

49. (A) The axillary portion of the ribs is best demonstrated in a 45° oblique position. The axillary ribs are demonstrated in the AP oblique projection with the affected side *adjacent to* the IR and in the PA oblique projection with the affected side *away from* the IR. Therefore, the *right* axillary ribs would be demonstrated in the RPO (AP oblique with affected side *adjacent to* the IR) and LAO (PA oblique with affected side *away from* the IR) positions.

50. (A) The *lateral oblique* demonstrates the interspaces between the first and second metatarsals and between the first and second cuneiforms. To best demonstrate *most* of the tarsals and intertarsal spaces (including the cuboid, sinus tarsi, and tuberosity of the fifth metatarsal), a *medial oblique projection* is required (plantar surface and IR form a 30° angle). A *weight-bearing lateral projection* of the feet is used to demonstrate the longitudinal arches.

51. (C) Surface landmarks, prominences, and depressions are very useful to the radiographer in locating anatomic structures that are not visible externally. The fifth thoracic vertebra is at approximately the same level as the sternal angle. The T2–T3 interspace is about at the same level as the manubrial (suprasternal) notch. The costal margin is about the same level as L3.

52. (A) The femur is the longest and strongest bone in the body. The femoral shaft/body is bowed slightly anteriorly and presents a long, narrow ridge posteriorly called the linea aspera. The *distal* femur is associated with two large *condyles* (medial and lateral); the deep depression separating them posteriorly is the intercondyloid fossa (Fig. 2-54). Just proximal/superior to the large condyles are the smaller *medial and lateral epicondyles.* Proximally, the femur presents a *head*, neck, and *greater and lesser trochanters.* Thus, from distal to proximal are lateral condyle, medial epicondyle, body/shaft, lesser trochanter, greater trochanter, head.

53. (A) Because sinus examinations are performed to evaluate the presence or absence of fluid, they must be performed in the *erect position with a horizontal x-ray beam.* The PA axial (Caldwell) projection demonstrates the frontal and ethmoidal sinus groups, and the parietoacanthial projection (Waters' method) shows the maxillary sinuses. The lateral position demonstrates all the sinus groups, and the SMV position is used frequently to demonstrate the sphenoidal sinuses.

54. (B) A PA oblique projection of the hand is shown in Figure 2-10. The correct degree of obliquity (45°) is evidenced by no overlap of midshaft third, fourth, and fifth metacarpals and minimal overlap of their heads. The phalanges are foreshortened and the interphalangeal joint spaces are not visualized because the fingers are not adjusted to be parallel to the IR.

55. (B) The *midsagittal* plane passes vertically through the midline of the body, dividing it into left and right halves. Any plane parallel to the MSP is termed a *sagittal* plane. The *midcoronal* plane is *perpendicular* to the MSP and divides the body into anterior and posterior halves. The *transverse* plane passes across the body, also *perpendicular* to a sagittal plane. These planes, especially the MSP, are very important reference points in radiographic positioning.

56. (C) The femur is the longest and strongest bone in the body. The femoral shaft is bowed slightly anteriorly and presents a long, narrow ridge posteriorly called the *linea aspera*. The distal femur is associated with two large condyles; the deep depression separating them posteriorly is the *intercondyloid fossa* (Fig. 2-54). Just superior to the large condyles are the smaller medial and lateral epicondyles. The posterior distal femoral surface presents the *popliteal surface,* whereas the distal anterior surface presents the patellar surface. Proximally, the femur presents a head, neck, and greater and lesser trochanters. The intertrochanteric crest is a prominent ridge of bone between the trochanters posteriorly; *anteriorly, the intertrochanteric line* is seen. The femoral head presents a roughened prominence, the fovea capitis femoris—ligaments attached here secure the femoral head to the acetabulum.

57. (D) Bilateral AP oblique hands are obtained using the Norgaard method or "ball-catcher position." The method is used to detect early rheumatoid arthritis changes or fracture to the base of the fifth metacarpal. The hands are positioned and supported in a 45° oblique, palm-up position.

The CR is directed to the level of the fifth metacarpophalangeal joint (MCP) midway between the hands—both hands are exposed simultaneously.

58. (C) *Pneumothorax* results from an accumulation of air in the pleural cavity, resulting in partial or complete collapse of the associated lung. The affected lung in this case can be seen displaced away from the chest wall. Pleural effusion is also demonstrated here by an accumulation of fluid in the pleural cavity. Air–fluid levels are well demonstrated in the erect position. In emphysema, however, air is trapped in the alveoli; it is a condition that is characterized by increased amount of air in the lungs, flattening of the hemidiaphragms, and widening of the intercostal spaces. Notice that Figure 2-11 has an *expiration* marker—recall that a pneumothorax diagnosis usually requires inspiration and expiration images.

59. (A) The inferior costal margin (inferior margin of the ribs) is located at the level of L2–L3. The ASIS is in the same transverse plane as S2. The ASIS and the pubic symphysis are the bony landmarks used to locate the hip joint, which is located midway between the two points. The uppermost portion of the iliac crest is at the approximate level of L4–L5. The most prominent part of the greater trochanter is at the same level as the pubic symphysis—both are valuable positioning landmarks.

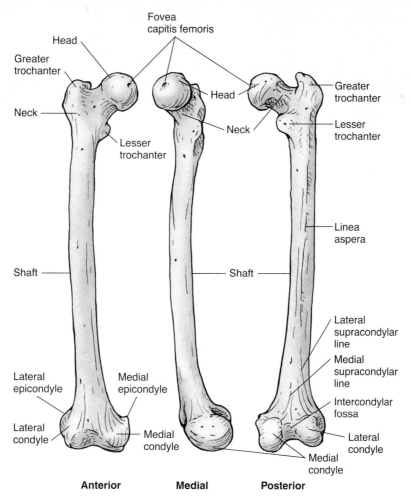

Figure 2-54

60. (C) Sacroiliac joints lie obliquely within the pelvis and open anteriorly at an angle of 25°–30° to the midsagittal plane. A 25°–30° oblique position places the joints perpendicular to the IR. The right sacroiliac joint may be demonstrated in the LPO and RAO positions with little magnification variation.

61. (D) The *scapular Y* projection is an oblique projection of the shoulder that is used to demonstrate anterior or posterior shoulder dislocation. The *inferosuperior axial* projection may be used to evaluate the glenohumeral joint when the patient is able to abduct the arm. The *transthoracic lateral* projection is used to evaluate the glenohumeral joint and upper humerus when the patient is unable to abduct the arm.

62. (C) The knee (femorotibial) joint is formed by the femur and tibia. The most superior aspect of the tibia is the *tibial plateau*—formed by the *tibial condyles just distal to it*. The proximal tibia also presents the *tibial tuberosity* on its anterior surface, just distal to the condyles. *Proximal* to the tibial plateau, and articulating with it, are the *femoral condyles*—the deep notch separating them is the *intercondyloid fossa*. The term *proximal* refers to a part located closer to the point of attachment; the term *distal* refers to a part located farther away from the point of attachment.

63. (C) The greater and lesser tubercles are prominences on the proximal humerus separated by the intertubercular (bicipital) groove. The lateral projection of the humerus places the shoulder in extreme internal rotation with the epicondyles perpendicular to the IR and superimposed. The lateral projection of the humerus should demonstrate the lesser tubercle in profile. The AP projection of the humerus/shoulder places the *epicondyles parallel to the IR* and the shoulder in *external rotation* and demonstrates the *greater tubercle in profile*.

64. (D) The mediastinum is the space between the lungs that contains the heart, great vessels, trachea, esophagus, and thymus gland. It is bounded anteriorly by the sternum and posteriorly by the vertebral column, and extends from the upper thorax to the diaphragm.

65. (C) A quality image of C1–C2 depends on adjusting the flexion of the neck *so that the maxillary occlusal plane and the base of the skull are superimposed.* Accurate adjustment of these structures usually demonstrates good visualization of the odontoid process and the atlantoaxial articulation. Figure 2-12 demonstrates the atlantoaxial articulation in its entirety; however, the odontoid process is incompletely visualized. The upper portion of the odontoid is superimposed by the base of the skull. With a little more flexion, the base of the skull will move upward and the lower edge of the maxillary incisors will move downward to superimpose on the base of the skull, thus demonstrating the odontoid process in its entirety.

66. (A) An *avulsion* fracture is a small, bony fragment pulled from a bony process as a result of a forceful pull of the attached ligament or tendon. A *comminuted* fracture is one in which the bone is broken or splintered into pieces. A *torus* fracture is a greenstick fracture with one cortex buckled and the other intact. A *compound* fracture is an open fracture in which the fractured ends have perforated the skin.

67. (D) The distal humerus articulates with the proximal radius and ulna to form the elbow joint. Specifically, the *semilunar/trochlear notch* of the proximal ulna articulates with the *trochlea* of the distal medial humerus. The *capitulum* is lateral to the trochlea and articulates with the *radial head* (Fig. 2-55).

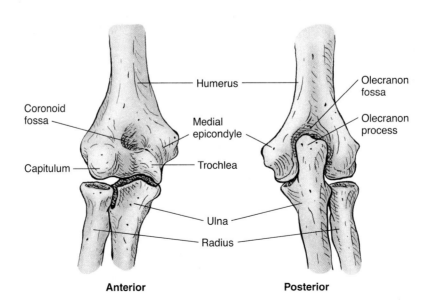

Anterior

Posterior

Figure 2-55

68. (C) To accurately position a lateral forearm, the elbow must form a 90° angle with the humeral epicondyles perpendicular to the IR and superimposed. The radius and ulna are superimposed distally. Proximally, the coronoid process and radial head are superimposed, and the radial tuberosity faces anteriorly. Failure of the elbow to form a 90° angle or the hand to be lateral results in a less than satisfactory lateral projection of the forearm.

69. (D) Generally, contrast medium is injected into the subarachnoid space between the third and fourth lumbar vertebrae (see Fig. 2-56). Because the spinal cord ends at the level of the first or second lumbar vertebra, this is considered to be a relatively safe injection site. The cisterna magna can be used, but the risk of contrast medium entering the ventricles and causing side effects increases. Diskography requires injection of contrast medium into the individual intervertebral disks.

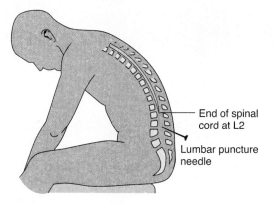

End of spinal cord at L2

Lumbar puncture needle

Figure 2-56

70. (C) The skull has two major parts: the *cranium*, which is composed of 8 bones and houses the brain, and the 14 irregularly shaped *facial bones* (Fig. 2-57). The inner and outer compact tables of the cranial skull are separated by cancellous tissue called *diploe*. The internal table has a number of branching meningeal grooves and larger sulci that house blood vessels. The bones of the skull are separated by immovable (synarthrotic) joints called *sutures*. The major sutures of the cranium are the *sagittal*, which separates the parietal bones; the *coronal*, which separates the frontal and parietal bones; the *lambdoidal*, which separates the parietal and occipital bones; and the *squamosal*, which separates the temporal and parietal bones. The sagittal and coronal sutures meet at the *bregma*, which corresponds to the fetal anterior fontanel. The sagittal and lambdoidal sutures meet posteriorly at the *lambda*, which corresponds to the fetal posterior fontanel. The parietal, frontal, and sphenoid bones meet at the *pterion*, the location of the anterolateral fontanel. The highest point of the skull is called the *vertex*.

71. (B) An accurately positioned right scapular Y is illustrated in Figure 2-13; this refers to the characteristic Y formed by the clearly visible humerus, acromion, and coracoid. The patient is positioned in a PA oblique position—in this case, an RAO of the right shoulder. The MCP is adjusted to approximately 45°–60° to the IR, and the affected arm is relaxed at the patient's side. The scapular Y position should demonstrate superimposition of the glenoid cavity and humeral head, the acromion process projected laterally, and the coracoid process free of superimposition and

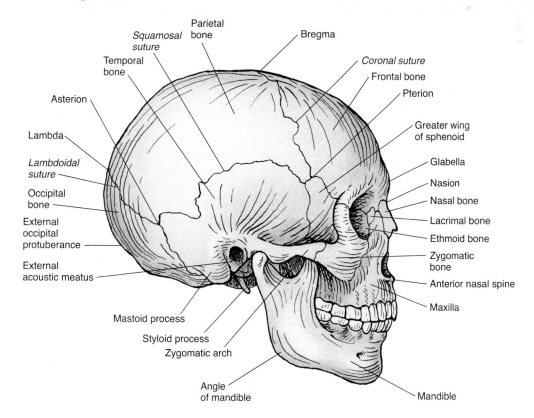

Figure 2-57

projected *below* the clavicle. The scapular Y position is used to demonstrate anterior or posterior humeral dislocation. The humerus is superimposed on the scapula in this position; any deviation from this may indicate dislocation.

72. (B) Typically, traumatic injury to the hip requires a cross-table (axiolateral) lateral projection, as well as an AP projection of the entire pelvis. Both of these are performed using minimal manipulation of the affected extremity, reducing the possibility of further injury. A physician should perform any required manipulation of the traumatized hip.

73. (B) The *zygapophyseal 45° oblique projection* of the lumbar spine generally is performed for demonstration of the *zygapophyseal joints.* In a correctly positioned oblique lumbar spine, "Scottie dog" images are demonstrated (Figs. 2-58 and 2-59). Scottie's *ear* corresponds to the superior articular process, its *nose* to the transverse process, its *eye* to the pedicle, its *neck* to the pars interarticularis, its *body* to the lamina, and its *front leg* to the inferior articular process.

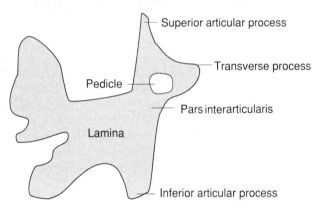

Figure 2-58

74. (C) The articular facets (zygapophyseal joints) of the *lumbosacral* (L5–S1) articulation form a 30° angle with the MSP; they are, therefore, well demonstrated in a 30° oblique position. The 45° oblique position demonstrates the zygapophyseal joints of L1–L4.

75. (B) Arranged from proximal to distal, the order is carpometacarpal joint, base of metacarpal, metacarpophalangeal joint, proximal interphalangeal joint, head of middle phalange, distal interphalangeal joint.

The hand is composed of five metacarpal bones, corresponding to the palm of the hand, and 14 *phalanges,* the fingers. The second through fifth fingers have three phalanges each; proximal, middle, and distal rows. The first finger, or thumb (pollex), has two phalanges (proximal and distal). The rows of phalanges articulate with each other forming proximal and distal interphalangeal joints, which permit flexion and extension motion. The proximal portion of each phalange and metacarpal is its base; its distal portion is its *head.* The most distal, flattened, portion of the phalanges is the ungual tuft.

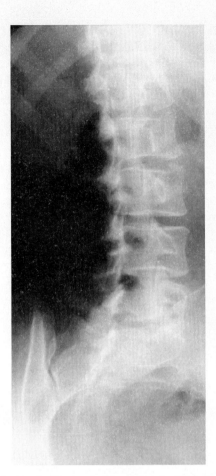

Figure 2-59. Used with permission of Stamford Hospital, Department of Radiology.

The *bases* of the proximal row of phalanges articulate with the heads of the metacarpals to form the *metacarpophalangeal joints,* which permit flexion and extension, abduction and adduction, and circumduction. The bases of the metacarpals articulate with each other and the distal row of carpals at the *carpometacarpal joints.* The first carpometacarpal joint is a saddle/sellar joint, permitting flexion and extension, abduction and adduction, and circumduction.

76. (B) *Ewing sarcoma* is a malignant bone tumor most common in young children. It attacks long bones and presents a characteristic "onion peel" appearance. *Osgood–Schlatter disease* is most common in adolescents, involving osteochondritis of the tibial tuberosity epiphysis. The large patellar tendon actually will pull the tibial tuberosity away from the tibia. Immobilization generally will resolve the issue. *Gout* is a type of arthritis that most commonly attacks the knee and first metatarsophalangeal joint, although other joints also can be involved. High levels of uric acid in the blood are deposited in the joint. *Exostosis* is a bony growth arising from the surface of a bone and growing away from the joint. It is a benign and sometimes painful condition.

77. (B) Synovial pivot joints are diarthrotic, that is, freely movable. Pivot joints permit rotation motion. Examples include the proximal radioulnar joint that permits supination and pronation of the hand. The atlantoaxial joint is the articulation between C1 and C2 and permits rotation of the head. The temporomandibular joint is diarthrotic, with both hinge and planar movements.

78. (C) The bony thorax consists of *12 pairs of ribs* and the structures to which they are attached anteriorly and posteriorly: the *sternum* (consisting of manubrium, body/gladiolus, and xiphoid/ensiform process) and the 12 *thoracic vertebrae* (Fig. 2-60). These structures form a bony cage that surrounds and protects the vital organs within (the heart, lungs, and great vessels). The scapulae, together with the clavicles, form the shoulder (pectoral) girdle of the upper extremity.

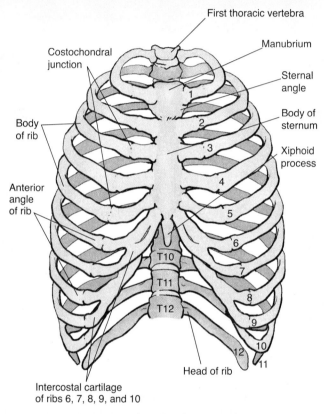

First thoracic vertebra

Costochondral junction

Manubrium

Sternal angle

Body of rib

Body of sternum

Xiphoid process

Anterior angle of rib

1
2
3
4
5
6
T10
7
T11
8
T12
9
12 10
11

Head of rib

Intercostal cartilage of ribs 6, 7, 8, 9, and 10

Anterior view

Figure 2-60

79. (A) Because the *right* main stem bronchus is *wider and more vertical,* aspirated foreign bodies are more likely to enter it than the left main stem bronchus, which is narrower and angles more sharply from the trachea. An *aspirated* foreign body does not enter the esophagus or the stomach because they are not respiratory structures. The esophagus and stomach are *digestive* structures; a foreign body would most likely be *swallowed* to enter these structures.

80. (B) A PA projection of the chest is shown in Figure 2-14. The shoulders are rolled forward, removing the *scapulae* from the lung fields. *Rotation* of the chest is demonstrated by the unequal distance between the sternum and medial extremities of the clavicles. Adequate *inspiration* is not

demonstrated because 10 posterior ribs are not visualized above the diaphragm. *Pulmonary apices* and *costophrenic angles* are demonstrated adequately. An *air-filled* trachea is seen in the lower cervical and upper thoracic region as an area of decreased brightness. Adequate *long-scale contrast* has been achieved, as indicated by visualization of pulmonary vascular markings.

81. (A) A PA projection of the chest is shown in Figure 2-14. The letter *A* indicates a left posterior rib, *B* represents a left anterior rib, and *C* represents the right costophrenic angle. Anterior ribs angle inferiorly and downward. *Rotation* of the chest is demonstrated by asymmetrical sternoclavicular joints. The apices and costophrenic angles should be included on every chest radiograph. Inadequate *inspiration* is demonstrated because 10 posterior ribs are not visualized above the diaphragm.

82. (B) The laryngeal prominence, or "Adam's apple," is formed by the *thyroid cartilage*—the principal cartilage of the larynx. The thyroid *gland,* one of the endocrine glands, is lateral and inferior to the thyroid cartilage. The *vocal cords* are within the laryngeal cavity. Portions of the *pharynx* serve as passages for both air and food.

83. (B) *Fibrous,* or immovable (synarthrotic), articulations are tightly joined by fibrous connective tissue and have no joint cavity. The articular surfaces in *cartilaginous* (amphiarthrotic) joints are held together by cartilage, offering them little movement. Only *synovial* (diarthrotic, freely movable) joints possess a joint cavity, thus permitting them free movement. Synovial type joints are the most numerous in the body.

84. (D) The thoracic zygapophyseal joints are demonstrated in an oblique position with the coronal plane 70° to the IR (MSP 20° to the IR). This may be accomplished by first placing the patient lateral and then obliquing the patient 20° "off lateral." The zygapophyseal joints closest to the IR are demonstrated in the PA oblique projection and those remote from the IR in the AP oblique projection. Comparable detail is obtained using either method because the OID is about the same. The thoracic intervertebral foramina are demonstrated in the lateral projection. This places the MSP of the patient parallel to the IR, and the coronal plane perpendicular to the IR.

85. (A) The dome of the acetabulum lies midway between the ASIS and the symphysis pubis. On an adult of average size, a line perpendicular to this point will parallel the plane of the femoral neck. In an AP projection of the hip, the CR should be directed to a point approximately 2 inches down the perpendicular line so as to enter the distal portion of the femoral head.

86–87. (86, A; 87, D) Figure 2-15 illustrates an anatomic lateral view of the paranasal sinuses. Number 1 points to the *frontal* sinuses and number 2 to the *ethmoidal* sinuses; both can be visualized using the PA projection (Caldwell method). Number 3 is the *sphenoidal* sinuses, which are well demonstrated in the SMV projection. Number 4 is the *maxillary* sinuses, which are best demonstrated using the parietoacanthial projection (Waters' method). The lateral projection demonstrates the four groups of paranasal sinuses with their left/right aspects *superimposed.*

88. (D) Surface landmarks, prominences, and depressions are very useful to the radiographer in locating anatomic structures that are not visible externally. The *costal margin* is at about the same level as L3. The *xiphoid tip* is at about the same level as T10. The *fourth lumbar vertebra* is at approximately the same level as the iliac crest. The *umbilicus* is at approximately the same level as the L3–L4 interspace, however can be somewhat variable and is not a recommended reference point.

89. (A) The radiograph shown in Figure 2-16 is a *medial oblique foot.* With the foot rotated medially so that the plantar surface forms a *30° angle* with the IR, the *sinus tarsi,* the *tuberosity* of the fifth metatarsal, and several *articulations* should be demonstrated—the articulations between the talus and the navicular, between the calcaneus and the cuboid, between the cuboid and the bases of the fourth and fifth metatarsals, and between the cuboid and the lateral (third) cuneiform.

90. (C) The AP projection of the radius and ulna in Figure 2-17 has anatomical features numbered from 1 to 12 (1, radial tuberosity; 2, neck of radius; 3, head of radius; 4, proximal radioulnar joint; 5, radius; 6, ulna; 7, base of fifth metacarpal; 8, lunate; 9, styloid process of ulna; 10, head of ulna; 11, scaphoid; 12, radial styloid process).

91. (B) Lumbar articular facets, forming the zygapophyseal joints, are demonstrated in the *oblique* position. L1–L4 are best demonstrated in a 45° oblique, whereas L5–S1 are best seen in the 30° oblique. The AP axial projection is used to demonstrate an AP projection of L5–S1.

92. (B) Chest positioning must be correct and accurate; thoracic structures are easily distorted. To avoid *superimposition on the upper medial apices,* the patient's chin should be sufficiently elevated. Movement of the diaphragm to its lowest position is a function of the erect position and of making the exposure after the second inspiration. The MSP is perpendicular to the IR in the PA projection and parallel to the IR in the lateral projection. The position of the chin has little to do with the MSP.

93. (C) Long bones are composed of a body/shaft, or diaphysis, and two extremities. The *diaphysis* is the *primary* ossification center. In the growing bone, the cartilaginous *epiphyseal plate* (located at the extremities of long bones) is gradually replaced by bone. The epiphyses are called the *secondary* ossification centers. The wider portion of bone adjacent to the epiphyseal plate is the *metaphysis*—that portion of long bone where lengthening/bone growth takes place. *Apophysis* refers to a bony projection without an independent ossification center.

94. (B) A *lateral* projection demonstrates the anterior and posterior relationships of structures. A *frontal* projection (AP or PA) demonstrates the *medial* and *lateral* relationships of structures. Two views, at right angles to each other, are generally required of most structures.

95. (A) The 45° oblique projection of the lumbar spine generally is performed for demonstration of the zygapophyseal joints. In a correctly positioned oblique lumbar spine, "Scottie dog" images are demonstrated. The Scottie's ear corresponds to the superior articular process, its nose to the transverse process, its eye to the pedicle, its neck to the pars interarticularis, its body to the lamina, and its front foot to the inferior articular process (Fig. 2-61).

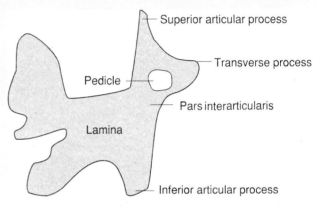

Figure 2-61

96. (A) Figure 2-18 shows the patient positioned on his left side with the IR behind his back. This is a *left lateral decubitus* position. Lying prone with a horizontal x-ray beam is termed a *ventral decubitus position.* The x-ray beam is directed *horizontally* in decubitus positions to demonstrate air–fluid levels. Air or fluid levels will be clearly delineated only if the CR is directed parallel to them. Fluid levels will be best detected on the *down* side (in this case, *left*); air levels will be best detected on the *up* side (in this case, *right*). If the patient were lying on the right side, it would be a *right lateral decubitus position.* If the patient were lying on his or her back with a horizontal x-ray beam, it would be a *dorsal decubitus position.*

97. (C) In the *AP* projection, the proximal fibula is at least partially superimposed on the lateral tibial condyle. *Medial rotation* of 45° will "open" the proximal tibiofibular articulation. *Lateral/external rotation* will obscure the articulation even more.

98. (D) The common carotid arteries function to supply oxygenated blood to the head and neck. Major branches of the common carotid arteries (internal carotids) function to supply the anterior brain, whereas the posterior brain is supplied by the vertebral arteries (branches of the subclavian). The carotid arteries bifurcate into internal and external carotid arteries at the level of C4. The foramen magnum and pharynx are superior to the level of bifurcation, and the larynx is inferior to the level of bifurcation.

99. (B) The position, shape, and motility of various organs can differ greatly from one body habitus to another. The *hypersthenic* individual is large and heavy; the lungs and heart are high, the stomach is high and transverse, the gallbladder is high and lateral, and the colon is high and peripheral. In contrast, the other habitus extreme is the *asthenic* individual. This patient is slender and light and has a long and narrow thorax, a low and long stomach, a low and medial gallbladder, and a low medial and redundant colon. The radiographer must consider these characteristic differences when radiographing individuals of various body types.

100. (C) Figure 2-19 shows a transthoracic lateral projection of the proximal humerus, most often used in trauma situations. The affected humerus is adjacent to the image receptor, the unaffected arm is elevated. The proximal humerus and shoulder joint are projected and visualized through the thorax. The unaffected shoulder is elevated as much as possible to avoid superimposition on the affected shoulder. If sufficient elevation of the unaffected shoulder is not possible, the CR can be directed cephalad 10°–15°. The use of "breathing technique" can further improve visualization of the proximal humerus, as seen in the current image.

101. (A) The hypersthenic body type is large and heavy. The thoracic cavity is short, the lungs are short with broad bases, and the heart is usually in an almost transverse position. The diaphragm is high; the stomach and gallbladder are high and transverse. The large bowel is positioned high and peripheral (and often requires that 14 × 17 inches IRs be placed cross-wise/landscape for imaging a BE).

102. (C) *Hydronephrosis* is a collection of urine in the renal pelvis owing to obstructed outflow, such as from a stricture or obstruction. If the obstruction occurs at the level of the bladder or along the course of the ureter, it will be accompanied by the condition of hydroureter above the level of obstruction. These conditions may be demonstrated during IVU. The term *pyelonephrosis* refers to some condition of the renal pelvis. *Nephroptosis* refers to drooping or downward displacement of the kidneys. This may be demonstrated using the erect position during IVU. *Cystourethritis* is inflammation of the bladder and urethra.

103. (B) The AP projection of the clavicle should demonstrate the clavicular *body/shaft* and its two extremities: the sternal extremity and its associated *sternoclavicular* articulation, and the acromial extremity and its associated *acromioclavicular* articulation. The sternocostal joint is the articulation between the sternum and rib and is not delineated in the AP clavicle image.

104. (C) Perhaps the most important prerequisite to a successful BE examination is a thoroughly clean large bowel. Any retained fecal material can simulate or obscure pathology. A single-contrast examination demonstrates the anatomy and contour of the large bowel, as well as anything that may project out *from* the bowel wall (e.g., diverticula). In a double-contrast examination, the bowel wall (*mucosa*) is coated with barium, and then the lumen is filled with air. This enables visualization of any *intraluminal lesions* such as polyps and tumor masses.

105. (D) To better visualize the joint space in the lateral projection of the knee, 20°–30° of flexion is recommended. The *femoral condyles are superimposed* so as to demonstrate the *patellofemoral joint* and the articulation between the femur and the tibia. The head of the fibula will be slightly superimposed on the proximal tibia. The correct degree of forward or backward body rotation is responsible for visualization of the patellofemoral joint. Cephalad tube angulation of 5°–7° is responsible for demonstrating the articulation between the femur and the tibia (by removing the magnified medial femoral condyle from superimposition on the joint space).

106. (C) Chest radiographs demonstrating *emphysema* will show the characteristic irreversible trapping of air that increases gradually and overexpands the lungs. This produces the characteristic "flattening" of the hemidiaphragms and widening of the intercostal spaces. The increased air content of the lungs requires a compensating decrease in technical factors. *Pneumonia* is inflammation of the lungs, usually caused by bacteria, virus, or chemical irritant. *Pneumothorax* is a collection of air or gas in the pleural cavity (outside the lungs), with an accompanying collapse of the lung. *Pleural effusion* is excessive fluid between the parietal and visceral layers of pleura.

107. (B) *Hematemesis* is the presence of blood in vomit—this can occur with gastric ulcers, gastritis, esophageal varices, and other conditions. The expectoration of blood from the larynx, trachea, bronchi, or lungs is termed *hemoptysis*. Hemoptysis can occur in several diseases, including pneumonia, bronchitis, pulmonary tuberculosis, and others.

108. (D) The walls of the digestive tract/alimentary canal from *outer to inner* are serosa, muscularis, submucosa, and mucosa. The outermost *serosa* is thin and membranous. The muscular layer assists with peristaltic activity and the formation of sphincter muscles. The submucosa is a fairly thick layer of loose connective tissue. The mucosa is the innermost layer, which forms folds called rugae in the stomach.

109. (C) The *external rotation* position is the true *AP position* and places the greater tubercle in profile laterally and places the lesser tubercle anteriorly. The *internal rotation* position demonstrates the lesser tubercle in profile medially and places the humerus in a true lateral position; the greater tubercle is seen superimposed on the humeral head. The epicondyles should be superimposed and perpendicular to the IR. The *neutral position* places the epicondyles about 45° to the IR and places the greater tubercle anteriorly but still lateral to the lesser tubercle.

110. **(C)** A PA projection of the hand is seen with seven anatomical features illustrated in Figure 2-20. Number 1 indicates the triquetrum; number 2 is the pisiform; number 3 is the base of the fifth metacarpal; number 4 is the head of the fifth metacarpal; number 5 is the fifth metacarpophalangeal joint; number 6 is the fifth proximal interphalangeal joint; number 7 is the fifth distal interphalangeal joint.

111. **(C)** The *external rotation* position is the true *AP* position and places the greater tubercle in profile laterally and places the lesser tubercle anteriorly. The *internal rotation* position demonstrates the lesser tubercle in profile medially and places the humerus in a true lateral position; the greater tubercle is seen superimposed on the humeral head. The epicondyles should be superimposed and perpendicular to the IR. The *neutral position* places the epicondyles about 45° to the IR and places the greater tubercle anteriorly but still lateral to the lesser tubercle.

112. **(C)** The PA axial projection (Camp–Coventry method) of the *intercondyloid fossa* (tunnel view) is shown in Figure 2-21. The knee is flexed about 40°, and the CR is directed caudally 40° and perpendicular to the tibia (Fig. 2-62). The patella and patellofemoral articulation are demonstrated in the axial/tangential view of the patella.

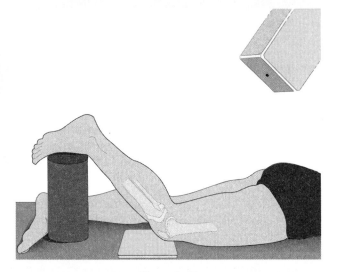

Figure 2-62

113. **(C)** The parietoacanthial projection (Waters' method) demonstrates a distorted view of the frontal and ethmoidal sinuses. The *maxillary sinuses* (number 4) are well demonstrated, projected free of the petrous pyramids. This is also the best single position for the demonstration of *facial bones*. The *mandibular angle* is illustrated by the number 1, the *zygomatic arch* by number 2, and the *coronoid process* by number 3 in Figure 2-22.

114. **(C)** *Diarthrotic,* or synovial, joints are freely movable. Most diarthrotic joints are associated with a joint capsule containing synovial fluid. Diarthrotic joints are the most numerous in the body and are subdivided according to the *type* of movement. Classifications of diarthrotic joints include plane/gliding, trochoid/pivot, ginglymus/hinge, spheroid/ball and socket, ellipsoid/condyloid, sellar/saddle, and bicondylar/modified hinge. *Amphiarthrotic* (cartilaginous) joints are partially movable joints whose articular surfaces are connected by cartilage, such as intervertebral joints. *Synarthrotic* fibrous joints, such as the cranial sutures and gomphosis (roots of teeth), are immovable.

115. **(C)** The carpal scaphoid is somewhat curved and consequently foreshortened radiographically in the PA position. To better separate it from the adjacent carpals, the ulnar flexion (ulnar deviation) maneuver is used frequently. In addition to correcting foreshortening of the scaphoid, ulnar flexion/deviation opens the interspaces between adjacent lateral carpals. Radial flexion/deviation is used to better demonstrate *medial* carpals.

116. **(B)** Figure 2-23 shows an AP projection of the shoulder. A plane passing through the epicondyles is parallel to the IR (and perpendicular to the CR). To project the coracoid process with less self-superimposition, the CR must be angled cephalad 15°. The amount of cephalad angulation depends on the degree of thoracic kyphosis; the greater the degree of kyphosis, the greater is the degree of cephalad angulation required. A 30° angle is used for the average patient.

117. **(B)** The posterior oblique positions (LPO and RPO) are used to demonstrate the zygapophyseal articulations of L1–L4. When correctly positioned, the classic "Scottie dog" should be visualized. If the zygapophyseal articulations are not clearly visualized, and the pedicle is seen on the *posterior* aspect of the vertebral body, patient rotation should be decreased. If the zygapophyseal articulations are not clearly visualized and the pedicle is seen on the *anterior* aspect of the vertebral body, patient rotation should be increased. Pelvic tilt is indicated when iliac crests are not opposite one another.

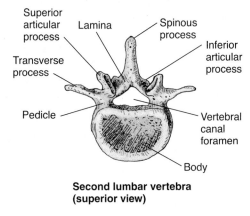

Second lumbar vertebra (superior view)

Figure 2-63

118. **(B)** The type of fracture in which the splintered ends of bone are forced through the skin is a *compound* fracture. In a *closed* fracture, no bone protrudes through the skin.

Compression fractures are seen in stressed areas, such as the vertebrae. A *depressed* fracture would not protrude but rather would be pushed in, for example, zygomatic arch or cranial fractures.

119. **(C)** If the x-ray photons can pass through/between structures such as joint spaces and foramina, these joint spaces and foramina must be situated perpendicular to the IR and parallel to the CR. The intervertebral foramina of the thoracic and lumbar vertebrae are perpendicular to the IR and, therefore, *parallel to the CR* in the *lateral* projection. The cervical intervertebral foramina are well demonstrated when placed 45° to the IR and CR.

120. **(B)** Electronic imaging (CR and DR) uses highly sensitive image-capture devices. Consideration must be given to the SR emerging from the patient and striking the IR. To reduce the amount of SR that reaches the IR, the x-ray beam should be tightly collimated, and a lead mat should be placed on the x-ray table just posterior to the patient's lumbosacral area. The x-ray photons that would have extended posterior to the patient's skin and simply struck the x-ray table—causing increased scattered radiation to reach the IR—will be absorbed by the lead mat. The SID is unrelated to scattered radiation production.

121. **(C)** A Colles fracture usually is caused by a fall onto an outstretched (extended) hand to "break" a fall. The wrist then suffers an impacted transverse fracture of the *distal* inch of the *radius* with an accompanying chip fracture of the *ulnar* styloid process. Because of the hand position at the time of the fall, the fracture usually is *displaced backward* approximately 30°.

122. **(B)** Obstruction of the small bowel is termed *ileus;* there are two types of ileus: paralytic/adynamic and mechanical. *Paralytic* or *adynamic ileus* is characterized by an absence of peristalsis. This can be caused by infection (e.g., appendicitis or peritonitis) or postoperative difficulty. *Mechanical ileus* is caused by some sort of physical obstruction such as tumor or adhesions.

123. **(D)** The tangential projection of the wrist, Gaynor–Hart method demonstrates the carpal canal and several carpals/portions of carpals. This position can be used to evaluate compression of median nerve and to detect carpal fractures. AP oblique hands/Norgaard method, often called the ball-catcher's position, is used to detect evidence of early rheumatoid arthritis. Radial deviation of the wrist is used to demonstrate medial carpals and their articulations. The PA axial projection wrist, Stecher method, is used to demonstrate scaphoid fracture.

124. **(C)** The lateral hand in extension, with appropriate technique adjustment, is recommended to evaluate foreign body location in soft tissue. A small lead marker frequently is taped to the spot thought to be the point of entry. The physician then uses this external marker and the radiograph to determine the exact foreign body location. Extension of the

hand in the presence of a fracture would cause additional and unnecessary pain and possibly additional injury.

125. **(B)** There are five fused sacral vertebrae; the fused transverse processes form the alae. The anterior and posterior sacral foramina transmit spinal nerves. The sacrum articulates superiorly with the fifth lumbar vertebra, forming the L5–S1 articulation, and inferiorly with the coccyx, forming the sacrococcygeal joint. The *sacrum curves posteriorly* and inferiorly, whereas the *coccyx curves anteriorly;* thus, they require different tube angles to "open them up." Figure 2-24A demonstrates an AP axial projection of the sacrum with CR angulation of 15° *cephalad.* Figure 2-24B is an AP axial projection of the coccyx using the required 10° *caudal* CR angle.

126. **(A)** The four types of body habitus describe differences in visceral shape, position, tone, and motility. One body type is *hypersthenic,* characterized by the very large individual with short and wide heart and lungs, and high transverse stomach. The hypersthenic habitus also has a high horizontal gallbladder and peripheral colon. The *sthenic individual* is the average, athletic, most predominant type. The *hyposthenic* patient is somewhat thinner and a little more frail, with organs positioned somewhat lower. The *asthenic* type is smaller in the extreme, with a long thorax, a very long, almost pelvic stomach, and a low medial gallbladder. The colon is medial and redundant. Hypersthenic patients usually demonstrate the greatest motility.

127. **(C)** When a cervical spine radiograph is requested to rule out subluxation or fracture, the patient will arrive in the radiology area on a stretcher. The patient should *not* be moved before a subluxation is ruled out. Any movement of the head and neck could cause serious damage to the spinal cord. A horizontal beam lateral projection is performed and evaluated. The physician then will decide what further images are required.

128. **(D)** The term *proximal* refers to structures closer to the point of attachment. For example, the elbow is described as being *proximal* to the wrist; that is, the elbow is closer to the point of attachment (the shoulder) than is the wrist. Referring to the question, then, the interphalangeal joints (both proximal and distal) and the metacarpals are both *distal* to the carpal bones. The radial styloid process is *proximal* to the carpals.

129. **(C)** The scapular Y projection requires that the *coronal* plane be about 60° to the IR (MSP is about 30°), thus resulting in an *oblique* projection of the shoulder. The vertebral and axillary *borders of the scapula are superimposed on the humeral shaft,* and the resulting relationship between the glenoid fossa and humeral head will demonstrate anterior or posterior dislocation. Lateral or medial dislocation is evaluated on the AP projection.

130. **(D)** An injury to a structure located on the side opposite of the primary injury is called a *contrecoup* injury. For example, a blow to the back of the head will injure frontal and

temporal lobes because they are forced forward against the irregularly shaped bones of the anterior cranial vault. *Blowout* fractures occur to the floor of the orbit on a direct blow. A *Le Fort* fracture involves severe bilateral maxillary fractures. *Contracture* refers to shortening of muscle fibers.

131. (A) The pharynx is the portion of the alimentary canal continuous with the oral cavity. Its three portions, from proximal to distal, are the nasopharynx, the oropharynx, and the laryngopharynx. The laryngopharynx is then continuous with the esophagus. The epiglottis covers the airway/laryngeal opening during swallowing.

132. (B) With the patient in the PA position, the *rami* are well visualized with a perpendicular ray or with 20°–25° of cephalad angulation. A portion of the mandibular body is demonstrated in this position, but most of it is superimposed over the cervical spine.

133. (B) The kidneys lie obliquely in the posterior portion of the trunk with their superior portion angled posteriorly and their *inferior portion and ureters angled anteriorly.* Therefore, to facilitate filling of the most anteriorly placed structures, the patient is examined in the prone position. Opacified urine then flows to the most dependent part of the kidney and ureter—*the ureteropelvic region, inferior calyces, and ureters.*

134. (B) The *median sagittal,* or *midsagittal,* plane (MSP) passes vertically through the midline of the body, dividing it into left and right halves. Any plane parallel to the MSP is termed a *sagittal* plane. The *midcoronal* plane is perpendicular to the MSP and divides the body into anterior and posterior halves. A *transverse* plane passes through the body at right angles to a sagittal plane. These planes, especially the MSP, are very important reference points in radiographic positioning (Fig. 2-64).

135. (C) The diaphragm is the major muscle of respiration. On inspiration/inhalation, the diaphragm and abdominal viscera are depressed, enabling the filling and expansion of the lungs, accompanied by upward movement of the sternum and ribs. During expiration/exhalation, air leaves the lungs and they deflate, and the diaphragm relaxes and moves to a more superior position along with the abdominal viscera. As the diaphragm relaxes and moves up, the sternum and ribs move inferiorly.

136. (B) The radiograph shown in Figure 2-25 illustrates an AP projection of the lumbar spine. The intervertebral disk spaces (number 3) are well visualized because the patient's knees were flexed with feet flat on the table. Number 2 points out the body/spinous process of the first lumbar vertebrae; number 4 is the transverse process

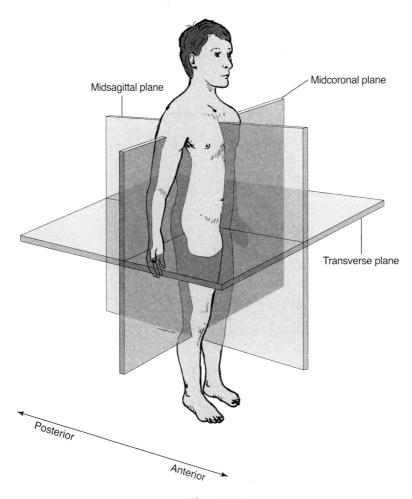

Midsagittal plane

Midcoronal plane

Transverse plane

Posterior

Anterior

Figure 2-64

of L3. Number 1 indicates the right 12th rib. Number 5 indicates the well-defined margins of the psoas muscle.

137. (A) The AP axial projection of the cervical spine demonstrates the bodies and intervertebral spaces of the last five vertebrae (C3–C7). The intervertebral foramina are 45° to the MSP and are therefore demonstrated in the oblique projection. The cervical zygapophyseal joints are 90° to the MSP and are demonstrated in the lateral projection.

138. (C) If structures are overlying or underlying the area to be demonstrated (e.g., the medial femoral condyle obscuring the joint space in the lateral knee projection), CR angulation is used (e.g., 5° cephalad angulation to see the joint space in the lateral knee).

If structures are likely to be foreshortened or self-superimposed (e.g., the scaphoid in a PA wrist), CR angulation may be used to place the structure more closely parallel with the IR.

Another example is the oblique cervical spine, where cephalad or caudad angulation is required to "open" the intervertebral foramina.

Magnification is controlled by object-to-image-receptor distance (OID) and SID; it is unrelated to CR angulation.

139. (C) In the dorsoplantar projection of the foot, the CR may be directed perpendicularly or angled 10° posteriorly. Angulation serves to "open" the tarsometatarsal joints that are not well visualized on the dorsoplantar projection with perpendicular ray. Inversion and eversion of the foot do not affect the tarsometatarsal joints.

140. (A) All of these are the terms used to describe particular body movements. *Eversion* refers to movement of the foot caused by turning the ankle outward. *Inversion* is foot motion caused by turning the ankle inward. *Abduction* is movement of a part away from the midline. *Adduction* is movement of a part toward the midline.

141. (A) The routine AP projection of the lumbar spine demonstrates the intervertebral disk spaces between the first four lumbar vertebrae. The space between L5 and S1, however, is angled with respect to the other disk spaces. Therefore, the CR must be directed 30°–35° cephalad to place it parallel to the disk space, and thus project it open onto the IR.

142. (C) A certain amount of object unsharpness is an inherent part of every radiographic image because of the position and shape of anatomic structures within the body. Structures within the three-dimensional human body lie in different *planes*. In addition, the three-dimensional *shape* of solid anatomic structures rarely coincides with the shape of the divergent beam. Consequently, some structures are imaged with more inherent distortion than others, and shapes of anatomic structures can be entirely misrepresented. Structures *farther* from the IR will be distorted (i.e., *magnified*) more than those *closer* to the IR; structures *closer* to the x-ray source will be distorted (i.e., magnified) more than those *farther* from the x-ray source.

For the *shape* of anatomic structures to be accurately recorded, the structures must be parallel to the x-ray tube and the IR, and aligned with the central ray (CR). *The shape of anatomic structures lying at an angle within the body or placed away from the CR will be misrepresented on the* IR. There are two types of shape distortion. If a linear structure is angled within the body, that is, not parallel with the long axis of the part/body and not parallel to the IR, then that anatomic structure will appear *smaller*—it will be *foreshortened*. On the contrary, *elongation* occurs when the x-ray tube is angled.

Image details placed away from the *path* of the CR will be exposed by more divergent rays, resulting in *rotation distortion*. This is why the CR must be directed to the part of greatest interest.

Unless the edges of a three-dimensional *object* conform to the shape of the x-ray beam, blur or unsharpness will occur at the partially attenuating edge of the object. This can be accompanied by changes in brightness, according to the thickness of areas traversed by the x-ray beam.

143. (C) Patients are instructed to remove all jewelry, hair clips, metal prostheses, coins, and credit cards before entering the room for MRI. MRI does not use radiation to produce images but instead uses a very strong magnetic field. All patients must be screened before entering the magnetic field to be sure that they do not have any metal on or within them. Proper screening includes questioning the patient about any eye injury involving metal, cardiac pacemakers, aneurysm clips, insulin pumps, heart valves, shrapnel, or any metal in the body. This is extremely important, and if there is any doubt, the patient should be rescheduled for a time after it has been determined that it is safe for him or her to enter the room. Patients who have done metalwork or welding are frequently sent to diagnostic radiology for screening images of the orbits to ensure that there are no metal fragments near the optic nerve. Any external metallic objects, such as bobby pins, hair clips, or coins in the pocket, must be removed, or they will be pulled by the magnet and can cause harm to the patient. Credit cards and any other plastic cards with a magnetic strip will be wiped clean if they come in contact with the magnetic field.

144. (C) A lateral projection generally is included in a routine skull series. The patient is placed in a PA oblique position. The *MSP* is positioned parallel to the IR, and the *IOML* is adjusted so as to be parallel to the long axis of the IR. The *interpupillary line* must be perpendicular to the IR. In a routine lateral projection of the skull, the CR should enter approximately 2 inches superior to the EAM.

145. (B) The radiograph shown in Figure 2-26 is a *prone recumbent* projection. If the patient were in the *supine recumbent* position, barium would be located in the fundus of the stomach because the fundus is more posterior, and barium would flow down to fill the posterior structure. If the patient were in the supine *Trendelenburg* position, barium flow to the fundus would be facilitated even more. If the patient were *erect,* air–fluid levels would be clearly defined. In addition, the barium-filled stomach tends to spread more horizontally in the prone position (as seen in the radiograph).

146. (C) The ductus arteriosus is a short fetal blood vessel connecting the aorta and pulmonary artery that usually closes within 10–15 h after birth. A *patent ductus arteriosus* is one that persists and requires surgical closure. *Atrial septal defect* is a small hole (the remnant of the fetal foramen ovale) in the interatrial septum. It usually closes spontaneously in the first months of life; if it persists or is unusually large, surgical repair is necessary. *Ventricular septal defect* is a congenital heart condition characterized by a hole in the interventricular septum that allows oxygenated and unoxygenated blood to mix. Some interventricular septal defects are small and close spontaneously; others require surgery. *Coarctation of the aorta* is a narrowing or constriction of the aorta.

147. (B) The fingers must be supported parallel to the IR (e.g., on a finger sponge) in order that the joint spaces parallel the x-ray beam. When the fingers are flexed or resting on the IR, the relationship between the joint spaces and the IR changes, and the joints appear "closed."

148. (B) Long bones are composed of a body/shaft, or diaphysis, and two extremities. The *diaphysis* is the *primary* ossification center. In the growing bone, the cartilaginous *epiphyseal plate* (located at the extremities of long bones) is gradually replaced by bone. The epiphyses are called the *secondary* ossification centers. The wider portion of bone adjacent to the epiphyseal plate is the *metaphysis*—that portion of long bone where lengthening/bone growth takes place. *Apophysis* refers to a bony projection without an independent ossification center.

149. (C) One of the most important principles in chest radiography is that it should be performed, whenever possible, in the erect position. It is in this position that the diaphragm can descend to its lowest position during inspiration, and any air–fluid levels can be detected. However, patients with mobile examinations can occasionally only be examined in the semi-upright position. If the patient is seated at a 70° angle, rather than 90°, the CR must be directed parallel to the floor. If the CR is angled caudally to compensate for the patients being only semierect, any air–fluid levels can be distorted or obliterated.

150. (A) The abdomen is divided into nine regions. The upper lateral regions are the left and right hypochondriac, with the epigastric separating them. The middle lateral regions are the left and right lumbar, with the umbilical region between them. The lower lateral regions are the left and right iliac, with the hypogastric region between them. The *ileocecal valve,* cecum, and appendix (if present) are located in the lower right abdomen—therefore, the *right iliac region.*

151. (B) Evaluation of the acromioclavicular joints requires *bilateral* AP or PA *erect* projections *with and without the use of weights.* Weights are used to emphasize the minute changes within a joint caused by *separation* or *dislocation.* Weights should be anchored from the patient's wrists rather than held in the patient's hands, because this encourages tightening of the shoulder muscles and obliteration of any small separation.

152. (A) *Ewing sarcoma* is a (primary) malignant bone tumor that arises from bone marrow and occurs in children and young adults. The disease is characterized by new bone formation in a layering effect, giving the bone the characteristic "onion peel" appearance radiographically. *Multiple myeloma* is also a cancerous bone tumor usually affecting adults between the ages of 40 and 70 years. Bone undergoes osteolytic changes, and radiographic demonstration appears as circular areas of bone loss. As their name implies (*chondr*), *enchondroma* and *osteochondroma* involve cartilage; they are both benign conditions.

153. (A) When the patient is recumbent with the head lower than the feet, he or she is said to be in the *Trendelenburg position.* The *decubitus position* is used to describe the patient who is recumbent (prone, supine, or lateral) with the CR directed horizontally. In the *Fowler position,* the patient's head is positioned higher than the feet. The *Sims position* is the (LAO) position assumed for enema tip insertion.

154. (D) The *SMV* projection is made with the patient's head resting on the vertex and the CR directed perpendicular to the IOML. This position may be used as part of a sinus survey to demonstrate the sphenoidal sinuses or as a view of the cranial base for the basal foramina (especially the foramina ovale and spinosum). It also demonstrates the bony part of the auditory (Eustachian) tubes. *AP or PA axial* projections are used frequently to demonstrate the occipital region or evaluate the sellar region. A *lateral* projection is usually part of a routine skull evaluation. The *parietoacanthial* projection is the single best position to demonstrate facial bones.

155. (B) The radiograph in Figure 2-27 illustrates a *lateral* projection of the *cervical spine;* all *seven* cervical vertebrae and the first thoracic vertebra are demonstrated. The zygapophyseal articulations, intervertebral disk spaces, spinous processes, and vertebral bodies are demonstrated. The air-filled structure is the *trachea.* An oblique cervical spine projection would demonstrate the intervertebral foramina.

156. (A) The femur is the longest and strongest bone in the body. The femoral shaft is bowed slightly anteriorly and presents a long, narrow ridge *posteriorly* called the *linea aspera.* The proximal femur consists of a head that is received by the pelvic acetabulum. The femoral neck, which joins the head and shaft, normally angles upward about 120° and forward (in anteversion) about 15°. The greater and lesser trochanters are large processes on the *posterior* proximal femur. The *intertrochanteric crest* runs obliquely between the trochanters; the intertrochanteric line parallels the intertrochanteric crest on the anterior femoral surface. The intercondyloid fossa, a deep notch, is found on the distal posterior femur between the large femoral condyles, and the *popliteal surface* is a smooth surface just superior to the intercondyloid fossa. Just opposite the popliteal surface, on the distal *anterior* femur is the *patellar surface*—a smooth surface for patellar motion during flexion and extension of the knee.

157. (A) The tangential axial projections of the patella are also often called *sunrise* or *skyline views.* The supine flexion 45° (Merchant) position requires a *special apparatus,* and the patellae can be examined bilaterally. This position also requires patient comfort *without muscle tension*—muscle tension can cause a subluxed patella to be pulled into the intercondylar sulcus, giving the appearance of a normal patella. The two prone positions differ according to the degree of flexion used. The 90° flexion (Settegast) position must not be used with suspected patellar fracture. The Hughston position requires the prone position, which can be uncomfortable with patellar injuries; positioning of the x-ray tube is also awkward/difficult in this position and can result in some part distortion.

158. (C) The typical vertebra is divided into two portions: the (anterior) *body* (number 11) and the (posterior) *vertebral arch.* The vertebral arch supports seven processes: two transverse (number 8), one spinous (number 1), two superior articular processes, and two inferior articular processes. A thoracic vertebra is shown in Figure 2-28. The thoracic vertebrae are unique in that they have downward-angling spinous processes and articulations for ribs. Numbers 5 and 10 illustrate the facets where the heads of ribs (number 7) articulate to form the costovertebral articulations (number 6). Number 2 illustrates the ribs' tubercle—it articulates with the transverse process facet (number 9) to form the costotransverse articulation (number 3).

159. (B) In a PA projection of the chest, there should be no rotation, as evidenced by *symmetry* of sternal extremities of clavicles equidistant from vertebral borders. The shoulders are rolled forward to remove the scapulae from the lung fields. Inspiration should be adequate to demonstrate 10 *posterior* ribs above the diaphragm. The air-filled *trachea* should be seen midline; the esophagus is unlikely to be visualized without a contrast agent.

160. (B) The talocalcaneal, or subtalar, joint is a three-faceted articulation formed by the talus and the os calcis (calcaneus). The plantodorsal and dorsoplantar projections of the os calcis should visualize the talocalcaneal joint (Fig. 2-65). This is the only "routine" projection that will demonstrate the talocalcaneal joint. If evaluation of the talocalcaneal joint is desired, special views (such as the Broden and Isherwood methods) are required.

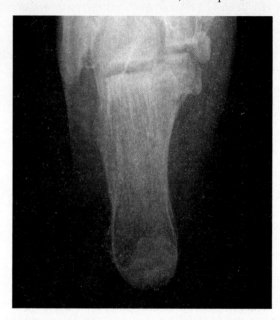

Figure 2-65. Used with permission of Orthopedic + Fracture Specialists, Portland, OR.

161. (C) In a lateral projection of the ankle, the tibia and fibula are superimposed, and the foot is somewhat dorsiflexed to better demonstrate the talotibial joint. The talofibular joint is not visualized because of superimposition with other bony structures. It may be well visualized in the medial oblique projection of the ankle.

162. (B) A double-contrast examination of the large bowel is performed to see through the bowel to its posterior wall and to visualize any intraluminal lesions or masses. Oblique projections are used to "open up" the flexures—the RAO for the hepatic flexure and the LAO for the splenic flexure. To view the redundant S-shaped sigmoid in the AP position, the CR is directed 30°–40° cephalad. The CR is reversed when the patient is in the PA position, that is, the CR is directed 30°–40° caudad.

163. (C) Radiographic examinations of the large bowel generally include the AP or PA axial position to "open" the S-shaped sigmoid colon, the lateral position especially for the rectum, and the LAO and RAO (or LPO and RPO) positions to "open" the colic flexures. The left and right decubitus positions usually are used only in double-contrast barium enemas to better demonstrate double contrast of the medial and lateral walls of the ascending and descending colon.

164. (A) The *15° medial oblique projection* is used to demonstrate the ankle mortise (joint). Although the joint is well demonstrated in the 15° medial oblique projection, there is some superimposition of the distal tibia and fibula, and greater obliquity is required to separate the bones. To best demonstrate the distal tibiofibular articulation, a *45° medial oblique projection* of the ankle is required.

165. (B) There are several types of Salter–Harris fractures. The fracture can be a transverse one through the growth plate or can involve the epiphysis and/or metaphysis as well. Hip dysplasia is a developmental abnormality. Talipes refers to a clubfoot deformity. Osgood–Schlatter disease involves inflammation of the patellar tendon and partial separation of the tibial tuberosity.

166. (A) Visualization of the scapular spine (number 13) indicates that this is a view of the *posterior* aspect of the scapula. The scapula's *anterior,* or *costal,* surface is that which is adjacent to the ribs. The scapula has no sternal articulation.

167–168. (167, A; 168, D) Figure 2-30 depicts a posterior view of the right scapula and its articulation with the humerus (number 4). The scapula presents two borders: the lateral or axillary border (number 7) and the medial or vertebral border (number 9). It also presents three angles: the apex or inferior angle (number 8), the superior angle (number 12), and the lateral angle (number 6). The processes of the scapula are the coracoid (number 2), the acromion (number 3), and the scapular spine (number 13). The scapula has a (supra) scapular notch (number 1), a supraspinatus fossa (number 11), and an infraspinatus fossa (number 10). Number 5 identifies the glenoid fossa—the articular surface for the humeral head, forming the glenohumeral articulation.

169. (C) For the PA projection of the skull, the OML is adjusted perpendicular to the IR, and the MSP must be perpendicular to the IR. The CR is directed so as to exit the nasion. In this position, the petrous pyramids should completely *fill* the orbits. When caudal angulation is used with this position, the petrous pyramids are projected in the *lower portion,* or out of, the orbits. If cephalad angulation is used with this position, the petrous pyramids are projected up toward the occipital region (as in the nuchofrontal projection).

170. (D) A PA axial projection of the skull with a 15° cau-dad angle will show the petrous pyramids in the lower third of the orbits. If *no* angulation is used, the petrous pyramids will fill the orbits. Either PA projection should demonstrate symmetrical petrous pyramids and an equal distance from the lateral border of the skull to the lateral border of the orbit on both sides. This determines that there is no rotation of the skull.

171. (A) The AP oblique positions (RPO and LPO) demonstrate the colonic structures farther from the IR. The LPO

position will demonstrate the hepatic/right colic flexure and ascending colon, whereas the RPO position demonstrates the splenic/left colic flexure and descending colon. In the prone oblique positions (RAO and LAO), the flexure disclosed is the one closer to the IR. Therefore, the LAO position will "open up" the left colic flexure, and the RAO position will demonstrate the right colic flexure.

172. (D) Hysterosalpingography may be performed for demonstration of uterine tubal patency, mass lesions in the uterine cavity, and uterine position. Although hysterosalpingography is often performed to check tubal patency, the uterine anatomy, position, and morphology are also exhibited. In addition, polyps, fibroids, or space-occupying lesions within the uterus are well demonstrated.

173. (B) A right lateral decubitus position will demonstrate a double-contrast visualization of left-sided bowel structures, that is, the lateral side of the descending colon and the medial side of the ascending colon. A left lateral decubitus position will demonstrate a double-contrast visualization of right-sided bowel structures, that is, the lateral side of the ascending colon and the medial side of the descending colon. With the patient in the erect position, barium moves inferiorly and air rises to provide double-contrast visualization of the hepatic and splenic flexures.

174. (A) The cervical intervertebral foramina lie 45° to the MSP and 15°–20° to a transverse plane. When the *PA axial* oblique position (LAO or RAO) is used, the cervical intervertebral foramina demonstrated are those *closer to* the IR. In the *AP axial* oblique position (LPO or RPO), the foramina disclosed are those *farther from* the IR. There is, therefore, some magnification of the foramina in the posterior oblique positions. The interarticular (zygapophyseal) joints and intervertebral joints are best visualized in the lateral projection.

175. (C) With inspiration, the diaphragm moves inferiorly and depresses the abdominal viscera. The ribs and sternum are elevated. As the ribs are elevated, their angle is decreased. Required technical factors can vary considerably depending on the phase of respiration during which the exposure is made.

176. (A) Femoral necks are nonpalpable bony landmarks. The ASIS, pubic symphysis, and greater trochanter are palpable bony landmarks used in radiography of the pelvis and for localization of the femoral necks.

177. (D) Figure 2-31 demonstrates the PA oblique sternum (*RAO* position). Minimal rotation succeeds in projecting the sternum free of superimposition with the vertebral column. The RAO position projects the sternum to the *left* side of the thorax. Superimposing the length of the sternum onto the heart and other mediastinal structures promotes more uniform exposure of the entire sternum. Exposure made during *shallow respiration* serves to obliterate pulmonary vascular markings.

178. (C) In the lateral projection of the knee, the joint space is obscured by the magnified medial femoral condyle unless the CR is angled 5°–7° cephalad. The degree of flexion of the knee is important when evaluating the knee for possible transverse patellar fracture. In such a case, the knee should not be flexed more than 10°. The knee normally should be flexed 20°–30° in the lateral position.

179. (A) During a double-contrast BE, barium and air will distribute themselves according to the position of parts of the colon within the body and according to body position. When the body is in the AP recumbent position, the most anterior structures will be air filled. Anterior structures include the transverse colon and a portion of the sigmoid colon. Both flexures would be air filled in the erect position.

180. (B) The base of the *first metacarpal,* on the lateral side of the hand, articulates with the most lateral carpal of the distal carpal row, the *trapezium*/greater multangular. This articulation forms a rather unique and very versatile *sellar/ saddle joint* named for the shape of its articulating surfaces.

181. (C) The PA (Caldwell) projection of the paranasal sinuses is used to demonstrate the frontal and ethmoidal sinuses. The patient's skull is placed PA, and the OML is elevated 15° from the horizontal. This projects the petrous pyramids into the lower third of the orbits, thus permitting optimal visualization of the frontal and ethmoidal sinuses.

182. (A) With an adult patient in the PA position and the OML perpendicular to the IR, a 15°–20° caudal angulation would place the petrous ridges in the lower third of the orbits. To achieve the same result in an infant or a small child, it is necessary to modify the angle to 10°–15° caudal.

183. (D) During GI radiography, the position of the stomach may vary depending on the respiratory phase, the body habitus, and the patient position. *Inspiration* causes the lungs to fill with air and the diaphragm to descend, thereby pushing the abdominal contents downward. On *expiration,* the diaphragm will rise, allowing the abdominal organs to ascend. Body *habitus* is an important factor in determining the size and shape of the stomach. An asthenic patient may have a long, J-shaped stomach, whereas the stomach of a hypersthenic patient may be transverse. The body habitus is an important consideration in determining the positioning and placement of the IR. The patient *position* also can alter the position of the stomach. If a patient turns from the RAO position to the AP position, the stomach will move to a more horizontal position. Although the cardiac sphincter and the pyloric sphincter are relatively fixed, the fundus is quite mobile and will vary in position.

184. (B) Operative cholangiography can play a vital role in biliary tract surgery. The contrast medium is injected, usually through the CBD, and images are usually made *following* the cholecystectomy. The procedure is used to investigate the patency of the bile ducts, the function of the hepatopancreatic sphincter (of Oddi), and the presence of previously undetected biliary tract calculi.

185. (A) Lateral projections of the barium-filled stomach (Fig. 2-66) may be performed recumbent or upright for demonstration of the retrogastric space. With the patient in the (usually right) lateral position, the CR is directed to a point midway between the midcoronal line and the anterior surface of the abdomen at the level of L1. When the patient is in the LPO or RAO position, the CR should be directed midway between the vertebral column (MCP) and the anterior surface of the abdomen. For the PA projection, the CR is directed perpendicular to the IR at the level of L2.

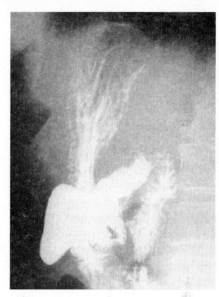

Figure 2-66. Used with permission of Stamford Hospital, Department of Radiology.

186. (B) When the foot is positioned for a lateral projection, the plantar surface should be perpendicular to the IR so as to superimpose the metatarsals. This may be accomplished with the patient lying on either the affected or the unaffected side (usually the affected), that is, mediolateral or lateromedial. The talofibular articulation is best demonstrated in the medial oblique projection of the ankle.

187. (C) When imaging a patient with a possible traumatic spine injury, it is appropriate either to maneuver the x-ray tube head or, if the patient must be moved, to use the logrolling method. This cannot be done by one person; the radiographer must summon assistance. If the patient is on a backboard and in a neck collar, as most patients with suspected spine injury are, it is never appropriate to ask the patient to turn, scoot, or slide over. The only movement that should be permitted is movement of the entire spine, body, and head together, as in logrolling. Any twisting could cause severe and permanent damage to the spinal cord, resulting in paralysis or even death.

188. (B) There are three important fat pads associated with the elbow. The anterior fat pad is located just anterior to the distal humerus. The posterior fat pad is located within the olecranon fossa at the distal posterior humerus. The supinator fat pad/stripe is located at the proximal radius just anterior to the head, neck, and tuberosity. The posterior fat pad is not visible radiographically in the *normal* elbow. All three fat pads can be demonstrated only in the lateral projection of the elbow.

189–190. (189, D; 190, A) The radiograph shown in Figure 2-33 is a lateral projection of the cervical spine taken in flexion. Flexion and extension views are useful in certain cervical injuries, such as whiplash, to indicate the degree of anterior and posterior motion. The structure labeled *number 1* is a *zygapophyseal joint;* because zygapophyseal joints form a 90° angle with the MSP, they are well visualized in the lateral projection. The structure labeled *number 2* is a *vertebral body.* Numbers 3–6 are various components of C1 (atlas) and C2 (axis). The large *body of C2 (number 6)* has a process superiorly, the *odontoid process/dens (number 4).* The odontoid process fits into, and articulates with C1. The superimposed *posterior arch of C1 (atlas)* is indicated by *number 3.* The dens (number 4) is articulated with the *anterior arch of C1 (number 5).*

191. (C) The voiding cystourethrogram (*VCUG*) is a functional study performed to evaluate the physiology of urination to demonstrate possible *vesicoureteral reflux* (backup of urine from bladder into ureters, causing repeated urinary tract infections). The retrograde urogram and retrograde cystogram demonstrate the anatomy (not function) of the urinary tract. The intravenous/excretory urogram does demonstrate function of the urinary tract but does not evaluate the urethra.

192. (C) All traumatic injuries require the radiographer to be particularly alert and observant. Patient status must be observed and monitored continually. The radiographer must speak calmly to the patient, *explaining the procedure* even if the patient appears unconscious or unresponsive. In the case of an injured limb, *both joints must be supported* if any movement is required. *Both joints also must be included* when examining long bones. The injured limb need not be placed in exact AP and lateral positions, but any two views of the part *at right angles to each other* must be obtained.

193. (C) The AP projection demonstrates superimposition of the distal fibula on the talus; the joint space is not well seen. The 15°–20° medial oblique position shows the entire mortise joint; the talofibular joint is well visualized, as well as the talotibial joint. There is considerable superimposition of the talus and fibula in the lateral and lateral oblique projections.

194. (B) To demonstrate the ankle joint space to best advantage, the plantar surface of the foot should be vertical in the AP projection of the ankle. Note that the fibula is the more distal of the two long bones of the lower leg and forms the lateral malleolus. The calcaneus is not well visualized in this projection because of superimposition with other tarsals.

195. (A) Blood is oxygenated in the lungs and carried to the left atrium by four pulmonary veins. From the left atrium, blood flows through the bicuspid (mitral) valve into the left ventricle. Blood leaving the left ventricle is bright red, oxygenated blood that travels through the systemic circulation, which delivers oxygenated blood via arteries and returns deoxygenated blood to the lungs via veins. From the left ventricle, blood first goes through the largest arteries and then goes to progressively smaller arteries (arterioles), to the capillaries, to the smallest veins (venules), and on to progressively larger veins.

196. (A) The sacroiliac joints angle posteriorly and medially 25° to the MSP. Therefore, to demonstrate the sacroiliac joints with the patient in the AP position, the *affected* side must be elevated 25°. This places the joint space perpendicular to the IR and parallel to the CR. Therefore, the RPO position will demonstrate the *left sacroiliac joint,* and the LPO position will demonstrate the *right sacroiliac joint.* When the examination is performed with the patient in the PA position, the *unaffected* side will be elevated 25°.

197. (D) AC joints usually are examined when separation or dislocation is suspected. They must be examined in the erect position, because in the recumbent position a separation appears to reduce itself. Both AC joints are examined simultaneously for comparison because separations may be minimal.

198. (B) *Geriatrics* deals with health care of the aging population; *gerontology* addresses health maintenance, quality of life, disease prevention, and management of this same population. The number of older adults is steadily increasing and health care professionals recognize the unique problems associated with this group. There is an increasing need for chronic care. The causes of death in 70% of people older than 65 years are *stroke, heart disease,* and *cancer.* Radiographers and all health care professionals must be prepared to meet the needs and challenges of this increasing population.

199. (C) The femoral head articulates with the acetabulum to form the hip joint. The femoral neck angles upward approximately 120° and forward (anteversion) approximately 15°. The *axiolateral inferosuperior projection* of the hip (also commonly called a cross-table lateral, horizontal beam lateral, or Danelius-Miller Method) is often used to evaluate suspected femoral neck fracture.

The patient is supine with unaffected leg elevated. If possible, the pelvis is elevated 1–2 inches from the stretcher/x-ray table and the affected leg rotated internally 15° to avoid anteversion; however, rotation must never be attempted when femoral neck fracture or destructive disease is suspected.

The top of the IR is placed just above the crest and adjusted to be parallel to the femoral neck and perpendicular to the CR.

The femoral neck is located 1–2 inches (3–5 cm) medial and 3–4 inches (8–10 cm) distal to the ASIS. The femoral neck is seen radiographically in the same transverse plane as the pubic symphysis and greater trochanters.

200. (C) Figure 2-34 shows an axial projection of the calcaneus. This position requires that the ankle be dorsiflexed. If the plantodorsal projection is used, the central ray is directed 40° cephalad. The calcaneal tuberosity is visualized as well as the talocalcaneal/subtalar joint and the sustentaculum tali. The sinus tarsi and tibiotalar joint are not visualized in this projection.

201. (B) Inhalation of a foreign substance such as water or food particles into the airway and/or bronchial tree is called *aspiration*. *Asphyxia* is caused by deprivation of oxygen as a result of interference with ventilation from trauma, electric shock, and so on. *Atelectasis* is incomplete expansion of a lung or portion of a lung. *Asystole* is cardiac standstill—failure of the heart muscle to contract and pump blood to vital organs.

202. (B) ERCP may be performed to investigate abnormalities of the biliary system or pancreas. The patient's throat is treated with a local anesthetic in preparation for the passage of the endoscope. The hepatopancreatic ampulla (of Vater) is located, and a cannula is passed through it so that contrast medium may be introduced into the common bile duct. Spot images of the common bile duct and pancreatic duct are taken frequently in the oblique position. Direct injection of barium mixture into the duodenum occurs during an enteroclysis procedure of the small bowel.

203. (C) The typical vertebra has two parts: the body and the vertebral arch. The body is the dense, anterior bony mass. The vertebral arch, a ring-like structure, is attached posteriorly. The vertebral arch is formed by two *pedicles* (short, thick processes projecting posteriorly from the body) and two *laminae* (broad, flat processes projecting posteriorly and medially from the pedicles).

204. (C) The IR for a cross-table (axiolateral or horizontal beam) lateral projection of the hip is placed in a vertical position. The top edge of the IR should be placed directly above the iliac crest and adjacent to the *lateral surface* of the affected hip. The IR is positioned *parallel* to the femoral neck; the CR is *perpendicular* to the femoral neck and IR.

205. (B) Radiation protection is exceedingly important in pediatric imaging. Immature tissues have higher radiosensitivity. Gonadal shielding should be used whenever possible; male reproductive organs can be more easily and effectively shielded. When upper extremities are being examined, the torso should be shielded. Radiography of the thorax and skull should be performed *PA* whenever possible to decrease dose to breast tissue and lens of eye. If fluoroscopy is required, pulsed systems with last-image-hold capability deliver less exposure.

206. (B) Radiologic interventional procedures function to *treat* pathologic conditions as well as provide diagnostic information. PTA uses an inflatable balloon catheter under fluoroscopic guidance to increase the diameter of a plaque-stenosed vessel. A *stent* is a cage-like metal device that can be placed in the vessel to provide support to the vessel wall. A PICC is also placed under fluoroscopic control. It is simply a venous access catheter that can be left in place for several months. It provides convenient venous access for patients requiring frequent blood tests, chemotherapy, or large amounts of antibiotics.

207. (C) Hysterosalpingography involves the introduction of a radiopaque contrast medium through a uterine cannula into the uterus and uterine (Fallopian) tubes. This examination is often performed to document patency of the uterine tubes in cases of infertility. A retrograde pyelogram requires cystoscopy and involves introduction of contrast medium through the vesicoureteral orifices and into the renal collecting system. A voiding cystourethrogram also requires cystoscopy and involves filling the bladder with contrast medium and documenting the voiding mechanism. A myelogram is performed to investigate the spinal canal.

208. (B) The *hilus* (hilum) is the slit-like opening on the medial aspect of the lung through which arteries, veins, and lymphatics enter and exit. The *carina* is an internal ridge located at the bifurcation of the trachea into right and left primary, or main stem, bronchi. The *epiglottis* is a flap of elastic cartilage that functions to prevent fluids and solids from entering the respiratory tract during swallowing. The *root* of the lung attaches the lung, via dense connective tissue, to the mediastinum. The root of the left lung is at the level of T6, and the root of the right lung is at T5.

209. (C) Because the heart contracts and relaxes while functioning to pump blood from the heart, arteries that are large and those that are in closest proximity to the heart will feel the effect of the heart's forceful contractions in their walls. The arterial walls pulsate in unison with the heart's contractions. This movement may be detected with the fingers in various parts of the body and is called the *pulse*.

210. (C) The AP axial projection (Towne method) of the skull requires that the CR be angled 30° caudad if the OML is perpendicular to the IR (37° caudad if the IOML is perpendicular to the IR). The frontal and facial bones are projected down and away from superimposition on the occipital bone. If positioning is accurate, the *dorsum sella* and *posterior clinoid processes* will be demonstrated within the foramen magnum. If the CR is angled excessively, the *posterior aspect of the arch of C1* will appear in the foramen magnum.

211. (D) The AP projection will give a general survey and show mediolateral and inferosuperior joint relationships. The scapular Y projection (LAO or RAO position) is used to demonstrate anterior (subcoracoid) or posterior (subacromial) humeral dislocation. The humerus is normally superimposed on the scapula in this position; any deviation from this may indicate dislocation. Rotational projections must be avoided in cases of suspected fracture. The AP and scapular Y combination is the closest to two projections at right angles to each other.

212. (A) The medial oblique projection requires that the leg be rotated medially until the plantar surface of the foot forms a 30° angle with the IR. This position demonstrates the navicular with minimal bony superimposition. The lateral oblique projection of the foot superimposes much of the navicular on the cuboid. The navicular is also superimposed on the cuboid in lateral projections.

213. (C) The *obturator foramen* is a large oval foramen below each acetabulum and is formed by the *ischium and pubis*. The acetabulum is the bony socket that receives the head of the femur to form the hip joint. The upper two-fifths of the acetabulum are formed by the ilium, the lower anterior one-fifth is formed by the pubis, and the lower posterior two-fifths are formed by the ischium. Thus, the acetabulum is formed by all three of the bones that form the pelvis—the ilium, the ischium, and the pubis.

214. (A) The knee is formed by three bones—the proximal tibia, the patella, and the distal femur—which form *two articulations*, the *femorotibial* (hinge joint) and *femoropatellar* (gliding joint). The femoral and tibial condyles articulate to form the *femorotibial joint*. Semilunar cartilages, the *menisci*, lie medially and laterally between these articulating bones and, together with the *cruciate* and *collateral ligaments*, help form the *articular capsule* of the knee.

The *patella* is a triangular bone with its *base* superior and *apex* inferior. The *patella* is the largest *sesamoid* bone and is attached to the tibial tuberosity by the patellar ligament and glides over the patellar surface of the distal femur (femoropatellar joint) during flexion and extension of the knee.

The labrum is a ring of fibrocartilage around the edge of the articular (joint) surface of a bone.

215. (C) The AP projection of the *sacrum* requires a 15° cephalad angle centered 2 inches superior to the pubic symphysis, approximately midway between the pubic symphysis and ASIS. The AP projection of the *coccyx* requires the CR to be directed 10° caudally and centered 2 inches superior to the pubic symphysis.

216. (C) Cartilage degeneration, arthritic changes, and other pathologies of the knee result in changes in the joint bony relationships. These bony relationships are best evaluated in the AP position. *Narrowing of the joint spaces* as a result of cartilage degeneration is readily detected more on AP *weight-bearing erect* projections than on recumbent projections.

217. (B) To avoid the possibility of rotation, weight should be evenly distributed on the feet. The chin should be elevated/extended to prevent its superimposition on pulmonary apices. The shoulders should be *depressed* and rolled forward to remove the scapula from the lung fields. In addition, in the case of large pendulous breasts, the patient should be requested to lift and move them laterally before leaning against the upright mechanism. The well-positioned PA chest should demonstrate scapulae away from lung fields, medial aspect of sternoclavicular joints equidistant from lateral aspect of adjacent vertebra, chin elevated away from lung apices, and inspiration adequate to demonstrate 10 posterior ribs.

218. (D) When the shoulder is placed in *internal rotation*, a greater portion of the glenoid fossa is superimposed by the humeral head, and the *lesser tubercle* is visualized, as in Figure 2-35B. *External rotation* (Figure 2-35A) removes the humeral head from a large portion of the glenoid fossa and better demonstrates the *greater tubercle*.

219. (B) The AP supine projection provides a general survey of the abdomen showing the size and shape of the liver, spleen, and kidneys. When performed erect, it should demonstrate both hemidiaphragms. The lateral projection is sometimes requested and is useful for evaluating the prevertebral space occupied by the aorta. Ventral and dorsal decubitus positions provide a lateral view of the abdomen that is useful for demonstration of air–fluid levels.

220. (C) The skull has two major parts: the cranium, which is composed of 8 bones and houses the brain, and the 14 irregularly shaped facial bones. The inner and outer compact tables of the skull are separated by cancellous tissue called diploe. The internal table has a number of branching meningeal grooves and larger sulci that house blood vessels. Sutures are the synarthrotic articulations between cranial bones. Canaliculi are tiny passages within the bony Haversian system.

221. (D) The patient is supine with the leg(s) *abducted* (drawn away from the midline) approximately 40°. This 40° abduction from the vertical places the long axes of the femoral necks parallel to the IR. The term *adduction* refers to drawing the extremity closer to the midline of the body.

222. (C) After forceful eversion or inversion injuries of the ankle, *AP stress studies* are valuable to confirm the presence of a ligament tear. Keeping the ankle in an AP position, the physician guides the ankle into inversion and eversion maneuvers. Characteristic changes in the relationship of the talus, tibia, and fibula will indicate ligament injury. Inversion stress demonstrates the lateral ligament, whereas eversion stress demonstrates the medial ligament. A fractured ankle would not be manipulated in this manner.

223. (C) When the arm is placed in the *AP* position, the epicondyles are parallel to the plane of the IR, and the shoulder is placed in external rotation. In this position, an AP projection of the humerus, elbow, and forearm can be obtained; it places the greater tubercle of the humerus in profile. For the *lateral* projection of the humerus and the internal rotation projection of the shoulder, the arm is *internally* rotated, elbow somewhat flexed, with the back of the hand against the thigh, and the *epicondyles are superimposed and perpendicular to the IR.* The lateral projections of the humerus, elbow, and forearm all require that the epicondyles be perpendicular to the plane of the IR.

224. (D) Correct and complete patient information about every radiograph is of paramount importance. Each radiographic image must be accurately labeled with patient information such as *name* or *identification number, institution name, date of examination,* and *side marker.* Other information may be included according to institution policy.

225. (D) Although routine elbow projections may be essentially negative, conditions may exist (such as an elevated fat pad) that seem to indicate the presence of a small fracture of the radial head. To demonstrate the entire circumference of the radial head, four exposures are made with the elbow flexed 90° and with the humeral epicondyles superimposed and perpendicular to the IR—one with the hand supinated as much as possible, one with the hand lateral, one with the hand pronated, and one with the hand in internal rotation, thumb down. Each maneuver changes the position of the radial head, and a different surface is presented for inspection.

226. (D) The radiograph shown in Figure 2-36 is made in the right lateral decubitus position. It is part of a series of radiographs made during an air-contrast (double-contrast) BE examination. A double-contrast examination of the large bowel is performed to see *through* the bowel to its posterior wall and to visualize any *intraluminal* (e.g., polypoid) *lesions* or *masses.* Various body positions are used to redistribute the barium and air. To demonstrate the medial and lateral walls of the bowel, decubitus positions are used. The radiograph shows a

right lateral decubitus position because the *barium has gravitated* to the right side (the side of the hepatic flexure). The *air rises* and delineates the medial side of the ascending colon and the lateral side of the descending colon. The posterior wall of the rectum could be visualized using the ventral decubitus position and a horizontal beam lateral to the rectum.

227. (C) Myelography is a radiologic examination of the spinal canal to demonstrate spinal cord impingement from herniated disks, bone fragments, or neoplasms. Water-soluble nonionic contrast material is injected into the subarachnoid space via L2/L3 or L3/L4 (Fig. 2-67). The patient is prone on the fluoroscopic table with footboard and shoulder support in place; the table is tilted to distribute the contrast to the desired vertebral level. The CDC requires that surgical masks be worn when the spinal canal or subdural space is being entered. The image intensifier must be in a locked position to avoid inadvertent intrusion on the spinal needle or sterile field.

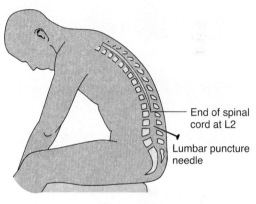

End of spinal cord at L2

Lumbar puncture needle

Figure 2-67

228. (D) Because the kidneys do not lie parallel to the IR in the AP position, the oblique positions are used during IVU to visualize them better. With the AP oblique projections (RPO and LPO positions), the kidney that is *farther* away is placed *parallel* to the IR, and the kidney that is *closer* is placed *perpendicular* to the IR. Therefore, in the LPO position, the *left kidney,* being closer, is *perpendicular* to the IR. The *right kidney,* the one farther away, is placed *parallel* to the IR.

229. (D) Spinal column studies often are required for evaluation of adolescent scoliosis, thus presenting a twofold problem—radiation exposure to youthful gonadal and breast tissues and significantly differing tissue densities/thicknesses. The PA projection reduces dose to the female breasts, the thyroid gland, and the reproductive organs. Electronic imaging (CR/DR) helps to reduce the exposure required for the examination. Exposure–dose concerns are also addressed with the use of a compensating filter (for more uniform receptor exposure) that also incorporates lead shielding for the breasts and gonads (Fig. 2-68).

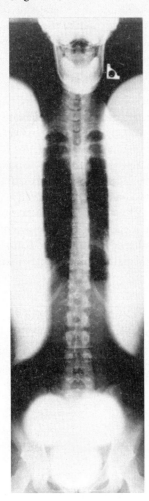

Figure 2-68. Used with permission of Nuclear Associates.

230. (B) *Diarthrodial* joints are freely movable joints that distinctively contain a joint capsule. Contrast medium is injected into this joint capsule to demonstrate the menisci, articular cartilage, bursae, and ligaments of the joint under investigation. *Synarthrodial* joints are immovable joints composed of either cartilage or fibrous connective tissue. *Amphiarthrodial* joints allow only slight movement.

231. (C) The axial trauma lateral (Coyle) position is described. If routine elbow projections in extension are not possible because of limited part movement, these positions can be used to demonstrate the coronoid process and/or radial head. With the elbow flexed *90°* and the CR directed to the elbow joint at an angle of 45° medially (i.e., toward the shoulder), the joint space between the *radial head* and capitulum should be revealed. With the elbow flexed *80°* and the CR directed to the elbow joint at an angle of 45° laterally (i.e., from the shoulder toward the elbow), the elongated *coronoid process* will be visualized.

232. (A) The erect position is used most often to demonstrate air–fluid levels in the chest or abdomen or both. However, patients with traumatic injuries frequently must be examined in the recumbent position. The recumbent position will not demonstrate air–fluid levels unless it is a decubitus position. If free air is being questioned, we will look for that quantity of air on the "up" side because air rises. However, because liver tissue is so homogenous, a small amount of air will be perceived more easily superimposed on it rather than on left-sided structures. Thus, an AP projection obtained in the left lateral decubitus position will best demonstrate a small amount of free air because that air will be superimposed on the liver.

233. (C) Wilms' tumor is a rapidly developing tumor of the kidney(s). It is the most common childhood renal tumor, usually affecting only one kidney. Newer treatments are effective in controlling about 90% of these tumors. Because the kidneys are affected, an *IVU* would be the most appropriate of the examinations listed. Other useful examinations would be CT scan and sonography.

234. (B) When placed in the recumbent lateral position, the average adult's lumbar spine will not be parallel to the x-ray tabletop. Because the shoulders and hips generally are wider than the waist, the vertebral column slopes downward in the central areas—making the lower thoracic and upper lumbar spine closer to the tabletop than the upper thoracic and lower lumbar spine. One solution is to place a radiolucent sponge under the patient's waist. This will elevate the sagging spinal area and make the *vertebral column parallel to the x-ray tabletop and IR*. It will also open the intervertebral disks better, placing more of them parallel to the path of the x-ray photons and *perpendicular to the IR*. This position also places the intervertebral foramina parallel with the path of the CR. The radiolucent sponge is strictly a positioning aid and has no impact on the amount of SR reaching the IR.

235. (D) This is a modification of the parietoacanthial projection (Waters' method) in which the patient is requested to open the mouth, and then the skull is positioned so that the OML forms a 37° angle with the IR. The CR is directed through the sphenoidal sinuses and exits the open mouth. The routine parietoacanthial projection (with mouth closed) is used to demonstrate the maxillary sinuses projected above the petrous pyramids. The frontal and ethmoidal sinuses are best visualized in the PA axial position (modified Caldwell method).

236. (A) Breast tissue is most dense, glandular, and radiographically homogenous in appearance in the postpubertal adolescent. Following pregnancy and lactation, changes occur within the breast that reduce the glandular tissue and replace it with fatty tissue (a process called *fatty infiltration*). Menopause causes further atrophy of glandular tissue.

237. **(D)** Standard radiographic protocols may be reduced to include two views, at right angles to each other, in emergency and trauma radiography. Department policy and procedure manuals include protocols for radiographic examinations. In the best interest of the patient, and to enable the radiologist to make an accurate diagnosis, standard radiographic protocols should be followed. If the radiographer must deviate from the protocol or believes that additional projections may be helpful, then this should be discussed with the radiologist. Emergency and trauma radiography occasionally is an exception to this rule. If the emergency department physician's request varies from the department protocol, the radiographer must respect this. A note should be added to the request so that the radiologist is informed of the reason for a change in protocol. For example, a patient who has been involved in a motor vehicle accident may need many radiographic studies, but the emergency department physician may order only an AP chest and an AP and cross-table lateral C-spine. Standard protocol may include a lateral chest and a cone-down view of the atlas and axis, as well as cervical oblique views. The emergency department physician has made a decision based on experience and expertise that overrules standard protocols. At a later time, when the patient has been stabilized, the patient may be sent back to radiology for additional views.

238. **(C)** The abdomen can be divided into four quadrants or nine regions. The liver, gallbladder, and hepatic/right colic flexure are all located in the RUQ. The stomach and spleen are both normally located in the LUQ.

239. **(B)** The *skull* has two major parts: the *cranium*, which is composed of 8 bones and houses the brain, and the 14 irregularly shaped *facial bones*. The 14 facial bones include the paired *nasal*, *lacrimal*, *palatine*, *inferior nasal conchae*, *maxillae*, and *zygomatic* bones and the unpaired *vomer* and *mandible*. The eight cranial bones are the paired *parietal* and *temporal* bones and the unpaired *frontal*, *occipital*, *ethmoid*, and *sphenoid* bones.

240. **(C)** In the direct PA projection of the wrist, the carpal pisiform is superimposed on the carpal triquetrum. The AP oblique projection (medial surface adjacent to the IR) separates the pisiform and triquetrum and projects the pisiform as a separate structure. The pisiform is the smallest and most palpable carpal.

241. **(C)** Myelography is used to demonstrate encroachment on and compression of the spinal cord as a result of disk herniation, tumor growth, or posttraumatic swelling of the cord. This is accomplished by injecting positive or negative contrast medium into the subarachnoid space. Myelography will demonstrate posterior protrusion of herniated intervertebral disks or spinal cord tumors. Anterior protrusion of a herniated intervertebral disk does not impinge on the spinal cord and is not demonstrated in myelography. Internal disk lesions can be demonstrated only by injecting contrast medium into the individual disks (*diskography*).

242. **(B)** The radiographer must check blood chemistry levels that are associated with renal function before beginning excretory urography. These levels are BUN and creatinine. Normal BUN range is 8–25 mg/100 mL. Normal creatinine range is 0.5–1.2 mg/100 mL. Elevated levels can indicate poor renal function.

243. **(B)** A trimalleolar fracture involves three separate fractures. The lateral malleolus is fractured in the "typical" fashion, but the medial malleolus is fractured on both its medial and posterior aspects. The trimalleolar fracture frequently is associated with subluxation of the articular surfaces.

244. **(B)** The term *supine* refers to being AP recumbent, lying on the back, face up. The AP recumbent position can be used to achieve a *dorsal decubitus* projection. However, to achieve a ventral decubitus projection, a prone position is required.

245. **(C)** Major branches of the common carotid arteries (internal carotids) function to supply the anterior brain, whereas the posterior brain is supplied by the vertebral arteries (branches of the subclavian artery). The brachiocephalic (innominate) artery is unpaired and is one of the three branches of the aortic arch, from which the right common carotid artery is derived. The left common carotid artery comes directly off the aortic arch.

246. **(D)** Barium sulfate suspension is the usual contrast medium of choice for investigation of the alimentary tract. There are, however, a few exceptions. Whenever there is a possibility of escape of contrast medium into the peritoneal cavity, barium sulfate is contraindicated, and a water-soluble iodinated medium is recommended because it is easily aspirated before surgery (or resorbed and excreted by the kidneys). Patients with a ruptured hollow viscus (e.g., perforated ulcer and diverticulitis), those with suspected large bowel obstruction, and those who are scheduled for surgery are examples of patients who should ingest only water-soluble iodinated media.

247. **(C)** There are many terms (with which the radiographer must be familiar) that are used to describe radiographic positioning techniques. *Cephalad* refers to that which is toward the head, and *caudad* refers to that which is toward the feet. Structures close to the source or beginning are said to be *proximal*, whereas those lying away from the source or origin are *distal*. Parts close to the midline are said to be *medial*, and those away from the midline are *lateral*.

248. **(C)** An oblique projection of the lumbar spine is shown in Figure 2-37. This is a 45° LPO projection demonstrating the zygapophyseal joints closest to the IR. The zygapophyseal joints are formed by the articulation of the inferior articular facets of one vertebra with the superior

articular facets of the vertebra below. Note the "Scottie dog" images that appear in the oblique lumbar spine. Intervertebral foramina are best visualized in the lateral lumbar position.

249. **(D)** The chest should be examined in the upright position whenever possible to demonstrate any air–fluid levels. For the lateral projection, the patient elevates the arms well enough to avoid upper-arm soft-tissue superimposition on the lung fields. In the left lateral position, the right posterior ribs, being remote from the IR, will be somewhat magnified and *very slightly* posterior to the left posterior ribs. The MSP must remain vertical to avoid "tilt" distortion, and the coronal plane must be vertical to avoid rotation distortion.

250. **(D)** A cross-sectional image of the abdomen is shown in Figure 2-38. The large structure on the right, labeled number 1, is the liver. The gallbladder is seen as a somewhat darker part on the medial border of the liver. The left kidney is labeled number 4; the right kidney is seen clearly on the other side. The vertebra is labeled number 5, and the psoas muscles are seen just posterior to the vertebra. Just anterior to the body of the vertebra is the circular aorta, labeled number 3 (some calcification can be seen as brighter densities). The somewhat flattened inferior vena cava (number 2) is seen to the left of and slightly anterior to the aorta.

251. **(B)** Statement number 1 describes the PA axial projection (Camp–Coventry method) for demonstration of the intercondyloid fossa. Statement number 2 describes the AP axial projection (Béclère method) for demonstration of the intercondyloid fossa. The positions are actually the reverse of each other. Statement number 3 describes the method of obtaining a PA projection of the patella.

252. **(A)** A lateral projection of the scapula superimposes its medial and lateral borders (vertebral and axillary, respectively). The coracoid and acromion processes should be readily identified separately (not superimposed) in the lateral projection. The entire scapula should be free of superimposition with the ribs. The erect position is probably the most comfortable position for a patient with scapular pain.

253. **(C)** The full length of the nasal septum is best demonstrated in the parietoacanthial (Waters' method) projection. This is also the single best view for facial bones. The PA axial (Caldwell method) projection superimposes the petrous structures over the nasal septum, whereas the lateral projection superimposes and obscures good visualization of the septum. The AP axial projection is used to demonstrate the occipital bone.

254. **(C)** Placing the patient in a 20°–30° AP Trendelenburg position during an upper GI examination helps to demonstrate the presence of a *hiatal hernia*. A 10°–15° Trendelenburg position with the patient rotated slightly to the right also will help demonstrate regurgitation and

hiatal hernia. Filling of the *duodenal bulb* and demonstration of the *duodenal loop* are best seen in the RAO position. *Congenital hypertrophic pyloric stenosis* is caused by excessive thickening of the pyloric sphincter. It is noted in infancy and characterized by projectile vomiting. The pyloric valve will let very little pass through, and as a result, the stomach becomes enlarged (hypertrophied).

255–256. **(255, B; 256, D)** Figure 2-39 illustrates a PA projection of the wrist. This projection best demonstrates visualization of the distal radioulnar joint, the proximal and distal rows of carpals, and the proximal metacarpals (more of the metacarpals should be seen here). The base of the fifth metacarpal is number 4. The trapezium (lateral carpal, distal row) is number 1; the base of the first metacarpal is seen articulating with the trapezium forming the (saddle) carpometacarpal articulation. Number 2 is the scaphoid—the most lateral carpal of the proximal carpal row. Number 3 is the radial styloid process. Number 5 is the pisiform, seen just lateral to, and partially superimposed upon, the triquetrum. Number 6 is the ulnar styloid process.

257. **(D)** A decubitus projection is obtained using a *horizontal* x-ray beam. The type of decubitus projection is dependent on the patient's recumbent position. When the patient is lying *AP recumbent* (i.e., *supine*), the patient is said to be in the dorsal decubitus position. When the patient is lying *prone,* he or she is in the ventral decubitus position. If the patient is lying in the *left or right lateral recumbent* position with the x-ray beam directed horizontally, the patient is said to be in the left or right lateral decubitus position, respectively. A *perpendicular* x-ray beam is used to obtain an AP or PA abdomen.

258. **(C)** The degree of anterior and posterior motion occasionally is diminished with a whiplash type of injury. Anterior (forward, flexion) and posterior (backward, extension) motion is evaluated in the lateral position, with the patient assuming the best possible flexion and extension. Left- and right-bending images of the thoracic and lumbar vertebrae are obtained frequently when evaluating scoliosis.

259. **(A)** When one cheekbone is depressed, a tangential projection is required to "open up" the zygomatic arch and draw it away from the overlying cranial bones. This is accomplished by placing the patient in the SMV position, rotating the head 15° toward the affected side, and centering to the zygomatic arch. A 30° rotation places the mandibular shadow over the zygomatic arch.

260. **(B)** Lisfranc injury is characterized by separation and/or avulsion fracture involving the bases of the first and second metatarsals and cuneiforms. It is a common soccer or football injury caused by falling onto a pointed downward foot. Osgood–Schlatter disease involves detachment of the tibial tuberosity by the patellar tendon; it is also a sports-related injury. A Jones fracture is

an avulsion fracture at the base of the fifth metatarsal; it is often caused by bending the foot inward when the toes are pointed. A Pott fracture is an avulsion fracture of the medial malleolus with lateral movement of the talus and possible fracture of lateral malleolus.

261. **(C)** Accurate positioning of the skull requires the use of several baselines. In Figure 2-40, line 1 represents the *glabellomeatal line* (GML), line 2 is the *orbitomeatal line* (OML), line 3 is the *infraorbitomeatal line* (IOML), and line 4 is the *acanthomeatal line* (AML). The OML and the IOML usually are separated by 7°. The OML and the GML usually are separated by 8°; therefore, there is a *15° difference between the GML and the IOML*. It is useful to remember these differences because CR angulation must be adjusted when using a baseline other than the one recommended for a particular position. For example, if it is recommended that the CR be angled *30° to the OML,* then the CR would be angled *37° to the IOML.*

262. **(D)** The lateral projection of the skull requires that the patient be in the prone oblique position with the MSP *parallel* to the IR and the interpupillary line perpendicular to the IR. This position requires that the IOML (line 3) be parallel to the long axis of the IR. The AP and PA axial projections of the skull require the OML or IOML to be *perpendicular* to the IR.

263. **(B)** The term *orthoroentgenography* is sometimes used to describe the radiographic measurement of long bone length. Long bone measurement can be required in adults or children with extremity length (especially leg) discrepancies. This can be performed most easily with the use of a special metallic ruler/scale (*Bell–Thompson scale*) secured to the x-ray tabletop adjacent to the limb being examined (or between both limbs for simultaneous bilateral examination). A 14 × 17 inches IR is in the Bucky tray (to permit movement of the IR between exposures), and three well-collimated exposures are made—at the hip joint, the knee joint, and the ankle joint. The visible ruler markings adjacent to the limb enable accurate limb measurements. A *cannula* is a tube placed in a cavity to introduce or withdraw material and is unrelated to long bone measurement.

264. **(C)** *Intervertebral joints* (occupied by the intervertebral disks) are well visualized in the lateral projection of all the vertebral groups. Cervical articular facets (forming *zygapophyseal/interarticular joints*) are 90° to the midsagittal plane and, therefore, are well demonstrated in the *lateral* projection. The cervical *intervertebral foramina* lie 45° to the midsagittal plane (and 15°–20° to a transverse plane) and, therefore, are demonstrated in the *oblique* position.

265. **(C)** The patient is placed in a true lateral position, and the CR is directed perpendicular to a point 1/2 inch distal to the nasion. An 8 × 10 inches IR divided in half may be used for this procedure.

266. **(B)** Within the body/shaft of a long bone is the medullary cavity, containing bone marrow and lined by a membrane called *endosteum*. In adults, *yellow marrow* is the most abundant and occupies the body/shaft, and *red marrow* is found within the *proximal* and *distal* extremities of long bones. Bone marrow, particularly red, is important in the production of blood cells—a process called *hematopoiesis*.

267. **(D)** X-ray arthrography requires the use of local anesthesia; sterile technique must be observed to avoid introducing infection into the joint. Fluoroscopy is used for proper placement of the needle and to obtain images immediately after the introduction of contrast medium. Many physicians follow up the x-ray arthrogram with a magnetic resonance (MR) arthrogram to visualize additional soft-tissue structures. Arthrography is performed to detect compromised knee capsule structures, meniscal damage, ligament tears, and Baker cysts.

268. **(D)** In the recumbent position, the upper portion of the stomach occupies a more posterior position in the body than the distal aspect of the stomach. Therefore, in the AP recumbent position (or LPO position), *barium* moves easily into the *fundus* of the stomach (from the more distal portions of the stomach), displacing/drawing the stomach somewhat superiorly. The fundus is filled with barium, whereas the *air* that had been in the fundus is now displaced into the *gastric body, pylorus,* and *duodenum,* illustrating them in *double contrast.* Double-contrast delineation of these structures allows us to see *through* the stomach to the retrogastric areas and structures. The RAO position demonstrates a *barium-filled* pylorus and duodenum. *Anterior and posterior aspects* of the stomach are visualized in the *lateral* position; medial and lateral aspects of the stomach are visualized in the AP projection.

269. **(D)** The phase of respiration is exceedingly important in thoracic radiography, because lung expansion and the position of the diaphragm strongly influence the appearance of the finished radiograph. Inspiration and expiration radiographs of the chest are taken to demonstrate air in the pleural cavity (*pneumothorax*), to demonstrate *atelectasis* (partial or complete collapse of one or more pulmonary lobes) or the degree of *diaphragm excursion,* or to detect the presence of a *foreign body.* The expiration image will require a somewhat greater exposure (6–8 kV more) to compensate for the diminished quantity of air in the lungs.

270. **(C)** Shoulder arthrograms (Fig. 2-69) are used to evaluate rotator cuff tear, glenoid labrum (a ring of fibrocartilaginous tissue around the glenoid fossa), and frozen shoulder. Routine radiographs demonstrate arthritis, and the addition of a transthoracic humerus or scapular Y projection would be used to demonstrate luxation (dislocation).

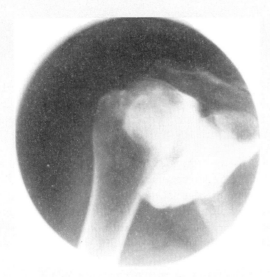

Figure 2-69. Used with permission of Stamford Hospital, Department of Radiology.

271. (D) In the *AP* projection of the elbow, the proximal radius and ulna are partially superimposed. In the *lateral* projection, the radial head is partially superimposed on the coronoid process, facing anteriorly. In the *medial oblique* projection, there is even greater superimposition. The *lateral oblique* projection completely separates the proximal radius and ulna, projecting the radial head, neck, and tuberosity free of superimposition with the proximal ulna.

272. (D) Bone tissue, or *osseous* (*os* = bone) tissue, is a specialized type of dense connective tissue. This tissue consists of bone cells (*osteocytes*) embedded in a nonliving matrix composed of calcium and collagen fibers. There are two types of osseous tissue: *cancellous* (spongy) and *compact* (hard, cortical).

Cancellous, or spongy, bone tissue has a reticular or latticework-type structure. This network of lattice-like bone is called *trabeculae.* These trabeculae form little spaces/septa filled with red bone marrow.

The structural unit of *compact* bone tissue is the Haversian (osteon) system. One Haversian system, or osteon, consists of a central Haversian canal surrounded by concentric cylinders of osteocytes within the calcium matrix.

273. (B) There are several surface landmarks and localization points that can help the radiographer in positioning various body structures. The *jugular notch,* located at the superior aspect of the manubrium, is approximately opposite the T2–T3 interspace. The *sternal angle* is located opposite the T4–T5 interspace. The *xiphoid* (or ensiform) *process* is located opposite T10.

274. (D) With the patient in the AP position, the scapula and upper thorax are normally superimposed. With the arm abducted, the elbow flexed, and the hand supinated, much of the scapula is drawn away from the ribs. The patient should not be rotated toward the affected side, because this causes superimposition of ribs on the scapula. The exposure is made during quiet breathing to obliterate pulmonary vascular markings.

275. (D) The two *innominate* bones (os coxae) make up the *pelvis.* Each innominate bone is made up of three bones: ilium, ischium, and pubis. These three bones contribute to the formation of the acetabulum. When the interior of the acetabulum is viewed, it shows that the ilium comprises its upper two-thirds, the ischium comprises its lower posterior two-thirds, and the pubis comprises the lower anterior one-third of the acetabulum.

276. (B) Traumatic fractures of the hand and wrist are common. A *boxer* fracture involves the distal end (neck) of the fourth or fifth metacarpal and often includes posterior displacement/angulation of the fractured metacarpals' proximal structures. The fracture is termed "boxer" because it is usually caused by the blow of a clenched fist (as in boxing) against a hard, unyielding object such as a muscular/bony body part or a structure such as a wall. A Colles fracture involves the distal portion of the radius. A Pott fracture is a complete fracture of the distal fibula. A Bennett fracture involves the base of the first metacarpal and carpometacarpal joint.

277. (C) Deoxygenated (venous) blood from the *upper* body (i.e., head, neck, thorax, and upper extremities) empties into the *superior vena cava.* Deoxygenated (venous) blood from the *lower* body (i.e., abdomen, pelvis, and lower extremities) empties into the *inferior vena cava.* The superior and inferior venae cavae empty into the right atrium. The coronary sinus, which returns venous blood from the heart, also empties into the right atrium. Deoxygenated blood passes from the right atrium through the tricuspid valve into the right ventricle. From the right ventricle, blood is pumped (during ventricular systole) through the pulmonary semilunar valve into the pulmonary artery—the only artery that carries deoxygenated blood. From the pulmonary artery, blood travels to the lungs, picks up oxygen, and is carried by the four pulmonary veins (the only veins carrying oxygenated blood) to the left atrium. The oxygenated blood passes through the mitral (or bicuspid) valve during atrial systole and into the left ventricle. During ventricular systole, oxygenated blood from the left ventricle passes through the aortic semilunar valve into the aorta and into the systemic circulation.

278. (C) The ribs below the diaphragm are best demonstrated with the diaphragm elevated. This is accomplished by placing the patient in a *recumbent* position and by taking the exposure at the end of *exhalation.* Conversely, the ribs above the diaphragm are best demonstrated with the diaphragm depressed. Placing the patient in the erect position and taking the exposure at the end of deep inspiration accomplishes this.

279. (A) Esophageal varices are tortuous dilatations of the esophageal veins. They are much less pronounced in the erect and semierect (Fowler) position and always must be examined with the patient recumbent. The recumbent position affords more complete filling of the veins because blood flows against gravity.

280. **(A)** The *plantodorsal* projection of the os calcis/calcaneus is described. It is performed *supine* and requires cephalad angulation. The CR enters the plantar surface and exits the dorsal surface. The axial *dorsoplantar* projection requires that the CR enters the dorsal surface of the foot and exits the plantar surface.

281. **(D)** To clearly demonstrate the atlas and axis without superimposition of the teeth or the base of the skull, a line between the maxillary occlusal plane (edge of upper teeth) and mastoid tip must be vertical. If the head is flexed too much, the teeth will be superimposed. If the head is extended too much, the cranial base will be superimposed on the area of interest. A line between the mentum and the mastoid tip is used to demonstrate the odontoid process only through the foramen magnum (Fuchs method).

282. **(A)** The respiratory passageways include the nose, pharynx, larynx (upper respiratory structures), trachea, bronchi, and lungs (lower structures). If obstruction of the breathing passageways occurs in the *upper* respiratory tract, above the larynx (i.e., in the nose or pharynx), *tracheotomy* may be performed to restore breathing. *Intubation* can be done into the *lower* structures, larynx, and trachea, moving aside any soft obstruction and restoring the breathing passageway.

283–284. **(283, A; 284, C)** Figure 2-41 illustrates the aortic arch (number 1) and its three main branches—the brachiocephalic artery (number 6), the left common carotid artery (number 4), and the left subclavian artery (number 2). The right common carotid artery (number 5) and the right subclavian artery (number 7) are branches of the brachiocephalic artery. The vertebral arteries are the first main branch of the subclavian arteries. The left vertebral artery is labeled number 3.

285. **(B)** When injury requires that the elbow be examined in partial flexion, the lateral projection offers little difficulty, but the AP projection requires special attention. If the AP radiograph is made with a perpendicular CR and the olecranon process resting on the tabletop, the articulating surfaces are obscured. With the elbow in partial flexion, *two exposures are necessary*. One is made with the forearm parallel to the IR (humerus elevated), which demonstrates the proximal forearm. The other is made with the humerus parallel to the IR (forearm elevated), which demonstrates the distal humerus. In both cases, the CR is perpendicular if the degree of flexion is not too great or is angled slightly into the joint space with greater degrees of flexion.

286. **(B)** The parietoacanthial (Waters' method) projection demonstrates the *maxillary* sinuses. The modified Waters' position, with the CR directed through the open mouth, will demonstrate the sphenoid sinuses through the open mouth. The PA axial projection demonstrates the *frontal and ethmoidal* sinus groups. The lateral projection, with the CR entering 1 inch posterior to the outer canthus, demonstrates *all* the paranasal sinuses. X-ray examinations of the sinuses always should be performed *erect* to demonstrate leveling of any fluid present.

287. **(B)** The typical vertebra, shown in Figure 2-70, is divided into two portions: the *body* (anteriorly) and the *vertebral arch* (posteriorly). The vertebral arch supports seven processes: two transverse, one spinous (number 3), two superior articular (number 4), and two inferior articular (number 2). The superior articular processes and the superjacent inferior articular processes join to form zygapophyseal joints. Pedicles (number 5) project posteriorly from the vertebral body (number 6). Their upper and lower surfaces form vertebral notches. Superjacent vertebral notches form intervertebral foramina. The *lamina* is represented by number 1. The transverse and spinous processes serve as attachments for muscles or articulations for ribs in the thoracic region. The superior and inferior surfaces of the vertebral body are covered with articular cartilage, and between the vertebral bodies lie the intervertebral disks.

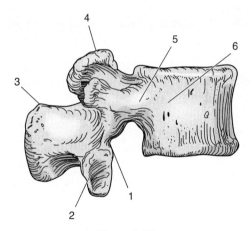

Figure 2-70

288. **(A)** The straight PA projection (0°), with CR directed perpendicular to the IR, effectively demonstrates the mandibular body. In this position, the rami and condyles are superimposed on the occipital bone and petrous portion of the temporal bone. To better visualize the rami and condyles, the CR is directed cephalad 20°–30°.

289. **(D)** A fluoroscopic unit with spot device and tilt table should be used for endoscopic retrograde pancreatography. The Trendelenburg position is sometimes necessary to fill the interhepatic ducts, and a semierect position may be necessary to fill the lower end of the common bile duct. A fiberoptic endoscope for locating the hepatopancreatic

ampulla and polyethylene catheters for the introduction of contrast medium are also necessary.

290. (B) Intussusception is a type of mechanical obstruction involving *telescoping* of a portion the pediatric large intestine, causing obstruction. Volvulus is a condition of the pediatric intestine involving *twisting* of intestinal loops, causing obstruction. These are described as mechanical conditions. Paralytic (adynamic) ileus is a type of obstruction caused as a result of loss of intestinal motility/contraction.

291. (A) In an AP projection of the shoulder, there is superimposition of the humeral head and glenoid fossa. With the patient obliqued 45° toward the affected side, the glenohumeral joint is open, and the glenoid fossa is seen in profile. The patient's arm is abducted somewhat and placed in internal rotation.

292. (C) An *intrathecal* injection is one made within the spinal meninges. A myelogram requires an intrathecal injection to introduce contrast medium into the subarachnoid space. An IVU requires an intravenous injection; a retrograde pyelogram requires that contrast medium be introduced into the ureters by way of cystoscopy. A cystogram requires that contrast medium be introduced via catheter into the urinary bladder.

293. (A) The vertebral/neural *arch* is formed by two pedicles and two laminae. The vertebral *foramen* is formed by two pedicles, two lamina, and vertebral body. The pedicles and laminae support the transverse processes, articular processes, and spinous process.

294. (C) The posterior oblique positions (LPO and RPO) of the lumbar vertebrae demonstrate the zygapophyseal joints closer to the IR. The left zygapophyseal joints are demonstrated in the LPO position, whereas the right zygapophyseal joints are demonstrated in the RPO position. The lateral position is useful to demonstrate the intervertebral disk spaces, intervertebral foramina, and spinous processes.

295–297. (295, B; 296, B; 297, B) An AP, external rotation, projection of the shoulder is pictured in Figure 2-43. The hand is supinated, and the arm is in the anatomical position. Therefore, the greater tubercle (number 3) is well visualized. The greater portion of the clavicle, the acromioclavicular joint (number 1), the acromion process (number 2), the coracoid process (number 4), and the glenohumeral joint (number 5) are seen.

298. (C) On the *AP* projection of the elbow, the radial head and ulna normally are somewhat superimposed. The *lateral oblique* projection demonstrates the radial head free of ulnar superimposition. The *lateral* projection demonstrates the olecranon process in profile. The *medial oblique* projection demonstrates considerable overlap of the proximal radius and ulna but should clearly demonstrate the

coronoid process free of superimposition and the olecranon process within the olecranon fossa.

299. (B) In the lateral position of the skull, the *midsagittal plane* must be *parallel* to the IR and the interpupillary line vertical. Flexion of the head is adjusted until the *IOML* is *parallel* to the IR. The CR should enter about *2 inches superior* to the EAM. The centering point for a lateral sella turcica is 3⁄4 inch anterior and superior to the EAM.

300. (C) For the lateral projections of the hand, wrist, forearm, and elbow, the elbow must be flexed 90° to superimpose the distal radius and ulna and humeral epicondyles. Although a lateral humerus can be performed with the elbow flexed, if flexion is not possible, the elbow may remain in the anteroposterior (AP) position and a transthoracic lateral projection of the upper one-half to two-thirds of the humerus may be obtained. Because a coronal plane passing through the epicondyles (interepicondylar line) is perpendicular to the IR in this position, the epicondyles will be superimposed. To obtain a lateral projection of the thumb (first digit), the patient's wrist must be somewhat internally rotated. Remember that an oblique projection of the thumb is obtained in a PA projection of the hand.

301. (C) The forward slipping of one vertebra on the one below it is called *spondylolisthesis*. *Spondylolysis* is the breakdown of the pars interarticularis; it may be unilateral or bilateral and results in forward slipping of the involved vertebra—the *condition* of spondylolisthesis. Inflammation of one or more vertebrae is called *spondylitis*. *Spondylosis* refers to degenerative changes occurring in the vertebra.

302. (C) Long bones are composed of a body/shaft, or diaphysis, and two extremities. The *diaphysis* is the *primary* ossification center. In the growing bone, the cartilaginous *epiphyseal plate* (located at the extremities of long bones) is gradually replaced by bone. The epiphyses are called the *secondary* ossification centers. The wider portion of bone adjacent to the epiphyseal plate is the *metaphysis*—that portion of long bone where lengthening/bone growth takes place. *Apophysis* refers to a bony projection without an independent ossification center.

303. (B) The male and female bony pelves have several differing characteristics; male/female pelvic anatomy differs more than any other body anatomy. An overview of comparisons is listed as follows:

Male pelvis
- The general structure is heavy and thick.
- The greater, or false, pelvis is deep.
- The pelvic brim, or inlet, is small and heart-shaped.
- The acetabulum is large and faces laterally.
- The pubic angle is less than 90°.
- The ilium is more vertical.

Female pelvis
- The general structure is light and thin.
- The greater, or false, pelvis is shallow.
- The pelvic brim, or inlet, is large and oval.
- The acetabulum is small and faces anteriorly.
- The pubic angle is more than 90°.
- The ilium is more horizontal.

304. (B) Note the relationship between the thigh, lower leg, patella, and CR. The CR is directed *parallel to the plane of the patella*, thereby providing a *tangential* projection of the patella (i.e., patella in profile) and an unobstructed view of the *patellofemoral articulation*. Figure 2-45 illustrates how the image is obtained with the patient in the prone position. Many patients may not be able to assume the prone position. The same relationship between the CR, part, and IR can be obtained in the lateral recumbent position or the seated position (Fig. 2-71A and B). The erect AP would superimpose the patella on other bony structures.

305. (D) Figure 2-46 illustrates a PA projection of the chest and the side marker correctly placed. The heart is seen on the *right* side—this is termed *dextrocardia*. Atelectasis (partial or complete collapse of lung) would be demonstrated as increased *tissue* density in the affected area. A classic pneumothorax (air within the thoracic cavity) would demonstrate an absence of lung markings in the affected area and flattening of the hemidiaphragm on the affected side. A small pneumothorax can be easily missed on a chest image with excessive or insufficient brightness.

306. (A) A lateral projection of the lumbar spine is illustrated. The intervertebral articulations (disk spaces) are well demonstrated. The intervertebral foramina are 90° to the MSP, forming the pedicles, and are well demonstrated in the lateral projection. The vertebral foramina, forming the space occupied by the spinal cord, can only be visualized via CT. The articular facets, forming the zygapophyseal joints, lie 30°–50° to the MSP and are visualized in the oblique position.

307. (D) When the clavicle is examined in the PA recumbent position, the CR must be directed 15°–30° caudad to project most of the clavicle's length above the ribs. The direction of the CR is reversed when examining the patient in the AP position.

308. (C) Diagnostic x-ray examinations that require contrast agents include upper GI series, lower GI series (BE), and IVU. Patient preparation is somewhat different for each of these examinations. The patient scheduled for an *upper GI series* must receive NPO (nothing by mouth) after midnight. A *lower GI series* (BE) requires that the large bowel be very clean prior to the administration of barium; this requires the administration of *cathartics* (laxatives) and cleansing enemas. Patient is usually allowed a light breakfast the morning of the exam.

Preparation for an IVU requires that the patient be NPO after midnight; some institutions also require that the large bowel be cleansed of gas and fecal material. Aftercare for barium examinations is very important. Patients typically are instructed to take Milk of Magnesia, increase their intake of fiber, drink plenty of water, and expect changes in stool color until all barium is evacuated and to call their physician if they do not have a bowel movement within 24 h. Because water is removed from the barium sulfate suspension in the large bowel, it is essential to make patients understand the importance of these instructions to avoid barium impaction in the large bowel. The use of barium sulfate suspensions is contraindicated when ruling out *visceral perforation*.

309. (C) The skeleton's design functions to *protect* vital internal organs such as the heart and lungs. Bone stores important *minerals* (e.g., calcium and phosphorus) and releases them into the blood as needed. Yellow bone marrow is mainly composed of fat cells and stores triglycerides for use as an energy reserve. The endocrine system is associated with hormone production; the integumentary system includes the skin that is important in protection and excretion; the muscular system is responsible for movement and heat production.

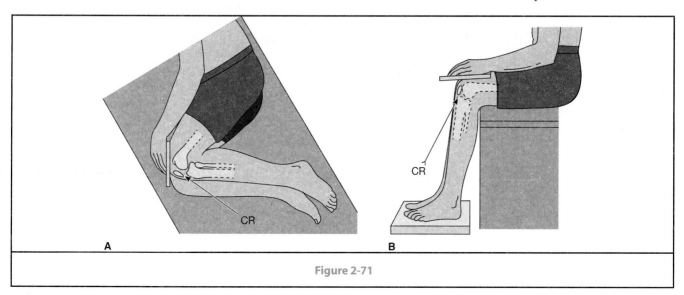

Figure 2-71

310. (B) *Intussusception* is the telescoping of one part of the intestinal tract into another. It is a major cause of bowel obstruction in children, usually in the region of the ileocecal valve, and is much less common in adults. Radiographically, intussusception appears as the classic "coil spring," with barium trapped between folds of the telescoped bowel. The diagnostic BE procedure occasionally can reduce the intussusception, although care must be taken to avoid perforation of the bowel. *Appendicitis* occurs when an obstructed appendix becomes inflamed. Distension of the appendix occurs, and if the appendix is left untended, gangrene and perforation can result. *Regional enteritis* (Crohn's disease) is a chronic granulomatous inflammatory disorder that can affect any part of the GI tract but generally involves the area of the terminal ilium. Ulceration and formation of fistulous tracts often occur. *Ulcerative colitis* occurs most often in young adults; its etiology is unknown, although psychogenic or autoimmune factors seem to be involved.

311. (B) Changes in hormone levels affect changes in the glandular tissue of the breast. These breast tissue changes are seen during breast development, during pregnancy and lactation, and during menopause. Women at higher risk of developing breast cancer include those who have experienced early menses (before age 12 years), late menopause (after age 52 years), and nulliparity (no full- or late-term pregnancies). Risks other than hormonal include family and personal history and age. The greatest single risk factor for breast cancer is gender—being female. Although occurrence of breast cancer in men is not unknown, it is fairly rare.

312. (C) The bony pelvis is shaped like a basin and the ilia are foreshortened in an AP projection. If the patient is obliqued 40°, affected side down, this places the iliac wing parallel to the IR. The hip of the affected side is centered to the midline and the CR is directed perpendicularly at the level of the ASIS. Sacroiliac joints can be demonstrated using AP oblique (25°–30°) projections (LPO and RPO positions), affected side up.

313. (C) In the PA position, portions of the barium-filled hypersthenic stomach superimpose on themselves. Thus, patients with a hypersthenic body habitus usually present a high transverse stomach with poorly defined curvatures. If the PA stomach is projected with a *35°–45° cephalad* CR, the stomach "opens up." That is, the curvatures, the antral portion, and the duodenal bulb all appear as a sthenic habitus stomach would appear. A 35°–40° *RAO* position is used to demonstrate many of these structures in the average, or sthenic, body habitus. A *lateral* position is used to demonstrate the anterior and posterior gastric surfaces and retrogastric space.

314. (C) The parietoacanthial projection (Waters' position) provides an oblique frontal projection of the facial bones. The maxilla (and antra), zygomatic arches, and orbits are well demonstrated. The patient is positioned PA with the head resting on the extended chin so that the OML forms a 37° angle with the IR. The position may be reversed if the patient is positioned AP and the CR is directed 30° cephalad to the IOML. This position is not preferred, however, because the facial bones are significantly magnified as a result of increased OID.

315. (C) The foot is composed of the 7 tarsal bones, 5 metatarsals, and 14 phalanges. The metatarsals and phalanges are miniature long bones; each has a shaft, base (proximal), and head (distal). The bases of the first to third metatarsals articulate with the three cuneiforms. The bases of the fourth and fifth metatarsals articulate with the cuboid. The heads of the metatarsals articulate with the bases of the first row of phalanges.

316. (B) The first cervical vertebra/atlas is a ring-like structure having no body. It consists of an anterior arch, a posterior arch, two lateral masses, and two transverse processes. The transverse processes have transverse foramina for the passage of the vertebral artery and vertebral vein. The odontoid process is part of the second cervical vertebra/axis, whose odontoid process projects behind the anterior arch of C1.

317. (B) Patient motion can present imaging and positioning difficulties for the radiographer. Involuntary motion is that over which the patient has little or no control. Causes of involuntary motion include tremors, chill, peristalsis, heart motion, pain, and spasm. Inability to control voluntary motion is sometimes encountered in those with mental illness, in young children and in the elderly. Patients who are excitable or nervous can experience difficulty with voluntary functions such as holding their breath or not moving.

318. (C) External body landmarks are used as an aid for accurate positioning. For example, C5 is at the level of the thyroid cartilage. The xiphoid process of the sternum is at the level of T9–T10. The jugular notch is at the level of T2–T3. The inferior costal margin is at the level of L2–L3. L4–L5 identifies the top of the iliac crest.

319. (C) Articulations are classified according to the type of connective tissue with which they are associated. *Cartilaginous* joints have no joint cavity; the structures are held together by fibrous or hyaline cartilage. They permit little or no motion. *Fibrous* articulations also have no joint cavity; their structures are held together by fibrous tissue that permits no motion. Synovial articulations are the most numerous in the body and they are freely movable.

320. (C) The humerus is a long bone having a body/shaft and two articular extremities. The parts of the humerus identified are correctly ordered from distal to proximal as trochlea, medial epicondyle, body/shaft, surgical neck, lesser tubercle, anatomical neck, and head. Additional features of the humerus with which the radiographer should be familiar are the capitulum, coronoid fossa, radial fossa, lateral epicondyle, lesser tubercle, and intertubercular groove.

SUBSPECIALTY LIST

Question Number and Subspecialty correspond to subcategories in each of the four ARRT examination specification sections

1. Extremity procedures
2. Extremity procedures/upper extremities
3. Extremity procedures/lower extremities
4. Extremity procedures/upper extremities
5. Head, spine and pelvis procedures/spine and pelvis
6. Extremity procedures/upper extremities
7. General procedural considerations
8. Thorax and abdomen procedures/thorax
9. Head, spine and pelvis procedures/head
10. Thorax and abdomen procedures/thorax
11. Thorax and abdomen procedures/thorax
12. Extremity procedures/lower extremities
13. Thorax and abdomen procedures/abdomen and GI studies
14. Thorax and abdomen procedures/abdomen and GI studies
15. Head, spine and pelvis procedures/head
16. Extremity procedures/lower extremities
17. Extremity procedures/lower extremities
18. Thorax and abdomen procedures/abdomen and GI studies
19. General procedural considerations
20. Head, spine and pelvis procedures/head
21. Extremity procedures/lower extremities
22. Thorax and abdomen procedures/thorax
23. Thorax and abdomen procedures/thorax
24. Extremity procedures
25. Extremity procedures/lower extremities
26. Thorax and abdomen procedures/thorax
27. Head, spine and pelvis procedures/spine and pelvis
28. Head, spine and pelvis procedures/head
29. Head, spine and pelvis procedures/head
30. Extremity procedures/upper extremities
31. Thorax and abdomen procedures/thorax
32. Extremity procedures
33. Head, spine and pelvis procedures/spine and pelvis
34. Thorax and abdomen procedures/abdomen and GI studies
35. Thorax and abdomen procedures/thorax
36. Extremity procedures/lower extremities
37. Extremity procedures/upper extremities
38. Extremity procedures/upper extremities
39. Head, spine and pelvis procedures/spine and pelvis
40. Extremity procedures/upper extremities
41. Head, spine and pelvis procedures/head
42. Head, spine and pelvis procedures/head
43. Thorax and abdomen procedures/thorax
44. Thorax and abdomen procedures/abdomen and GI studies
45. Thorax and abdomen procedures/abdomen and GI studies
46. Head, spine and pelvis procedures/spine and pelvis
47. Extremity procedures/upper extremities
48. Thorax and abdomen procedures/abdomen and GI studies
49. Thorax and abdomen procedures/thorax
50. Extremity procedures/lower extremities
51. Thorax and abdomen procedures/thorax
52. Extremity procedures/lower extremities
53. Head, spine and pelvis procedures/head
54. Extremity procedures/upper extremities
55. General procedural considerations
56. Extremity procedures/lower extremities
57. Extremity procedures/upper extremities
58. Thorax and abdomen procedures/thorax
59. Head, spine and pelvis procedures/spine and pelvis
60. Head, spine and pelvis procedures/spine and pelvis
61. Extremity procedures/upper extremities
62. Extremity procedures/lower extremities
63. Extremity procedures/upper extremities
64. Thorax and abdomen procedures/thorax
65. Head, spine and pelvis procedures/spine and pelvis
66. Extremity procedures
67. Extremity procedures/upper extremities
68. Extremity procedures/upper extremities
69. Head, spine and pelvis procedures/spine and pelvis
70. Head, spine and pelvis procedures/head
71. Extremity procedures/upper extremities
72. Head, spine and pelvis procedures/spine and pelvis
73. Head, spine and pelvis procedures/spine and pelvis
74. Head, spine and pelvis procedures/spine and pelvis
75. Extremity procedures/upper extremities

76. Extremity procedures/lower extremities
77. Head, spine and pelvis procedures/spine and pelvis
78. Thorax and abdomen procedures/thorax
79. Thorax and abdomen procedures/thorax
80. Thorax and abdomen procedures/thorax
81. Thorax and abdomen procedures/thorax
82. Thorax and abdomen procedures/thorax
83. Extremity procedures
84. Head, spine and pelvis procedures/spine and pelvis
85. Head, spine and pelvis procedures/spine and pelvis
86. Head, spine and pelvis procedures/head
87. Head, spine and pelvis procedures/head
88. Head, spine and pelvis procedures/spine and pelvis
89. Extremity procedures/lower extremities
90. Extremity procedures/upper extremities
91. Head, spine and pelvis procedures/spine and pelvis
92. Thorax and abdomen procedures/thorax
93. Extremity procedures
94. Extremity procedures/lower extremities
95. Head, spine and pelvis procedures/spine and pelvis
96. Thorax and abdomen procedures/thorax
97. Extremity procedures/lower extremities
98. Head, spine and pelvis procedures/head
99. Thorax and abdomen procedures/abdomen and GI studies
100. Extremity procedures/lower extremities
101. General procedural considerations
102. Thorax and abdomen procedures/abdomen and GI studies
103. Extremity procedures/upper extremities
104. Thorax and abdomen procedures/abdomen and GI studies
105. Extremity procedures/lower extremities
106. Thorax and abdomen procedures/thorax
107. Thorax and abdomen procedures/abdomen and GI studies
108. Thorax and abdomen procedures/abdomen and GI studies
109. Extremity procedures/upper extremities
110. Extremity procedures/upper extremities
111. Extremity procedures/upper extremities
112. Extremity procedures/lower extremities
113. Head, spine and pelvis procedures/head
114. Extremity procedures
115. Extremity procedures/upper extremities
116. Extremity procedures/upper extremities
117. Head, spine and pelvis procedures/spine and pelvis
118. Extremity procedures
119. Head, spine and pelvis procedures/spine and pelvis
120. Head, spine and pelvis procedures/spine and pelvis
121. Extremity procedures/upper extremities
122. Thorax and abdomen procedures/abdomen and GI studies
123. Extremity procedures/upper extremities
124. Extremity procedures/upper extremities
125. Head, spine and pelvis procedures/spine and pelvis
126. General procedural considerations
127. Head, spine and pelvis procedures/spine and pelvis
128. Extremity procedures/upper extremities
129. Extremity procedures/upper extremities
130. General procedural considerations
131. Thorax and abdomen procedures/thorax
132. Head, spine and pelvis procedures/head
133. Thorax and abdomen procedures/abdomen and GI studies
134. General procedural considerations
135. Thorax and abdomen procedures/thorax
136. Head, spine and pelvis procedures/spine and pelvis
137. Head, spine and pelvis procedures/spine and pelvis
138. General procedural considerations
139. Extremity procedures/lower extremities
140. Extremity procedures/lower extremities
141. Head, spine and pelvis procedures/spine and pelvis
142. General procedural considerations
143. General procedural considerations
144. Head, spine and pelvis procedures/head
145. Thorax and abdomen procedures/abdomen and GI studies
146. Thorax and abdomen procedures/thorax
147. Extremity procedures/upper extremities
148. Extremity procedures
149. Thorax and abdomen procedures/thorax
150. Thorax and abdomen procedures/abdomen and GI studies
151. Extremity procedures/upper extremities
152. Extremity procedures
153. General procedural considerations
154. Head, spine and pelvis procedures/head
155. Head, spine and pelvis procedures/spine and pelvis
156. Extremity procedures/lower extremities
157. Extremity procedures/lower extremities
158. Head, spine and pelvis procedures/spine and pelvis
159. Thorax and abdomen procedures/thorax
160. Extremity procedures/lower extremities
161. Extremity procedures/lower extremities
162. Thorax and abdomen procedures/abdomen and GI studies
163. Thorax and abdomen procedures/abdomen and GI studies
164. Extremity procedures/lower extremities
165. Extremity procedures

166. Extremity procedures/upper extremities
167. Extremity procedures/upper extremities
168. Extremity procedures/upper extremities
169. Head, spine and pelvis procedures/head
170. Head, spine and pelvis procedures/head
171. Thorax and abdomen procedures/abdomen and GI studies
172. Head, spine and pelvis procedures/spine and pelvis
173. Thorax and abdomen procedures/abdomen and GI studies
174. Head, spine and pelvis procedures/spine and pelvis
175. Thorax and abdomen procedures/thorax
176. Head, spine and pelvis procedures/spine and pelvis
177. Thorax and abdomen procedures/thorax
178. Extremity procedures/lower extremities
179. Thorax and abdomen procedures/abdomen and GI studies
180. Extremity procedures/upper extremities
181. Head, spine and pelvis procedures/head
182. Head, spine and pelvis procedures/head
183. Thorax and abdomen procedures/abdomen and GI studies
184. Thorax and abdomen procedures/abdomen and GI studies
185. Thorax and abdomen procedures/abdomen and GI studies
186. Extremity procedures/lower extremities
187. Head, spine and pelvis procedures/spine and pelvis
188. Extremity procedures/upper extremities
189. Head, spine and pelvis procedures/spine and pelvis
190. Head, spine and pelvis procedures/spine and pelvis
191. Thorax and abdomen procedures/abdomen and GI studies
192. Extremity procedures/upper extremities
193. Extremity procedures/lower extremities
194. Extremity procedures/lower extremities
195. Thorax and abdomen procedures/thorax
196. Head, spine and pelvis procedures/spine and pelvis
197. Extremity procedures/upper extremities
198. General procedural considerations
199. Head, spine and pelvis procedures/spine and pelvis
200. Extremity procedures/lower extremities
201. Thorax and abdomen procedures/thorax
202. Thorax and abdomen procedures/abdomen and GI studies
203. Head, spine and pelvis procedures/spine and pelvis
204. Head, spine and pelvis procedures/spine and pelvis
205. General procedural considerations
206. Thorax and abdomen procedures/abdomen and GI studies
207. Thorax and abdomen procedures/abdomen and GI studies
208. Thorax and abdomen procedures/thorax
209. Thorax and abdomen procedures/thorax
210. Head, spine and pelvis procedures/head
211. Extremity procedures/upper extremities
212. Extremity procedures/lower extremities
213. Head, spine and pelvis procedures/spine and pelvis
214. Extremity procedures/lower extremities
215. Head, spine and pelvis procedures/spine and pelvis
216. Extremity procedures/lower extremities
217. Thorax and abdomen procedures/thorax
218. Extremity procedures/upper extremities
219. Thorax and abdomen procedures/abdomen and GI studies
220. Head, spine and pelvis procedures/head
221. Head, spine and pelvis procedures/spine and pelvis
222. Extremity procedures/lower extremities
223. Extremity procedures/upper extremities
224. General procedural considerations
225. Extremity procedures/upper extremities
226. Thorax and abdomen procedures/abdomen and GI studies
227. Head, spine and pelvis procedures/spine and pelvis
228. Thorax and abdomen procedures/abdomen and GI studies
229. Head, spine and pelvis procedures/spine and pelvis
230. Extremity procedures
231. Extremity procedures/upper extremities
232. Thorax and abdomen procedures/abdomen and GI studies
233. Thorax and abdomen procedures/abdomen and GI studies
234. Head, spine and pelvis procedures/spine and pelvis
235. Head, spine and pelvis procedures/head
236. General procedural considerations
237. General procedural considerations
238. Thorax and abdomen procedures/abdomen and GI studies
239. Head, spine and pelvis procedures/head
240. Extremity procedures/upper extremities
241. Head, spine and pelvis procedures/spine and pelvis
242. Thorax and abdomen procedures/abdomen and GI studies
243. Extremity procedures/lower extremities
244. General procedural considerations
245. Head, spine and pelvis procedures/head
246. Thorax and abdomen procedures/abdomen and GI studies
247. General procedural considerations
248. Head, spine and pelvis procedures/spine and pelvis

CHAPTER 2 • PROCEDURES

249. Thorax and abdomen procedures/thorax
250. Head, spine and pelvis procedures/spine and pelvis
251. Extremity procedures/lower extremities
252. Extremity procedures/upper extremities
253. Head, spine and pelvis procedures/head
254. Thorax and abdomen procedures/abdomen and GI studies
255. Extremity procedures/upper extremities
256. Extremity procedures/upper extremities
257. Thorax and abdomen procedures/abdomen and GI studies
258. Head, spine and pelvis procedures/spine and pelvis
259. Head, spine and pelvis procedures/head
260. Extremity procedures/lower extremities
261. Head, spine and pelvis procedures/head
262. Head, spine and pelvis procedures/head
263. Extremity procedures
264. Head, spine and pelvis procedures/spine and pelvis
265. Head, spine and pelvis procedures/head
266. Extremity procedures
267. Extremity procedures/lower extremities
268. Thorax and abdomen procedures/abdomen and GI studies
269. Thorax and abdomen procedures/thorax
270. Extremity procedures/upper extremities
271. Extremity procedures/upper extremities
272. Extremity procedures
273. Head, spine and pelvis procedures/spine and pelvis
274. Extremity procedures/upper extremities
275. Head, spine and pelvis procedures/spine and pelvis
276. Extremity procedures/lower extremities
277. Thorax and abdomen procedures/thorax
278. Thorax and abdomen procedures/thorax
279. Thorax and abdomen procedures/abdomen and GI studies
280. Extremity procedures/lower extremities
281. Head, spine and pelvis procedures/spine and pelvis
282. Thorax and abdomen procedures/thorax
283. Thorax and abdomen procedures/thorax
284. Thorax and abdomen procedures/thorax
285. Extremity procedures/upper extremities

286. Head, spine and pelvis procedures/head
287. Head, spine and pelvis procedures/spine and pelvis
288. Head, spine and pelvis procedures/head
289. Thorax and abdomen procedures/abdomen and GI studies
290. Thorax and abdomen procedures/abdomen and GI studies
291. Extremity procedures/upper extremities
292. Head, spine and pelvis procedures/spine and pelvis
293. Extremity procedures/lower extremities
294. Head, spine and pelvis procedures/spine and pelvis
295. Extremity procedures/upper extremities
296. Extremity procedures/upper extremities
297. Extremity procedures/upper extremities
298. Extremity procedures/upper extremities
299. Head, spine and pelvis procedures/head
300. Extremity procedures/upper extremities
301. Head, spine and pelvis procedures/spine and pelvis
302. Extremity procedures
303. Head, spine and pelvis procedures/spine and pelvis
304. Extremity procedures/lower extremities
305. Thorax and abdomen procedures/thorax
306. Head, spine and pelvis procedures/spine and pelvis
307. Extremity procedures/upper extremities
308. Thorax and abdomen procedures/abdomen and GI studies
309. General procedural considerations
310. Thorax and abdomen procedures/abdomen and GI studies
311. Thorax and abdomen procedures/thorax
312. Head, spine and pelvis procedures/spine and pelvis
313. Thorax and abdomen procedures/abdomen and GI studies
314. Head, spine and pelvis procedures/head
315. Head, spine and pelvis procedures/spine and pelvis
316. Head, spine and pelvis procedures/spine and pelvis
317. General procedural considerations
318. Thorax and abdomen procedures/thorax
319. Extremity procedures
320. Extremity procedures/upper extremities

TARGETED READING

Lampignano JP, Kendrick LE. *Bontrager's Textbook of Radiographic Positioning and Related Anatomy.* 9th ed. St Louis, MO: Mosby Elsevier; 2018.

Long BW, Rollins JH, Smith BJ. *Merrill's Atlas of Radiographic Positioning and Procedures.* Vols 1-3. 13th ed. St Louis, MO: Mosby; 2016.

Mills WR. The relation of bodily habitus to visceral form, tonus, and motility. *Am J Roentgenol.* 1917;4:155-169.

Peart O. *Lange Radiographic Positioning Flashcards.* New York, NY: McGraw Hill; 2014.

Saia DA. *Radiography PREP.* 9th ed. New York, NY: McGraw Hill; 2018.

Saladin KS. *Anatomy and Physiology: The Unity of Form and Function.* 7th ed. New York, NY: McGraw Hill; 2015.

Safety

QUESTIONS

DIRECTIONS: Each of the numbered items or incomplete statements in this section is followed by answers or by completions of the statement. Select the appropriate letter answer(s) or completion(s) for each of the numbered items or incomplete statements in this section.

1. What type of personnel radiation monitoring device has a gas-filled ionization chamber and provides a reading at any time via Internet connection?
   - ❏ A. Pocket dosimeter
   - ❏ B. Direct ion storage dosimeter
   - ❏ C. Optically stimulated luminescence dosimeter
   - ❏ D. Thermoluminescent dosimeter

2. Figure 3-1 is representative of
   - ❏ A. the production of Compton scatter
   - ❏ B. the photoelectric effect
   - ❏ C. the production of Bremsstrahlung x-ray photons
   - ❏ D. the production of characteristic x-rays

3. A time of 5 min is required for a particular fluoroscopic examination, whose exposure rate is 150 mGy$_a$/h. What is the approximate radiation exposure for the radiologic staff present in the fluoroscopy room during the examination?
   - ❏ A. 75 mGy$_a$
   - ❏ B. 37.5 mGy$_a$
   - ❏ C. 12.5 mGy$_a$
   - ❏ D. 3.75 mGy$_a$

4. Stochastic/probabilistic effects of radiation are those that
   1. have a threshold
   2. may be described as "all-or-nothing" effects
   3. are late effects
      - ❏ A. 1 only
      - ❏ B. 1 and 2 only
      - ❏ C. 2 and 3 only
      - ❏ D. 1, 2, and 3

5. The uppermost collimator shutter functions to eliminate
   - ❏ A. off-focus radiation
   - ❏ B. leakage radiation
   - ❏ C. scatter radiation
   - ❏ D. primary radiation

6. *Somatic effects* of radiation refer to effects that are manifested
   - ❏ A. in the descendants of the exposed individual
   - ❏ B. during the life of the exposed individual
   - ❏ C. in the exposed individual and his or her descendants
   - ❏ D. in the reproductive cells of the exposed individual

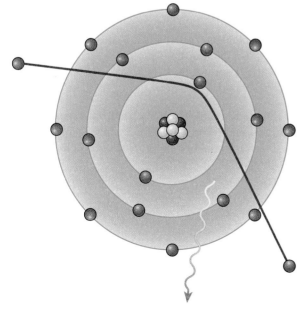

Figure 3-1

7. Guidelines for the use of protective shielding state that gonadal shielding should be used
   1. if the patient has reasonable reproductive potential
   2. when the gonads are within 5 cm of the collimated field
   3. when tight collimation is not possible
   - ❏ A. 1 only
   - ❏ B. 1 and 2 only
   - ❏ C. 1 and 3 only
   - ❏ D. 2 and 3 only

8. The skin response to radiation exposure, which appears as reddening of the irradiated skin area, is known as
   - ❏ A. dry desquamation
   - ❏ B. moist desquamation
   - ❏ C. erythema
   - ❏ D. epilation

9. Increasing field size, while leaving technical factors unchanged, will
   - ❏ A. decrease the DAP
   - ❏ B. decrease SR production
   - ❏ C. increase the DAP
   - ❏ D. increase the EFS size

10. The single most important source of scattered radiation in both radiography and fluoroscopy is the
    - ❏ A. x-ray table
    - ❏ B. x-ray tube
    - ❏ C. patient
    - ❏ D. IR

11. Which acute radiation syndrome requires the largest exposure before the associated effects become apparent?
    - ❏ A. Hematopoietic
    - ❏ B. Gastrointestinal
    - ❏ C. Cerebrovascular
    - ❏ D. Skeletal

12. How are kV and HVL related?
    - ❏ A. Directly
    - ❏ B. Inversely
    - ❏ C. Inverse squared
    - ❏ D. Direct squared

13. Occupational radiation monitoring is required when it is possible that the individual might receive more than
    - ❏ A. 0.05 mSv
    - ❏ B. 0.1 mSv
    - ❏ C. 5 mSv
    - ❏ D. 50 mSv

14. Sources of natural background radiation contributing to whole-body radiation dose include
    1. dental x-rays
    2. terrestrial radionuclides
    3. internal radionuclides
    - ❏ A. 1 only
    - ❏ B. 1 and 2 only
    - ❏ C. 2 and 3 only
    - ❏ D. 1, 2, and 3

15. Which of the following tissues is/are considered to be particularly radiosensitive?
    1. Intestinal mucous membrane
    2. Epidermis of extremities
    3. Optic nerves
    - ❏ A. 1 only
    - ❏ B. 1 and 2 only
    - ❏ C. 2 and 3 only
    - ❏ D. 1, 2, and 3

16. Diagnostic x-radiations are correctly described as
    - ❏ A. low energy, low LET
    - ❏ B. low energy, high LET
    - ❏ C. high energy, low LET
    - ❏ D. high energy, high LET

17. What is used to account for differences in tissue characteristics when determining effective dose to biologic material?
    1. Tissue weighting factors (W_t)
    2. Radiation weighting factors (W_r)
    3. Absorbed dose
    - ❏ A. 1 only
    - ❏ B. 1 and 2 only
    - ❏ C. 2 and 3 only
    - ❏ D. 1, 2, and 3

18. The x-ray interaction with matter that is responsible for the majority of scattered radiation reaching the image receptor (IR) is
    - ❏ A. the photoelectric effect
    - ❏ B. Compton scatter
    - ❏ C. classical scatter
    - ❏ D. Thompson scatter

19. The exposure rate to a body 5 m from a source of radiation is 50 mGy$_a$/h. Which of the following distances would best decrease the exposure to 10 mGy$_a$/h?
    - ❏ A. 2.2 m
    - ❏ B. 5 m
    - ❏ C. 11 m
    - ❏ D. 25 m

20. Types of secondary radiation barriers include
   1. the control booth
   2. lead aprons
   3. the x-ray tube housing
   ❏ A. 2 only
   ❏ B. 1 and 2 only
   ❏ C. 2 and 3 only
   ❏ D. 1, 2, and 3

21. Late radiation–induced somatic effects include
   1. thyroid cancers
   2. cataractogenesis
   3. reduced fertility
   ❏ A. 1 only
   ❏ B. 1 and 2 only
   ❏ C. 2 and 3 only
   ❏ D. 1, 2, and 3

22. Each time an x-ray photon scatters, its intensity at 1 m from the scattering object is what fraction of its original intensity?
   ❏ A. 1/10
   ❏ B. 1/100
   ❏ C. 1/500
   ❏ D. 1/1000

23. The law of Bergonié and Tribondeau states that cells are more radiosensitive if they are
   1. highly proliferative
   2. highly differentiated
   3. immature
   ❏ A. 1 only
   ❏ B. 1 and 2 only
   ❏ C. 1 and 3 only
   ❏ D. 1, 2, and 3

24. A thermoluminescent dosimetry system uses which of the following crystals?
   ❏ A. Silver halide
   ❏ B. Sodium thiosulfate
   ❏ C. Lithium fluoride
   ❏ D. Aluminum oxide

25. A controlled area is one that is occupied by
   1. radiology personnel
   2. patients
   3. anyone
   ❏ A. 1 only
   ❏ B. 2 only
   ❏ C. 1 and 2 only
   ❏ D. 3 only

26. All of the following have an effect on patient dose, *except*
   ❏ A. kilovoltage
   ❏ B. milliampere seconds
   ❏ C. focal spot size
   ❏ D. inherent filtration

27. The degree of x-ray attenuation is directly related to what quality of the radiographed part?
   ❏ A. Valence electrons
   ❏ B. Binding energy
   ❏ C. Atomic number
   ❏ D. Electron shells

28. An increase in total filtration of the x-ray beam will increase
   ❏ A. patient skin dose
   ❏ B. beam HVL
   ❏ C. image contrast
   ❏ D. milliroentgen (mR) output

29. In radiation protection, the product of absorbed dose, tissue weighting factor, and radiation weighting factor is used to determine
   ❏ A. C/kg
   ❏ B. mR
   ❏ C. EfD
   ❏ D. QF

30. Which of the following is recommended for the pregnant radiographer?
   ❏ A. Change dosimeters weekly
   ❏ B. Wear a second dosimeter under the lead apron
   ❏ C. Wear two dosimeters and switch their positions appropriately
   ❏ D. Leave radiation areas for duration of the pregnancy

31. The annual dose limit for medical imaging personnel includes radiation from
   1. occupational exposure
   2. background radiation
   3. medical x-rays
   ❏ A. 1 only
   ❏ B. 1 and 2 only
   ❏ C. 2 and 3 only
   ❏ D. 1, 2, and 3

32. Neurologic anomalies will most likely occur if an exposure dose of 40 mGy (40 rad) was delivered to a pregnant uterus during the
   ❏ A. 3rd week of pregnancy
   ❏ B. 9th week of pregnancy
   ❏ C. 15th week of pregnancy
   ❏ D. 24th week of pregnancy

33. If a quantity of ionizing radiation is delivered to a body over a long period of time, the effect
   ❏ A. will be greater than if it were delivered all at one time
   ❏ B. will be less than if it were delivered all at one time
   ❏ C. has no relation to how it is delivered in time
   ❏ D. depends solely on the radiation quality

34. Moving the image intensifier closer to the patient during fluoroscopy
1. decreases patient dose
2. improves image quality
3. decreases the SID
   ❏ A. 1 only
   ❏ B. 1 and 2 only
   ❏ C. 1 and 3 only
   ❏ D. 1, 2, and 3

35. Which of the following types of radiation is/are considered electromagnetic?
1. X-ray
2. Visible light
3. Gamma
4. Ultraviolet light
5. Beta
   ❏ A. 1, 3, and 5
   ❏ B. 2, 3, 4, and 5
   ❏ C. 1, 2, 3, and 4
   ❏ D. 2, 3, and 5
   ❏ E. 3, 4, and 5

36. How does filtration affect the primary beam?
1. It increases the average energy of the primary beam
2. It decreases the average energy of the primary beam
3. It makes the useful beam more penetrating
4. It increases the intensity of the primary beam
5. It decreases x-ray beam quality
6. It decreases patient dose
   ❏ A. 1, 4, and 5
   ❏ B. 1, 3, and 6
   ❏ C. 2, 3, and 5
   ❏ D. 3, 5, and 6
   ❏ E. 4, 5, and 6

37. What is the minimum lead requirement for lead aprons, according to the NCRP?
   ❏ A. 1.0-mm Pb equivalent
   ❏ B. 0.25-mm Pb equivalent
   ❏ C. 0.50-mm Pb equivalent
   ❏ D. 0.05-mm Pb equivalent

38. Calculation of effective dose (EfD) requires:
1. absorbed dose (D)
2. type of radiation (W_r)
3. tissue exposed (W_t)
   ❏ A. 1 only
   ❏ B. 2 only
   ❏ C. 1 and 2 only
   ❏ D. 1 and 3 only
   ❏ E. 1, 2, and 3

39. Immature cells are called
1. undifferentiated cells
2. stem cells
3. genetic cells
   ❏ A. 1 only
   ❏ B. 1 and 2 only
   ❏ C. 1 and 3 only
   ❏ D. 1, 2, and 3

40. What is the term used to describe x-ray photon interaction with matter and the transference of part of the photon's energy to matter?
   ❏ A. Absorption
   ❏ B. Scattering
   ❏ C. Differential absorption
   ❏ D. Divergence

41. Advantages of anatomic compression during imaging include
1. decreased patient dose
2. improved contrast resolution
3. improved spatial resolution
   ❏ A. 1 only
   ❏ B. 1 and 2 only
   ❏ C. 2 and 3 only
   ❏ D. 1, 2, and 3

42. To be in compliance with radiation safety standards, the fluoroscopy exposure switch must
   ❏ A. sound during fluoro-on time
   ❏ B. be on a 6-foot-long cord
   ❏ C. terminate exposure after 5 min
   ❏ D. be the "dead-man" type

43. Any wall that the useful x-ray beam may be directed toward must be a
   ❏ A. secondary barrier
   ❏ B. primary barrier
   ❏ C. leakage barrier
   ❏ D. scattered barrier

44. The annual dose limit for occupationally exposed individuals is valid for
   ❏ A. alpha, beta, and x-radiations
   ❏ B. x- and gamma radiations only
   ❏ C. beta, x-, and gamma radiations
   ❏ D. all ionizing radiations

45. The interaction between x-ray photons and matter shown in Figure 3-2 is associated with

1. an inner-shell electron
2. photoelectric effect
3. partial energy transfer from photon to electron
   ❏ A. 1 only
   ❏ B. 1 and 2 only
   ❏ C. 1 and 3 only
   ❏ D. 2 and 3 only

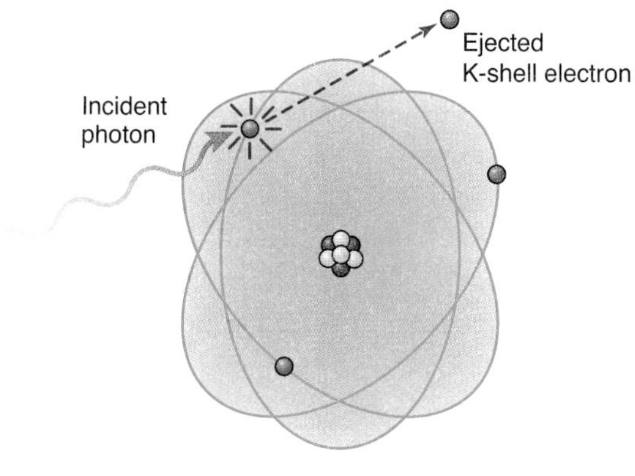

Figure 3-2

46. Patient dose increases as fluoroscopic
   ❏ A. FOV increases
   ❏ B. FOV decreases
   ❏ C. FSS increases
   ❏ D. FSS decreases

47. Types of gonadal shielding include which of the following?

1. Flat contact
2. Shaped contact (contour)
3. Shadow
   ❏ A. 1 only
   ❏ B. 1 and 2 only
   ❏ C. 2 and 3 only
   ❏ D. 1, 2, and 3

48. What unit of measure is used to express ionizing radiation dose to biologic material?
   ❏ A. Air kerma (Gy_a)
   ❏ B. Gy_t
   ❏ C. Sv
   ❏ D. RBE

49. LET is best defined as

1. a method of expressing radiation quality
2. a measure of the rate at which radiation energy is transferred to soft tissue
3. transmission of polyenergetic radiation
   ❏ A. 1 only
   ❏ B. 1 and 2 only
   ❏ C. 1 and 3 only
   ❏ D. 1, 2, and 3

50. For exposure to 10 mGy of each of the following ionizing radiations, which would result in the greatest dose to the individual?
   ❏ A. External source of 1-MeV x-rays
   ❏ B. External source of diagnostic x-rays
   ❏ C. Internal source of alpha particles
   ❏ D. Internal source of beta particles

51. The skin response to radiation exposure that appears as hair loss is known as
   ❏ A. dry desquamation
   ❏ B. moist desquamation
   ❏ C. erythema
   ❏ D. epilation

52. Irradiation of macromolecules in vitro can result in

1. cleaved chromosome
2. cross-linking
3. mutation
   ❏ A. 1 only
   ❏ B. 1 and 2 only
   ❏ C. 2 and 3 only
   ❏ D. 1, 2, and 3

53. The reduction in the intensity of an x-ray beam as it passes through material is termed
   ❏ A. absorption
   ❏ B. scattering
   ❏ C. attenuation
   ❏ D. divergence

54. Which type of dose–response relationship represents radiation-induced leukemia and genetic effects?
   ❏ A. Linear, threshold
   ❏ B. Nonlinear, threshold
   ❏ C. Linear, nonthreshold
   ❏ D. Nonlinear, nonthreshold

55. Which of the following groups of technical factors will deliver the *least* amount of exposure to the patient?
   ❏ A. 400 mA, 0.25 s, 100 kVp
   ❏ B. 600 mA, 0.33 s, 90 kVp
   ❏ C. 800 mA, 0.5 s, 80 kVp
   ❏ D. 800 mA, 1.0 s, 70 kVp

56. Late effects of radiation, whose incidence is dose related and for which there is no threshold dose, are called
   ❏ A. nonstochastic/deterministic
   ❏ B. stochastic/probabilistic
   ❏ C. chromosomal aberration
   ❏ D. hematologic depression

57. Which of the following statements is/are true regarding the human gonadal cells?

1. The female oogonia reproduce only during fetal life
2. The male spermatogonia reproduce continuously
3. Both male and female stem cells reproduce only during fetal life
   - ❏ A. 1 only
   - ❏ B. 2 only
   - ❏ C. 1 and 2 only
   - ❏ D. 3 only

58. Classify the following tissues in order of *increasing* radiosensitivity.

1. Liver cells
2. Intestinal crypt cells
3. Muscle cells
   - ❏ A. 1, 3, 2
   - ❏ B. 2, 3, 1
   - ❏ C. 2, 1, 3
   - ❏ D. 3, 1, 2

59. The largest amount of diagnostic x-ray absorption is most likely to occur in which of the following tissues?

- ❏ A. Lung
- ❏ B. Adipose
- ❏ C. Muscle
- ❏ D. Bone

60. According to NCRP regulations, leakage radiation from the x-ray tube must not exceed

- ❏ A. 0.1 mGy$_a$/h (10 mR/h)
- ❏ B. 1.0 mGy$_a$/h (100 mR/h)
- ❏ C. 0.1 mGy$_a$/min (10 mR/min)
- ❏ D. 1.0 mGy$_a$/min (100 mR/min)

61. The interaction between x-ray photons and tissue that can impact radiographic contrast but that contributes significantly to patient dose is

- ❏ A. the photoelectric effect
- ❏ B. Compton scatter
- ❏ C. coherent scatter
- ❏ D. pair production

62. Which of the following statements is/are true with respect to radiation safety in fluoroscopy?

1. Tabletop radiation intensity must not exceed 21 mGy$_a$/min/mA
2. Tabletop radiation intensity must not exceed 100 mGy$_a$/min
3. In high-level fluoroscopy, tabletop intensity should be up to 200 mGy$_a$/min
   - ❏ A. 1 only
   - ❏ B. 1 and 2 only
   - ❏ C. 2 and 3 only
   - ❏ D. 1, 2, and 3

63. In the production of characteristic radiation at the tungsten target, the incident electron

- ❏ A. ejects an inner-shell tungsten electron
- ❏ B. ejects an outer-shell tungsten electron
- ❏ C. is deflected, with resulting energy loss
- ❏ D. is deflected, with resulting energy gain

64. Which of the following account(s) for an x-ray beam's heterogeneity?

1. Incident electrons interacting with several layers of tungsten target atoms
2. Energy differences among incident electrons
3. Electrons moving to fill different shell vacancies
   - ❏ A. 1 only
   - ❏ B. 1 and 2 only
   - ❏ C. 1 and 3 only
   - ❏ D. 1, 2, and 3

65. Patient dose in diagnostic radiography is usually expressed as

- ❏ A. genetically significant dose
- ❏ B. mean marrow dose
- ❏ C. entrance skin exposure
- ❏ D. gonadal dose

66. Which of the following contributes *most* to occupational exposure?

- ❏ A. The photoelectric effect
- ❏ B. Compton scatter
- ❏ C. Classic scatter
- ❏ D. Thompson scatter

67. The likelihood of adverse radiation effects to any radiographer whose dose is kept below the recommended guideline is

- ❏ A. very probable
- ❏ B. possible
- ❏ C. very remote
- ❏ D. zero

68. Primary radiation barriers must be *at least* how high?

- ❏ A. 5 feet (1.5 m)
- ❏ B. 6 feet (1.8 m)
- ❏ C. 7 feet (2.1 m)
- ❏ D. 8 feet (2.4 m)

69. For radiographic examinations of the skull, it is generally preferred that the skull be examined in the

- ❏ A. AP projection
- ❏ B. PA projection
- ❏ C. erect position
- ❏ D. supine position

70. According to the NCRP, the annual occupational dose-equivalent limit to the thyroid, skin, and extremities is
- ❏ A. 50 mSv
- ❏ B. 150 mSv
- ❏ C. 500 mSv
- ❏ D. 1500 mSv

71. The majority of occupational radiation exposure is received during
1. bedside radiography
2. general radiography
3. fluoroscopy
- ❏ A. 1 only
- ❏ B. 2 only
- ❏ C. 1 and 2 only
- ❏ D. 1 and 3 only

72. Which of the dose–response curve(s) shown in Figure 3-3 illustrate(s) a linear threshold response to radiation exposure?
1. Dose–response curve *A*
2. Dose–response curve *B*
3. Dose–response curve *C*
- ❏ A. 1 only
- ❏ B. 2 only
- ❏ C. 1 and 2 only
- ❏ D. 2 and 3 only

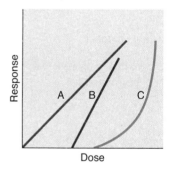

Figure 3-3

73. The NCRP recommends an annual effective occupational whole-body dose-equivalent limit of
- ❏ A. 25 mSv
- ❏ B. 50 mSv
- ❏ C. 100 mSv
- ❏ D. 200 mSv

74. Which of the following formulas is a representation of the inverse-square law of radiation used to determine x-ray intensity at different distances?
- ❏ A. $\dfrac{I_1}{I_2} = \dfrac{D_2^2}{D_1^2}$
- ❏ B. $\dfrac{I_1}{I_2} = \dfrac{D_1^2}{D_2^2}$
- ❏ C. $\dfrac{kVp_1}{kVp_2} = \dfrac{D_2^2}{D_1^2}$
- ❏ D. $\dfrac{kVp_1}{kVp_2} = \dfrac{D_1^2}{D_2^2}$

75. An increase of 1.0-mm added aluminum filtration of the x-ray beam would have which of the following effects?
1. Increase in average energy of the beam
2. Increase in patient skin dose
3. Increase in mGy_a output
- ❏ A. 1 only
- ❏ B. 1 and 2 only
- ❏ C. 2 and 3 only
- ❏ D. 1, 2, and 3

76. Which of the following projections would deliver the largest thyroid dose?
- ❏ A. AP skull
- ❏ B. PA skull
- ❏ C. AP abdomen
- ❏ D. PA chest

77. The amount of time that x-rays are being produced and directed toward a particular wall is called the
- ❏ A. workload
- ❏ B. use factor
- ❏ C. occupancy factor
- ❏ D. controlling factor

78. The operation of personnel radiation monitoring devices can depend on which of the following?
1. Ionization
2. Luminescence
3. Thermoluminescence
- ❏ A. 1 only
- ❏ B. 1 and 2 only
- ❏ C. 2 and 3 only
- ❏ D. 1, 2, and 3

79. Which of the following cell types has the greatest radiosensitivity in the adult human?
- ❏ A. Nerve cells
- ❏ B. Muscle cells
- ❏ C. Spermatids
- ❏ D. Lymphocytes

80. How will x-ray photon intensity be affected if the source-to-image-receptor distance (SID) is doubled?
- ❏ A. Its intensity increases 2 times
- ❏ B. Its intensity increases 4 times
- ❏ C. Its intensity decreases 2 times
- ❏ D. Its intensity decreases 4 times

81. Which of the following terms refers to the period between conception and birth?
- ❏ A. Gestation
- ❏ B. Congenital
- ❏ C. Neonatal
- ❏ D. In vitro

82. Referring to the nomogram in Figure 3-4, what is the approximate patient ESE from an AP projection of the abdomen made at 105 cm using 80 kVp, 300 mA, 50 ms, and 2.5 mm Al total filtration?
- ❏ A. 18 mGy
- ❏ B. 9 mGy
- ❏ C. 180 mGy
- ❏ D. 90 mGy

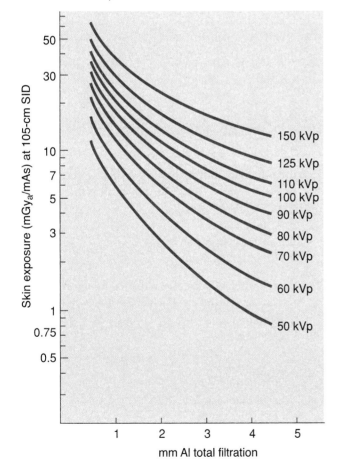

Figure 3-4. Reproduced, with permission, from McCullough EC, Cameron JR. Exposure rates from diagnostic x-ray units. *Br J Radiol.* 1970;43:448–451.

83. The unit of measurement used to express occupational exposure is
- ❏ A. Gy_a
- ❏ B. Gy
- ❏ C. Sv
- ❏ D. RBE

84. Which of the following refers to a regular program of evaluation that ensures the proper functioning of x-ray equipment, thereby protecting both radiation workers and patients?
- ❏ A. Sensitometry
- ❏ B. Quality assurance
- ❏ C. Quality control
- ❏ D. Modulation transfer function

85. The Bucky slot cover is in place to protect the
1. patient
2. fluoroscopist
3. technologist
- ❏ A. 1 only
- ❏ B. 1 and 2 only
- ❏ C. 2 and 3 only
- ❏ D. 1, 2, and 3

86. Which type of personnel radiation monitor can provide an immediate reading?
- ❏ A. Thermoluminescent dosimeter (TLD)
- ❏ B. Optically stimulated luminescence (OSL)
- ❏ C. Film badge
- ❏ D. Ionization chamber

87. Which of the following terms is correctly used to describe x-ray beam quality?
- ❏ A. mA
- ❏ B. HVL
- ❏ C. Intensity
- ❏ D. Dose rate

88. The most effective type of shield for anterior and lateral male gonadal protection during fluoroscopy is
- ❏ A. flat contact
- ❏ B. shaped contact (contour)
- ❏ C. shadow
- ❏ D. cylindrical

89. Isotopes are atoms that have the same
- ❏ A. mass number but a different atomic number
- ❏ B. atomic number but a different mass number
- ❏ C. atomic number but a different neutron number
- ❏ D. atomic number and mass number

90. If the ESE for a particular exposure is 1.1 mGy, what will be the intensity of the scattered beam perpendicular to and 1 m from the patient?
- ❏ A. 1.0 mGy
- ❏ B. 0.1 mGy
- ❏ C. 0.01 mGy
- ❏ D. 0.001 mGy

91. Primary radiation barriers usually require which thickness of lead shielding?
- ❏ A. 1/4-inch lead equivalent
- ❏ B. 1/8-inch lead equivalent
- ❏ C. 1/16-inch lead equivalent
- ❏ D. 1/32-inch lead equivalent

92. Factors that contribute to the amount of scattered radiation produced include
1. radiation quality
2. field size
3. grid ratio
- ❏ A. 1 only
- ❏ B. 1 and 2 only
- ❏ C. 2 and 3 only
- ❏ D. 1, 2, and 3

93. The SSD in mobile fluoroscopy must be
- ❏ A. a minimum of 38 cm
- ❏ B. a maximum of 38 cm
- ❏ C. a minimum of 30 cm
- ❏ D. a maximum of 30 cm

94. The automatic exposure device that is located immediately under the x-ray table is the
- ❏ A. ionization chamber
- ❏ B. scintillation camera
- ❏ C. photomultiplier
- ❏ D. photocathode

95. According to the NCRP, the annual occupational whole-body dose-equivalent limit is
- ❏ A. 1 mSv
- ❏ B. 50 mSv
- ❏ C. 150 mSv
- ❏ D. 500 mSv

96. It is necessary to question a female patient of childbearing age regarding her
1. date of last menstrual period
2. possibility of being pregnant
3. age at her first pregnancy
- ❏ A. 1 only
- ❏ B. 1 and 2 only
- ❏ C. 1 and 3 only
- ❏ D. 2 and 3 only

97. Which of the dose–response curves seen in Figure 3-5 represents possible genetic effects of ionizing radiation?
- ❏ A. Dose–response curve *A*
- ❏ B. Dose–response curve *B*
- ❏ C. Dose–response curve *C*
- ❏ D. None of these

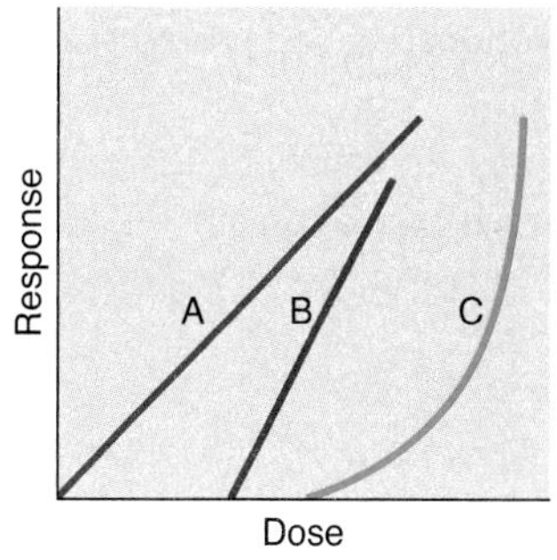

Figure 3-5

98. What is the effect on RBE as LET increases?
- ❏ A. As LET increases, RBE increases
- ❏ B. As LET increases, RBE decreases
- ❏ C. As LET increases, RBE stabilizes
- ❏ D. LET has no effect on RBE

99. Which of the following would *most likely* result in the greatest skin dose?
- ❏ A. Short SID
- ❏ B. High kVp
- ❏ C. Increased filtration
- ❏ D. Increased mA

100. Which of the following radiation-induced conditions is most likely to have the *longest* latent period?
- ❏ A. Leukemia
- ❏ B. Temporary infertility
- ❏ C. Erythema
- ❏ D. Acute radiation lethality

101. Which of the following ionizing radiations is described as having an RBE of 1.0?
- ❏ A. 10 MeV protons
- ❏ B. 5 MeV alpha particles
- ❏ C. Diagnostic x-rays
- ❏ D. Fast neutrons

102. If an individual receives 50 mGy while standing 4 feet from a source of ionizing radiation for 2 min, which of the following option(s) will *most effectively* reduce his or her radiation exposure to that source of ionizing radiation?
- ❏ A. Standing 3 feet from the source for 2 min
- ❏ B. Standing 8 feet from the source for 2 min
- ❏ C. Standing 5 feet from the source for 1 min
- ❏ D. Standing 6 feet from the source for 2 min

103. An optically stimulated luminescence dosimeter contains which of the following detectors?
- ❏ A. Gadolinium
- ❏ B. Aluminum oxide
- ❏ C. Lithium fluoride
- ❏ D. Photographic film

104. How do fractionation and protraction affect radiation dose effects?
1. They reduce the effect of radiation exposure
2. They permit cellular repair
3. They allow tissue recovery
- ❏ A. 1 only
- ❏ B. 1 and 2 only
- ❏ C. 2 and 3 only
- ❏ D. 1, 2, and 3

105. The photoelectric effect is an interaction between an x-ray photon and
- ❏ A. an inner-shell electron
- ❏ B. an outer-shell electron
- ❏ C. a nucleus
- ❏ D. another photon

106. Filters used in radiographic x-ray tubes generally are composed of
- ❏ A. aluminum
- ❏ B. copper
- ❏ C. tin
- ❏ D. lead

107. All of the following function to reduce patient dose, *except*
- ❏ A. beam restriction
- ❏ B. high kVp, low mAs factors
- ❏ C. a high-speed grid
- ❏ D. a high-speed imaging system

108. In the production of Bremsstrahlung radiation
- ❏ A. the incident photon ejects an inner-shell tungsten electron
- ❏ B. the incident photon is deflected, with resulting energy loss
- ❏ C. the incident electron ejects an inner-shell tungsten electron
- ❏ D. the incident electron is deflected, with resulting energy loss

109. All of the following radiation-exposure responses exhibit a nonlinear threshold dose–response relationship, *except*
- ❏ A. skin erythema
- ❏ B. hematologic depression
- ❏ C. radiation lethality
- ❏ D. leukemia

110. Which of the following may be used to express exposure in air?
- ❏ A. Air kerma
- ❏ B. Gy
- ❏ C. Sv
- ❏ D. RBE

111. The purpose of filters in a film badge is
- ❏ A. to eliminate harmful rays
- ❏ B. to measure radiation quality
- ❏ C. to prevent exposure by alpha particles
- ❏ D. as a support for the film contained within

112. How many HVLs are required to reduce the intensity of a beam of monoenergetic photons to less than 15% of its original value?
- ❏ A. 2
- ❏ B. 3
- ❏ C. 4
- ❏ D. 5

113. Which of the following has/have an effect on the amount and type of radiation-induced tissue damage?
1. Quality of radiation
2. Type of tissue being irradiated
3. Fractionation
- ❏ A. 1 only
- ❏ B. 1 and 2 only
- ❏ C. 1 and 3 only
- ❏ D. 1, 2, and 3

114. Radiation dose to personnel is reduced by which of the following exposure control cord guidelines?
1. Exposure cords on fixed equipment must be very short
2. Exposure cords on mobile equipment should be fairly long
3. Exposure cords on fixed and mobile equipment should be of the coiled, expandable type
- ❏ A. 1 only
- ❏ B. 1 and 2 only
- ❏ C. 2 and 3 only
- ❏ D. 1, 2, and 3

115. Which of the following groups of technical factors will deliver the least patient dose?
- ❏ A. 300 mA, 250 ms, 70 kVp
- ❏ B. 300 mA, 125 ms, 80 kVp
- ❏ C. 400 mA, 90 ms, 80 kVp
- ❏ D. 600 mA, 30 ms, 90 kVp

116. Which of the following body parts is/are included in whole-body dose?
1. Gonads
2. Blood-forming organs
3. Extremities
   - ❏ A. 1 only
   - ❏ B. 1 and 2 only
   - ❏ C. 1 and 3 only
   - ❏ D. 1, 2, and 3

117. Aluminum filtration has its greatest effect on
- ❏ A. low-energy x-ray photons
- ❏ B. high-energy x-ray photons
- ❏ C. low-energy scattered photons
- ❏ D. high-energy scattered photons

118. Which of the following personnel monitoring devices used in diagnostic radiography is considered to be the *most* sensitive and accurate?
- ❏ A. TLD
- ❏ B. Film badge
- ❏ C. OSL dosimeter
- ❏ D. Pocket dosimeter

119. Types of structural damage to a DNA molecule by ionizing radiation include which of the following?
1. Single-side-rail scission
2. Double-side-rail scission
3. Cross-linking
   - ❏ A. 1 only
   - ❏ B. 2 only
   - ❏ C. 1 and 2 only
   - ❏ D. 1, 2, and 3

120. Which of the following radiation situations is potentially the *most* harmful?
- ❏ A. A large dose to a specific area all at once
- ❏ B. A small dose to the whole body over a period of time
- ❏ C. A large dose to the whole body all at one time
- ❏ D. A small dose to a specific area over a period of time

121. As field size decreases
- ❏ A. DAP decreases
- ❏ B. SR production increases
- ❏ C. DAP is unchanged
- ❏ D. EFS size increases

122. Occupational radiation monitoring is required when it is likely that an individual will receive more than what fraction of the annual dose limit?
- ❏ A. 1/2
- ❏ B. 1/4
- ❏ C. 1/10
- ❏ D. 1/40

123. The interaction illustrated in Figure 3-6
1. can pose a safety hazard to personnel
2. can have a negative impact on image quality
3. occurs with low-energy incident photons
   - ❏ A. 1 only
   - ❏ B. 1 and 2 only
   - ❏ C. 2 and 3 only
   - ❏ D. 1, 2, and 3

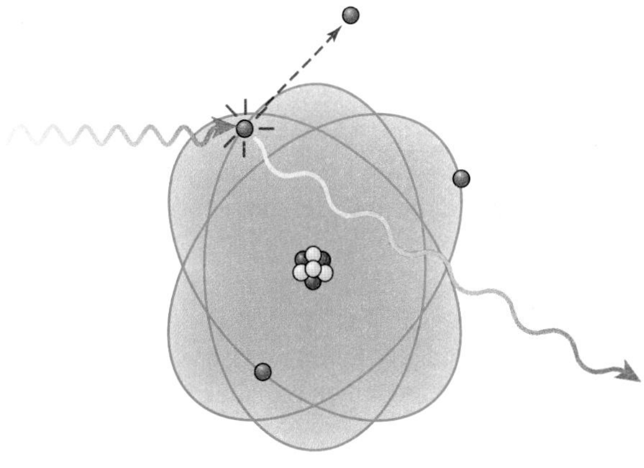

Figure 3-6

124. Biologic material is *least* sensitive to irradiation under which of the following conditions?
- ❏ A. Anoxic
- ❏ B. Hypoxic
- ❏ C. Oxygenated
- ❏ D. Hyperoxia

125. Which of the following cells are the *most* radiosensitive?
- ❏ A. Myelocytes
- ❏ B. Erythroblasts
- ❏ C. Megakaryocytes
- ❏ D. Myocytes

126. Which of the following statements is/are true regarding the pregnant radiographer?
1. She should declare her pregnancy to her supervisor
2. She should be assigned a second personnel monitor
3. Her radiation history should be reviewed
   - ❏ A. 1 only
   - ❏ B. 1 and 2 only
   - ❏ C. 2 and 3 only
   - ❏ D. 1, 2, and 3

127. Select the *three* correct statements regarding deviation index (DI).

1. DI indicates the difference between the ideal exposure and the actual exposure
2. A negative DI indicates overexposure
3. The ideal receptor exposure has a DI of 0.0
4. DI functions to indicate receptor underexposure/overexposure
5. A DI of +1 indicates 50% overexposure

   ❏ A. 1, 2, and 5
   ❏ B. 1, 3, and 4
   ❏ C. 2, 3, and 4
   ❏ D. 3, 4, and 5

128. Which of the following contributes *most* to the patient dose?

   ❏ A. The photoelectric effect
   ❏ B. Compton scatter
   ❏ C. Classic scatter
   ❏ D. Thompson scatter

129. Which of the following statements is/are true with respect to the dose–response curve shown in Figure 3-7?

1. The quantity of radiation is directly related to the dose received
2. No threshold is required for effects to occur
3. A minimum amount of radiation is required for manifestation of effects

   ❏ A. 1 only
   ❏ B. 1 and 2 only
   ❏ C. 1 and 3 only
   ❏ D. 2 and 3 only

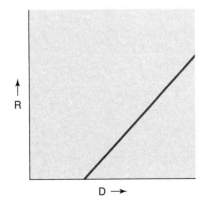

Figure 3-7

130. The classifications of acute radiation syndrome include all of the following, *except*

   ❏ A. cerebrovascular
   ❏ B. gastrointestinal
   ❏ C. neonatal
   ❏ D. hematologic

131. The symbols $^{130}_{56}Ba$ and $^{138}_{56}Ba$ are examples of which of the following?

   ❏ A. Isotopes
   ❏ B. Isobars
   ❏ C. Isotones
   ❏ D. Isomers

132. What is the effect on relative biologic effectiveness (RBE) as linear energy transfer (LET) decreases?

   ❏ A. As LET decreases, RBE increases
   ❏ B. As LET decreases, RBE decreases
   ❏ C. As LET decreases, RBE stabilizes
   ❏ D. LET has no effect on RBE

133. If an exposure dose of 1.5 mGy/h is delivered from a distance of 3 feet, what would be the dose delivered after 20 min at a distance of 5 feet from the source?

   ❏ A. 0.18 mGy
   ❏ B. 0.54 mGy
   ❏ C. 13.5 mGy
   ❏ D. 25 mGy

134. The term *effective dose* refers to

   ❏ A. whole-body dose
   ❏ B. localized organ dose
   ❏ C. genetic effects
   ❏ D. somatic and genetic effects

135. Potential ionizing radiation damage to tissue is dependent on the

1. *Z* number of the tissue
2. type of ionizing radiation
3. mass density of the tissue

   ❏ A. 1 only
   ❏ B. 1 and 2 only
   ❏ C. 2 and 3 only
   ❏ D. 1, 2, and 3

136. The operation of personnel radiation monitoring devices can be based on stimulated luminescence. Which of the following personnel radiation monitors function(s) in that manner?

1. OSL dosimeter
2. TLD
3. Pocket dosimeter

   ❏ A. 1 only
   ❏ B. 1 and 2 only
   ❏ C. 1 and 3 only
   ❏ D. 1, 2, and 3

137. If a patient received 0.014 Gy during a 7-min fluoroscopic examination, what was the dose rate?

   ❏ A. 1.4 mGy/min
   ❏ B. 0.14 mGy/min
   ❏ C. 0.02 mGy/min
   ❏ D. 2.0 mGy/min

138. The least radiosensitive stage of human cell mitosis is

❏ A. M
❏ B. G_1
❏ C. S
❏ D. G_2

139. Which interaction between ionizing radiation and the target molecule involves formation of a free radical?

❏ A. Direct effect
❏ B. Indirect effect
❏ C. Target effect
❏ D. Random effect

140. The term used to express kinetic energy released in matter is

❏ A. erg
❏ B. gray
❏ C. kerma
❏ D. rad

141. All of the following statements regarding TLDs are true, *except*

❏ A. TLDs are reusable
❏ B. a TLD is a personnel radiation monitor
❏ C. TLDs use a lithium fluoride phosphor
❏ D. after x-ray exposure, TLDs emit heat in response to stimulation by light

142. A student radiographer who is younger than 18 years must not receive an annual occupational dose of greater than

❏ A. 1 mSv
❏ B. 5 mSv
❏ C. 50 mSv
❏ D. 100 mSv

143. Sources of medical radiation exposure include

1. computed tomography
2. sonography
3. magnetic resonance imaging
  ❏ A. 1 only
  ❏ B. 1 and 2 only
  ❏ C. 1 and 3 only
  ❏ D. 1, 2, and 3

144. Which of the following is/are likely to improve image quality *and* decrease patient dose?

1. Beam restriction
2. Low-kilovolt *and* high-microampere-second factors
3. Grids
  ❏ A. 1 only
  ❏ B. 1 and 3 only
  ❏ C. 2 and 3 only
  ❏ D. 1, 2, and 3

145. Protective devices such as lead aprons function to protect the user from

1. scattered radiation
2. the primary beam
3. remnant radiation
  ❏ A. 1 only
  ❏ B. 1 and 2 only
  ❏ C. 1 and 3 only
  ❏ D. 1, 2, and 3

146. Which of the following radiation protection concepts/measures apply to mobile radiography?

1. The radiographer should be at least 6 feet from the patient and the x-ray tube during the exposure
2. The least amount of scattered radiation is perpendicular to the scattering object
3. At least one lead apron should be assigned to each mobile unit
  ❏ A. 1 and 2 only
  ❏ B. 1 and 3 only
  ❏ C. 2 and 3 only
  ❏ D. 1, 2, and 3

147. Examples of late effects of ionizing radiation on humans include

1. leukemia
2. local tissue damage
3. malignant disease
  ❏ A. 1 only
  ❏ B. 1 and 2 only
  ❏ C. 1 and 3 only
  ❏ D. 1, 2, and 3

148. Which of the following can be an effective means of reducing radiation exposure?

1. Barriers
2. Distance
3. Time
  ❏ A. 1 only
  ❏ B. 2 only
  ❏ C. 1 and 2 only
  ❏ D. 1, 2, and 3

149. The effects of radiation on biologic material depend on several factors. If a large quantity of radiation is delivered to a body over a short period of time, the effect

❏ A. will be greater than if it were delivered in increments
❏ B. will be less than if it were delivered in increments
❏ C. has no relation to how it is delivered in time
❏ D. solely depends on the radiation quality

150. Which of the following result(s) from restriction of the x-ray beam?

1. Less scattered radiation production
2. Less patient hazard
3. Less radiographic contrast
   - ❏ A. 1 only
   - ❏ B. 1 and 2 only
   - ❏ C. 2 and 3 only
   - ❏ D. 1, 2, and 3

151. What minimum total amount of filtration (inherent plus added) is required in x-ray equipment operated above 70 kVp?

- ❏ A. 2.5-mm Al equivalent
- ❏ B. 3.5-mm Al equivalent
- ❏ C. 2.5-mm Cu equivalent
- ❏ D. 3.5-mm Cu equivalent

152. The dose of radiation that will cause a noticeable skin reaction is called the

- ❏ A. LET
- ❏ B. SSD
- ❏ C. SED
- ❏ D. SID

153. What is the intensity of scattered radiation perpendicular to and 1 m from a patient compared with the useful beam at the patient's surface?

- ❏ A. 0.01%
- ❏ B. 0.1%
- ❏ C. 1.0%
- ❏ D. 10.0%

154. Some patients, such as infants and children, are unable to maintain the necessary radiographic position without assistance. If mechanical restraining devices cannot be used, who of the following should be the first choice to help immobilize the patient?

- ❏ A. Transporter
- ❏ B. Patient's father
- ❏ C. Patient's mother
- ❏ D. Student radiographer

155. A *controlled area* is defined as one

1. that is occupied by people trained in radiation safety
2. that is occupied by people who wear radiation monitors
3. whose occupancy factor is 1
   - ❏ A. 1 and 2 only
   - ❏ B. 2 only
   - ❏ C. 1 and 3 only
   - ❏ D. 1, 2, and 3

156. Early symptoms of acute radiation syndrome include

1. leukopenia
2. nausea and vomiting
3. cataracts
   - ❏ A. 1 and 2 only
   - ❏ B. 2 only
   - ❏ C. 1 and 3 only
   - ❏ D. 2 and 3 only

157. Somatic effects resulting from radiation exposure can

1. have possible consequences on the exposed individual
2. have possible consequences on future generations
3. cause temporary infertility
   - ❏ A. 1 only
   - ❏ B. 1 and 3 only
   - ❏ C. 2 and 3 only
   - ❏ D. 1, 2, and 3

158. Which of the following is/are considered especially radiosensitive tissues?

1. Bone marrow
2. Intestinal crypt cells
3. Erythroblasts
   - ❏ A. 1 and 2 only
   - ❏ B. 1 and 3 only
   - ❏ C. 2 and 3 only
   - ❏ D. 1, 2, and 3

159. In which type of monitoring device do photons release electrons by their interaction with air?

- ❏ A. Film badge
- ❏ B. TLD
- ❏ C. Pocket dosimeter
- ❏ D. OSL dosimeter

160. The biologic effect on an individual depends on which of the following?

1. Type of tissue interaction(s)
2. Amount of interactions
3. Biologic differences
   - ❏ A. 1 and 2 only
   - ❏ B. 1 and 3 only
   - ❏ C. 2 and 3 only
   - ❏ D. 1, 2, and 3

161. The person responsible for ascertaining that all radiation guidelines are adhered to and that personnel understand and use radiation safety measures is the

- ❏ A. radiology department manager
- ❏ B. radiation safety officer
- ❏ C. chief radiologist
- ❏ D. chief technologist

162. Which of the following dose–response curves appears to be valid for genetic and some somatic effects?

1. Linear
2. Nonlinear
3. Nonthreshold
   - ❏ A. 1 only
   - ❏ B. 1 and 3 only
   - ❏ C. 2 and 3 only
   - ❏ D. 1, 2, and 3

163. Which of the following is used to illustrate the relationship between exposure to ionizing radiation and possible resultant biologic responses?

- ❏ A. Ionization chamber
- ❏ B. Thermoluminescent dosimeter
- ❏ C. Dose–response curve
- ❏ D. Electromagnetic spectrum

164. With milliamperes (mA) increased to maintain output intensity, how is the ESE affected as the source-to-skin distance (SSD) is increased?

- ❏ A. The ESE increases
- ❏ B. The ESE decreases
- ❏ C. The ESE remains unchanged
- ❏ D. ESE is unrelated to SSD

165. The primary function of filtration is to reduce

- ❏ A. patient skin dose
- ❏ B. operator dose
- ❏ C. image noise
- ❏ D. scattered radiation

166. Which of the following factors can affect the amount or the nature of radiation damage to biologic tissue?

1. Radiation quality
2. Absorbed dose
3. Size of irradiated area
   - ❏ A. 1 only
   - ❏ B. 2 only
   - ❏ C. 1 and 2 only
   - ❏ D. 1, 2, and 3

167. Examples of stochastic/probabilistic effects of radiation exposure include

1. radiation-induced malignancy
2. genetic effects
3. leukemia
   - ❏ A. 1 only
   - ❏ B. 1 and 2 only
   - ❏ C. 2 and 3 only
   - ❏ D. 1, 2, and 3

168. Irradiation of water molecules within the body and their resulting breakdown is termed as

- ❏ A. epilation
- ❏ B. radiolysis
- ❏ C. proliferation
- ❏ D. repopulation

169. A dose of 250 mGy (25 rad) to the fetus during the 7th or 8th week of pregnancy is likely to cause which of the following?

- ❏ A. Spontaneous abortion
- ❏ B. Skeletal anomalies
- ❏ C. Neurologic anomalies
- ❏ D. Organogenesis anomalies

170. If the exposure rate to an individual standing 4.0 m from a source of radiation is 0.7 mGy/h, what will be the dose received after 20 min at a distance of 6 m from the source?

- ❏ A. 11.2 mGy/h
- ❏ B. 0.46 mGy/h
- ❏ C. 0.311 mGy/h
- ❏ D. 0.103 mGy/h

171. Methods of decreasing patient exposure during fluoroscopic procedures include

1. using a low pulse rate
2. minimizing the use of boost mode
3. using high kilovoltage/low milliampere combination
   - ❏ A. 1 only
   - ❏ B. 1 and 2 only
   - ❏ C. 2 and 3 only
   - ❏ D. 1, 2, and 3

172. Under what circumstances is a radiographer required to wear two dosimeters?

1. During pregnancy
2. While performing vascular procedures
3. While performing mobile radiography
   - ❏ A. 1 and 2 only
   - ❏ B. 2 only
   - ❏ C. 2 and 3 only
   - ❏ D. 1, 2, and 3

173. What quantity of radiation exposure to the reproductive organs is required to cause temporary infertility?

- ❏ A. 1 Gy
- ❏ B. 2 Gy
- ❏ C. 3 Gy
- ❏ D. 4 Gy

174. Which of the following personnel radiation monitors uses Bluetooth technology?

- ❏ A. TLD
- ❏ B. OSL
- ❏ C. DIS
- ❏ D. PBL

175. Biologic material irradiated under hypoxic conditions is
- ❏ A. more sensitive than when irradiated under oxygenated conditions
- ❏ B. less sensitive than when irradiated under anoxic conditions
- ❏ C. less sensitive than when irradiated under oxygenated conditions
- ❏ D. unaffected by the presence or absence of oxygen

176. Which of the dose–response curves shown in Figure 3-8 is/are representative of radiation-induced skin erythema?
1. Dose–response curve *A*
2. Dose–response curve *B*
3. Dose–response curve *C*
- ❏ A. 1 only
- ❏ B. 1 and 2 only
- ❏ C. 3 only
- ❏ D. 2 and 3 only

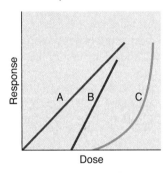

Figure 3-8

177. If the exposure rate at 91 cm from the fluoroscopic table is 1.5 mGy/h, what will be the exposure rate for 30 min at a distance of 152 cm from the table?
- ❏ A. 0.27 mGy
- ❏ B. 0.54 mGy
- ❏ C. 20.9 mGy
- ❏ D. 13.5 mGy

178. Lead aprons are worn during fluoroscopy to protect the radiographer from exposure to radiation from
- ❏ A. the photoelectric effect
- ❏ B. Compton scatter
- ❏ C. classic scatter
- ❏ D. pair production

179. Radiation that passes through the tube housing in directions other than that of the useful beam is termed as
- ❏ A. scattered radiation
- ❏ B. secondary radiation
- ❏ C. leakage radiation
- ❏ D. remnant radiation

180. The deviation index (DI) indicates exposure data
- ❏ A. to the patient's surface
- ❏ B. to midline of part
- ❏ C. as entrance dose
- ❏ D. to the IR

181. Possible responses to irradiation in utero include
1. spontaneous abortion
2. congenital anomalies
3. childhood malignancies
- ❏ A. 1 only
- ❏ B. 1 and 2 only
- ❏ C. 2 and 3 only
- ❏ D. 1, 2, and 3 only

182. What should be the radiographer's main objective regarding personal radiation safety?
- ❏ A. Not to exceed his or her dose limit
- ❏ B. To keep personal exposure as far below the dose limit as possible
- ❏ C. To avoid whole-body exposure
- ❏ D. To wear protective apparel when "holding" patients for exposures

183. Referring to the nomogram in Figure 3-9, what is the approximate patient ESE from a particular projection made at 105 cm using 110 kVp, 300 mA, 5 ms, and 2.5 mm Al total filtration?
- ❏ A. 18 mGy
- ❏ B. 12 mGy
- ❏ C. 8 mGy
- ❏ D. 4 mGy

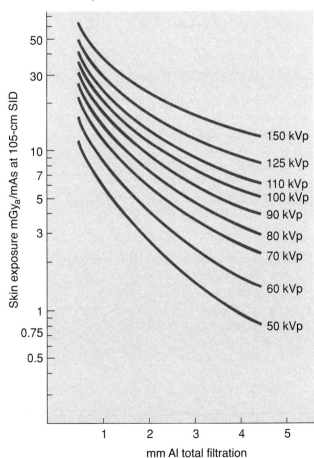

Figure 3-9. Reproduced, with permission, from McCullough EC, Cameron JR. Exposure rates from diagnostic x-ray units. *Br J Radiol.* 1970;43:448–451.

184. If the exposure rate to a body standing 7 feet from a radiation source is 1.5 mGy, what will be the dose to that body at a distance of 8 feet from the source in 30 min?

❏ A. 0.57 mGy
❏ B. 1.14 mGy
❏ C. 1.31 mGy
❏ D. 13.1 mGy

185. Which of the following is/are composed of nondividing, differentiated cells?

1. Neurons and neuroglia
2. Epithelial tissue
3. Lymphocytes

❏ A. 1 only
❏ B. 1 and 2 only
❏ C. 1 and 3 only
❏ D. 1, 2, and 3

186. Which of the following features of fluoroscopic equipment is/are designed especially to eliminate unnecessary radiation exposure to the patient and/or personnel?

1. Bucky slot cover
2. Exposure switch/foot pedal
3. Cumulative exposure timer

❏ A. 1 only
❏ B. 1 and 2 only
❏ C. 2 and 3 only
❏ D. 1, 2, and 3

187. Radiation output from a diagnostic x-ray tube is measured in which of the following units of measurement?

❏ A. Sievert
❏ B. Gray
❏ C. Air kerma
❏ D. Becquerel

188. If the image intensifier is moved farther from the patient

1. SID increases
2. patient dose decreases
3. image quality improves

❏ A. 1 only
❏ B. 1 and 2 only
❏ C. 1 and 3 only
❏ D. 1, 2, and 3

189. Which of the following safeguards is/are taken to prevent inadvertent irradiation in early pregnancy?

1. Patient postings
2. Patient questionnaire
3. Elective booking

❏ A. 1 and 2 only
❏ B. 1 and 3 only
❏ C. 2 and 3 only
❏ D. 1, 2, and 3

190. Patient dose during fluoroscopy is affected by the

1. distance between the patient and the input phosphor
2. amount of magnification
3. tissue density

❏ A. 1 only
❏ B. 3 only
❏ C. 2 and 3 only
❏ D. 1, 2, and 3

191. Which of the following is/are acceptable way(s) to monitor the radiation exposure of those who are occupationally employed?

1. TLD
2. OSL dosimeter
3. Quarterly blood cell count

❏ A. 1 only
❏ B. 1 and 2 only
❏ C. 1 and 3 only
❏ D. 1, 2, and 3

192. The genetic dose of radiation borne by each member of the reproductive population is called the

❏ A. genetically related dose
❏ B. genetically significant dose
❏ C. somatic related dose
❏ D. somatic significant dose

193. According to the NCRP, the pregnant radiographer's gestational dose-equivalent limit for a 1-month period is

❏ A. 1 mSv
❏ B. 5 mSv
❏ C. 0.1 mSv
❏ D. 0.5 mSv

194. What percentage of the SID must the collimator light and actual irradiated area be accurate?

❏ A. 2%
❏ B. 5%
❏ C. 10%
❏ D. 15%

195. The correct way(s) to check for cracks in lead aprons is/are

1. to fluoroscope them once a year
2. to radiograph them at low kilovoltage twice a year
3. by visual inspection

❏ A. 1 only
❏ B. 1 and 2 only
❏ C. 2 and 3 only
❏ D. 1, 2, and 3

196. The target *theory applies* to

❏ A. spermatogonia
❏ B. oocytes
❏ C. lymphocytes
❏ D. DNA molecules

197. Which of the following is/are features of fluoroscopic equipment designed especially to eliminate unnecessary radiation to patient and/or personnel?

1. Protective curtain
2. Filtration
3. Collimation
   - ❑ A. 1 only
   - ❑ B. 1 and 2 only
   - ❑ C. 1 and 3 only
   - ❑ D. 1, 2, and 3

198. Which of the following has/have been identified as source(s) of radon exposure?

1. Indoors, in houses
2. Smoking cigarettes
3. Radiology departments
   - ❑ A. 1 only
   - ❑ B. 1 and 2 only
   - ❑ C. 2 and 3 only
   - ❑ D. 1, 2, and 3

199. The interaction between ionizing radiation and the target molecule that is *most likely* to occur is the

- ❑ A. direct effect
- ❑ B. indirect effect
- ❑ C. target effect
- ❑ D. random effect

200. The advantages of beam restriction include which of the following?

1. Less scattered radiation is produced
2. Less biologic material is irradiated
3. Less total filtration will be necessary
   - ❑ A. 1 only
   - ❑ B. 1 and 2 only
   - ❑ C. 2 and 3 only
   - ❑ D. 1, 2, and 3

201. The tabletop exposure rate during fluoroscopy shall *not* exceed

- ❑ A. 2.1 mGy$_a$/min at 80 kVp
- ❑ B. 2.1 mGy$_a$/h at 80 kVp
- ❑ C. 21 mGy$_a$/min at 80 kVp
- ❑ D. 21 mGy$_a$/h at 80 kVp

202. What percentage of public exposure to ionizing radiation is from medical sources?

- ❑ A. 5%
- ❑ B. 10%
- ❑ C. 25%
- ❑ D. 50%

203. According to the National Council on Radiation Protection and Measurements (NCRP), the gestational dose-equivalent limit for embryo/fetus of a pregnant radiographer is

- ❑ A. 0.1 mSv
- ❑ B. 0.5 mSv
- ❑ C. 1.0 mSv
- ❑ D. 5.0 mSv

204. What is the established annual occupational dose-equivalent limit for the extremities?

- ❑ A. 500 mSv
- ❑ B. 200 mSv
- ❑ C. 50 mSv
- ❑ D. 10 mSv

205. The photoelectric effect is more likely to occur with

1. absorbers having a high Z number
2. high-energy incident photons
3. positive contrast media
   - ❑ A. 1 and 2 only
   - ❑ B. 1 and 3 only
   - ❑ C. 2 and 3 only
   - ❑ D. 1, 2, and 3

206. The most radiosensitive portion of the GI tract is the

- ❑ A. upper esophagus
- ❑ B. stomach
- ❑ C. small bowel
- ❑ D. cecum and ascending colon

207. Sources of secondary radiation include

1. background radiation
2. leakage radiation
3. scattered radiation
   - ❑ A. 1 only
   - ❑ B. 1 and 2 only
   - ❑ C. 2 and 3 only
   - ❑ D. 1, 2, and 3

208. Which of the following factors will affect both the quality and the quantity of the primary beam?

1. Half-value layer (HVL)
2. Kilovoltage (kV)
3. Milliamperes (mA)
   - ❑ A. 1 only
   - ❑ B. 1 and 2 only
   - ❑ C. 1 and 3 only
   - ❑ D. 1, 2, and 3

209. The average annual patient dose from medical imaging procedures in 1990 was 0.6 mSv. In 2017, the average annual patient dose was

- ❑ A. 0.6 mSv
- ❑ B. 1.2 mSv
- ❑ C. 2.2 mSv
- ❑ D. 3.2 mSv

210. Effects of deoxyribonucleic acid (DNA) irradiation include

1. mitotic delay
2. reproductive death
3. chromosome breakage
   - ❏ A. 1 only
   - ❏ B. 1 and 2 only
   - ❏ C. 2 and 3 only
   - ❏ D. 1, 2, and 3

211. The properties/characteristics of x-rays include which of the following?

1. Not perceptible by the senses
2. Ionizing action on air
3. Travel at the speed of sound
4. Homogeneous nature
5. Penetrating effect on all forms of matter
6. Behave both as waves and particles
7. Electrically charged
8. Luminescent effect on living tissue
9. Travel in straight lines
   - ❏ A. 1, 2, 4, 7, and 8
   - ❏ B. 1, 2, 5, 6, and 9
   - ❏ C. 2, 3, 5, 8, and 9
   - ❏ D. 2, 6, 7, 8, and 9
   - ❏ E. 3, 4, 5, 7, and 8

212. The production of x-ray photons by the sudden deceleration of high-speed electrons is termed:

- ❏ A. characteristic radiation
- ❏ B. Bremsstrahlung
- ❏ C. photoelectric effect
- ❏ D. Compton production

213. Which of the following will impact the x-ray beam HVL?

1. mAs
2. kV
3. Filtration
4. SID
   - ❏ A. 1 and 2 only
   - ❏ B. 1, 2, and 3 only
   - ❏ C. 2 and 3 only
   - ❏ D. 2, 3, and 4 only

214. Calculation of equivalent dose (EqD) requires:

1. absorbed dose (D)
2. type of radiation (W_r)
3. tissue exposed (W_t)
   - ❏ A. 1 only
   - ❏ B. 2 only
   - ❏ C. 1 and 2 only
   - ❏ D. 1 and 3 only
   - ❏ E. 1, 2, and 3

215. The NCRP states that x-ray tubes must be "ray-proof," that is, leakage radiation must not exceed

- ❏ A. 1 mGy_a/h at 1 m
- ❏ B. 5 mGy_a/h at 1 m
- ❏ C. 10 mGy_a/h at 1 m
- ❏ D. 20 mGy_a/h at 1 m

216. How much protection is provided from a 100-kVp x-ray beam when using a 0.50-mm lead equivalent apron?

- ❏ A. 40%
- ❏ B. 75%
- ❏ C. 88%
- ❏ D. 99%

217. What is the equivalent occupational annual dose limit for the lens of the eye?

- ❏ A. 50 mSv
- ❏ B. 10 mSv
- ❏ C. 150 mSv
- ❏ D. 500 mSv

218. The whole-body LD 50/60 for the adult human population is approximately:

- ❏ A. 1 Gy_t
- ❏ B. 2 Gy_t
- ❏ C. 3.5 Gy_t
- ❏ D. 5 Gy_t
- ❏ E. 10 Gy_t

219. The dose area product (DAP) meter is generally placed

- ❏ A. between the part and ionization chamber
- ❏ B. between the anode and cathode
- ❏ C. between the ionization chamber and grid
- ❏ D. below the collimators

220. The required thickness of a primary barrier is usually expressed as

- ❏ A. 1.2 mm (3/64 inch) Pb
- ❏ B. 1.6 mm (1/16 inch) Pb
- ❏ C. 0.8 mm (1/32 inch) Al
- ❏ D. 0.4 mm (1/64 inch) Al

221. If a particular x-ray beam intensity was reduced by four half-value layers, the resulting beam would be what percentage of its original value?

- ❏ A. 75
- ❏ B. 50
- ❏ C. 25
- ❏ D. 12.5
- ❏ E. 6.25

222. What can be done to reduce their occupational exposure when the radiographer is required to assist during fluoroscopy?
1. Wear a lead apron
2. Wear a dosimeter
3. Stand behind the radiologist
4. Increase distance from fluoroscopy tube
   - ❏ A. 1 and 2 only
   - ❏ B. 2, 3, and 4 only
   - ❏ C. 1, 2, and 4 only
   - ❏ D. 1, 3, and 4 only
   - ❏ E. 1, 2, 3, and 4

223. If the effective dose to the part was 0.2 mSv at 36-inch SID, what would the dose be at twice that distance?
- ❏ A. 0.8 mSv
- ❏ B. 0.4 mSv
- ❏ C. 0.1 mSv
- ❏ D. 0.05 mSv

224. The protective curtain used during fluoroscopic procedures must have a lead equivalent of at least what thickness?
- ❏ A. 0.15 mm
- ❏ B. 0.25 mm
- ❏ C. 0.5 mm
- ❏ D. 0.7 mm

225. Where should a radiographer wear his or her dosimeter while assisting in a fluoroscopic procedure?
- ❏ A. At waist level under lead apron
- ❏ B. At collar level under lead apron
- ❏ C. At collar level outside of lead apron
- ❏ D. At waist level outside of lead apron

226. The control dosimeter/monitor records background radiation received during
1. storage
2. handling
3. transportation
   - ❏ A. 1 and 2 only
   - ❏ B. 1 and 3 only
   - ❏ C. 2 and 3 only
   - ❏ D. 1, 2, and 3

227. How is effective dose calculated?
- ❏ A. EfD = $W_r \times W_t \times D$
- ❏ B. EfD = $D \times W_r$
- ❏ C. EfD = $W_t \times D$
- ❏ D. EfD = $W_t \times W_r$

228. An equivalent dose of 0.5 mSv was delivered to a part when image is at 36-inch SID. What would be the approximate equivalent dose if the part were imaged at 54-inch SID?
- ❏ A. 3 mSv
- ❏ B. 1.12 mSv
- ❏ C. 0.33 mSv
- ❏ D. 0.22 mSv

229. What type of dose–response curve is used to predict probabilistic effect?
- ❏ A. Nonlinear, nonthreshold
- ❏ B. Nonlinear, threshold
- ❏ C. Linear, nonthreshold
- ❏ D. Linear, threshold

230. How are wavelength and energy related?
- ❏ A. Inversely
- ❏ B. Directly
- ❏ C. Chemically
- ❏ D. Electrically

231. Which of the following defines the gonadal dose that, if received by every member of the population, would be expected to produce the same total genetic effect on that population as the actual doses received by each of the individuals?
- ❏ A. Genetically significant dose
- ❏ B. Somatically significant dose
- ❏ C. Maximum permissible dose
- ❏ D. Lethal dose

232. Which of the following account(s) for x-ray beam heterogeneity?
1. Incident electrons interacting with several layers of tungsten target atoms
2. Electrons moving to fill different shell vacancies
3. Its nuclear origin
   - ❏ A. 1 only
   - ❏ B. 1 and 2 only
   - ❏ C. 1 and 3 only
   - ❏ D. 1, 2, and 3

233. Which of the following statements regarding fluoroscopy are true?
1. The Bucky slot cover must have at least 0.5-mm lead equivalent
2. The protective curtain should be positioned between the fluoroscopist and the patient
3. A thyroid shield should have at least 0.25-mm lead equivalent
4. Protective aprons with lead equivalent of 0.5 mm are recommended
5. The lowest amount of scatter radiation is 90° from the patient
6. The protective curtain must have at least 0.25-mm lead equivalent
- A. 1, 2, 4, and 6
- B. 2, 3, 4, and 5
- C. 2, 4, 5, and 6
- D. 1, 3, 4, and 5

234. Methods of decreasing patient exposure during fluoroscopic procedures include
1. positioning the image intensifier as far from the patient as possible
2. using the last-image-hold feature
3. using the smallest FOV
- A. 1 only
- B. 1 and 2 only
- C. 2 and 3 only
- D. 1, 2, and 3

235. The protective control booth from which the radiographer makes the x-ray exposure is a
- A. primary barrier
- B. secondary barrier
- C. useful beam barrier
- D. leakage radiation barrier

236. Which of the following groups of technical factors will deliver the *least* exposure to the patient?
- A. 5 mAs, 90 kV
- B. 10 mAs, 80 kV
- C. 20 mAs, 68 kV
- D. 40 mAs, 66 kV

237. Which of the following are possible late tissue reactions resulting from excessive ionizing radiation exposure?
1. Sterility
2. Cataractogenesis
3. Epilation
4. Blood changes
5. Erythema
6. Reduced fertility
- A. 1, 2, and 6
- B. 2, 3, and 4
- C. 3, 4, and 5
- D. 1, 3, and 4

238. What is the annual dose limit for a student radiographer who is younger than 18 years and beginning clinical assignments?
- A. 1 mSv
- B. 5 mSv
- C. 50 mSv
- D. 100 mSv

239. What is the established monthly fetal dose-limit guideline for pregnant radiographers?
- A. 0.5 mSv
- B. 5 mSv
- C. 50 mSv
- D. 100 mSv

240. According to the NCRP, what is the annual dose limit (DL) to the extremities?
- A. 50 mSv
- B. 100 mSv
- C. 200 mSv
- D. 500 mSv

1. **(B)** The newest type of personnel monitoring device is the *direct ion storage dosimeter* (DIS); it is a digital ionization dosimeter. The DIS eliminates the need to collect and send dosimeters for monthly or quarterly processing. The user wears the DIS, which looks like a small flash drive, in the same way as other monitors such as an OSL (optically stimulated luminescence) dosimeter. The DIS has a gas-filled ionization chamber within and uses Bluetooth technology to relate its raw data via mobile device or any computer with Internet access and a USB connection. Occupational exposure can be read, and reread, at any time without loss of information.

   The pocket dosimeter, or pocket ionization chamber, resembles a penlight and has a thimble ionization chamber within. Ions are counted and radiation quantity is registered in milliroentgens (mR). The use of the pocket dosimeter is indicated when working with high exposures or large quantities of radiation for short periods of time, so that an immediate reading is available to the user. The pocket dosimeter is sensitive and accurate but has limited application in diagnostic radiography.

2. **(C)** Bremsstrahlung (braking or Brems) radiation is one of the two types of x-ray photons produced at the x-ray tube tungsten target. When high-speed electrons coming from the cathode filament pass near or through a tungsten atom, they can be attracted by the positively charged nucleus, slowed down/braked, and *deflected from their course with a resulting loss of energy.* This energy is given up in the form of an x-ray photon.

3. **(C)** If the exposure rate for the examination is 150 mGy$_a$/h (60 min), then a 5-min examination would be proportionally less—as the following equation illustrates:

$$\frac{150 \, mGy_a}{60 \, min} = \frac{x \, mGy_a}{5.0 \, min}$$

$$60x = 750$$

   Thus, $x = 12.5$ mGy$_a$ dose in 5 min.

4. **(C)** Late effects of radiation can occur in cells that have survived a previous irradiation months or years earlier. These late effects, such as carcinogenesis and genetic effects are "all-or-nothing" effects—either the organism develops cancer or it does not. Most late effects do not have a threshold dose; that is, *any* dose, however small, theoretically can induce an effect. Increasing that dose *will* increase the *likelihood* of the occurrence but *will not* affect its *severity;* these effects are termed *stochastic/ probabilistic. Nonstochastic/deterministic effects* are those that will not occur below a particular threshold dose and that increase in severity as the dose increases.

5. **(A)** The collimator is the most practical and efficient beam-restricting device; the collimator box is attached to the tube head. Adjustable lead shutter collimators are used to define the size and shape of the x-ray field that emerge from the x-ray tube port window. The fixed diaphragm located just outside the x-ray tube's port window functions to significantly reduce the effect of *off-focus* radiation. Off-focus (extrafocal or stem) radiation is produced when electrons strike surfaces other than the focal track.

   The next set/stage of lead shutters consists of two pairs of adjustable shutters—one pair for field length and another pair for field width. These shutters are used to regulate the length and width of the irradiated field.

6. **(B)** *Somatic effects* of radiation refer to those effects experienced directly by the exposed individual, such as erythema, epilation, and cataracts. *Genetic effects* of radiation exposure are caused by irradiation of the reproductive cells of the exposed individual and are transmitted from one generation to the next.

7. **(B)** It is our professional responsibility to minimize exposure dose to both patients and ourselves, and one of the most important ways is with a closely collimated radiation field. Gonadal shielding should be used when the patient is of reproductive age or younger, when the gonads are in or within 5 cm of the collimated field, and when the clinical objectives will not be compromised.

8. **(C)** The first noticeable skin response to excessive irradiation would be *erythema,* a reddening of the skin very much like sunburn. *Dry desquamation,* a dry peeling of the skin, may follow. *Moist desquamation* is peeling with associated pus-like fluid. *Epilation,* or hair loss, may be temporary or permanent depending on sensitivity and dose.

9. **(C)** Dose area product (DAP) expresses the dose of radiation to a particular volume of tissue, thereby being a potentially better indicator of risk than dose values alone. DAP is expressed in terms of cGy-cm². An *increased* field size will *increase* the DAP even if the technical factors (dose) remain unchanged. As field size decreases, the amount of exposed tissue decreases, and DAP is decreased.

   DAP can be monitored using a DAP meter in both radiographic and fluoroscopic procedures. The DAP meter is radiolucent and is mounted just below the radiographic collimator, measuring x-radiation before it reaches the part. Skin dose can be determined by dividing the skin area exposed by the DAP measurement. This value represents potential deterministic effect to that tissue.

Increasing field size increases the production of scattered radiation. Focal spot size is unrelated to dose.

10. (C) The patient, as the first scatterer, is the most important scatterer. At 1 m from the patient, the intensity of the scattered beam is 0.1% of the intensity of the primary beam. Compton scatter emerging from the patient is almost as energetic as the primary beam entering the patient.

11. (C) Radiation effects that appear days or weeks following exposure (early effects) are in response to high radiation doses; this is called *acute radiation syndrome*. These effects should never occur in diagnostic radiology; they occur only in response to much greater, usually whole-body, doses. Sufficient exposure of the *hematologic* system to ionizing radiation can result in nausea, vomiting, diarrhea, decreased blood cells count, and infection. Very large exposure of the *GI system* (6–10 Gy) causes severe damage to the (stem) cells lining the GI tract. This can result in nausea, vomiting, diarrhea, blood changes, and hemorrhage. Exposure greater than 50 Gy is required to cause cerebrovascular syndrome, affecting the normally resilient CNS and cardiovascular systems.

12. (A) HVL is defined as the thickness of any absorber that will reduce x-ray beam intensity to one-half of its original value. It is influenced by the type of rectification, total filtration, and kilovoltage. As kilovoltage increases, half-value layer increases—thus making it a direct relationship. An x-ray tube HVL should remain almost constant. If HVL decreases, it is an indication of a decrease in the actual kilovoltage. If the HVL increases, it indicates the deposition of vaporized tungsten on the inner surface of the glass envelope (as a result of tube aging) or an increase in the actual kilovoltage.

13. (C) Different types of monitoring devices are available for the occupationally exposed, and anyone who might receive more than *one-tenth the annual dose limit* (of 50 mSv, i.e., 5 rem) must be monitored. Ionization is the fundamental principle of operation of both the film badge (film emulsion) and the pocket dosimeter (air chamber). TLDs are radiation monitors that use lithium fluoride crystals. Once exposed to ionizing radiation and then heated, these crystals give off light in proportion to the amount of radiation received. OSL dosimeters are radiation monitors that use aluminum oxide crystals. These crystals, once exposed to ionizing radiation and then subjected to a laser, give off luminescence proportional to the amount of radiation received.

14. (C) The entire population of the world is exposed to varying amounts of background (environmental) radiation. Sources of background radiation are either *natural* or *man-made*. Exposure to *natural* background radiation is a result of cosmic radiation from space (*external terrestrial*) and naturally radioactive elements *within the earth's crust* (internal terrestrial) and our own bodies (internal sources, from ingested materials). Naturally, the closer we are to the cosmic radiations from space, the greater our personal exposure will be; living at higher elevations and air travel expose us to greater amounts of radiation. Living or working in a building made of materials derived from the ground exposes us to some background radiation from the naturally radioactive elements found in the earth's crust. The food we eat, the water we drink, and the air we breathe all contribute to the quantity of radiation we ingest and inhale. Man-made radiation, however, is the type of background radiation over which we have some control. Medical and dental x-rays, nuclear power plant environs, and nuclear medicine contribute to our exposure to *man-made* background radiation. According to the BEIR VII report, medical and dental x-rays and nuclear medicine studies account for approximately 79% of the man-made radiation exposure in the United States. In addition, NCRP Reports No. 160 and 184 indicate that *medical radiation exposure now contributes 50% of the public's exposure to ionizing radiation*. NRC (Nuclear Regulatory Commission) regulations and radiation exposure limits are published in Title 10 of the Code of Federal Regulations (CFR), Part 20.

15. (A) The most radiosensitive portion of the GI tract is the small bowel. Projecting from the lining of the small bowel are villi, from the epithelial crypts of Lieberkühn, which are responsible for the absorption of nutrients into the bloodstream. Because the epithelial cells of the villi are continually being cast off, new cells must continually arise from the crypts of Lieberkühn. These new cells are highly mitotic undifferentiated stem cells and therefore very radiosensitive. Thus, the small bowel is the most radiosensitive portion of the GI tract. In adults, the CNS is the most radioresistant system, and the epidermis is composed of radioresistant, mature postmitotic cells.

16. (A) X-radiation used for diagnostic purposes is of relatively *low energy*. Kilovoltages of up to 150 kV are used, as compared with radiations having energies of up to several million volts. *Linear energy transfer* (LET) refers to the rate at which energy is transferred from ionizing radiation to soft tissue. Particulate radiations, such as alpha particles, have mass and charge and, therefore, lose energy rapidly as they penetrate only a few centimeters of air. X- and gamma radiations, having no mass or charge, are *low-LET* radiations.

17. (A) The *tissue weighting factor* (W_t) represents the relative tissue radiosensitivity of irradiated material (e.g., muscle vs. intestinal epithelium vs. bone). The *radiation weighting factor* (W_r) is a number assigned to different types of ionizing radiations to better determine their effect on tissue (e.g., x-ray vs. alpha particles). The W_r of different ionizing radiations depends on the LET of that particular radiation. The following formula is used to determine *effective dose (EfD)*:

Effective dose *(EfD)* = radiation weighting factor (W_r)
× tissue weighting factor (W_t)
× absorbed dose

18. **(B)** In the *photoelectric effect,* a relatively low-energy photon uses all its energy to eject an inner-shell electron, leaving a vacancy. An electron from the shell above drops down to fill the vacancy and in so doing gives up a characteristic ray. This type of interaction is most harmful to the patient because all the photon energy is transferred to the tissue. In *Compton scatter,* a high-energy incident photon ejects an outer-shell electron. In so doing, the incident photon is deflected with reduced energy, but it *usually retains most of its energy and exits the body as an energetic scattered ray.* This scattered ray will either contribute to image fog or pose a radiation hazard to personnel depending on its direction of exit. In *classic scatter,* a low-energy photon interacts with an atom but causes no ionization; the incident photon disappears into the atom and then is released immediately as a photon of identical energy but with changed direction. *Thompson scatter* is another name for classic scatter.

19. **(C)** The relationship between x-ray intensity and distance from the source is expressed by the inverse-square law of radiation. The formula is

$$\frac{I_1}{I_2} = \frac{D_2^2}{D_1^2}$$

Substituting known values:

$$\frac{50\,\text{mGy}_a/\text{h}}{10\,\text{mGy}_a/\text{h}} = \frac{x^2}{5^2}$$

$$10\,x^2 = 1250$$

$$x^2 = 125$$

$$x = 11.1 \text{ m}$$

Thus, $x = 11.1$ m (36 feet) is necessary to decrease the exposure to 10 mGy$_a$/h. Note that in order for the exposure rate to decrease, the distance from the source of radiation must increase; as distance decreases, exposure rate increases.

20. **(D)** *Secondary* radiation includes *leakage and scattered radiation.* Secondary barriers are those that should never be struck by the primary beam. The control booth wall is a secondary barrier; therefore, the primary beam must never be directed toward it. The x-ray tube housing must reduce leakage radiation to less than 1 mGy$_a$/h (100 mR/h) at a distance of 1 m from the housing. Lead aprons, lead gloves, portable x-ray barriers, and so on are also designed to protect the user from exposure to *scattered* radiation and will not protect the individual from the primary beam.

21. **(D)** Late somatic effects are those that can occur years after initial exposure and are caused by low, chronic exposures. Occupationally, exposed personnel are concerned with the late effects of radiation exposure. Bone malignancies, thyroid cancers, leukemia, and skin cancers are examples of *carcinogenic* somatic effects of radiation. Another example of somatic effects of radiation is *cataract* formation in the lenses of eyes of individuals accidentally exposed to sufficient quantities of radiation. The lives of many of the early radiation workers were several years shorter than the lives of the general population. Statistics revealed that radiologists, for example, had a shorter life span than physicians of other specialties. *Life span shortening,* then, *was* another somatic effect of radiation. Certainly, these effects should *never be experienced nowadays.* The human reproductive organs are particularly radiosensitive. *Fertility* and *heredity* can be greatly affected by the *germ cells* produced within the testes (*spermatogonia*) and ovaries (*oogonia*). Excessive radiation exposure to the gonads can cause *reduced fertility or permanent sterility* and/or *genetic mutations.*

22. **(D)** One of the radiation protection guidelines for the occupationally exposed is that x-ray photons should scatter twice before reaching the operator. Each time an x-ray photon scatters, its intensity at 1 m from the scattering object is *one-thousandth* of its original intensity. Of course, the operator should be behind a protective shield while making the exposure, but multiple scatterings further reduce the danger of exposure from the scattered radiation.

23. **(C)** Bergonié and Tribondeau were French scientists who, in 1906, theorized what has now become verified law. Cells are more radiosensitive if they are *immature* (undifferentiated or stem) cells, if they are *highly mitotic* (having a high rate of proliferation), and if the irradiated tissue is young. Cells and tissues that are still undergoing development are more radiosensitive than fully developed tissues.

24. **(C)** TLDs are personnel radiation monitors that use *lithium fluoride* crystals. Once exposed to ionizing radiation and then heated, these crystals give off light proportional to the amount of radiation received. TLDs are very accurate personnel monitors. Even more accurate are optically stimulated luminescence (OSL) dosimeters. OSL dosimeters use *aluminum oxide* as their sensitive crystal. Silver halide is in film emulsion and sodium thiosulfate is in fixer solution.

25. **(C)** A *controlled area* is occupied by radiology personnel and patients. The radiology personnel are trained in radiation safety and wear radiation monitors. The radiation barriers in a controlled area must keep the weekly dose to radiation workers to less than 1 mSv/week (100 mrem). That limit is based on the annual occupational dose limit of 50 mSv/year. The occupancy factor in a controlled area is considered to be 1, indicating that the area may always be occupied and, therefore, requires maximum shielding.

An *uncontrolled area* is one that is occupied by anyone; the maximum exposure permitted in an uncontrolled area is 20 μSv (2 mrem)/week. That limit is based on the recommended annual dose limit to the general population of 1 mSv (100 mrem)/year. Shielding requirements vary according to several factors, one being occupancy factor.

26. **(C)** The selected milliampere seconds are directly related to patient dose, that is, if milliampere seconds are doubled, patient dose is doubled. Similarly, if milliampere seconds are cut in half, patient dose is cut in half. The selected kilovolts peak is inversely related to patient dose, that is, if the kilovolts peak is increased, patient dose can be decreased because more x-ray photons are transmitted through the patient rather than being absorbed. Inherent filtration is provided by materials that are a permanent part of the tube housing, that is, the glass envelope of the x-ray tube and the oil coolant. Added filtration, usually thin sheets of aluminum, is present to make a total of 2.5-mm Al equivalent for equipment operated above 70 kVp. Filtration is used to decrease patient dose by removing the weak x-rays that have no value but contribute to the skin dose. The effect of focal spot size is principally on radiographic sharpness; it has no effect on patient dose.

27. **(C)** The radiologic image is obtained as a result of the attenuation processes occurring in the body. Tissues having a *high atomic number* (e.g. bone) are very dense and will allow little or no passage of x-rays. Those tissues appear white or light on the image as a result of photoelectric interactions. Other tissues are easier for x-ray photons to penetrate—those tissues appear darker because a greater number of photons reached the IR.

Valence electrons are those in the outermost atomic shell. Electron binding energy is related to its proximity to the atomic nucleus; inner-shell electrons have a higher binding energy than outer electrons.

28. **(B)** Aluminum filters are used to decrease patient skin dose by absorbing the low-energy photons (therefore, *decreased* mGy$_a$ output) that *do not contribute to the image* but *do contribute to patient skin dose*. HVL is defined as that thickness of any absorber that will decrease the intensity of a particular beam to one-half of its original value. As filtration of an x-ray beam is increased, the overall *average energy of the resulting beam is greater* (because the low-energy photons have been removed)—and, therefore, the HVL thickness required would be greater.

29. **(C)** The *tissue weighting factor* (W_t) represents the relative tissue radiosensitivity of irradiated material (e.g., muscle vs. intestinal epithelium vs. bone). The *radiation weighting factor* (W_r) is a number assigned to different types of ionizing radiations to better determine their effect on tissue (e.g., x-ray vs. alpha particles). The W_r of different ionizing radiations depends on the LET of that particular radiation. The following formula is used to determine *effective dose* (EfD):

Effective dose (EfD) = radiation weighting factor (W_r) × tissue weighting factor (W_t) × absorbed dose

30. **(B)** Special arrangements are required for occupational monitoring of the pregnant radiographer. The pregnant radiographer will wear two dosimeters—one in its usual place at the collar and the other, a baby/fetal dosimeter, worn over the abdomen and *under* the lead apron during fluoroscopy. The baby/fetal dosimeter must be identified as such and always must be worn in the same place. Care must be taken not to mix the positions of the two dosimeters. The dosimeters are read monthly, as usual. The pregnant radiographer may not be made to leave the radiation area/department because of her pregnancy.

31. **(A)** Occupationally, exposed individuals are required to use devices that will record and provide documentation of the radiation they receive over a given period of time, traditionally 1 month. The most commonly used personnel dosimeters are the OSL, the TLD, DOS dosimeter, and the film badge. These devices must be worn *only* for documentation of occupational exposure. They must not be worn for any medical or dental x-rays one receives as a patient, and they are not used to measure naturally occurring background radiation.

32. **(B)** Irradiation during *pregnancy,* especially in early pregnancy, must be avoided. The fetus is particularly radiosensitive during the first trimester, during much of which time pregnancy may not even be suspected. High-risk examinations include pelvis, hip, femur, lumbar spine, cystograms and urograms, and upper and lower gastrointestinal (GI) series. During the first trimester, specifically the 2nd to 10th weeks of pregnancy (i.e., during major organogenesis), if the radiation dose is sufficient, fetal anomalies can be produced. *Skeletal and/or organ anomalies* can appear if irradiation occurs in the *early* part of this time period, and *neurologic anomalies* can be formed in the *latter* part; mental retardation and childhood malignant diseases, such as cancers or leukemia, and retarded growth/development also can result from irradiation during the first trimester. Fetal irradiation during the second and third trimesters is not likely to produce anomalies but rather, with sufficient dose, some type of childhood malignant disease. Fetal irradiation during the first 2 weeks of gestation can result in embryonic resorption or spontaneous abortion. It must be emphasized, however, that the likelihood of producing fetal anomalies at doses less than 200 mGy (20 rad) is exceedingly small and that most general diagnostic examinations are likely to deliver fetal doses of less than 10–20 mGy (1–2 rad).

33. **(B)** The effects of a quantity of radiation delivered to a body depend on the amount of radiation received, the size of the irradiated area, and how the radiation is delivered in time. If the radiation is delivered in portions over a period of time, it is said to be *fractionated* and has a less harmful effect than if it were delivered all at once because cells have an opportunity to repair, and some recovery occurs between doses.

34. (B) X-ray intensity is inversely related to SID; as SID increases, x-ray intensity decreases. The x-ray intensity at the image intensifier also depends on the SID. Moving the image intensifier *closer* to the patient *decreases* the patient entrance dose and increases x-ray beam intensity at the input phosphor. The automatic brightness control (ABC) then *decreases the milliamperes* again decreasing the patient dose. Moving the image intensifier closer to the patient also results in a *shorter OID,* therefore decreased magnification and improved image quality.

35. (C) *Gamma and x-radiations are electromagnetic,* having wavelike fluctuations like other radiations of the electromagnetic spectrum (e.g., visible light, radio waves, ultraviolet, and infrared). Alpha and beta radiations are *particulate* radiations; alpha is composed of two protons and two neutrons, and beta is identical to an electron.

36. (B) X-rays produced at the tungsten target make up a heterogeneous primary beam. Filtration serves to eliminate the softer, less penetrating, low-energy photons, leaving an x-ray beam of higher average energy. Because x-ray photons were removed from the beam, it has a decreased intensity/quantity. The overall x-ray beam is now more penetrating. Filtration is important in patient protection, because unfiltered, low-energy photons that are not energetic enough to reach the IR stay in the body and contribute to total patient dose.

37. (C) Lead aprons are secondary radiation barriers and *must* contain at least 0.25-mm Pb equivalent (*according to CFR 20*), usually in the form of lead-impregnated vinyl. Many radiology departments routinely use lead aprons containing 0.5 mm Pb (the NCRP *recommends* 0.5-mm Pb equivalent minimum). These aprons are heavier, but they attenuate a higher percentage of scattered radiation.

38. (E) The term *effective dose* (EfD) refers to the dose from radiation sources internal and/or external to the body and is expressed in units of Sievert or rem. The factors used to determine effective dose (*EfD*) are as follows:

$$\text{EfD} = \text{radiation weighting factor } (W_r)$$
$$\times \text{ tissue weighting factor } (W_t)$$
$$\times \text{ absorbed dose } (D)$$

The term *equivalent dose* (EqD) refers simply to the product of the absorbed dose (Gy/rad) and its radiation weighting factor (W_r).

39. (B) Cells are frequently identified by their stage of development. *Immature* cells may be called *undifferentiated* or *stem* cells. Immature cells are much more radiosensitive than mature cells.

40. (B) *Scattering* occurs when there is partial transfer of the proton's energy to matter, as in the Compton effect. *Absorption* occurs when an x-ray photon interacts with matter and disappears, such as in the photoelectric effect. *Differential absorption* describes the absorption characteristics of various tissues such as bone, muscle, and soft tissue. The reduction in the intensity (quantity) of an x-ray beam as it passes through matter is termed *attenuation. Divergence* refers to a directional characteristic of the x-ray beam as it is emitted from the focal spot.

41. (D) Part compression, when possible, can improve spatial resolution by reducing part thickness and decreasing OID. Contrast resolution is improved because less scattered radiation will be generated in a thinner part. Because the part is essentially thinner, technical factors can be reduced thereby decreasing patient dose.

42. (D) For radiation safety, the fluoroscopy exposure switch must be of the "*dead-man*" type. When the foot is removed from the fluoro pedal, the "dead-man" switch will terminate the exposure immediately. There must also be a fluoroscopy cumulative timer that will either *sound or interrupt* (it will not terminate/stop exposure) exposure after 5 min of fluoroscopy.

43. (B) Protective barriers are classified as either primary or secondary. *Primary* barriers protect from the useful, or primary, x-ray beam and consist of a certain thickness of lead. They are located anywhere that the primary beam can possibly be directed, for example, the walls of the x-ray room. The walls of the x-ray room usually require a 1/16 inch (1.6 mm) thickness of lead and should be 7 feet high. Secondary barriers protect from secondary (scattered and leakage) radiation. Secondary barriers are control booths, lead aprons, gloves, and the wall of the x-ray room above 7 feet. Secondary barriers require much less lead than primary barriers.

44. (C) The occupational dose limit is valid for beta, x-, and gamma radiations. Because alpha radiation is so rapidly ionizing, traditional personnel monitors will not record alpha radiation. However, because alpha particles are capable of penetrating only a few centimeters of air, they are practically harmless as an external source.

45. (B) Diagnostic x-ray photons interact with tissue in a number of ways, but most frequently they are involved in the production of *Compton scatter* or in a *photoelectric* interaction. The *photoelectric effect* is shown in Figure 3-10; it occurs when a relatively *low-energy* x-ray photon *uses all its energy* to eject an *inner-shell electron.* That electron is ejected (photoelectron) from the innermost (K) shell, leaving a "hole" in the K shell and producing a positive ion. An L-shell electron then drops down to fill the K vacancy and in so doing emits a *characteristic ray* whose energy is equal to the difference between the binding energies of the K and L shells. The photoelectric effect occurs with high–atomic-number absorbers, such as bone and positive contrast media and is responsible for the production of contrast. Therefore, its occurrence is helpful for the production of the radiographic image, but it contributes significantly to the dose received by the patient (because it involves complete absorption of the incident photon). Scattered radiation, which produces a radiation hazard to the radiographer (as in fluoroscopy), is a product of the Compton scatter interaction occurring with higher energy x-ray photons.

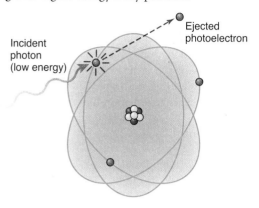

Figure 3-10

46. (B) During fluoroscopic procedures, as field of view (FOV) decreases, magnification of the output screen image increases, and contrast and resolution improve. The focal point on an image intensifier's 6-inch field/mode is further away from the output phosphor than the focal point on the normal mode; therefore, the output image is magnified. Because less minification takes place, the *image is not as bright. Exposure factors are increased automatically to compensate for the loss in brightness with smaller FOVs.* Focal spot size (FSS) is unrelated to patient dose.

47. (D) Gonadal shielding should be used whenever appropriate and possible during radiographic and fluoroscopic examinations. *Flat contact* shields are useful for simple recumbent (AP and PA) studies, but when the examination necessitates obtaining oblique, lateral, or erect projections, they become less efficient. *Shaped contact (contour)* shields are best because they enclose the male reproductive organs and remain in position in oblique, lateral, and erect positions. *Shadow* shields that attach to the tube head are particularly useful for surgical sterile fields.

48. (C) The Sievert (Sv) is the unit radiation dose to biologic material, and is used to express occupational exposure and effective dose. The traditional unit *rem* is an acronym for *radiation equivalent man*; it includes the RBE specific to the tissue irradiated and can be used as a unit of measurement for the dose to biologic tissue. The traditional unit *rad* is an acronym for *radiation absorbed dose*; it measures the energy deposited in any material. The SI unit used to express radiation dose is Gy_t. Air kerma (Gy_a) is the SI unit of radiation exposure. *Roentgen* is a unit of exposure; it can be used to express the quantity of ionizations in air as a traditional unit of measure.

49. (B) When biologic material is irradiated, there are a number of modifying factors that determine what kind and how much response will occur in the material. One of these factors is LET, which expresses the *rate at which*

particulate or photon energy is transferred to the absorber. Because different kinds of radiation have different degrees of penetration in different materials, it is also a useful way of expressing the quality of the radiation.

50. (C) Electromagnetic radiations, such as x-rays and gamma rays are considered low-LET radiations because they produce fewer ionizations than the highly ionizing particulate radiations, such as alpha particles. *Alpha particles* are large and heavy (two protons and two neutrons), and although they possess a great deal of kinetic energy (approximately 5 MeV), their energy is lost rapidly through multiple ionizations (approximately 40,000 atoms/cm of air). As an *external* source, alpha particles are almost harmless because they ionize the air very quickly and never reach the individual. As *internal sources,* however, they ionize tissues and are potentially the most harmful. It may be stated that the alpha particle has one of the highest LETs of all ionizing radiations.

51. (D) The various skin responses to irradiation include all four choices. The first noticeable response would be *erythema,* a reddening of the skin very much like sunburn. *Dry desquamation* could follow; it is a dry peeling of the skin. *Moist desquamation* is peeling with associated pus-like fluid. *Epilation* is hair loss; it can be temporary or permanent depending on sensitivity and dose.

52. (D) Irradiation damage is a result of either the effects of irradiation on water (radiolysis) or its effects on macromolecules. Effects on macromolecules include cleaved chromosomes, cross-linking, and mutations. *Cleaved/broken chromosome* is the result of a double-strand break on the same DNA "rung." *Cross-linking* is incorrect joining of broken DNA fragments. A *mutation* is the result of damage/alteration of nitrogenous base sequence as a result of irradiation. Because 80% of the body is made up of water, radiolysis of water is the predominant radiation interaction in the body.

53. (C) The reduction in the intensity (quantity) of an x-ray beam as it passes through matter as a result of absorption and scatter is called *attenuation. Absorption* occurs when an x-ray photon interacts with matter and disappears, such as in the *photoelectric effect. Scattering* occurs when there is partial transfer of energy to matter, such as in the *Compton effect.*

54. (C) Radiation-induced malignancy, leukemia, and genetic effects are late effects (or stochastic/probabilistic effects) of radiation exposure. These can occur years after survival of an acute radiation dose or after exposure to low levels of radiation over a long period of time. Radiation workers need to be especially aware of the late effects of radiation because their exposure to radiation is usually low level over a long period of time. Occupational radiation protection guidelines, therefore, are based on late effects of radiation according to a *linear, nonthreshold dose–response curve.*

55. (A) The milliampere second setting regulates the quantity of radiation delivered to the patient, and the kilovolts peak setting regulates the quality (i.e., penetration) of the radiation delivered to the patient. Therefore, higher energy (i.e., more penetrating) radiation (which is more likely to exit the patient), accompanied by lower milliampere seconds, is the safest combination for the patient.

56. (B) *Late* or *long-term effects* of radiation can occur in tissues that have survived a previous irradiation months or years earlier. These late effects, such as carcinogenesis and genetic effects are "all-or-nothing" effects—either the organism develops cancer or it does not. Most late effects *do not have a threshold dose,* that is, any dose, however small, can induce an effect. Increasing that dose will increase the *likelihood* of the occurrence but will not affect its severity; these effects are termed *stochastic/ probabilistic. Nonstochastic/deterministic effects* (most currently called *tissue responses*) are those that will not occur below a particular threshold dose and that increase in severity as the dose increases. *Early* effects of radiation exposure are in response to relatively high radiation doses. These should never occur in diagnostic radiology; they occur only in response to doses much greater than those used in diagnostic radiology. One of the effects that may be noted in such a circumstance is the *hematologic effect*—reduced numbers of white blood cells, red blood cells, and platelets in the circulating blood. Immediate local tissue effects can include effects on the gonads (temporary infertility) and on the skin (epilation, erythema). Acute radiation lethality, or radiation death, occurs after an acute exposure and results in death in weeks or days.

57. (C) The development of male and female reproductive stem cells has important radiation protection implications. Male stem cells reproduce continuously. However, female stem cells develop only during fetal life; women are born with all the reproductive cells they will ever have. It is exceedingly important to shield children whenever possible because they have their reproductive futures ahead of them.

58. (D) According to Bergonié and Tribondeau, the most radiosensitive cells are undifferentiated, rapidly dividing cells, such as lymphocytes, intestinal crypt (of Lieberkühn) cells, and spermatogonia. Liver cells are among the types of cells that are somewhat differentiated and capable of mitosis. These characteristics render them somewhat radiosensitive. Muscle cells, as well as nerve cells and red blood cells, are highly differentiated and do not divide. Therefore, in order of *increasing* sensitivity (from least to greatest sensitivity), the cells are muscle, liver, and then intestinal crypt cells.

59. (D) Our bodies contain a variety of tissues having a variety of *tissue densities.* These tissue densities afford differing degrees of resistance to the passage of x-ray photons. Tissues having *greater density absorb more* of the x-ray beam (recall the photoelectric effect). Soft tissues are fairly easily penetrated to varying degrees, that is, lung and adipose are easier to penetrate than muscle. *Bone* has much higher tissue mass density and, therefore, absorbs more of the x-ray beam.

60. (B) X-ray photons produced in the x-ray tube can radiate in directions other than the one desired. The *tube housing,* therefore, is constructed so that very little of this leakage radiation is permitted to escape. The regulation states that leakage radiation must not exceed 1 mGy$_a$/h (100 mR/h) at 1 m while the tube is operated at maximum potential.

61. (A) In the photoelectric effect, the incident (low-energy) photon is completely absorbed and thus is responsible for producing contrast and contributing to patient dose. The photoelectric effect is the interaction between x-ray and tissue that predominates in the diagnostic range. In Compton scatter, only partial absorption occurs, and most energy emerges as scattered photons. In coherent scatter, no energy is absorbed by the part; it all emerges as scattered photons. Pair production occurs only at very high energy levels, at least 1.02 MeV.

62. (D) In fluoroscopy, the source of x-rays is 30–38 cm below the x-ray tabletop. Because the source-to-object distance (SOD) is so short, patient skin dose can be quite high. Consequently, the x-ray intensity at the tabletop is limited to keep patient dose (ESE) within safe limits. The radiation protection guidelines state that x-ray intensity at tabletop must not exceed *21 mGy$_a$/min/mA at 80 kVp.* In equipment *without* high-level fluoroscopy capability, the guideline is *100 mGy$_a$/min* tabletop limit. In equipment with high-level fluoroscopy capability, the tabletop limit is *200 mGy$_a$/min.*

63. (A) Characteristic radiation is one of two kinds of x-rays produced at the tungsten target of the x-ray tube. The incident, or incoming, high-speed electron ejects a K-shell tungsten electron. This leaves a hole in the K shell, and an L-shell electron drops down to fill the K vacancy. Because L electrons are at a higher energy level than K-shell electrons, the L-shell electron gives up the difference in binding energy in the form of a photon, a *characteristic x-ray* (characteristic of the K shell).

64. (D) The x-ray photons produced at the tungsten target make up a heterogeneous beam, a spectrum of photon energies. This is accounted for by the fact that the incident electrons have differing energies. Also, the incident electrons travel through several layers of tungsten target material, lose energy with each interaction, and, therefore, produce increasingly weaker photons. During characteristic x-ray production, vacancies may be filled in the K, L, or M shells, which differ from each other in binding energies, and, therefore, photons with varying amounts of energy are emitted.

65. (C) Entrance skin exposure (ESE) is generally used to express patient dose in diagnostic radiography because it is fairly simple to measure. Genetically significant dose (GSD) is used to express gonadal exposure; gonadal dose is related to possible genetic responses. Mean marrow dose (MMD) is used to express dose to bone marrow because of its relationship to radiation-induced leukemia.

66. (B) In the *photoelectric effect,* a relatively low-energy photon uses all its energy to eject an inner-shell electron, leaving a vacancy. An electron from the shell above drops down to fill the vacancy and in so doing gives up a characteristic ray. This type of interaction is most harmful to the patient because all the photon energy is transferred to tissue. In *Compton scatter,* a high-energy incident photon uses some of its energy to eject an outer-shell electron. In so doing, the incident photon is deflected with reduced energy, but it usually retains most of its energy and exits the body as an energetic scattered ray. *This scattered ray will either contribute to image fog or pose a radiation hazard to personnel* depending on its direction of exit; thus, Compton scatter contributes the most to occupational exposure. In *classic scatter,* a low-energy photon interacts with an atom but causes no ionization; the incident photon disappears into the atom and then is released immediately as a photon of identical energy but with changed direction. *Thompson scatter* is another name for classic scatter.

67. (C) The likelihood of radiation effects to occupationally exposed individuals whose dose is kept below the recommended limits is very remote. Exposure to ionizing radiation always carries some risk, but studies have indicated that the risk is a very small one if established guidelines are followed. Potential hazards must be understood and proper precautions must be taken.

68. (C) Radiation protection guidelines have established that primary radiation barriers must be 7 feet high. *Primary radiation barriers* are walls toward which the primary beam may be directed. These walls usually contain 1.6 mm (about 1/16 inch) of lead, but this can vary depending on use factor, and so on. *Secondary* radiation barriers include the portion of the walls *above* 2.1 m (7 feet) in height; this area requires only 0.8 mm (1/32 inch) of lead. The control booth is also a secondary barrier, toward which the primary beam must never be directed.

69. (B) Because the primary x-ray beam has a polyenergetic (heterogeneous) nature, *the entrance or skin dose is significantly greater than the exit dose.* This principle may be used in radiation protection by placing particularly radiosensitive organs away from the primary beam. To place the gonads further from the primary beam and reduce gonadal dose, abdominal radiography should be performed in the posteroanterior (PA) position whenever possible. Dose to the *lens* is decreased significantly when skull radiographs are performed in the PA position.

70. (C) According to the NCRP, the annual occupational *whole-body* dose-equivalent limit is 50 mSv (5 rem or 5000 mrem). The annual occupational whole-body dose-equivalent limit for *students* younger than 18 years is 1 mSv (100 mrem or 0.1 rem). The annual occupational dose-equivalent limit for the *lens of eye* is 150 mSv (15 rem). The annual occupational dose-equivalent limit for the *thyroid, skin,* and *extremities* is 500 mSv (50 rem). The total gestational dose-equivalent limit for *embryo/fetus* of a pregnant radiographer is 5 mSv (500 mrem), not to exceed 0.5 mSv in 1 month.

71. (D) The majority of a radiographer's occupational exposure comes from fluoroscopy and bedside radiography. The protection afforded by walls and control booths, available during general radiography, is absent during these procedures. It is therefore essential that radiographers make use of protective lead aprons during bedside and fluoroscopic procedures.

72. (B) Dose–response curves are used to illustrate the relationship between exposure to ionizing radiation and possible resultant biologic responses. Figure 3-3 illustrates three dose–response curves. *Curve A* begins at zero, indicating that there is no safe dose, that is, *no threshold.* Even one x-ray photon theoretically can cause a response. It is a straight (*linear*) line, indicating that *response is proportional to dose,* that is, as dose increases, response increases. *Curve B* is another *linear* curve, but this one illustrates a situation in which a particular dose of radiation must be received before the response will occur—that is, there is a *threshold dose,* and this is a linear threshold curve. *Curve C* is another threshold curve, but this curve is nonlinear. It illustrates that once the minimum dose is received, a response occurs slowly initially and then increases sharply as exposure increases.

73. (B) In the past few decades, ICRP and NCRP studies have indicated that radiation-induced cancer risks are greater than radiation-induced genetic risks—contrary to previous thought. Their philosophy then grew to be concerned with the probability of radiation-induced cancer mortality in the occupational radiation industry in comparison with annual accidental mortality in "safe" (radiation-free) industries. The NCRP reexamined its 1987 recommendations, and in NCRP Report No. 116, it reiterates its *annual effective whole-body occupational DL (dose limit) as 50 mSv (5 rem).*

74. (A) As an x-ray source moves away from a detector, the x-ray intensity (quantity) decreases. Conversely, as the source of x-rays moves closer to the detector, the intensity increases. This is a predictable relationship that may be calculated using the inverse-square law, which states that the intensity (exposure rate) of radiation at a given distance from a point source is inversely proportional to the square of the distance. For example, if the distance from an x-ray source were doubled, the intensity of x-rays at the detector would be one-fourth of its original value. This relationship is represented by the formula:

$$\frac{I_1}{I_2} = \frac{D_2^2}{D_1^2}$$

75. **(A)** Aluminum filters are used to *decrease* patient skin dose by absorbing the low-energy photons (therefore, *decreased* milliroentgen output) that *do not contribute to the image* but *do contribute to patient skin dose.* HVL is defined as that thickness of any absorber that will decrease the intensity of a particular beam to one-half of its original value. As filtration of an x-ray beam is increased, the overall *average energy of the resulting beam is greater* (because the low-energy photons have been removed) and, therefore, the HVL thickness required would be greater.

76. **(A)** Exposure dose to patients can be expressed as *entrance skin exposure* (ESE), sometimes called *skin entrance exposure* (SEE). Exposure can also be expressed in terms of *organ dose.* Organ doses to the gonads, bone marrow, breast, thyroid, lens, and lung can be determined. Patient position and beam restriction often make a significant difference in patient dose. Examinations performed PA, rather than AP, often decrease exposure to sensitive organs. This is so because the lower energy x-ray photons will be absorbed by the anatomic structures closer to the x-ray source, and the higher energy photons will penetrate and exit the part (penetrating the sensitive part rather than being absorbed by it). PA abdomen radiographs deliver less quantity dose to the reproductive organs than do AP abdomen radiographs. An AP skull, head, and neck projection (80 kVp) delivers about 0.9 mGy (90 mrad) to the thyroid, whereas a PA skull, head, and neck (80 kVp) radiograph projection delivers about 0.8 mGy (8 mrad); a PA esophagus (110 kVp) image delivers 0.09 mGy (9 mrad), and the PA chest (120 kVp) delivers about 0.008 mGy (0.8 mrad).

77. **(B)** *Use factor* describes the percentage of time that the primary beam is directed toward a particular wall. The use factor is one of the factors considered in determining protective barrier thickness. Another is *workload,* which is determined by the number of x-ray exposures made per week. *Occupancy factor* is a reflection of who occupies particular areas (radiation workers or nonradiation workers) and is another factor used in determining radiation barrier thickness.

78. **(D)** *Ionization* is the fundamental principle of operation of both the film badge and the pocket dosimeter. In the film badge, the film's silver halide emulsion is ionized by x-ray photons. The pocket dosimeter contains an ionization chamber, and the number of ionizations taking place may be equated to the exposure dose. TLDs contain lithium fluoride crystals that undergo characteristic changes on irradiation. When the crystals are subsequently *heated,* they emit a quantity of visible (thermo) *luminescence/light* in proportion to the amount of radiation absorbed. OSL dosimeters contain aluminum oxide crystals that also undergo characteristic changes on irradiation. When the Al_2O_3 crystals are *stimulated by a laser,* they emit (optically stimulated) *luminescence/light* in proportion to the amount of radiation absorbed.

79. **(D)** *Lymphocytes,* a type of white blood cell concerned with the immune system, have the *greatest* radiosensitivity of all body cells. *Spermatids* are also highly radiosensitive, although not to the same degree as lymphocytes. *Muscle* cells have a fairly low radiosensitivity, and *nerve* cells are the *least* radiosensitive in the body (in fetal life, however, nerve cells are highly radiosensitive).

80. **(D)** Source-to-image-receptor distance (SID) has a significant impact on x-ray beam *intensity* (other terms we could use are *exposure rate* and *dose*). *As the distance between the x-ray tube and IR increases, exposure rate/intensity/dose (and, therefore, receptor exposure) decreases according to the inverse-square law.* According to the inverse-square law, the exposure rate is *inversely* proportional to the *square* of the distance—that is, if the SID is *doubled,* the resulting beam intensity will be one-fourth of the original intensity; if the SID is cut in half, the resulting beam intensity will be 4 times greater than the original intensity.

81. **(A)** The length of time from conception to birth, that is, pregnancy, is called *gestation.* The term *congenital* refers to a condition existing at birth. *Neonatal* relates to the time immediately after birth and the first month of life. *In vitro* refers to something living outside a living body (as in a test tube), as opposed to *in vivo* (within a living system).

82. **(D)** An approximate ESE can be determined using the nomogram illustrated in Figure 3-4. First, mark 2.5 mm Al on the *x* (horizontal) axis. Next, mark where a line drawn up from that point intersects the 80-kVp line. Draw a line straight across to the *y* (vertical) axis; this should approximately reach the 6 mGy/mAs (mGy × mAs) point. Because 15 mAs were used for the exposure, the approximate ESE is 90 mGy (6 × 15).

83. **(C)** The Sievert (Sv) is the unit radiation dose to biologic material, and is used to express occupational exposure and effective dose. *Rem* is an acronym for *r*adiation *e*quivalent *m*an; it includes the RBE specific to the tissue irradiated and can be used as a unit of measurement for the dose to biologic tissue. *Rad* is an acronym for *r*adiation *a*bsorbed *d*ose; it measures the energy deposited in any material. The SI unit used to express radiation dose is Gy_t. Air kerma (Gy_a) is the SI unit of radiation exposure. *Roentgen* is a unit of exposure; it can be used to express the quantity of ionizations in air as a traditional unit of measure.

84. **(C)** Quality control involves testing and maintenance of equipment, whereas quality assurance involves direct patient-related factors.

Sensitometry was used as a portion of a complete QC program when x-ray film processors were used.

Modulation transfer function (MTF) is used to express spatial resolution—another component of the QC program. A complete QC program includes testing, monitoring, and maintenance of all equipment components of the imaging system—filtration (HVL), collimation, focal spot, x-ray timers, beam alignment, and so on.

85. **(C)** All *fluoroscopic* equipment has protective devices and protocols to protect the patient and user. Fluoroscopic equipment must provide at least 12 inches (30 cm), and preferably 15 inches (38 cm), between the x-ray source (focal spot) and the x-ray tabletop (patient), according to NCRP Report No. 102. The tabletop intensity of the fluoroscopic beam must not exceed 10 R/min or 2.1 R/min/mA. With undertable fluoroscopic tubes, a *Bucky slot closer/cover* having at least the equivalent of 0.25 mm Pb must be available to attenuate scattered radiation coming from the patient, *posing a radiation hazard to the fluoroscopist and radiographer.* Fluoroscopic milliamperes must not exceed 5 mA. Because the image intensifier functions as a primary barrier, it must have a lead equivalent of at least 2.0 mm. A cumulative timing device must be available to signal the fluoroscopist when a maximum of 5 min of fluoroscopy time has elapsed. Because occupational exposure to scattered radiation is of considerable importance in fluoroscopy, a protective curtain/drape of at least 0.25-mm Pb equivalent must be placed between the patient and fluoroscopist.

86. **(D)** The pocket dosimeter, or *pocket ionization chamber,* resembles a penlight. Within the dosimeter is a thimble ionization chamber. In the presence of ionizing radiation, a particular quantity of air will be ionized and cause the fiber indicator to register radiation quantity in milliroentgen (mR). The self-reading type may be "read" by holding the dosimeter up to the light and, looking through the eyepiece, observing the fiber indicator, which indicates a quantity of 0–200 mR. Although it provides an immediate reading whereas other personnel monitors require "processing," the disadvantage of the pocket dosimeter is that it does not provide a permanent legal record of exposure.

87. **(B)** Kilovoltage (kV) and the HVL effect a change in both the quantity and the quality of the primary beam. *The principal qualitative factor of the primary beam is kilovoltage* but an increase in kilovoltage will also increase the *number* of photons produced at the target. HVL, defined as *the amount of material necessary to decrease the intensity of the beam to one-half,* therefore changes both beam quality and beam quantity. Milliamperage is directly proportional to x-ray intensity (i.e., quantity/dose rate) but is unrelated to the quality of the beam.

88. **(B)** Gonadal shielding should be used whenever appropriate and possible during radiographic and fluoroscopic examinations. *Flat contact shields* are useful for simple recumbent studies, but when the examination necessitates obtaining oblique, lateral, or erect projections, flat contact shields are easily displaced and become less efficient. *Shaped contact* (contour) *shields* are best because they enclose the male reproductive organs (principally the anterior and lateral portions) and remain in position for oblique, lateral, and erect projections. *Shadow shields* that attach to the tube head are particularly useful for surgical sterile fields.

89. **(B)** *Isotopes* are atoms of the same element (the same atomic number or number of protons) but a different mass number. They differ, therefore, in their number of neutrons. Atoms having the same mass number but different atomic number are *isobars.* Atoms having the same neutron number but different atomic number are *isotones.* Atoms with the same atomic number and mass number are *isomers.*

90. **(D)** The patient is the most important radiation scatterer during both radiography and fluoroscopy. In general, at 1 m from the patient, *the intensity is reduced by a factor of 1000,* that is, 0.1% of the original intensity. Successive scatterings can reduce the intensity to unimportant levels. Calculate that 0.1% of 1.1 mGy is 0.001 mGy.

91. **(C)** Examples of *primary* barriers are the lead walls and doors of a radiographic room, that is, any surface that could be struck by the useful beam. Primary protective barriers of typical installations generally consist of walls with 1.6 mm (1/16 *inch*) of lead and 2.1 m (7 feet) high. *Secondary radiation* is defined as leakage and/or scattered radiation. The x-ray tube housing protects from leakage radiation, as stated earlier. The patient is the source of most scattered radiation. *Secondary radiation barriers* include the portion of the walls *above* 7 feet in height; this area requires only 0.8 mm (1/32 *inch*) of lead. The control booth is also a secondary barrier, toward which the primary beam must never be directed.

92. **(B)** The amount of scattered radiation produced depends first on the kilovoltage (beam quality) selected; *the higher the kilovolts peak,* the more scattered radiation is produced. The size of the irradiated field also has a great deal to do with the amount of scattered radiation produced; *the larger the field size,* the greater is the amount of scattered radiation. Thickness and condition of tissue are also important considerations; *the thicker and/or denser the tissue,* the more scatter is produced. If the condition of the tissue is such that *pathology* makes it more difficult to penetrate, more scattered radiation will be produced. Grid ratio has no effect on the amount of scattered radiation *produced* but does significantly impact the amount of scattered radiation *reaching the IR.*

93. (C) Lead and distance are the two most important ways to protect from radiation exposure. Fluoroscopy can be particularly hazardous because the *source-to-skin distance* (SSD) is so much shorter in overhead radiography. Therefore, it has been established that *fixed* (stationary) *and mobile* fluoroscopic equipment must provide at least 30 cm (12 inches) of SSD for protection of the patient.

94. (A) Automatic exposure control (AEC) devices are used in equipment nowadays and serve to produce consistent and comparable radiographic results. In one type of AEC, there is an *ionization chamber* just beneath the tabletop above the IR. The part to be examined is centered on it (the sensor) and radiographed. When a predetermined quantity of ionization has occurred (equal to the correct exposure), the exposure terminates automatically. In the other type of AEC, the *phototimer/ photomultiplier,* a small fluorescent screen is positioned beneath the IR. When remnant radiation emerging from the patient exposes the IR and exits the IR, the fluorescent screen emits light. Once a predetermined amount of fluorescent light is "seen" by the photocell sensor, the exposure is terminated. A *scintillation camera* is used in nuclear medicine. A *photocathode* is an integral part of the image intensification system.

95. (B) According to the NCRP, the annual occupational *whole-body* dose-equivalent limit is 50 mSv (5 rem or 5000 mrem). The annual occupational whole-body dose-equivalent limit for *students* younger than 18 years is 1 mSv (100 mrem or 0.1 rem). The annual occupational dose-equivalent limit for the *lens of eye* is 150 mSv (15 rem). The annual occupational dose-equivalent limit for the *thyroid, skin, and extremities* is 500 mSv (50 rem). The total gestational dose-equivalent limit for embryo/ fetus of a pregnant radiographer is 5 mSv (500 mrem), not to exceed 0.5 mSv in 1 month.

96. (B) It is our ethical responsibility to minimize radiation exposure to ourselves and our patients, particularly during early pregnancy. One way to do this is to inquire about the *possibility of* our female patients *being pregnant* or for the *date of their last menstrual* period (to determine the possibility of irradiating a newly fertilized ovum). The safest time for a woman of childbearing age to have elective radiographic examinations is during the first 10 days following the onset of menstruation.

97. (A) Figure 3-5 illustrates three dose–response curves. Dose–response curves are used to illustrate the relationship between exposure to ionizing radiation and possible resultant biologic responses. *Curve A* begins at zero, indicating that there is no safe dose, that is, *no threshold.* Even one x-ray photon theoretically can cause a response. It is a straight (*linear*) line, indicating that *response is proportional to dose;* as dose increases, response increases.

Radiation-induced cancer, leukemia, and *genetic effects* follow a linear nonthreshold dose–response relationship. *Curve B* is another linear curve (*response is proportional to dose*), but this one illustrates that a particular dose of radiation must be received before a response will occur— that is, there is a *threshold dose;* this is called a *linear threshold curve. Curve C* is another threshold curve, but this curve is nonlinear. It illustrates that once the minimum dose is received, a response occurs slowly initially and then increases sharply as exposure increases. This threshold, nonlinear (sigmoid) dose–response curve, illustrates the effect to skin from exposure to high levels of ionizing radiation.

98. (A) LET increases with the *ionizing* potential of the radiation; for example, alpha particles are more ionizing than x-radiation; therefore, they have a higher LET. As ionizations and LET increase, there is greater possibility of an effect on living tissue; therefore, the RBE increases. The RBE (sometimes called *quality factor*) of diagnostic x-rays is 1; the RBE of fast neutrons is 10; and the RBE of 5-MeV alpha particles is 20.

99. (A) *The shorter the SID, the greater is the skin dose;* that is why there are specific SSD restrictions in fluoroscopy. High kilovolt peak produces more penetrating photons, thereby decreasing skin dose. Filtration is used to remove the low-energy photons from the primary beam, which contribute to skin dose.

100. (A) Radiation effects that appear days or weeks following exposure (early effects) are in response to relatively high radiation doses. These should never occur in diagnostic radiology nowadays; they occur only in response to doses much greater than those used in diagnostic radiology. One of the effects that may be noted in such a circumstance is the hematologic effect—reduced numbers of white blood cells, red blood cells, and platelets in the circulating blood. Immediate local tissue effects can include effects on the gonads (i.e., temporary infertility) and on the skin (e.g., epilation and erythema). Acute radiation lethality, or radiation death, occurs after an acute exposure and results in death in weeks or days. Radiation-induced malignancy, leukemia, and genetic effects are late effects (or stochastic/probabilistic effects) of radiation exposure. These can occur years after survival of an acute radiation dose or after exposure to low levels of radiation over a long period of time. Radiation workers need to be especially aware of the late effects of radiation because their exposure to radiation is usually low level over a long period of time. Occupational radiation protection guidelines, therefore, are based on late effects of radiation according to a linear, nonthreshold dose–response curve.

101. (C) LET increases with the *ionizing* potential of the radiation; for example, alpha particles are more ionizing than x-radiation, and, therefore, they have a higher LET. As ionizations and LET increase, there is greater possibility of an effect on living tissue; therefore, the RBE increases. The RBE (sometimes called *quality factor* [QF]) of diagnostic x-rays is 1; the RBE of fast neutrons is 10; the RBE of 5-MeV alpha particles is 20; and the RBE of 10-MeV protons is 5.0.

102. **(B)** A quick survey of the distractors reveals that option (A) will increase exposure dose and thus is eliminated as a possible correct answer. Options (B), (C), and (D) will serve to reduce radiation exposure because, in each case, either time is decreased or distance is increased. It remains to be seen, then, which is the more effective. Using the inverse-square law of radiation for option (B), at a distance of 8 feet, the individual will receive *12.5 mGy in 2 min* (double distance from source = one-fourth of the original intensity). At 5 feet, the individual will receive 16 mGy in 1 min:

$$\frac{50(I_1)}{x(I_2)} = \frac{25(D_2^2)}{16(D_1^2)}$$
$$25x = 800$$
$$x = 32 \text{ mGy}$$

Thus, $x = 32$ mGy in 2 min at 5 feet and, therefore, 16 mGy in 1 min. At 6 feet, the individual will receive 22.2 mGy in 2 min:

$$\frac{50(I_1)}{x(I_2)} = \frac{36(D_2^2)}{16(D_1^2)}$$
$$36x = 800$$
$$x = 22.2 \text{ mGy}$$

Thus, $x = 22.2$ mGy in 2 min at 6 feet. Therefore, the most effective option is (B), *12.5 mGy in 2 min at 8 feet.*

103. **(B)** Different types of monitoring devices are available for the occupationally exposed. The film badge has *photographic film;* the pocket dosimeter contains an ionization chamber; TLDs use *lithium fluoride* crystals. *OSL dosimeters* are personnel radiation monitors that use *aluminum oxide* crystals. These crystals, once exposed to ionizing radiation and then subjected to a laser, give off luminescence proportional to the amount of radiation received.

104. **(D)** Fractionation and protraction influence the effect of radiation on tissue. Larger quantities, of course, increase tissue effect. The energy (i.e., quality and penetration) of the radiation determines whether the effects will be superficial (erythema) or deep (organ dose). Certain tissues (e.g., blood-forming organs and the gonads) are more radiosensitive than others (e.g., muscle and nerve). If the dose is delivered in *portions (fractionation)* and/or delivered over a *length of time (protraction), effects on the tissue are less.*

105. **(A)** In the *photoelectric effect,* a relatively low-energy incident photon uses all its energy to eject an inner-shell electron, leaving a vacancy. An electron from the next shell will drop to fill the vacancy, and *a characteristic ray is given up* in the transition. This type of interaction has a greater potential to contribute to patient dose and cause biological damage because all the photon energy is transferred to tissue.

106. **(A)** Filters are used in radiography to remove soft (low-energy) radiation that contributes only to patient dose. The filters usually are made of aluminum. Equipment operating above 70 kVp must have *total filtration* of 2.5-mm Al equivalent (inherent + added).

107. **(C)** The use of a *grid* requires an increase in milliampere seconds and, therefore, patient dose; the higher the grid ratio, the greater is the increase in milliampere seconds required. *Collimation* (beam restriction) restricts the amount of tissue being irradiated and, therefore, reduces patient dose. *High kilovoltage* reduces the amount of radiation absorbed by the patient's tissues (recall the photoelectric effect), and low milliampere seconds reduces the quantity of radiation delivered to the patient. The higher the speed of the *imaging system* (e.g., film–screen combination), the less are the required milliampere seconds.

108. **(D)** Bremsstrahlung (or Brems) radiation is one of the two kinds of x-rays produced at the tungsten target of the x-ray tube during interaction between high-speed electrons coming from the filament and the anodes' tungsten atoms. The incident high-speed electron, passing through a tungsten atom, is attracted by the positively charged nucleus and, therefore, is *deflected from its course, with a resulting loss of energy.* This energy is given up in the form of an x-ray photon.

109. **(D)** Dose–response curves are used to illustrate the relationship between exposure to ionizing radiation and possible resultant biologic responses. The genetic effects of radiation and some somatic effects, such as leukemia, are plotted on a *linear* dose–response curve. The linear dose–response curve has *no threshold,* that is, *there is no dose below which radiation is absolutely safe.* The *nonlinear/sigmoidal* dose–response curve has a *threshold* and is thought to be generally correct for most *somatic* effects—such as *skin erythema, epilation, hematologic depression,* and *radiation lethality* (death).

110. **(A)** Air kerma (Gy_a) is the SI unit of radiation exposure. *Roentgen* is a unit of exposure; it had been used to express the quantity of ionizations in air as a traditional unit of measure.

The Sievert (Sv) is the unit radiation dose to biologic material, and is used to express occupational exposure and effective dose. Personnel dosimeters still use the rem to report occupational exposure; however, the unit has been largely replaced by the Sievert. *Rem* is an acronym for radiation *e*quivalent *m*an; it includes the RBE specific to the tissue irradiated and can be used as a unit of measurement for the dose to biologic tissue. *Rad* is an acronym for *r*adiation *a*bsorbed *d*ose; it measures the energy deposited in any material. The SI unit used to express radiation dose is Gy_t.

111. **(B)** The filters (usually aluminum and copper) serve to help measure radiation quality (i.e., energy). Only the most energetic radiation will penetrate the copper; radiation of lower levels of energy will penetrate the aluminum, and the lowest energy radiation will pass readily through the unfiltered area. Thus, radiation of different energy levels can be recorded, measured, and reported.

112. **(B)** An HVL may be defined as the amount and thickness of absorber necessary to reduce the radiation intensity to half its original value. Thus, the first HVL would reduce the intensity to 50% of its original value, the second to 25%, the third to 12.5%, and the fourth to 6.25% of its original value.

113. **(D)** All the factors listed influence the effect of radiation on tissue. Larger *quantities,* of course, increase radiation's effect on tissue. The *energy* (i.e., quality and penetration) of the radiation determines whether the effects will be superficial (erythema) or deep (organ dose). *Certain tissues* (e.g., blood-forming organs and the gonads) are more radiosensitive than others (e.g., muscle and nerve). The *length of time* over which the exposure is spread (*fractionation*) is important; the longer the period of time, the less are the tissue effects.

114. **(B)** Radiographic and fluoroscopic equipment is designed to help decrease the exposure dose to patient and operator. One of the design features is the exposure cord. Exposure cords on *fixed* equipment must be short enough or fixed to the control panel to prevent the exposure from being made outside the control booth. Exposure cords on *mobile* equipment must be long enough to permit the operator to stand at least 6 feet away from the x-ray tube.

115. **(D)** Selection of exposure factors has a significant impact on patient dose. Remember that milliampere seconds are used to regulate the *quantity* of radiation delivered to the patient and kilovolts peak determines the *penetrability* of the x-ray beam. As kilovoltage is increased, more high-energy photons are produced, and the overall average energy of the beam is increased. An increase in milliampere seconds increases the number of photons produced at the target, but milliampere seconds are unrelated to photon energy. Generally speaking, then, in an effort to keep radiation dose to a minimum, it makes sense to use the lowest milliampere second setting and the highest kilovolts peak setting that will produce the desired radiographic results. An added benefit is that at high kilovolts peak and low milliampere second values, the heat delivered to the x-ray tube is lower, and tube life is extended. In this example, (A) = 75 mAs, (B) = 37.5 mAs, (C) = 36 mAs, and (D) = 18 mAs. Decreasing

the milliampere seconds and increasing the kilovolts peak appropriately is the most effective combination for reducing patient dose.

116. **(B)** Whole-body dose is calculated to include all the especially radiosensitive organs. The gonads and the blood-forming organs are particularly radiosensitive. Some body parts, such as the skin and extremities, have a higher annual dose limit.

117. **(A)** X-ray photons emerging from the focal spot comprise a *heterogeneous* primary beam. There are many low-energy x-rays that, if not removed, would contribute significantly to patient *skin dose.* These low-energy photons are too weak to penetrate the patient and expose the IR; they simply penetrate a small thickness of tissue before being absorbed. Filters, usually made of aluminum, are used in radiography to reduce patient dose by removing this low-energy radiation (i.e., *decreased* beam intensity), and resulting in an x-ray beam of *higher average energy. Total filtration* is composed of *inherent filtration* plus *added filtration.* X-ray photons scatter only after they have interacted with the absorber/patient; scatter is unrelated to filtration.

118. **(C)** Ionization is the fundamental principle of operation of both the film badge and the pocket dosimeter. In the film badge, the film's silver halide emulsion is ionized by x-ray photons. The pocket dosimeter contains an ionization chamber, and the number of ionizations taking place may be equated to exposure dose; it is accurate, but it is used principally to detect larger amounts of radiation exposure. The pocket dosimeter is considered the most sensitive and accurate, though it must be handled carefully; if dropped, the pocket dosimeter can lose some or all of its data. The TLD can measure exposures as low as 5 mrem, whereas film badges cannot express exposure less than 10 mrem. TLDs contain lithium fluoride crystals that undergo characteristic changes on irradiation. When the crystals are subsequently heated, they emit a quantity of visible (thermo) luminescence/light in proportion to the amount of radiation absorbed. The relatively new OSL dosimeters contain aluminum oxide crystals that also undergo characteristic changes on irradiation. When the Al_2O_3 crystals are stimulated by a laser, they emit (optically stimulated) luminescence/light in proportion to the amount of radiation absorbed. OSL dosimeters can measure exposures as low as 1 mrem.

119. **(D)** The principal interactions that occur between x-ray photons and body tissues in the diagnostic x-ray range, the photoelectric effect and Compton scatter, are ionization processes producing photoelectrons and recoil electrons that traverse tissue and subsequently ionize molecules. These interactions occur randomly but can lead to molecular damage in the form of *impaired function* or *cell death.* The *target theory* specifies that DNA molecules are the targets of greatest importance and sensitivity, that is, DNA is the key sensitive molecule.

However, as the body is 65%–80% water, most interactions between ionizing radiation and body cells will involve radiolysis of water rather than direct interaction with DNA. The two major types of effects that occur are the direct effect and the indirect effect. The *direct effect* usually occurs with high-LET radiations and when ionization occurs at the DNA molecule itself. The *indirect effect,* which occurs most frequently, happens when ionization takes place away from the DNA molecule in cellular water. However, the energy from the interaction can be transferred to the molecule via a free radical (formed by radiolysis of cellular water).

Possible damage to the DNA molecule is diverse. A single main-chain/side-rail scission (break) on the DNA molecule is repairable. A double main-chain/side-rail scission may be repaired with difficulty or may result in cell death. A double main-chain/side-rail scission on the same rung of the DNA ladder results in irreparable damage or cell death. Faulty repair of main-chain breakage can result in cross-linking. Damage to the nitrogenous bases, that is, damage to the base itself or to the rungs connecting the main chains, can result in alteration of base sequences, causing a molecular lesion/point mutation. Any subsequent divisions result in daughter cells with incorrect genetic information.

120. (C) The greatest effect–response from irradiation is brought about by a *large dose of radiation to the whole body delivered all at one time.* Whole-body radiation can depress many body functions. With a fractionated dose, the effects would be less severe because the body would have an opportunity to repair between doses.

121. (A) Dose area product (DAP) expresses the dose of radiation to a particular volume of tissue, thereby being a potentially better indicator of risk than dose values alone. DAP can be determined by multiplying the dose by the field size, and is expressed in terms of cGy-cm². *An increased field size will increase the DAP even if the technical factors (dose) remain unchanged.* As field size *decreases,* the amount of exposed tissue decreases, and DAP is *decreased.*

DAP can be monitored by using a DAP meter in both radiographic and fluoroscopic procedures. The DAP meter is radiolucent and is mounted just below the radiographic collimator, measuring x-radiation before it reaches the part. Skin dose can be determined by dividing the skin area exposed by the DAP measurement. This value represents potential deterministic effect to that tissue.

122. (C) Different types of monitoring devices are available for the occupationally exposed, and anyone who might receive more than *one-tenth the annual dose limit must* be monitored. Ionization is the fundamental principle of operation of both the film badge and the pocket dosimeter. In the film badge, the film's silver halide emulsion is ionized by x-ray photons. The pocket dosimeter contains an ionization chamber (containing air), and the number of ions formed (of either sign) is equated to exposure dose. TLDs are radiation monitors that use lithium fluoride crystals. Once exposed to ionizing radiation and then heated, these crystals give off light proportional to the amount of radiation received. OSL dosimeters are radiation monitors that use aluminum oxide crystals. These crystals, once exposed to ionizing radiation and then subjected to a laser, give off luminescence proportional to the amount of radiation received.

123. (B) The principal interactions that occur between x-ray photons and body tissues in the diagnostic x-ray range, the *photoelectric effect* and *Compton scatter,* are ionization processes producing photoelectrons and recoil electrons that traverse tissue and subsequently ionize molecules. In the *illustrated Compton* scatter (see Fig. 3-6), a fairly *high*-energy x-ray photon ejects an *outer-shell* electron. Although the x-ray photon is deflected with reduced energy (modified scatter), it retains most of its original energy and exits the body as an energetic scattered photon. Because the scattered photon exits the body, it does not pose a radiation hazard to the patient. It can, however, contribute to *image fog* and pose a *radiation hazard to personnel* (as in fluoroscopic procedures). In the photoelectric effect, a *low*-energy x-ray photon uses all its energy to eject an *inner-shell* electron, leaving an orbital vacancy. An electron from the shell above fills the vacancy and in so doing gives up energy in the form of a characteristic ray. The photoelectric effect is more likely to occur in absorbers having high atomic number and contributes significantly to patient dose because all the photon energy is absorbed by the patient. Coherent (unmodified) scatter does not involve ionization.

124. (A) Tissue is most sensitive to radiation when it is oxygenated *and least sensitive when it is devoid of oxygen. Anoxic* refers to tissue without oxygen; *hypoxic* refers to tissue with little oxygen. Anoxic and hypoxic tumors typically are avascular (with little or no blood supply) and, therefore, more radioresistant. Hyperoxia refers to an *excess* of oxygen.

125. (B) Bergonié and Tribondeau theorized in 1906 that all precursor cells are particularly radiosensitive (e.g., stem cells found in bone marrow). There are several types of stem cells in bone marrow, and the different types differ in degree of radiosensitivity. Of these, red blood cell precursors, or erythroblasts, are the most radiosensitive. White blood cell precursors, or myelocytes, follow. Platelet precursor cells or megakaryocytes are the least radiosensitive. Myocytes are mature muscle cells that are fairly radioresistant.

126. (D) The pregnant radiographer *should* (not *shall*, and has the right to rescind the declaration if she chooses) declare her pregnancy to her supervisor; at that time, her radiation exposure history can be reviewed and appropriate assignments made. Special arrangements are required for occupational monitoring of the pregnant radiographer. The pregnant radiographer will wear two dosimeters—one in its usual place at the collar and the other, a baby/fetal dosimeter, worn over the abdomen and *under* the lead apron during fluoroscopy. The baby/fetal dosimeter must be identified as such and always must be worn in the same place. Care must be taken not to mix the positions of the two dosimeters. The dosimeters are read monthly as usual.

127. **(B)** Exposure indicators (EI) are helpful but vary greatly among manufacturers. Therefore, a standardized DI that is consistent among manufacturers has been established. The DI indicates the *difference* between the ideal exposure (EI_T) and the actual exposure (EI) at the image receptor (*not* at, or within, the *part*). The ideal/correct receptor exposure has a DI of *0.0*. The DI functions to indicate receptor underexposure/overexposure. A negative DI indicates *under*exposure; a positive DI indicates overexposure. A DI of +1 indicates 25% excessive exposure; a DI of −1 indicates 20% insufficient exposure. The formula to calculate DI: $DI = 10\log_{10}(EI/EI_T)$.

128. **(A)** In the *photoelectric effect,* a relatively low-energy photon uses all its energy to eject an inner-shell electron, leaving a vacancy. An electron from the shell above drops down to fill the vacancy and in so doing emits a characteristic ray. This type of interaction is most harmful to the patient because *all the photon energy is transferred to tissue.* In *Compton scatter,* a high-energy incident photon uses some of its energy to eject an outer-shell electron. In so doing, the incident photon is deflected with reduced energy but usually retains most of its energy and exits the body as an energetic scattered ray. The scattered radiation will either contribute to image fog or pose a radiation hazard to personnel depending on its direction of exit. In *classic scatter,* a low-energy photon interacts with an atom but causes no ionization; the incident photon disappears in the atom and then reappears immediately and is released as a photon of identical energy but with changed direction. *Thompson scatter* is another name for classic scatter.

129. **(C)** Dose–response curves are used to illustrate the relationship between exposure to ionizing radiation and possible resultant biologic responses. Figure 3-7 shows a linear threshold dose–response curve. Its linear aspect indicates that the response/effect is related directly to the dose received, that is, as the dose increases, the response increases. The fact that this is a threshold curve indicates that a particular dose is required before any response/effect will occur.

130. **(C)** Early somatic effects are manifested within minutes, hours, days, or weeks of irradiation and occur only following a very large dose of ionizing radiation. It must be emphasized that doses received from diagnostic radiologic procedures are not sufficient to produce these early effects. An exceedingly *high dose of radiation delivered to the whole body in a short period of time* is required to produce early somatic effects. These whole-body responses are grouped into three categories—reflecting the system(s) affected and the resulting symptoms: *hematologic, gastrointestinal,* and *cerebrovascular system.*

131. **(A)** $^{130}_{56}Ba$ and $^{138}_{56}Ba$ are isotopes of the same element, barium (Ba), because they have the *same atomic number* but different mass numbers (numbers of neutrons). *Isobars* are atoms with the same mass number but different atomic numbers. *Isotones* have the *same number of neutrons* but different atomic numbers. *Isomers* have the *same atomic number and mass number;* they are identical atoms existing at different energy states.

132. **(B)** LET expresses the rate at which photon or particulate energy is transferred to (absorbed by) biologic material (through ionization processes) and is dependent on radiation type and tissue absorption characteristics. RBE describes the degree of response or amount of biologic change we can expect of the irradiated material, and is *directly related to LET.* As the amount of transferred energy (LET) *increases* (from interactions occurring between radiation and biologic material), the amount of biologic effect or damage (RBE) will also *increase;* as the amount of LET *decreases,* the RBE will also *decrease.*

133. **(A)** The relationship between x-ray intensity and distance from the source is expressed by the *inverse-square law of radiation.* The formula is

$$\frac{I_1}{I_2} = \frac{D_2^2}{D_1^2}$$

Substituting known values:

$$\frac{1.5}{x} = \frac{25}{9}$$
$$25x = 13.5$$

Thus, $x = 0.54$ mGy in 60 min and, therefore, 0.18 mGy in 20 min. Distance has a profound effect on dose received and, therefore, is one of the cardinal rules of radiation protection. *As distance from the source increases, dose received decreases.*

134. **(A)** Every radiographic examination involves an ESE, which can be determined fairly easily. It also involves a gonadal dose and a marrow dose, which, if needed, can be calculated by the radiation physicist. If the ESE of a particular examination were calculated to determine the *equivalent whole-body dose,* this would be termed the *effective dose.* For example, the ESE of a PA chest radiograph is approximately 70 mrem, whereas the effective dose is 10 mrem. The effective (whole-body) dose is much less because much of the body is not included in the primary beam.

135. (D) Absorbed dose refers to the amount of energy deposited per unit mass and is strongly related to chemical change and biologic damage. The amount of energy deposited and, thus, the amount of possible biologic damage are dependent on the *type of ionizing radiation,* the *atomic (Z) number of the tissue,* the *mass density of the tissue,* and the *energy of the radiation.*

A radiation weighting factor (W_r) is a number assigned to different types of ionizing radiations so that their effect(s) may be better determined. The W_r of different ionizing radiations is dependent on the LET of that particular radiation. A tissue weighting factor (W_t) represents the relative tissue radiosensitivity of the irradiated material.

LET is another means of expressing radiation quality and determining the W_r. As the LET of radiation increases, the radiation's ability to produce biologic damage also increases. This is described quantitatively by RBE; LET and RBE are directly related.

Most sources of ionizing radiation have a mixture of high- and low-LET radiations. Low-LET radiations deposit less energy in cells/tissues along their path than high-LET radiations, and are considered less destructive as they traverse tissues.

136. (B) Occupationally exposed individuals are required to use devices to record and document the radiation they receive over a given period of time, traditionally 1 month. The most commonly used personnel dosimeters are the OSL dosimeter, the TLD, and the film badge. These devices are worn *only* for documentation of occupational exposure, not for any medical or dental x-rays received as a patient. TLDs are radiation monitors that use lithium fluoride crystals. Once exposed to ionizing radiation and then heated, these crystals give off light proportional to the amount of radiation received. OSL dosimeters are radiation monitors that use aluminum oxide crystals. These crystals, once exposed to ionizing radiation and then subjected to a laser, give off luminescence proportional to the amount of radiation received. The pocket dosimeter contains an ionization chamber (containing air), and the number of ions formed (of either sign) is equated to exposure dose.

137. (D) The quantity 0.014 Gy is equal to 14 mGy. If 14 mGy were delivered in 7 min, then the dose rate would be 2.0 mGy/min:

$$\frac{14\,\text{mGy}}{7\,\text{min}} = \frac{x\,\text{mGy}}{1\,\text{min}}$$
$$7x = 14$$
$$x = 2\,\text{mGy/min}$$

138. (C) The four phases of the human cell cycle are **G**ap 1, **S**ynthesis, **G**ap 2 and **M**itosis. Mitosis is the division phase and has four parts. Synthesis is the phase in which DNA is synthesized. Mitosis is the most radiosensitive (least radioresistant) stage and the latter part of synthesis is the most radioresistant (least radiosensitive) stage.

139. (B) The principal interactions that occur between x-ray photons and body tissues in the diagnostic x-ray range, the photoelectric effect and Compton scatter, are ionization processes producing photoelectrons and recoil electrons that traverse tissue and subsequently ionize molecules. These interactions occur randomly but can lead to molecular damage in the form of *impaired function* or *cell death.* The *target theory* specifies that DNA molecules are the targets of greatest importance and sensitivity, that is, DNA is the key sensitive molecule. However, as the body is 65%–80% water, most interactions between ionizing radiation and body cells will involve radiolysis of water rather than direct interaction with DNA. The two major types of effects that occur are the direct effect and the indirect effect. The *direct effect* usually occurs with high-LET radiations and when ionization occurs at the DNA molecule itself. The *indirect effect,* which occurs most frequently, happens when ionization takes place away from the DNA molecule in cellular water. However, the energy from the interaction can be transferred to the molecule via a free radical (formed by radiolysis of cellular water).

Possible damage to the DNA molecule is diverse. A single main-chain/side-rail scission (break) on the DNA molecule is repairable. A double main-chain/side-rail scission may be repaired with difficulty or may result in cell death. A double main-chain/side-rail scission on the same rung of the DNA ladder results in irreparable damage or cell death. Faulty repair of main-chain breakage can result in cross-linking. Damage to the nitrogenous bases, that is, damage to the base itself or to the rungs connecting the main chains, can result in alteration of base sequences, causing a molecular lesion/point mutation. Any subsequent divisions result in daughter cells with incorrect genetic information.

140. (C) The term *kerma* is used to express *k*inetic *e*nergy *r*eleased in *ma*tter. X-rays expend kinetic energy as they ionize the air or matter. Joule/kilogram is used to measure air kerma and 1 J/kg = 1 Gy_a. The subscript *a* represents *air* as the absorber. The mGy_a is the Standard International (SI) unit of measure of radiation intensity. The rad has been described as equivalent to *100 ergs* of energy deposited *per gram* of irradiated material. The SI unit is *Gray* (Gy_t)—the subscript *t* representing *tissue.*

141. (D) A TLD is a sensitive and accurate device used in radiation dosimetry. It may be used as a personnel dosimeter or to measure patient dose during radiographic examinations and therapeutic procedures. The TLD uses a thermoluminescent phosphor, usually lithium fluoride. When used as a personnel monitor, the TLD is worn for 1 month. During this time, it stores information about the radiation to which it has been exposed. It is then returned to the commercial supplier. In the laboratory, the phosphors are heated. They respond by emitting a particular quantity of light (not heat) that is in proportion to the quantity of radiation delivered to it. After they are cleared of stored information, they are returned for reuse.

142. (A) Because the established dose-limit formula guideline is used for occupationally exposed persons 18 years of age and older, guidelines had to be established to cover the event that a student entered the clinical component of a radiography educational program prior to age 18. The guideline states that the occupational dose limit for students *younger than 18* years is 1 mSv in any given year.

143. (A) Medical imaging includes diagnostic x-ray, computed tomography (CT), interventional procedures, diagnostic sonography, magnetic resonance imaging (MRI), nuclear medicine, and so on. Some forms of medical imaging use ionizing radiation, others do not. Diagnostic x-ray, fluoroscopy and interventional procedures, CT, nuclear medicine, and positron emission tomography (PET) all use ionizing radiation. Sonography uses sound waves; MRI uses magnetic fields.

144. (A) The use of beam restrictors limits the amount of tissue being irradiated, thus decreasing patient dose *and* decreasing the production of scattered radiation. High milliampere second factors increase patient dose. Patient dose is reduced by using high kilovolt and low milliampere second combinations. Although the use of a grid improves image quality by decreasing the amount of scattered radiation reaching the IR, it always requires an increase in exposure factor (usually milliampere seconds) and, therefore, results in increased patient dose.

145. (A) Protective apparel functions to protect the occupationally exposed person *from scattered radiation only.* Lead aprons and lead gloves do not protect from the primary beam. No one in the radiographic room except the patient must ever be exposed to the primary beam. The occupationally exposed and those (family and friends) who might assist a patient during an examination must wear protective apparel and keep out of the way of the primary beam.

146. (D) Mobile radiography (along with fluoroscopy and special procedures) is an area of *higher occupational exposure.* With no lead barrier to retreat behind, distance becomes the best source of protection. The exposure switch of mobile equipment must be manufactured to allow the technologist to stand *at least 6 feet* away from the patient and the x-ray tube. The least amount of scattered radiation is perpendicular to the scattering object; however, lead and distance have the greatest impact on personal protection during mobile imaging. At least one lead apron must be assigned to each mobile unit, and worn by the radiographer during the exposure.

Hospital personnel, visitors, and patients also must be protected from unnecessary radiation exposure. Therefore, the radiographer must request that persons leave the immediate area until after the exposure is made and *announce* in a loud voice when the exposure is about to be made, allowing time for individuals to leave the area. A second lead apron is often available for visitors/staff/patient who are unable to leave the area.

147. (D) Occupationally exposed individuals are concerned principally with *late* (i.e., *long-term* or *delayed*) effects of ionizing radiation, such as radiation-induced *genetic effects, leukemia,* and *cancers* (e.g., bone, lung, thyroid, and breast), as well as *local effects,* such as skin erythema, infertility, and cataracts—these can occur many years following initial exposure to low levels of ionizing radiation. The long-term/delayed effects usually are *chronic,* and many are represented by the linear, nonthreshold dose–response curve.

148. (D) As the amount of time one spends in a controlled area decreases, radiation exposure should decrease. Radiation exposure is affected considerably by one's proximity to the radiation source, as defined by the inverse-square law. Barriers (shielding) are an effective means of reducing radiation exposure; primary barriers, such as walls, protect one from the primary beam, and secondary barriers, such as lead aprons, are used to protect one from secondary radiation.

149. (A) The effects of a quantity of radiation delivered to a body depend on a few factors, including the amount of radiation received, the size of the irradiated area, and how the radiation is delivered in time. If the radiation is delivered in portions over a period of time, it is said to be *fractionated* and has a less harmful effect than if the radiation were delivered all at once. Cells have an opportunity to repair, and some recovery occurs between doses.

150. (B) As the size of the irradiated field decreases, scattered radiation production and patient hazard decrease. If the amount of scattered radiation decreases, then radiographic contrast is higher (shorter scale).

151. (A) The x-ray tube's glass envelope and oil coolant are considered inherent (built-in) filtration. Thin sheets of aluminum are added to make *a total of at least 2.5-mm Al equivalent filtration in equipment operated above 70 kVp.* This is done to remove the low-energy photons that serve only to contribute to patient skin dose.

152. (C) *Erythema* is the reddening of skin as a result of exposure to large quantities of ionizing radiation. It was one of the first somatic responses to irradiation demonstrated to the early radiology pioneers. The effects of radiation exposure to the skin follow a *nonlinear, threshold dose–response relationship.* An individual's response to skin irradiation depends on the dose received, the period of time over which it was received, the size of the area irradiated, and the individual's sensitivity. The dose that it takes to bring about a noticeable erythema is called the *SED*.

153. (B) The patient is the most important source of scattered radiation during both radiography and fluoroscopy. In general, at 1 m from the patient, *the intensity is reduced by a factor of 1000* to about 0.1% of the original intensity. Successive scatterings can reduce the intensity to unimportant levels.

154. (B) If mechanical restraint is impossible, a relative or friend accompanying the patient may be requested/permitted to hold the patient. If a parent is to perform this task, it is preferable to elect the father so as to avoid the possibility of subjecting a newly fertilized ovum to even scattered radiation. If a friend or relative is not available, a nurse or transporter may be asked for help. Protective apparel, such as lead apron and gloves, must be provided to the person(s) holding the patient. *It is the protocol of many radiology departments that radiology personnel must never assist in holding patients. In any case, the individual assisting must never be in the path of the primary beam.*

155. (D) A *controlled area* is one that is occupied by radiation workers who are trained in radiation safety and who wear radiation monitors. The exposure rate in a controlled area must not exceed 100 mR/week; its occupancy factor is considered to be 1, indicating that the area may always be occupied and, therefore, requires maximum shielding. An *uncontrolled area* is one occupied by the general population; the exposure rate there must not exceed 10 mR/week. Shielding requirements vary according to several factors, one being *occupancy factor*.

156. (A) Occupationally, exposed individuals generally receive small amount of low-energy radiation over a long period of time. These individuals, therefore, are concerned with the potential *long-term* effects of radiation, such as *carcinogenesis* (including *leukemia*) and *cataractogenesis*. However, if a large amount of radiation is delivered to the whole body at one time, the short-term early somatic effects must be considered. If the whole body receives 600 rad at one time, *acute radiation syndrome* is likely to occur. Early signs of acute radiation syndrome include *nausea, vomiting, diarrhea, fatigue,* and *leukopenia* (decreased white blood cells count); these occur in the first (*prodromal*) stage of acute radiation syndrome.

157. (B) It is well established that sufficient quantities of ionizing radiation can cause a number of serious somatic and/or genetic effects. *Somatic effects* of radiation are those that affect the *irradiated body itself.* Somatic effects are described as being *early* or *late* depending on the length of time between irradiation and manifestation of effects. The human reproductive organs are particularly radiosensitive. *Fertility* and *heredity* are greatly affected by the *germ cells* produced within the testes (spermatogonia) and ovaries (oogonia). Excessive radiation exposure

to the gonads can cause *temporary or permanent infertility* and/or *genetic mutations*. Infertility is somatic because it affects the exposed individual; genetic mutations affect future generations.

158. (D) All the tissues listed are considered especially radiosensitive. The intestinal *crypt cells of Lieberkühn* are responsible for the absorption of nutrients into the bloodstream. Because these cells are continually being cast off, new cells must continually arise. Being highly mitotic undifferentiated stem cells, they are very radiosensitive. Excessive radiation to the *blood-forming organs* (e.g., *bone marrow*) can cause leukemia or life span shortening. Young, immature embryonic cells, such as *erythroblasts* are listed among the most radiosensitive. Lymphocytes are the most radiosensitive cells in the body.

159. (C) Different types of monitoring devices are available for the occupationally exposed. Ionization is the fundamental principle of operation of both the film badge and the pocket dosimeter. The pocket dosimeter contains an ionization chamber (containing air), and the number of ions formed (of either sign) is equated to exposure dose. In the film badge, the film's silver halide emulsion is ionized by x-ray photons. TLDs are radiation monitors that use lithium fluoride crystals. Once exposed to ionizing radiation and then heated, these crystals emit a quantity of light proportional to the amount of radiation received. OSL dosimeters are radiation monitors that use aluminum oxide crystals. These crystals, once exposed to ionizing radiation and then subjected to a laser, emit luminescence proportional to the amount of radiation received.

160. (D) *Photoelectric* interaction in tissue involves complete absorption of the incident photon, whereas *Compton* interactions involve only partial transfer of energy. The larger the *quantity* of radiation and the greater the number of photoelectric interactions, the greater is the patient dose. Radiation to more *radiosensitive tissues,* such as gonadal tissue or blood-forming organs is more harmful than the same dose to muscle tissue.

161. (B) Radiation safety guidelines are valuable only if they are followed by radiation personnel. The radiation safety officer (RSO) is responsible for being certain that established guidelines are enforced and that personnel understand and use radiation safety measures to protect themselves and their patients. The RSO is also responsible for performing routine equipment checks to ensure that all equipment meet radiation safety standards.

162. (B) The genetic effects of radiation and some somatic effects, such as leukemia, are plotted on a linear dose–response curve. The linear dose–response curve has *no threshold,* that is, *there is no dose below which radiation is absolutely safe.* The nonlinear/sigmoidal dose–response curve has a threshold and is thought to be generally correct for most somatic effects.

163. (C) Although humans are exposed to ionizing radiation from both natural and man-made sources, very high doses of *man-made* ionizing radiation can cause tissue damage that can manifest within *days* after exposure. Late effects, such as cancer, which can occur after more ordinary doses, may take many *years* to develop. The association between a dose of ionizing radiation and the magnitude of the resulting response or effect is called a *dose–response, or dose-effect, relationship.* Dose–response curves are used to illustrate the relationship between exposure to ionizing radiation and possible resultant biologic responses. Ionization chambers and thermoluminescent dosimeters are used to detect and quantify an individual's exposure to ionizing radiation. The electromagnetic spectrum identifies the various types of wavelike fluctuations of electric and magnetic fields.

164. (B) As an x-ray source moves away from an absorber, the x-ray intensity (quantity) decreases. Conversely, as the source of x-rays moves closer to the absorber, the intensity increases. In fluoroscopy, the source of x-rays is 12–15 inches below the x-ray tabletop. Because the source-to-object distance (SOD) is so short, patient skin dose can be quite high. Simply increasing the SID will decrease ESE, but milliamperes will have to be increased to maintain the required exit exposure. Although milliamperes is increased to maintain required exit exposure, because of the characteristic *divergence* of the x-ray beam, ESE will *still* be less at longer SIDs.

Distance has a profound effect on dose received and, therefore, is one of the cardinal rules of radiation protection. *As distance from the source increases, dose received decreases.*

165. (A) It is our ethical responsibility to minimize the radiation dose to our patients. X-rays produced at the tungsten target make up a heterogeneous primary beam. There are many "soft" (low-energy) photons that, if not removed by filters, would only contribute to greater patient skin dose. They are too weak to penetrate the patient and contribute to the image-forming radiation; they penetrate a small thickness of tissue and are absorbed.

166. (D) *Radiation quality* determines degree of penetration and the amount of energy transferred to the irradiated tissue (LET). Certainly, the larger the absorbed radiation dose, the greater is the effect. Biologic effect is increased as the size of the irradiated area is increased. The nature of the effect is influenced by the location of irradiated tissue (bone marrow vs. gonads).

167. (D) Radiation effects that appear days or weeks following exposure (early effects) are in response to relatively high radiation doses. These should never occur in diagnostic radiology nowadays; they occur only in response to doses much greater than those used in diagnostic radiology. One of the effects that may be noted in such a circumstance is the hematologic effect—reduced numbers of white blood

cells, red blood cells, and platelets in the circulating blood. Immediate local tissue effects can include effects on the gonads (i.e., temporary infertility) and on the skin (e.g., epilation and erythema). Acute radiation lethality, or radiation death, occurs after an acute exposure and results in death in weeks or days. Radiation-induced malignancy, leukemia, and genetic effects are late effects (or stochastic/probabilistic effects) of radiation exposure. These can occur years after survival of an acute radiation dose or after exposure to low levels of radiation over a long period of time. Radiation workers need to be especially aware of the late effects of radiation because their exposure to radiation is usually low level over a long period of time. Occupational radiation protection guidelines, therefore, are based on late effects of radiation according to a linear, nonthreshold dose–response curve.

168. (B) *Radiolysis* has to do with the irradiation of water molecules and the formation of free radicals. Free radicals contain enough energy to damage other molecules some distance away. They can migrate to and damage a DNA molecule (indirect hit theory).

169. (C) During the first trimester, specifically the 2nd through 8th week of pregnancy (during major organogenesis), if the radiation dose is at least 250 mGy (20 rad), fetal anomalies can be produced. *Skeletal anomalies* usually appear if irradiation occurs in the early part of this time period, and *neurologic anomalies* are formed in the latter part; mental retardation and childhood malignant diseases, such as cancers or leukemia, also can result from irradiation during the first trimester. Fetal irradiation during the second and third trimesters is not likely to produce anomalies but rather, with sufficient dose, some type of childhood malignant disease. Fetal irradiation during the first 2 weeks of gestation can result in *spontaneous abortion.* It must be emphasized that the likelihood of producing fetal anomalies at doses less than 250 mGy (20 rad) is exceedingly small and that most general diagnostic examinations are likely to deliver fetal doses of less than 10–20 mGy (1–2 rad).

170. (D) The relationship between x-ray intensity and distance from the source is expressed in the inverse-square law of radiation. The formula is

$$\frac{I_1}{I_2} = \frac{D_2^2}{D_1^2}$$

Substituting known values:

$$\frac{0.7}{x} = \frac{36}{16}$$
$$36x = 11.2$$
$$x = 0.311$$

Thus, $x = 0.311$ mGy in *60 min* and, therefore, 0.103 mGy in *20 min*. Distance has a profound effect on dose received and, therefore, is one of the cardinal rules of radiation protection. As distance from the source increases, dose received decreases.

171. (D) Fluoroscopic examinations have the potential to deliver significant patient dose, but there are a number of ways to keep that dose as low as possible: keeping the length of the fluoroscopic exposure/procedure to a minimum, using the last-image-hold feature, keeping the image intensifier as close to the patient as possible, using ABC settings with highest kilovoltage and lowest milliampere combinations, keeping the use of "boost" and magnification modes to a minimum, using the smallest practical FOV, using the lowest practical pulse rate, and adjusting tube angle/patient position to spread exposure dose over a larger area.

172. (A) Radiographers usually are required to wear one dosimeter, positioned at their collar and worn *outside* a lead apron. Special circumstances, however, warrant the use of a second monitor. During pregnancy, a second "baby monitor" is worn at the abdomen, *under* any lead apron. During special vascular procedures, the dose to the radiographer can increase significantly. This is so because the leaded protective curtain is often absent from the fluoro tower and because of the extensive use of cineradiography. As a result, the radiographer's upper extremities can receive a greater exposure (e.g., when assisting during catheter introduction), and a *ring* or *bracelet badge* is often recommended. A second dosimeter is not required when performing mobile radiography.

173. (B) The reproductive cells are considered among the most radiosensitive cells in the body. The immature female sex cells are the oogonia; they mature to ova. The immature male sex cells are the spermatogonia; they mature to sperm. Different amounts of ionizing radiation to these cells can cause differing levels/degrees of response. Doses as low as 10 rad can cause menstrual changes in women and decrease the number of sperm in men. At 200 rad, temporary infertility is likely, and at 500 rad, sterility will result.

174. (C) The newest type of personnel monitoring device is the *direct ion storage dosimeter (DIS)*; it is a digital ionization dosimeter. The DIS eliminates the need to collect and send dosimeters for monthly or quarterly processing. The user wears the DIS, which looks like a small flash drive, in the same way as other monitors such as an OSL (optically stimulated luminescence) dosimeter. The DIS has a gas-filled ionization chamber within and uses Bluetooth technology to relate its raw data via mobile device or any computer with Internet access and a USB connection. Occupational exposure can be read, and reread, at any time without loss of information. *TLDs* (thermoluminescent dosimeters) are radiation monitors that use lithium fluoride crystals. Once exposed to ionizing radiation and then heated, these crystals give off light in proportion to the amount of radiation received. *OSL*

(optically stimulated luminescence) dosimeters are radiation monitors that use aluminum oxide crystals. These crystals, once exposed to ionizing radiation and then subjected to a laser, give off luminescence proportional to the amount of radiation received. PBL refers to positive beam limitation.

175. (C) Biologic tissue is more sensitive to radiation when it is in an oxygenated state. A characteristic of many avascular (and, therefore, hypoxic) tumors is their resistance to treatment with radiation. Hyperbaric (high-pressure oxygen) therapy is used in some therapy centers in an effort to increase the sensitivity of the tissues being treated.

176. (C) *Erythema* is the reddening of skin as a result of exposure to large quantities of ionizing radiation. It was one of the first somatic responses to irradiation demonstrated to the early radiology pioneers. Figure 3-8 illustrates three dose–response curves. *Curve A* begins at zero, indicating that there is no safe dose, that is, *no threshold*. Even one x-ray photon theoretically can cause a response. It is a straight (linear) line, indicating that *response is directly related to dose;* as dose increases, response increases. *Radiation-induced cancer, leukemia,* and *genetic effects* follow a linear nonthreshold dose–response relationship. *Curve B* is another linear curve (response is *directly related* to dose), but this one illustrates that a particular dose of radiation must be received before a response will occur—that is, there is a *threshold dose;* this is called a *linear threshold curve. Curve C* is another threshold curve, but this curve is nonlinear. It illustrates that once the minimum dose is received, a response occurs slowly initially and then increases sharply as exposure increases. This threshold, nonlinear (sigmoid) dose–response curve, illustrates the effect to *skin* from exposure to high levels of ionizing radiation. An individual's response to skin irradiation depends on the dose received, the period of time over which it was received, the size of the area irradiated, and the individual's sensitivity. The dose that it takes to bring about a noticeable erythema is called the *SED.*

177. (A) The intensity/exposure rate of radiation at a given distance from a point source is inversely proportional to the square of the distance. This is the inverse-square law of radiation, and it is expressed in the following equation:

$$\frac{I_1}{I_2} = \frac{D_2^2}{D_1^2}$$

Substituting known values:

$$\frac{1.5 \text{ mGy}_a/\text{h}}{x \text{ mR/h}} = \frac{152^2}{91^2}$$

$$23104x = 12421.5$$

$$x = 0.537 \text{ mGy/h (60 min)}$$

Thus, $x = 0.537$ mGy/h and, therefore, 0.268 mGy in 30 min.

178. (B) In the *photoelectric effect,* a relatively low-energy photon uses all its energy to eject an inner-shell electron, leaving a vacancy. An electron from the shell above drops down to fill the vacancy and in so doing gives up a characteristic ray. This type of interaction is most harmful to the patient because all the photon energy is transferred to tissue. In *Compton scatter,* a high-energy incident photon ejects an outer-shell electron. The incident photon is deflected with reduced energy, but it usually retains most of its energy and exits the body as an energetic scattered ray. This scattered ray will either contribute to image fog or *pose a radiation hazard to personnel* depending on its direction of exit. In *classic scatter,* a low-energy photon interacts with an atom but causes no ionization; the incident photon disappears into the atom and then is released immediately as a photon of identical energy but with changed direction. *Pair production* is an interaction that occurs only at energies of 1.02 MeV, and therefore, it does not occur in diagnostic radiography.

179. (C) *Scattered and secondary radiations* are those that have deviated in direction while passing through a part. *Leakage radiation* is the radiation that emerges from the leaded tube housing in directions other than that of the useful beam. Tube head construction must keep leakage radiation to less than 1 mGy$_a$/h (100 mR/h) at 1 m from the tube. *Remnant radiation* is the radiation that emerges from the patient to form the radiographic image.

180. (D) A standardized DI that is consistent among manufacturers has been established. The DI indicates the difference between the ideal exposure (EI$_T$) and the actual exposure (EI) *at the image receptor* (*not* at, or within, the part). The ideal/correct receptor exposure has a DI of *0.0.* The DI functions to indicate receptor underexposure/overexposure. A negative DI indicates *under*exposure; a positive DI indicates overexposure. A DI of +1 indicates 25% excessive exposure; a DI of −1 indicates 20% insufficient exposure. The formula to calculate DI: DI = $10\log_{10}$ (EI/EI$_T$).

181. (D) Irradiation during pregnancy, especially in early pregnancy, is avoided because the fetus is particularly radiosensitive during the first trimester. Especially high-risk examinations include pelvis, hip, femur, lumbar spine, cystograms and urograms, upper GI series, and barium enema (BE) examinations. During the 2nd through 10th week of pregnancy (i.e., during major organogenesis), fetal anomalies can be produced. *Skeletal and/or organ anomalies* can appear if irradiation occurs early on, and *neurologic* anomalies can be formed in the latter part; *mental retardation* and *childhood malignant diseases* can also result from irradiation during the first trimester. Fetal irradiation during the second and third trimesters, with sufficient dose, can cause some type of childhood malignant disease. Fetal irradiation during the first 2 weeks of gestation most likely will result in *embryonic resorption* or *spontaneous abortion.* It must be emphasized that the likelihood of producing fetal anomalies at doses less than 20 rad is exceedingly small and that most general diagnostic examinations are likely to deliver fetal doses of less than 1–2 rad.

182. (B) Even the smallest exposure to radiation can be harmful. It, therefore, must be every radiographer's objective to keep his or her occupational exposure as far below the dose limit as possible. Radiology personnel never should hold patients during an x-ray examination.

183. (A) An approximate ESE can be determined using the nomogram illustrated in Figure 3-9. First, mark 2.5 mm Al on the *x* (horizontal) axis. Next, mark where a line drawn up from that point intersects the 110 kVp line. Draw a line straight across to the *y* (vertical) axis; this should approximately reach the 12 mGy/mAs (mGy × mAs) point. Because 1.5 mAs was used for the exposure, the approximate ESE is 18 mGy (12 × 1.5).

184. (A) The relationship between x-ray intensity and distance from the source is expressed in the inverse-square law of radiation. The formula is

$$\frac{I_1}{I_2} = \frac{D_2^2}{D_1^2}$$

Substituting known values:

$$\frac{1.5}{x} = \frac{64}{49}$$
$$64x = 73.5$$

Thus, x = 1.14 mGy in 1 h (60 min) and, therefore, 0.57 mGy in 30 min. Note the inverse relationship between distance and dose. As distance from the source of radiation increases, dose rate decreases significantly.

185. (A) Nondividing, differentiated cells are specialized, mature cells that *do not undergo mitosis.* Having these qualities, they are rendered radioresistant, according to the theory proposed by Bergonié and Tribondeau. The adult nervous system is composed of nondividing, differentiated cells, and thus is the most radioresistant system in the adult. Epithelial tissue and lymphocytes contain many precursor stem cells and hence are among the most radiosensitive cells in the body.

186. (D) The *Bucky slot cover* shields the opening at the side of the table because the Bucky tray is parked at the end of the table for the fluoroscopy procedure; this is important because the opening created otherwise would allow scattered radiation to emerge at approximately the level of the operator's gonads. The *exposure switch* (usually a foot pedal) must be of the "dead-man" type, that is, when the foot is released from the switch, there is immediate termination of exposure. The *cumulative exposure timer* sounds or interrupts the exposure after 5 min of fluoro time, thus making the fluoroscopist aware of accumulated fluoro time. In addition, *source-to-tabletop distance* is restricted to at least 15 inches for stationary equipment and at least 12 inches for mobile equipment. Increased source-to-tabletop distance increases source-to-patient distance, thereby decreasing patient dose.

187. (C) The Sievert (Sv) is the unit radiation dose to biologic material, and is used to express occupational exposure and effective dose. *Rem* is an acronym for *radiation equivalent man*; it includes the RBE specific to the tissue irradiated and can be used as a unit of measurement for the dose to biologic tissue. *Rad* is an acronym for *radiation absorbed dose*; it measures the energy deposited in any material. The SI unit used to express radiation dose is Gy_t. *Air kerma* (Gy_a) is the SI unit of radiation exposure. As x-ray photons emerge from the x-ray tube, they immediately encounter air—before being intercepted by any material. The Gy_a is the unit of measure describing this quantitatively. Roentgen is the former unit of exposure expressing the quantity of ionization in air.

Becquerel is the SI unit of measurement for radioactivity.

188. (A) X-ray intensity is inversely related to SID; as SID increases, x-ray intensity decreases. The x-ray intensity at the image intensifier also depends on the SID. Moving the image intensifier *farther from* the patient *increases* the SID and decreases x-ray beam intensity at the input phosphor. The automatic brightness control (ABC) would then *increase* the *milliamperes* thereby increasing patient dose. Moving the image intensifier farther from the patient also results in a *longer OID,* thereby increasing magnification and diminishing image quality.

189. (D) Elective booking of a radiologic examination after inquiring about the patient's previous menstrual cycle is the most effective means of preventing accidental exposure of a recently fertilized ovum. Patient questionnaires obtain this information from the patient and are also used often in an informed consent form. Patient postings in waiting and changing areas alert patients to advise the radiographer if there is any chance of pregnancy. These three safeguards replace the earlier 10-day rule, which is now obsolete.

190. (D) Moving the image intensifier closer to the patient during fluoroscopy decreases the SID and patient dose (as SID is reduced, the intensity of the x-ray photons at the image intensifier's input phosphor increases; the automatic brightness control then automatically decreases the milliamperage and, therefore, the patient dose). Moving the image intensifier closer to the patient during fluoroscopy also decreases the OID and, therefore, magnification. As tissue density increases, a greater exposure dose is required.

191. (B) The OSL dosimeter and TLD are used frequently to measure the radiation exposure of radiographers. The pocket dosimeter may be used by radiation workers who are exposed to higher doses of radiation and need a daily reading. A blood test is an unacceptable method of monitoring radiation dose effects because a very large dose would have to be received before blood changes would occur.

192. (B) The genetically significant dose (GSD) illustrates that large exposures to a few people are cause for little concern when diluted by the total population. On the contrary, we all share the burden of that radiation received by the total population, especially as the use of medical radiation increases, so each individual's share of the total exposure increases.

193. (D) According to the NCRP, the annual occupational *whole-body* dose-equivalent limit is 50 mSv (5 rem or 5000 mrem). The annual occupational whole-body dose-equivalent limit for *students* younger than 18 years is 1 mSv (100 mrem or 0.1 rem). The annual occupational dose-equivalent limit for the *lens of the eye* is 150 mSv (15 rem). The annual occupational dose-equivalent limit for the *thyroid, skin,* and *extremities* is 500 mSv (50 rem). The total gestational dose-equivalent limit for the *embryo/fetus* of a pregnant radiographer is 5 mSv (500 mrem), not to exceed 0.5 mSv in 1 month.

194. (A) Restriction of field size is one important method of patient protection. However, the accuracy of the light field must be evaluated periodically as part of a quality assurance (QA) program. Guidelines for patient protection state that the collimator light and actual irradiated area must be accurate to within 2% of the SID.

195. (A) Lead aprons require certain maintenance and care if they are to continue to provide protection from ionizing radiation. They can be kept clean with a damp cloth. It is very important that they be hung when not in use rather than being folded or left in a heap between examinations. A folded or crumpled position encourages the formation of cracks in the leaded vinyl. Lead aprons should be fluoroscoped or radiographed (at about 120 kVp) at least once a year to check for development of any cracks.

196. (D) The principal interactions that occur between x-ray photons and body tissues in the diagnostic x-ray range, the photoelectric effect and Compton scatter, are ionization processes producing photoelectrons and recoil electrons that traverse tissue and subsequently ionize molecules. These interactions occur randomly but can lead to molecular damage in the form of *impaired function* or *cell death*. The *target theory* specifies that DNA molecules are the targets of greatest importance and sensitivity, that is, DNA is the key sensitive molecule. However, as the body is 65%–80% water, most interactions between ionizing radiation and body cells will involve radiolysis of water rather than direct interaction with DNA. The two major types of effects that occur are the direct effect and the indirect effect. The *direct effect* usually occurs with high-LET radiations and when ionization occurs at the DNA molecule itself. The *indirect effect,* which occurs most frequently, happens when ionization takes place away from the DNA molecule in cellular water. However, the energy from the interaction can be transferred to the molecule via a free radical (formed by radiolysis of cellular water).

197. (D) The *protective curtain,* which is usually made of leaded vinyl with at least 0.25-mm Pb equivalent, must be positioned between the patient and the fluoroscopist to greatly reduce the exposure of the fluoroscopist to energetic scatter from the patient. As with overhead equipment, fluoroscopic total *filtration* must be at least 2.5-mm Al equivalent to reduce excessive exposure to soft radiation. *Collimator–beam* alignment must be accurate to within 2%.

198. (B) Because minerals in rocks and the earth can emanate radioactivity, high levels of radon gas inside homes have been of recent concern. Another source of radon gas is from burning cigarettes, whether as a smoker or as passive exposure. Uranium miners have been identified with a much higher incidence of lung cancer; many of these individuals also were smokers. Radiology departments are not known as a source of radon gas exposure.

199. (B) The principal interactions that occur between x-ray photons and body tissues in the diagnostic x-ray range, the photoelectric effect and Compton scatter, are ionization processes producing photoelectrons and recoil electrons that traverse tissue and subsequently ionize molecules. These interactions occur randomly but can lead to molecular damage in the form of *impaired function* or *cell death.* The *target theory* specifies that DNA molecules are the targets of greatest importance and sensitivity, that is, DNA is the key sensitive molecule. However, as the body has 65%–80% water, most interactions between ionizing radiation and body cells will involve radiolysis of water rather than direct interaction with DNA. The two major types of effects that occur are the *direct effect* and the *indirect effect.* The direct effect usually occurs with high-LET radiations and when ionization occurs at the DNA molecule itself. The indirect effect, which occurs most frequently, happens when ionization takes place away from the DNA molecule in cellular water. However, the energy from the interaction can be transferred to the molecule via a *free radical* (formed by *radiolysis of cellular water*). Possible damage to the DNA molecule is diverse. A single main-chain/side-rail scission (break) on the DNA molecule is *repairable.* A double main-chain/side-rail scission may repair with difficulty or may result in *cell death.* A double main-chain/side-rail scission on the same "rung" of the DNA ladder results in *irreparable* damage or *cell death.* Faulty repair

of main-chain breakage can result in *cross-linking.* Damage to the nitrogenous bases, that is, damage to the base itself or to the rungs connecting the main chains, can result in alteration of base sequences, causing a *molecular lesion/point mutation.* Any subsequent divisions result in daughter cells with incorrect genetic information.

200. (B) With greater beam restriction, less biologic material is irradiated, thereby reducing the possibility of harmful effects. If less tissue is irradiated, less scattered radiation is produced, resulting in improved IR contrast. The total filtration is not a function of beam restriction but rather is a radiation protection guideline aimed at reducing patient skin dose.

201. (C) It is important to limit tabletop exposure during undertable fluoroscopy because the SSD is much less in overhead radiography; therefore, a much higher skin dose is delivered to the patient. For this reason, the tabletop exposure rate during fluoroscopy should not exceed 21 mGy$_a$/min/mA at 80 kV. During high-level-control fluoroscopy, the maximum permissible tabletop intensity is 200 mGy$_a$/min.

202. (D) Humans have always been exposed to ionizing radiation. Some ionizing radiations occur naturally in the earth's crust and in its atmosphere. These radiations are present in the structures in which we live and in the food we consume; radioactive gas is present in the air that we breathe, and there are traces of radioactive minerals in our bodies. These radiations are called external and internal sources of *natural background* (environmental) *radiation.* Our largest source of natural background radiation exposure is radon and thoron gases.

We are also exposed to sources of radiation created by humans. *Artificial* or *man-made* radiation contributes to the dose received by the US population. According to the BEIR VII report, medical and dental x-rays and nuclear medicine studies account for approximately 79% of the man-made radiation exposure in the United States. In addition, NCRP Reports No. 160 and 184 indicate that *medical radiation exposure now contributes 50% of the public's exposure to ionizing radiation.* NRC (Nuclear Regulatory Commission) regulations and radiation exposure limits are published in Title 10 of the Code of Federal Regulations (CFR), Part 20.

203. (D) The pregnant radiographer poses a special radiation protection consideration for the safety of the unborn individual. It must be remembered that the developing fetus is particularly sensitive to radiation exposure. Therefore, established guidelines state that the occupational gestational dose-equivalent limit for *embryo/fetus* of a pregnant radiographer is 5 mSv (500 mrem), not to exceed 0.5 mSv in 1 month. According to the NCRP, the annual occupational *whole-body* dose-equivalent limit is 50 mSv (5 rem or 5000 mrem). The annual occupational whole-body dose-equivalent limit for *students* younger than 18 years is 1 mSv (100 mrem or 0.1 rem). The annual occupational dose-equivalent limit for the *lens of eye* is 150 mSv (15 rem). The annual occupational dose-equivalent limit for the *thyroid, skin,* and *extremities* is 500 mSv (50 rem).

204. (A) According to the NCRP, the annual occupational *whole-body* dose-equivalent limit is 50 mSv (5 rem or 5000 mrem). The annual occupational whole-body dose-equivalent limit for *students* younger than 18 years is 1 mSv (100 mrem or 0.1 rem). The annual occupational whole-body dose-equivalent limit for the *lens of eye* is 150 mSv (15 rem). The annual occupational dose-equivalent limit for the *skin, hands,* and *feet* is 500 mSv (50 rem).

205. (B) The photoelectric effect is the interaction between x-ray photons and matter that is largely responsible for patient dose. The photoelectric effect occurs when a relatively *low*-energy photon uses *all* its energy to eject an *inner-shell* electron. That electron is ejected from the atom, leaving a hole in, for example, the K shell. An L-shell electron then drops down to fill the K vacancy and in so doing emits a characteristic ray whose energy equals the difference in binding energies for the K and L shells. The photoelectric effect occurs with *high*–atomic-number (*Z*) absorbers, such as bone and with positive contrast media.

206. (C) The most radiosensitive portion of the GI tract is the small bowel. Projecting from the lining of the small bowel are villi, from the intestinal crypt cells of Lieberkühn, which are responsible for the absorption of nutrients into the bloodstream. Because the cells of the villi are continually being cast off, new cells must continually arise from the crypts of Lieberkühn. Being highly mitotic undifferentiated stem cells, they are very radiosensitive. Thus, the small bowel is the most radiosensitive portion of the GI tract.

207. (C) *Secondary* radiation consists of *leakage and scattered* radiation. Leakage radiation can be emitted when a defect exists in the tube housing. A significant quantity of scattered radiation is generated within, and emitted from, the patient. *Background* radiation is naturally occurring radiation that is emitted from the earth and that also exists within our bodies.

208. (B) Kilovoltage (kV) and the HVL effect a change in both the quantity and the quality of the primary beam. *The principal qualitative factor of the primary beam is kilovoltage,* but an increase in kilovoltage will also increase the *number* of photons produced at the target. HVL, defined as the *amount of material necessary to decrease the intensity of the beam to one-half,* therefore changes both beam quality and beam quantity. Milliamperage is directly proportional to x-ray intensity (quantity) but is unrelated to the quality of the beam.

209. (D) The use of diagnostic imaging has increased dramatically the past few decades resulting in significant increase in patient dose. The increased use of diagnostic x-ray, and especially computed tomography and nuclear medicine, has more than tripled the average annual patient dose to the current average of 3.2 mSv. There are several reasons for this increase but radiographers must recognize their responsibility in practicing ALARA principles.

210. (D) Irradiation of cellular DNA has the potential to produce a number of effects that can have an impact on the structure and/or function of the cell. The cell's mitotic potential can be delayed or completely stopped. Most chromosome breakage/damage is an indirect consequence of irradiation. If the damage happens to the DNA of a germ cell, the radiation response may not occur until one or more generations later.

211. (B) X-rays are very useful in obtaining medical images. We also use their properties in dosimetry, image intensification, radiobiology, and so on. The outstanding characteristics/properties of x-rays are as follows:

o not perceptible by the senses
o ionizing action on air
o photographic effect on film emulsion
o physiological effect on living tissue
o luminescent effect on certain crystals
o penetrating effect on all forms of matter
o classified as electromagnetic, but behave as both waves and particles
o electrically neutral
o polyenergetic and heterogeneous
o travel in straight lines
o travel at the speed of light

212. (B) A high-speed electron is accelerated from the heated filament toward a tungsten atom within the anode focal track. The negative electron is attracted by the positive nucleus of the tungsten atom and, as a result, is pulled off course and redirected toward the nucleus. The electron's deflection from its original course caused by the "braking" (slowing down) results in a loss of energy. This energy loss is given up in the form of an x-ray photon: Bremsstrahlung (Brems or braking) radiation (Fig. 3-11). The electron does not generally lose all its kinetic energy in one such interaction; it goes on to have several more interactions with tungsten atoms deeper within the target, each time producing an x-ray photon having less and less energy. This is one reason the x-ray beam is heterogeneous (polyenergetic), that is, has a spectrum of energies. Brems radiation comprises 70%–90% of the primary x-ray beam.

Characteristic radiation is produced when an electron transits from a higher energy level (outer shell) to a lower energy level (inner shell). Photoelectric and Compton are interactions between x-ray photons and tissue. (*Saia, PREP, 9th ed,* p. 240)

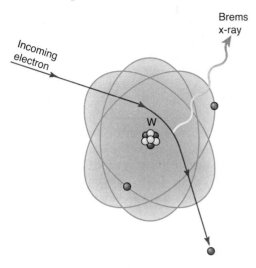

Figure 3-11

213. (C) Half-value layer (HVL) testing provides beam quality information. HVL is defined as the thickness of any absorber that will reduce x-ray beam intensity to one-half of its original value. It is determined by measuring the beam intensity without an absorber and then recording the intensity as successive millimeters of aluminum are added to the radiation field. *It is influenced by the type of rectification, total filtration, and kV.* An x-ray tube HVL should remain almost constant. If HVL decreases, it is an indication of a decrease in the actual kV. If the HVL increases, it indicates the deposition of vaporized tungsten on the inner surface of the glass envelope (as a result of tube aging) or an increase in the actual kV. HVL is tested periodically to evaluate x-ray beam quality and should remain almost constant.

214. (C) Similar absorbed doses of different kinds of ionizing radiation can cause different biologic effects to tissues of differing radiosensitivity. A *radiation weighting factor* (W_r) is a number assigned to different types of ionizing radiations so that their effect(s) may be better determined (e.g., x-rays vs. alpha particles). The W_r of different ionizing radiations is dependent on the LET of that particular radiation.

The term *equivalent dose* (EqD) refers to the product of the absorbed dose (Gy/rad) and its radiation weighting factor (W_r).

A *tissue* weighting factor (W_t) represents the relative tissue radiosensitivity of the irradiated material (e.g., muscle vs. intestinal epithelium vs. bone).

215. (A) Secondary radiation is defined as leakage and/or scattered radiation. The x-ray tube housing is the secondary radiation barrier that protects from leakage radiation. The patient is the source of most scattered radiation.

Leakage radiation is that which is emitted from the x-ray to housing in directions other than that of the primary beam. NCRP guidelines state that leakage radiation from the lead-lined x-ray tube must not exceed 1 mGy$_a$/h (100 mR/h) when measured at a distance of 1 m from the x-ray tube.

216. (B) Lead aprons are worn by occupationally exposed individuals during fluoroscopic procedures. Lead aprons are available with various lead equivalents; 0.25, 0.5, and 1.0 mm of lead are the most common. The 1.0-mm lead equivalent apron will provide close to 100% protection at most kilovoltage levels, but it is rarely used because it weighs anywhere from 12 to 24 pounds. A 0.25-mm lead equivalent apron will attenuate about 97% of a 50-kVp x-ray beam, 66% of a 75-kVp beam, and 51% of a 100-kVp beam. A 0.5-mm apron will attenuate about 99% of a 50-kVp beam, 88% of a 75-kVp beam, and 75% of a 100-kVp beam.

217. (C) According to the NCRP, the annual occupational *whole-body* dose-equivalent limit is 50 mSv (5 rem or 5000 mrem). The annual occupational whole-body dose-equivalent limit for *students* younger than 18 years is 1 mSv (100 mrem or 0.1 rem). The annual occupational dose-equivalent limit for the *lens of the eye* is 150 mSv (15 rem). The annual occupational dose-equivalent limit for the *thyroid, skin,* and *extremities* is 500 mSv (50 rem). The total gestational dose-equivalent limit for the *embryo/fetus* of a pregnant radiographer is 5 mSv (500 mrem), not to exceed 0.5 mSv in 1 month.

218. (C) The whole-body radiation dose that would cause 50% of those irradiated to die within 60 days is termed the LD 50/60. The approximate LD 50/60 for humans is 3.5 Gy$_t$. The LD 50/60 varies with the species. Many species have a higher LD 50/60 (goldfish, rabbit, turtle, etc.).

219. (D) DAP expresses the dose of radiation to a particular volume of tissue, thereby being a potentially better indicator of risk than dose values alone. DAP can be monitored using a DAP meter in both radiographic and fluoroscopic procedures. The DAP meter is radiolucent and is mounted just below the radiographic collimator, measuring x-radiation before it reaches the part. Skin dose can be determined by dividing the skin area exposed by the DAP measurement. This value represents potential deterministic effect to that tissue.

DAP can be determined by multiplying the dose by the field size, and is expressed in terms of cGy-cm². *An increased field size will increase the DAP even if the technical factors (dose) remain unchanged.* As field size decreases, the amount of exposed tissue decreases, and DAP is decreased.

220. (B) The required lead thickness of a primary barrier is usually expressed as 1.6 mm or 1/16 inch of lead (Pb).

Secondary barriers must never have the primary beam directed toward them and can be made of materials such as gypsum board, glass, or lead acrylic. Aluminum is used for x-ray beam filtration, not as an x-ray barrier.

221. **(E)** The thickness of any material that will reduce the intensity of the x-ray beam to half of its original value is called the half-value later (HVL). In this case, the first HVL would reduce the intensity from 100% to 50%. The second HVL would reduce the intensity from 50% to 25%. The third HVL would reduce the intensity from 25% to 12.5%. The fourth HVL would reduce the intensity from 12.5% to 6.25%.

222. **(D)** When the radiographer is present during the fluoroscopic examination, he or she must wear a lead apron. Occupational exposure can be further reduced by moving away from the fluoroscopic tube and/or standing behind the radiologist. Although a dosimeter must be worn appropriately to record occupational exposure, it does nothing to *reduce* occupational exposure.

223. **(D)** The inverse-square law of radiation states that "the intensity or exposure rate of radiation at a given distance from a point source is inversely proportional to the square of the distance." Then, according to the inverse-square law if the distance is doubled, one-fourth of the original dose will be delivered to the part. Conversely, if the distance were halved, 4 times the original dose would be delivered to the part.

224. **(B)** The *protective curtain,* which is usually made of leaded vinyl must be at least the equivalent of 0.25 mm Pb. It is positioned between the patient and the fluoroscopist to greatly reduce the exposure of the fluoroscopist to energetic scatter from the patient. The patient is the most significant scatterer.

225. **(C)** The personnel radiation monitor should be worn at collar level outside of the lead apron for fluoroscopy, and in the same position for a general radiography. When worn in this position for radiography, the dosimeter report is considered accurate for effective dose.

Because we are very well shielded during fluoroscopic examinations, the collar monitor overestimates effective dose and a conversion/correction factor of 0.1 can be used to more accurately identify occupational fluoroscopic effective dose.

226. **(D)** The control monitor received with each new batch of radiation dosimeters must be kept far away from all sources of ionizing radiation, in a distant safe area. Its function is to measure any background radiation exposure it receives during handling, storage, and transportation. The background radiation received by the control monitor is subtracted from each individual personnel monitor so that only occupational exposure is reported.

227. **(A)** The term *effective dose* (EfD) *equivalent* refers to the dose from radiation sources internal and/or external to the body and is expressed in units of Sievert or rem. The factors used to determine effective dose (*EfD*) are as follows:

EfD = radiation weighting factor (W_r) × tissue weighting factor (W_t) × absorbed dose (D)

The term *equivalent dose* (EqD) refers simply to the product of the absorbed dose (Gy/rad) and its radiation weighting factor (W_r).

228. **(D)** The inverse-square law of radiation states that "the intensity or exposure rate of radiation at a given distance from a point source is inversely proportional to the square of the distance." The equation is expressed as:

$$\frac{I_1}{I_2} = \frac{D_2^2}{D_1^2}$$

Substituting known factors:

$$\frac{0.5}{x} = \frac{54^2}{36^2}$$
$$2916x = 648$$
$$x = 0.22 \text{ mSv}$$

229. **(C)** The linear, nonthreshold curve is used to illustrate responses such as leukemia, cancer, and genetic effects. These are also called probabilistic/stochastic effects. Probabilistic/stochastic effects occur randomly and are "all-or-nothing" type effects, that is, they do not occur with degrees of severity. Remember that in a *nonthreshold curve there is no safe dose,* that is, no dose below which there will definitely be no biologic response. Theoretically, even one x-ray photon can cause a biologic response. The linear, nonthreshold curve is the curve of choice to predict effects of low level (e.g., medical and occupational) exposure to ionizing radiation.

230. **(A)** Frequency and wavelength are closely associated with the relative energy of electromagnetic radiations. *More energetic radiations have shorter wavelengths and higher frequency;* thus, they are inversely related. The relationship between frequency, wavelength, and energy is illustrated in the electromagnetic spectrum. Some radiations are energetic enough to rearrange atoms in materials through which they pass, and can therefore be hazardous to living tissue.

231. **(A)** The genetically significant dose (GSD) illustrates that large exposures to a few people are cause for little concern when diluted by the total population. On the contrary, we all share the burden of that radiation received by the total population, especially as the use of medical radiation increases, each individual's share of the total exposure increases.

232. (B) The x-ray photons produced at the tungsten target comprise a heterogeneous beam, that is, a spectrum of photon energies. This is accounted for by the fact that the incident electrons have different energies. Also, the incident electrons travel through several layers of tungsten target material, lose energy with each interaction, and therefore produce increasingly weaker x-ray photons. During characteristic x-ray production, vacancies may be filled in the K, L, or M shells, differing with each other in binding energies, and, therefore, a variety of energy photons are emitted.

233. (C) Potentially high occupational exposure is possible in fluoroscopy, mobile radiography, vascular procedures, and interventional surgery. Time, distance, and shielding are the cardinal principles of radiation protection. The following is a list of radiation safety guidelines in fluoroscopy:

The Bucky slot cover must have at least 0.25-mm lead equivalent to reduce gonadal level exposure to radiologist and radiographer.

The protective curtain must have at least 0.25-mm lead equivalent and be positioned between the fluoroscopist and the patient to absorb scatter from the tabletop.

Thyroid shields having at least 0.5-mm lead equivalent should be worn.

Protective lead aprons must be worn; lead equivalent of 0.5 mm is recommended.

The lowest amount of scatter radiation is 90° (perpendicular) from the patient.

234. (C) Fluoroscopic examinations have the potential to deliver significant patient dose, but there are a number of ways to keep that dose as low as possible: keeping the length of the fluoroscopic exposure/procedure to a minimum, using the last-image-hold feature, keeping the image intensifier as close to the patient as possible, using ABC settings with highest kilovoltage and lowest milliampere combinations, keeping the use of "boost" and magnification modes to a minimum, using the smallest practical FOV, using the lowest practical pulse rate, and adjusting tube angle/patient position to spread exposure dose over a larger area.

235. (B) *Primary barriers* are those that protect us from the primary or useful beam. They have much greater attenuation capability than secondary barriers that protect only from leakage and scattered radiation. The radiographic room walls are therefore considered primary barriers because the primary beam is often directed toward them, such as in chest radiography. Most control booth barriers, however, are *secondary barriers* and the primary beam is never directed toward them. They are usually constructed of four thicknesses of gypsum board and/or 0.5–1 inch of plate glass. Leakage radiation is reduced by the x-ray tube housing.

236. (A) Milliampere seconds regulate the *quantity* of radiation delivered to the patient. Kilovoltage regulates the *quality* (penetration) of the radiation delivered to the patient. Therefore, higher energy (more penetrating) radiation—which is more likely to exit the patient—accompanied by lower milliampere seconds is the safest combination for the patient, delivering the *lowest* dose. Higher milliampere seconds at lower kilovoltage values *increases* patient dose.

237. (A) Examples of tissue reactions (formally called deterministic effect) can be early or late. Examples of *early* tissue reactions include epilation, erythema, and decreased white blood cell count. More severe early effects include radiation sickness/acute radiation syndrome. *Late* effects of radiation include reduced fertility, sterility, cataract formation, organ atrophy, and fibrosis.

238. (A) Because the established dose limit formula guideline is used for occupationally exposed persons 18 years of age and older, guidelines had to be established in the event a student entered training prior to age 18 years. The guideline states that the occupational dose limit for students younger than 18 years is 1 mSv (0.1 rem or 100 mrem) in any given year.

239. (A) The declared pregnant radiographer poses a special radiation protection consideration because the safety of the unborn individual must be considered. It must be remembered that the developing fetus is particularly sensitive to radiation exposure. Therefore, established guidelines state that the occupational radiation exposure to the fetus must not exceed 5 mSv (0.5 rem/500 mrem) during the entire gestation period; the *monthly* fetal dose must not exceed 0.5 mSv (0.05 rem).

240. (D) The annual whole-body dose established by the NCRP takes into account sensitivities of numerous organs and tissues. However, some body tissues and organs have a higher DL. During fluoroscopic and interventional procedures, the upper extremities might receive greater occupational exposure than the trunk. The annual DL for the extremities is 500 mSv/year. (*Bushong, 11th ed. p. 604*)

Question Number and Subspecialty correspond to subcategories in each of the four ARRT examination specification sections

1. Radiation protection/personnel protection
2. Radiation physics and radiobiology/principles of radiation physics
3. Radiation protection/personnel protection
4. Radiation physics and radiobiology/biological aspects of radiation
5. Radiation protection/minimizing patient exposure
6. Radiation physics and radiobiology/biological aspects of radiation
7. Radiation protection/minimizing patient exposure
8. Radiation physics and radiobiology/biological aspects of radiation
9. Radiation protection/minimizing patient exposure
10. Radiation protection/personnel protection
11. Radiation physics and radiobiology/biological aspects of radiation
12. Radiation physics and radiobiology/principles of radiation physics
13. Radiation protection/personnel protection
14. Radiation physics and radiobiology/biological aspects of radiation
15. Radiation physics and radiobiology/biological aspects of radiation
16. Radiation physics and radiobiology/biological aspects of radiation
17. Radiation physics and radiobiology/biological aspects of radiation
18. Radiation physics and radiobiology/principles of radiation physics
19. Radiation physics and radiobiology/principles of radiation physics
20. Radiation protection/personnel protection
21. Radiation physics and radiobiology/biological aspects of radiation
22. Radiation physics and radiobiology/principles of radiation physics
23. Radiation physics and radiobiology/biological aspects of radiation
24. Radiation protection/personnel protection
25. Radiation protection/personnel protection
26. Radiation protection/minimizing patient exposure
27. Radiation physics and radiobiology/principles of radiation physics
28. Radiation protection/minimizing patient exposure
29. Radiation physics and radiobiology/biological aspects of radiation
30. Radiation protection/personnel protection
31. Radiation protection/personnel protection
32. Radiation protection/personnel protection
33. Radiation physics and radiobiology/biological aspects of radiation
34. Radiation protection/minimizing patient exposure
35. Radiation physics and radiobiology/principles of radiation physics
36. Radiation physics and radiobiology/principles of radiation physics
37. Radiation protection/personnel protection
38. Radiation physics and radiobiology/biological aspects of radiation
39. Radiation physics and radiobiology/biological aspects of radiation
40. Radiation physics and radiobiology/principles of radiation physics
41. Radiation protection/minimizing patient exposure
42. Radiation protection/minimizing patient exposure
43. Radiation protection/personnel protection
44. Radiation protection/personnel protection
45. Radiation physics and radiobiology/principles of radiation physics
46. Radiation protection/minimizing patient exposure
47. Radiation protection/minimizing patient exposure
48. Radiation physics and radiobiology/biological aspects of radiation
49. Radiation physics and radiobiology/biological aspects of radiation
50. Radiation physics and radiobiology/principles of radiation physics
51. Radiation protection/minimizing patient exposure
52. Radiation physics and radiobiology/biological aspects of radiation
53. Radiation physics and radiobiology/principles of radiation physics
54. Radiation physics and radiobiology/biological aspects of radiation
55. Radiation protection/minimizing patient exposure
56. Radiation physics and radiobiology/biological aspects of radiation
57. Radiation physics and radiobiology/biological aspects of radiation
58. Radiation physics and radiobiology/biological aspects of radiation

59. Radiation physics and radiobiology/biological aspects of radiation
60. Radiation protection/personnel protection
61. Radiation physics and radiobiology/principles of radiation physics
62. Radiation protection/minimizing patient exposure
63. Radiation physics and radiobiology/principles of radiation physics
64. Radiation physics and radiobiology/principles of radiation physics
65. Radiation physics and radiobiology/biological aspects of radiation
66. Radiation protection/personnel protection
67. Radiation protection/personnel protection
68. Radiation protection/personnel protection
69. Radiation protection/minimizing patient exposure
70. Radiation protection/personnel protection
71. Radiation protection/personnel protection
72. Radiation physics and radiobiology/biological aspects of radiation
73. Radiation protection/personnel protection
74. Radiation physics and radiobiology/principles of radiation physics
75. Radiation physics and radiobiology/principles of radiation physics
76. Radiation physics and radiobiology/biological aspects of radiation
77. Radiation physics and radiobiology/principles of radiation physics
78. Radiation protection/personnel protection
79. Radiation physics and radiobiology/biological aspects of radiation
80. Radiation physics and radiobiology/principles of radiation physics
81. Radiation protection/minimizing patient exposure
82. Radiation physics and radiobiology/principles of radiation physics
83. Radiation protection/personnel protection
84. Radiation protection/minimizing patient exposure
85. Radiation protection/personnel protection
86. Radiation protection/personnel protection
87. Radiation physics and radiobiology/principles of radiation physics
88. Radiation protection/minimizing patient exposure
89. Radiation physics and radiobiology/principles of radiation physics
90. Radiation physics and radiobiology/principles of radiation physics
91. Radiation protection/personnel protection
92. Radiation protection/minimizing patient exposure
93. Radiation protection/minimizing patient exposure
94. Radiation protection/minimizing patient exposure
95. Radiation protection/personnel protection
96. Radiation protection/minimizing patient exposure
97. Radiation physics and radiobiology/biological aspects of radiation
98. Radiation physics and radiobiology/biological aspects of radiation
99. Radiation physics and radiobiology/biological aspects of radiation
100. Radiation physics and radiobiology/biological aspects of radiation
101. Radiation physics and radiobiology/biological aspects of radiation
102. Radiation physics and radiobiology/principles of radiation physics
103. Radiation protection/personnel protection
104. Radiation physics and radiobiology/principles of radiation physics
105. Radiation physics and radiobiology/principles of radiation physics
106. Radiation physics and radiobiology/principles of radiation physics
107. Radiation protection/minimizing patient exposure
108. Radiation physics and radiobiology/principles of radiation physics
109. Radiation physics and radiobiology/biological aspects of radiation
110. Radiation physics and radiobiology/principles of radiation physics
111. Radiation protection/personnel protection
112. Radiation physics and radiobiology/principles of radiation physics
113. Radiation physics and radiobiology/biological aspects of radiation
114. Radiation protection/personnel protection
115. Radiation protection/minimizing patient exposure
116. Radiation protection/personnel protection
117. Radiation physics and radiobiology/principles of radiation physics
118. Radiation protection/personnel protection
119. Radiation physics and radiobiology/biological aspects of radiation
120. Radiation physics and radiobiology/biological aspects of radiation
121. Radiation physics and radiobiology/principles of radiation physics
122. Radiation protection/personnel protection
123. Radiation physics and radiobiology/principles of radiation physics
124. Radiation physics and radiobiology/biological aspects of radiation
125. Radiation physics and radiobiology/biological aspects of radiation
126. Radiation protection/personnel protection

127. Radiation protection/minimizing patient exposure
128. Radiation protection/minimizing patient exposure
129. Radiation physics and radiobiology/biological aspects of radiation
130. Radiation physics and radiobiology/biological aspects of radiation
131. Radiation physics and radiobiology/principles of radiation physics
132. Radiation physics and radiobiology/biological aspects of radiation
133. Radiation physics and radiobiology/principles of radiation physics
134. Radiation physics and radiobiology/biological aspects of radiation
135. Radiation physics and radiobiology/principles of radiation physics
136. Radiation protection/personnel protection
137. Radiation protection/minimizing patient exposure
138. Radiation physics and radiobiology/biological aspects of radiation
139. Radiation physics and radiobiology/biological aspects of radiation
140. Radiation physics and radiobiology/biological aspects of radiation
141. Radiation protection/personnel protection
142. Radiation protection/personnel protection
143. Radiation physics and radiobiology/principles of radiation physics
144. Radiation protection/minimizing patient exposure
145. Radiation protection/personnel protection
146. Radiation protection/personnel protection
147. Radiation physics and radiobiology/biological aspects of radiation
148. Radiation protection/personnel protection
149. Radiation physics and radiobiology/biological aspects of radiation
150. Radiation protection/minimizing patient exposure
151. Radiation protection/minimizing patient exposure
152. Radiation physics and radiobiology/biological aspects of radiation
153. Radiation physics and radiobiology/principles of radiation physics
154. Radiation protection/personnel protection
155. Radiation protection/personnel protection
156. Radiation physics and radiobiology/biological aspects of radiation
157. Radiation physics and radiobiology/biological aspects of radiation
158. Radiation physics and radiobiology/biological aspects of radiation
159. Radiation protection/personnel protection

160. Radiation physics and radiobiology/biological aspects of radiation
161. Radiation protection/personnel protection
162. Radiation physics and radiobiology/biological aspects of radiation
163. Radiation physics and radiobiology/biological aspects of radiation
164. Radiation protection/minimizing patient exposure
165. Radiation protection/minimizing patient exposure
166. Radiation physics and radiobiology/biological aspects of radiation
167. Radiation physics and radiobiology/biological aspects of radiation
168. Radiation physics and radiobiology/biological aspects of radiation
169. Radiation physics and radiobiology/biological aspects of radiation
170. Radiation physics and radiobiology/principles of radiation physics
171. Radiation protection/minimizing patient exposure
172. Radiation protection/personnel protection
173. Radiation physics and radiobiology/biological aspects of radiation
174. Radiation protection/personnel protection
175. Radiation physics and radiobiology/biological aspects of radiation
176. Radiation physics and radiobiology/biological aspects of radiation
177. Radiation physics and radiobiology/principles of radiation physics
178. Radiation protection/personnel protection
179. Radiation protection/personnel protection
180. Radiation protection/minimizing patient exposure
181. Radiation physics and radiobiology/biological aspects of radiation
182. Radiation protection/personnel protection
183. Radiation physics and radiobiology/principles of radiation physics
184. Radiation physics and radiobiology/principles of radiation physics
185. Radiation physics and radiobiology/biological aspects of radiation
186. Radiation protection/minimizing patient exposure
187. Radiation physics and radiobiology/biological aspects of radiation
188. Radiation protection/minimizing patient exposure
189. Radiation protection/minimizing patient exposure
190. Radiation protection/minimizing patient exposure
191. Radiation protection/personnel protection
192. Radiation physics and radiobiology/biological aspects of radiation
193. Radiation protection/personnel protection

194. Radiation protection/minimizing patient exposure
195. Radiation protection/personnel protection
196. Radiation physics and radiobiology/biological aspects of radiation
197. Radiation protection/minimizing patient exposure
198. Radiation physics and radiobiology/principles of radiation physics
199. Radiation physics and radiobiology/biological aspects of radiation
200. Radiation protection/minimizing patient exposure
201. Radiation protection/minimizing patient exposure
202. Radiation protection/minimizing patient exposure
203. Radiation protection/personnel protection
204. Radiation protection/personnel protection
205. Radiation physics and radiobiology/principles of radiation physics
206. Radiation physics and radiobiology/biological aspects of radiation
207. Radiation physics and radiobiology/principles of radiation physics
208. Radiation physics and radiobiology/principles of radiation physics
209. Radiation protection/minimizing patient exposure
210. Radiation physics and radiobiology/biological aspects of radiation
211. Radiation physics and radiobiology/principles of radiation physics
212. Radiation physics and radiobiology/principles of radiation physics
213. Radiation physics and radiobiology/principles of radiation physics
214. Radiation physics and radiobiology/biological aspects of radiation
215. Radiation protection/personnel protection
216. Radiation protection/personnel protection
217. Radiation protection/personnel protection
218. Radiation protection/personnel protection
219. Radiation protection/minimizing patient exposure
220. Radiation protection/personnel protection
221. Radiation physics and radiobiology/principles of radiation physics
222. Radiation protection/personnel protection
223. Radiation physics and radiobiology/principles of radiation physics
224. Radiation protection/personnel protection
225. Radiation protection/personnel protection
226. Radiation protection/personnel protection
227. Radiation physics and radiobiology/biological aspects of radiation
228. Radiation physics and radiobiology/principles of radiation physics
229. Radiation physics and radiobiology/biological aspects of radiation
230. Radiation physics and radiobiology/principles of radiation physics
231. Radiation physics and radiobiology/biological aspects of radiation
232. Radiation physics and radiobiology/principles of radiation physics
233. Radiation protection/minimizing patient exposure
234. Radiation protection/minimizing patient exposure
235. Radiation protection/personnel protection
236. Radiation protection/minimizing patient exposure
237. Radiation physics and radiobiology/biological aspects of radiation
238. Radiation protection/personnel protection
239. Radiation protection/personnel protection
240. Radiation protection/personnel protection

Bushong SC. *Radiologic Science for Technologists.* 11th ed. St Louis, MO: Mosby; 2017.

Carlton RR, Adler AM, Balas V. *Principles of Radiographic Imaging.* 6th ed. Albany, NY: Delmar; 2020.

Johnston JN, Fauber TL. *Essentials of Radiographic Physics and Imaging.* 3rd ed. St Louis, MO: Mosby Elsevier; 2020.

NCRP Report No. 99. *Quality Assurance for Diagnostic Imaging.* NCRP; 1990.

NCRP Report No. 102. *Medical X-Ray, Electron Beam and Gamma-Ray Protection for Energies up to 50 MeV (Equipment Design, Performance and Use).* NCRP; 1989.

NCRP Report No. 116. *Recommendations on Limits for Exposure to Ionizing Radiation.* NCRP; 1987.

NCRP Report No. 160. *Ionizing Radiation Exposure of the Population of the United States.* NCRP; 2009.

NCRP Report No. 184. *Medical Radiation Exposure of Patients in the United States.* NCRP, 2019

Saia DA. *Radiography PREP.* 9th ed. New York, NY: McGraw Hill; 2018.

Seeram E, Brennan PC. *Radiation Protection in Diagnostic X-Ray Imaging.* Burlington, MA: Jones and Bartlett Learning; 2017.

Statkiewicz-Sherer MA, Visconti PJ, Ritenour ER, Haynes KW. *Radiation Protection in Medical Radiography.* 8th ed. St Louis, MO: Mosby; 2018.

Wolbarst AB. *Physics of Radiology.* 2nd ed. Madison, WI: Medical Physics Publishing; 2005.

Image Production: Image Acquisition and Technical Evaluation

QUESTIONS

DIRECTIONS: Each of the numbered items or incomplete statements in this section is followed by answers or by completions of the statement. Select the *one* letter answer or completion that is *best* in each case.

1. The fixed spatial resolution characteristic of direct digital systems is determined by the
   - ❑ A. TFT and DEL size
   - ❑ B. sampling frequency
   - ❑ C. laser scanner
   - ❑ D. PSP thickness

2. Which of the following control the subject contrast of the exit/remnant x-ray signal in digital imaging?
   1. Rescaling
   2. Lookup table
   3. Kilovoltage
   4. Windowing
   5. Photon energy
      - ❑ A. 1 and 3 only
      - ❑ B. 3 and 5 only
      - ❑ C. 1, 2, and 4 only
      - ❑ D. 2, 4, and 5 only

3. Which of the following pathologic conditions probably will require a decrease in exposure factors?
   - ❑ A. Osteomyelitis
   - ❑ B. Osteoporosis
   - ❑ C. Osteosclerosis
   - ❑ D. Osteochondritis

4. An algorithm, as used in x-ray imaging, is/are
   - ❑ A. a geometric formula
   - ❑ B. specific exposure factors
   - ❑ C. a series of variable instructions
   - ❑ D. predetermined exposure factors

5. The chest radiograph shown in Figure 4-1 demonstrates
   - ❑ A. part motion
   - ❑ B. aliasing artifact
   - ❑ C. double exposure
   - ❑ D. grid cutoff

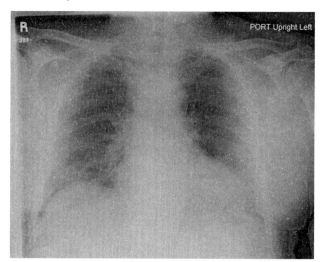

Figure 4-1. Used with permission of Stamford Hospital, Department of Radiology.

6. The components of a detector element (DEL) include which three of the following?
   1. Sensing area
   2. TFT
   3. Capacitor
   4. ADC
   5. CCD
      - ❑ A. 1, 2, and 3
      - ❑ B. 1, 2, and 5
      - ❑ C. 2, 4, and 5
      - ❑ D. 2, 3, and 4

167

7. Geometric sharpness is *inversely* influenced by
1. OID
2. SOD
3. SID
   - ❏ A. 1 only
   - ❏ B. 1 and 2 only
   - ❏ C. 1 and 3 only
   - ❏ D. 1, 2, and 3

8. The part of a detector element (DEL) that stores electrical charges is the
   - ❏ A. capacitor
   - ❏ B. TFT
   - ❏ C. sensing area
   - ❏ D. CCD

9. The radiograph shown in Figure 4-2 demonstrates an example of
   - ❏ A. motion blur
   - ❏ B. underexposure
   - ❏ C. scanner/reader artifact
   - ❏ D. exposure artifact

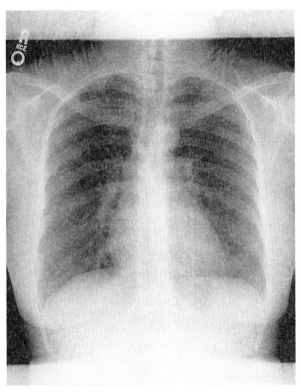

Figure 4-2. Used with permission of Stamford Hospital, Department of Radiology.

10. An increase in kilovoltage will have which of the following effects on the remnant beam/signal?
1. Increased production of scattered radiation
2. Increased exposure rate
3. Increased image contrast
   - ❏ A. 1 only
   - ❏ B. 1 and 2 only
   - ❏ C. 2 and 3 only
   - ❏ D. 1, 2, and 3

11. Factors that can impact image spatial resolution/image sharpness include
1. patient factors
2. focal spot size
3. SID
   - ❏ A. 1 only
   - ❏ B. 1 and 2 only
   - ❏ C. 2 and 3 only
   - ❏ D. 1, 2, and 3

12. The x-ray image seen in Figure 4-3 is most likely the result of
   - ❏ A. an off-level grid
   - ❏ B. pronounced anode heel effect
   - ❏ C. insufficient mAs factors
   - ❏ D. insufficient kVp factors

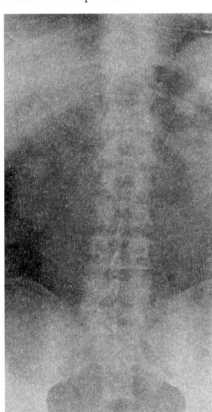

Figure 4-3. Used with permission of Stamford Hospital, Department of Radiology.

13. The function of the backup timer in automatic exposure control devices is to
1. prevent patient overexposure
2. prevent x-ray tube overheating
3. adjust programmed receptor exposure
   - ❏ A. 1 only
   - ❏ B. 1 and 2 only
   - ❏ C. 2 and 3 only
   - ❏ D. 1, 2, and 3

14. Which of the following groups of exposure factors will produce the greatest receptor exposure?
- ❏ A. 100 mA, 50 ms
- ❏ B. 200 mA, 40 ms
- ❏ C. 400 mA, 70 ms
- ❏ D. 600 mA, 30 ms

15. Which of the following is/are directly related to photon energy?
1. Kilovoltage
2. Milliamperes
3. Wavelength
- ❏ A. 1 only
- ❏ B. 1 and 2 only
- ❏ C. 1 and 3 only
- ❏ D. 1, 2, and 3

16. An x-ray image of the ankle was made at 40-inch SID, 200 mA, 50 ms, 70 kV, 0.6-mm focal spot, and minimal OID. Which of the following modifications would result in the greatest increase in magnification?
- ❏ A. 1.2-mm focal spot
- ❏ B. 36-inch SID
- ❏ C. 44-inch SID
- ❏ D. 4-inch OID

17. Grid cutoff due to off-centering would result in
- ❏ A. overall loss of receptor exposure
- ❏ B. both sides of the image receptor underexposed
- ❏ C. overexposure under the anode end
- ❏ D. underexposure under the anode end

18. The postprocessing function that removes high frequency noise from the x-ray image is
- ❏ A. windowing
- ❏ B. smoothing
- ❏ C. edge enhancement
- ❏ D. aliasing

19. An exposure of 500 mA and 70 kV has been selected for an AP projection of the abdomen using AEC. If 90 ms has been selected for the backup time, and the minimum response time is 25 ms, the milliampere seconds exposure will be *at least*
- ❏ A. 45
- ❏ B. 12.5
- ❏ C. 450
- ❏ D. 125

20. The lateral coccyx image shown in Figure 4-4 was made using AEC but is overexposed. This is most likely a result of
- ❏ A. incorrect selection of the small focal spot
- ❏ B. insufficient backup time
- ❏ C. selection of the center photocell
- ❏ D. incorrect centering of the part

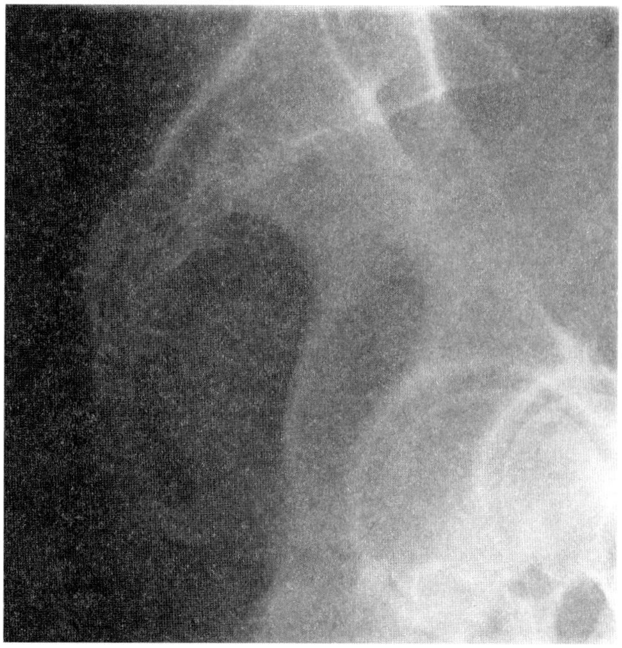

Figure 4-4. Reproduced, with permission, from Shephard CT. *Radiographic Image Production and Manipulation*. New York, NY: McGraw Hill; 2003.

21. Which of the following units is/are used to express resolution?
1. Line-spread function
2. Line pairs per millimeter
3. Line-focus principle
- ❏ A. 1 only
- ❏ B. 1 and 2 only
- ❏ C. 2 and 3 only
- ❏ D. 1, 2, and 3

22. If an IR exposed using a 12:1 ratio grid exhibits loss of signal at its lateral edges, it is probably because the
- ❏ A. SID was too great
- ❏ B. grid failed to move during the exposure
- ❏ C. x-ray tube was angled in the direction of the lead strips
- ❏ D. central ray was off-center

23. Foreshortening can be caused by
- ❏ A. the radiographic object being placed at an angle to the IR
- ❏ B. excessive distance between the object and the IR
- ❏ C. insufficient distance between the focus and the IR
- ❏ D. excessive distance between the focus and the IR

24. Acceptable method(s) of minimizing motion unsharpness is/are
1. suspended respiration
2. short exposure time
3. patient instruction
- ❏ A. 1 only
- ❏ B. 1 and 2 only
- ❏ C. 1 and 3 only
- ❏ D. 1, 2, and 3

25. Using fixed milliampere seconds and variable kilovoltage technical factors, each centimeter increase in patient thickness requires what adjustment in kilovoltage?

❏ A. Increase 2 kV
❏ B. Decrease 2 kV
❏ C. Increase 4 kV
❏ D. Decrease 4 kV

26. In which of the following systems does the radiographer select the anatomic part from the console menu?

❏ A. AEC
❏ B. APR
❏ C. TFT
❏ D. CCD

27. Which of the following statements is/are true regarding the location of the artifact seen in the erect PA chest shown in Figure 4-5?

❏ A. The object is located within the patient
❏ B. The object is located within the IP
❏ C. The object is located between the patient and the x-ray tube
❏ D. The object is located between the patient and the IP

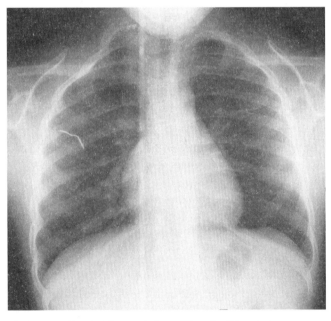

Figure 4-5. Used with permission of Stamford Hospital, Department of Radiology.

28. Which of the following can impact the remnant signal?

1. Tissue density
2. Pathology
3. Beam restriction

❏ A. 1 and 2 only
❏ B. 1 and 3 only
❏ C. 2 and 3 only
❏ D. 1, 2, and 3

29. X-ray photon energy is inversely related to

1. photon wavelength
2. applied milliamperes (mA)
3. applied kilovoltage (kV)

❏ A. 1 only
❏ B. 1 and 2 only
❏ C. 1 and 3 only
❏ D. 1, 2, and 3

30. The PA chest image shown in Figure 4-6 exhibits which of the following qualities?

1. Adequate penetration of the heart
2. Long-scale contrast
3. Adequate inspiration

❏ A. 1 only
❏ B. 1 and 2 only
❏ C. 2 and 3 only
❏ D. 1, 2, and 3

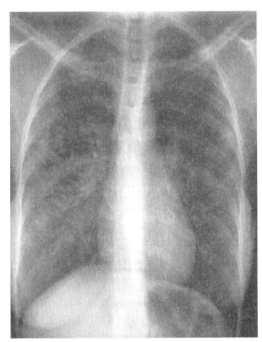

Figure 4-6. Used with permission of Stamford Hospital, Department of Radiology.

31. The device that functions to terminate the x-ray exposure following ionization of a particular quantity of an air is the

❏ A. image intensifier AEC
❏ B. output screen
❏ C. grid
❏ D. AEC

32. Compared with a low-ratio grid, a high-ratio grid will

1. allow more centering latitude
2. absorb more scattered radiation
3. absorb more primary radiation

❏ A. 1 only
❏ B. 1 and 2 only
❏ C. 2 and 3 only
❏ D. 1, 2, and 3

33. A decrease in kilovoltage will result in
1. a decrease in sharpness/image resolution
2. a decrease in photon energy
3. a decrease in receptor exposure
   - ❏ A. 1 only
   - ❏ B. 1 and 2 only
   - ❏ C. 2 and 3 only
   - ❏ D. 1, 2, and 3

34. Select the true statement(s) regarding Figure 4-7.
1. Excessive receptor exposure and insufficient visualization of the cervical vertebra
2. The image demonstrates motion unsharpness
3. The airway is adequately demonstrated
4. Receptor exposure is insufficient for adequate vertebrae visualization
   - ❏ A. 1, 2, and 3
   - ❏ B. 2 and 4
   - ❏ C. 1, 3, and 4
   - ❏ D. 3 and 4

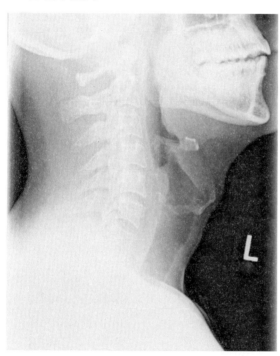

Figure 4-7

35. The primary function of x-ray beam filtration is to
   - ❏ A. reduce operator dose
   - ❏ B. reduce image noise
   - ❏ C. reduce patient skin dose
   - ❏ D. reduce scattered radiation

36. The exposure factors of 400 mA, 70 ms, and 78 kV were used to produce a particular image receptor exposure. A similar image could be produced using 500 mA, 90 kV, and
   - ❏ A. 14 ms
   - ❏ B. 28 ms
   - ❏ C. 56 ms
   - ❏ D. 70 ms

37. An exposure was made at a 36-inch SID using 300 mA, a 30-ms exposure, and 80 kV and an 8:1 grid. It is desired to repeat the radiograph using a 40-inch SID and 70 kV. With all other factors remaining constant, what new exposure time will be required?
   - ❏ A. 0.03 s
   - ❏ B. 0.07 s
   - ❏ C. 0.14 s
   - ❏ D. 0.36 s

38. The part of a detector element (DEL) that functions as a switch/gate to release charges for readout is the
   - ❏ A. capacitor
   - ❏ B. TFT
   - ❏ C. sensing area
   - ❏ D. CCD

39. An exposure was made using 300 mA, 40 ms exposure, and 85 kV. Each of the following changes will decrease the receptor exposure by one-half, *except* a change to
   - ❏ A. 0.02 s
   - ❏ B. 72 kV
   - ❏ C. 10 mAs
   - ❏ D. 150 mA

40. Which of the following groups of digital technical factors would be *most appropriate* for the radiographic examination shown in Figure 4-8?
   - ❏ A. 400 mA, 0.03 s, 72 kV
   - ❏ B. 300 mA, 20 ms, 84 kV
   - ❏ C. 300 mA, 8 ms, 97 kV
   - ❏ D. 50 mA, 0.25 s, 72 kV

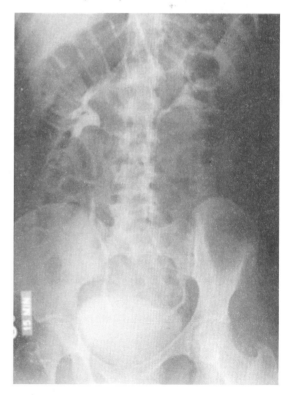

Figure 4-8. Used with permission of Stamford Hospital, Department of Radiology.

41. All of the following affect the exposure rate of the primary beam, *except*

- ❑ A. milliamperage
- ❑ B. kilovoltage
- ❑ C. distance
- ❑ D. field size

42. Which of the following has the greatest effect on radiographic IR exposure?

- ❑ A. Aluminum filtration
- ❑ B. Kilovoltage
- ❑ C. SID
- ❑ D. Scattered radiation

43. Subject contrast is related to

1. differential tissue absorption
2. atomic number of tissue being traversed
3. proper regulation of milliampere seconds
   - ❑ A. 1 only
   - ❑ B. 1 and 2 only
   - ❑ C. 1 and 3 only
   - ❑ D. 1, 2, and 3

44. What grid ratio is represented in Figure 4-9?

- ❑ A. 3:1
- ❑ B. 5:1
- ❑ C. 10:1
- ❑ D. 16:1

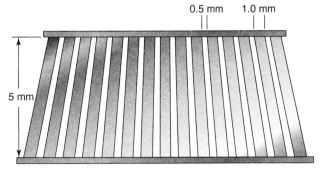

Figure 4-9

45. A 5-inch object to be radiographed at a 44-inch SID lies 6 inches from the IR. What will be the image width?

- ❑ A. 5.1 inches
- ❑ B. 5.7 inches
- ❑ C. 6.1 inches
- ❑ D. 6.7 inches

46. An image demonstrating many brightness levels, or shades of gray, with only slight difference between the levels/shades is said to possess

1. long-scale contrast
2. low contrast
3. short-scale contrast
   - ❑ A. 1 only
   - ❑ B. 2 only
   - ❑ C. 1 and 2 only
   - ❑ D. 2 and 3 only

47. The term *pixel* is associated with all of the following, *except*

- ❑ A. two dimensional
- ❑ B. picture element
- ❑ C. measured in *xy* direction
- ❑ D. how much of the part is included in the matrix

48. Spatial resolution/detail sharpness can be improved by decreasing

1. the SID
2. the OID
3. patient/part motion
   - ❑ A. 1 only
   - ❑ B. 3 only
   - ❑ C. 2 and 3 only
   - ❑ D. 1, 2, and 3

49. Which of the following devices is used to overcome severe variation in patient anatomy or tissue density, providing more uniform receptor exposure?

- ❑ A. Compensating filter
- ❑ B. Grid
- ❑ C. Collimator
- ❑ D. Added filtration

50. The tiny increased brightness, dropout artifacts, seen in the proximal portion of the CR image of the radius shown in Figure 4-10 are representative of

- ❑ A. backscatter
- ❑ B. skipped scan lines
- ❑ C. dust/dirt on the PSP
- ❑ D. image fading

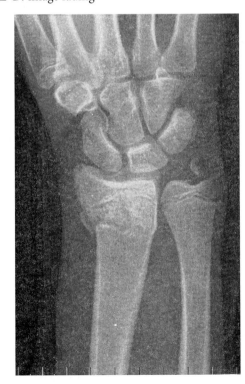

Figure 4-10. Reproduced, with permission, from Shephard CT. *Radiographic Image Production and Manipulation.* New York: McGraw Hill; 2003.

51. Radiographic images, for medicolegal reasons, are required to include the following information:

1. the patient's name and/or identification number
2. a left- or right-side marker
3. the patient's birth date
   - ❑ A. 1 only
   - ❑ B. 1 and 2 only
   - ❑ C. 1 and 3 only
   - ❑ D. 1, 2, and 3

52. Special considerations/conditions that often require increase from typical technical factors include

1. excessive BMI
2. skeletal sclerosis
3. osteomalacia
   - ❑ A. 1 only
   - ❑ B. 1 and 2 only
   - ❑ C. 2 and 3 only
   - ❑ D. 1, 2, and 3

53. The distance between the center of one pixel and the center of an adjacent pixel is termed

- ❑ A. picture element
- ❑ B. volume element
- ❑ C. pixel pitch
- ❑ D. bit depth

54. Because of the anode heel effect, the intensity of the x-ray beam is greatest at the

- ❑ A. path of the central ray
- ❑ B. anode end of the beam
- ❑ C. cathode end of the beam
- ❑ D. transverse axis of the IR

55. The differences between CR and DR include

1. CR uses IPs
2. CR has higher DQE and lower patient dose
3. CR images are displayed immediately
   - ❑ A. 1 only
   - ❑ B. 1 and 2 only
   - ❑ C. 2 and 3 only
   - ❑ D. 1, 2, and 3

56. Which two of the following are associated with the term "voxel"?

1. Bit depth
2. Volume element
3. Measure in Z direction
4. Field of view
   - ❑ A. 1 and 2
   - ❑ B. 2 and 4
   - ❑ C. 2 and 3
   - ❑ D. 1 and 3

57. Using a 48-inch SID, how much OID must be introduced to magnify an object 2 times?

- ❑ A. 8-inch OID
- ❑ B. 12-inch OID
- ❑ C. 16-inch OID
- ❑ D. 24-inch OID

58. A particular radiograph was produced using 12 mAs and 85 kV with a 16:1 ratio grid. The radiograph is to be repeated using an 8:1 ratio grid. What should be the new milliampere seconds value?

- ❑ A. 3
- ❑ B. 6
- ❑ C. 8
- ❑ D. 10

59. Pathologic or abnormal conditions that would require a *decrease* in exposure factors include all of the following, *except*

- ❑ A. osteoporosis
- ❑ B. osteomalacia
- ❑ C. emphysema
- ❑ D. pneumonia

60. Analog-to-digital conversion is required in which of the following imaging system?

- ❑ A. CR
- ❑ B. DR
- ❑ C. SF
- ❑ D. Direct conversion

61. The photostimulable phosphor (PSP) plates used in CR are constructed in layers that include

1. light shield layer
2. support layer
3. electroconductive layer
   - ❑ A. 1 only
   - ❑ B. 1 and 2 only
   - ❑ C. 2 and 3 only
   - ❑ D. 1, 2, and 3

62. For the same field of view (FOV), spatial resolution will be improved using

- ❑ A. a smaller matrix
- ❑ B. a larger matrix
- ❑ C. fewer pixels
- ❑ D. shorter SID

63. Which of the following are methods of limiting the production of scattered radiation?

1. Using moderate ratio grids
2. Using the prone position for abdominal examinations
3. Restricting the field size to the smallest practical size
   - ❑ A. 1 and 2 only
   - ❑ B. 1 and 3 only
   - ❑ C. 2 and 3 only
   - ❑ D. 1, 2, and 3

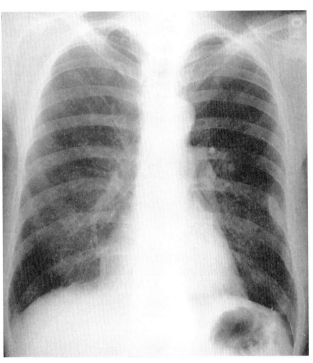
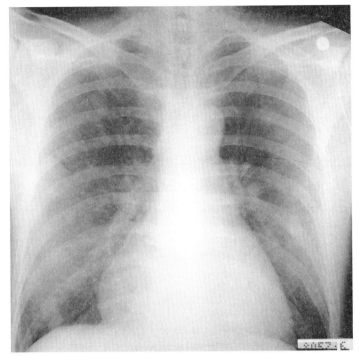

A   B

Figure 4-11

64. The PA erect chest images seen in Figure 4-11 were made of the same patient within 24 h. Which of the following statements are true regarding the images?
1. Figure 4-11B demonstrates insufficient inspiration
2. Figure 4-11A was performed at 6 feet, whereas Figure 4-11B was performed at much shorter SID
3. Figure 4-11A is underexposed
4. Figure 4-11B demonstrates magnification of the heart shadow
5. Figure 4-11B was performed at 6 feet, whereas Figure 4-11A was performed at much shorter SID
6. Figure 4-11A demonstrates better resolution/ sharpness
   - ❏ A. 1, 2, and 3
   - ❏ B. 1, 3, and 5
   - ❏ C. 2, 4, and 6
   - ❏ D. 4, 5, and 6

65. Exposure factors of 90 kV and 3 mAs are used for a particular nongrid exposure. What should be the new milliampere seconds (mAs) value if a 12:1 grid is added?
   - ❏ A. 86
   - ❏ B. 9
   - ❏ C. 12
   - ❏ D. 15

66. Which of the images in Figure 4-12 has the smallest matrix size?
   - ❏ A. Image #1
   - ❏ B. Image #2
   - ❏ C. Image #3
   - ❏ D. Image #4

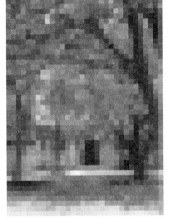
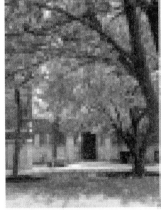

1   2

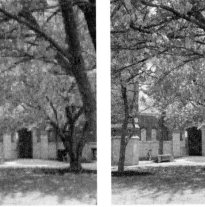
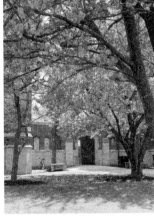

3   4

Figure 4-12

67. Types of shape distortion include
1. magnification
2. elongation
3. foreshortening
   - ❑ A. 1 only
   - ❑ B. 1 and 2 only
   - ❑ C. 2 and 3 only
   - ❑ D. 1, 2, and 3

68. For the same FOV, as the matrix size increases
1. spatial resolution increases
2. image quality increases
3. pixel size decreases
   - ❑ A. 1 only
   - ❑ B. 1 and 2 only
   - ❑ C. 2 and 3 only
   - ❑ D. 1, 2, and 3

69. If a duration of 0.05 s was selected for a particular exposure, what milliamperage would be necessary to produce 30 mAs?
   - ❑ A. 900
   - ❑ B. 600
   - ❑ C. 500
   - ❑ D. 300

70. In which of the following ways does SID affect sharpness of image details?
   - ❑ A. Image detail sharpness is directly related to SID
   - ❑ B. Image detail sharpness is inversely related to SID
   - ❑ C. As SID increases, image detail sharpness decreases
   - ❑ D. SID is not an image detail sharpness factor

71. A satisfactory radiograph was made using a 36-inch SID, 12 mAs, and a 12:1 grid. If the examination will be repeated at a distance of 42 inches and using a 5:1 grid, what should be the new milliampere seconds value to maintain the original receptor exposure?
   - ❑ A. 5.6
   - ❑ B. 6.5
   - ❑ C. 9.7
   - ❑ D. 13

72. Of the following groups of exposure factors, which will produce the most receptor exposure?
   - ❑ A. 400 mA, 30 ms, 72-inch SID
   - ❑ B. 200 mA, 30 ms, 36-inch SID
   - ❑ C. 200 mA, 60 ms, 36-inch SID
   - ❑ D. 400 mA, 60 ms, 72-inch SID

73. Image resolution improves as
1. scintillation increases
2. DEL size decreases
3. fill factor increases
   - ❑ A. 1 only
   - ❑ B. 1 and 2 only
   - ❑ C. 2 and 3 only
   - ❑ D. 1, 2, and 3

74. All of the following statements regarding digital imaging are true, *except*
   - ❑ A. window level adjustments are associated with image brightness
   - ❑ B. brightness is related to IR exposure
   - ❑ C. image visibility is a function of IR exposure
   - ❑ D. brightness and density are not interchangeable terms

75. In digital imaging, kilovoltage selection has an effect on
1. photon energy
2. penetration
3. image contrast
   - ❑ A. 1 only
   - ❑ B. 1 and 2 only
   - ❑ C. 2 and 3 only
   - ❑ D. 1, 2, and 3

76. The quality assurance term used to describe consistency in exposure at adjacent mA stations is
   - ❑ A. automatic exposure control
   - ❑ B. positive beam limitation
   - ❑ C. linearity
   - ❑ D. reproducibility

77. Exposure factors of 2 mAs and 75 kV were used for a particular part. Which of the following changes would result in twice the exposure to the image receptor?
   - ❑ A. 1 mAs
   - ❑ B. 4 mAs
   - ❑ C. 76 kV
   - ❑ D. 64 kV

78. Factors impacting spatial resolution include
1. focal spot size
2. subject motion
3. SOD
   - ❑ A. 1 and 2 only
   - ❑ B. 1 and 3 only
   - ❑ C. 2 and 3 only
   - ❑ D. 1, 2, and 3

79. A grid usually is used in which of the following circumstances?
1. When radiographing a large or dense body part
2. When using high kilovoltage
3. When a lower patient dose is required
   - ❑ A. 1 only
   - ❑ B. 3 only
   - ❑ C. 1 and 2 only
   - ❑ D. 1, 2, and 3

80. Which of the following errors is illustrated in Figure 4-13?

❑ A. Patient not centered to IR
❑ B. X-ray tube not centered to grid
❑ C. Inaccurate collimation
❑ D. Unilateral grid cutoff

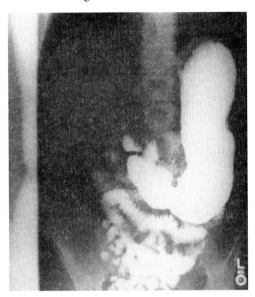

Figure 4-13. Used with permission of Stamford Hospital, Department of Radiology.

81. How are milliampere seconds and patient dose related?

❑ A. Milliampere seconds and patient dose are inversely proportional
❑ B. Milliampere seconds and patient dose are directly proportional
❑ C. Milliampere seconds and patient dose are unrelated
❑ D. Milliampere seconds and patient dose are inversely related

82. Image plate front material can be made of which of the following?

1. Carbon fiber
2. Magnesium
3. Lead
   ❑ A. 1 only
   ❑ B. 1 and 2 only
   ❑ C. 1 and 3 only
   ❑ D. 1, 2, and 3

83. Which of the following pathologic conditions would require a decrease in exposure factors?

❑ A. Congestive heart failure
❑ B. Pneumonia
❑ C. Emphysema
❑ D. Pleural effusion

84. What pixel size has a 512 × 512 matrix with a 20-cm field of view (FOV)?

❑ A. 0.07 mm/pixel
❑ B. 0.40 mm/pixel
❑ C. 0.04 mm/pixel
❑ D. 4.0 mm/pixel

85. Practice(s) that enable the radiographer to reduce the exposure time required for a particular image include

1. use of a higher milliamperage
2. use of a higher kilovoltage
3. use of a higher ratio grid
   ❑ A. 1 only
   ❑ B. 1 and 2 only
   ❑ C. 2 and 3 only
   ❑ D. 1, 2, and 3

86. All of the following statements regarding kilovoltage are correct, *except*

❑ A. increased kilovoltage increases beam intensity
❑ B. receptor exposure can be doubled or halved by using the 15% rule
❑ C. increased kilovoltage can decrease absorbed dose
❑ D. kilovoltage and wavelength are directly proportional

87. Factors impacting spatial resolution in CR digital imaging include

1. pixel pitch
2. sampling frequency
3. DEL size of the TFT
   ❑ A. 1 only
   ❑ B. 1 and 2 only
   ❑ C. 2 and 3 only
   ❑ D. 1, 2, and 3

88. Which of the following statements are true regarding Figure 4-14?

1. Line A indicates greater dynamic range
2. Line A is representative of CR
3. Line B represents a linear relationship between exposure and luminance
4. Line B represents film emulsion response
   ❑ A. 1, 3, and 4
   ❑ B. 1 and 2
   ❑ C. 1, 2, and 4
   ❑ D. 1, 3, and 4

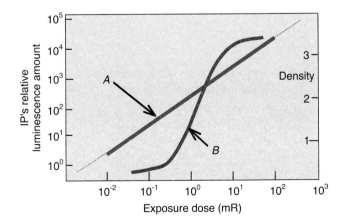

Figure 4-14. Used with permission of FUJIFILM Medical Systems USA, Inc.

89. Exposure artifacts include
1. double exposure
2. motion
3. image fading
❏ A. 1 only
❏ B. 1 and 2 only
❏ C. 2 and 3 only
❏ D. 1, 2, and 3

90. An increase in the kilovoltage applied to the x-ray tube increases the
1. x-ray wavelength
2. exposure rate
3. patient absorption
❏ A. 1 only
❏ B. 2 only
❏ C. 2 and 3 only
❏ D. 1, 2, and 3

91. Foreshortening of the radiographic image is a result of
❏ A. tube angulation
❏ B. increased OID
❏ C. decreased SID
❏ D. improper part alignment

92. Misalignment of the tube–part–IR relationship results in
❏ A. shape distortion
❏ B. size distortion
❏ C. magnification
❏ D. blur

93. If the radiographer is unable to achieve a short OID because of the structure of the body part or patient condition, which of the following adjustments can be made to minimize magnification distortion?
❏ A. A smaller focal spot size should be used
❏ B. A longer SID should be used
❏ C. A shorter SID should be used
❏ D. A lower ratio grid should be used

94. The exposure factors used for a particular nongrid x-ray image were 300 mA, 4 ms, and 90 kV. Another image, using an 8:1 grid, is requested. Which of the following groups of factors is *most appropriate*?
❏ A. 400 mA, 3 ms, 110 kV
❏ B. 400 mA, 12 ms, 90 kV
❏ C. 300 mA, 8 ms, 100 kV
❏ D. 200 mA, 240 ms, 90 kV

95. Which of the radiographs shown in Figure 4-15 most likely required less exposure?
❏ A. Image A
❏ B. Image B
❏ C. No difference in exposure was required

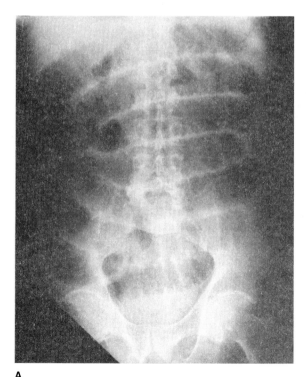

A

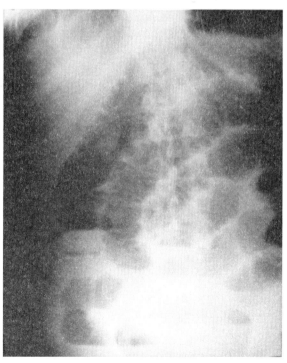

B

Figure 4-15. From the American College of Radiology Learning File. Used with permission of the ACR.

96. Exposure rate will decrease with an increase in
1. SID
2. kilovoltage
3. focal spot size
   - ❏ A. 1 only
   - ❏ B. 1 and 2 only
   - ❏ C. 2 and 3 only
   - ❏ D. 1, 2, and 3

97. As digital image matrix size increases
1. pixel size decreases
2. resolution decreases
3. pixel depth decreases
   - ❏ A. 1 only
   - ❏ B. 2 only
   - ❏ C. 1 and 2 only
   - ❏ D. 2 and 3 only

98. Distortion can be caused by
1. tube angle
2. the position of the organ or structure within the body
3. the radiographic positioning of the part
   - ❏ A. 1 only
   - ❏ B. 1 and 2 only
   - ❏ C. 2 and 3 only
   - ❏ D. 1, 2, and 3

99. If a 6-inch OID is introduced during a particular radiographic examination, what change in SID will be necessary to overcome objectionable magnification?
   - ❏ A. The SID must be increased by 6 inches
   - ❏ B. The SID must be increased by 18 inches
   - ❏ C. The SID must be decreased by 6 inches
   - ❏ D. The SID must be increased by 42 inches

100. Decreasing field size from 14 × 17 inches to 8 × 10 inches, with no other changes, will
   - ❏ A. decrease the amount of scattered radiation generated within the part
   - ❏ B. increase the amount of scattered radiation generated within the part
   - ❏ C. increase x-ray penetration of the part
   - ❏ D. decrease x-ray penetration of the part

101. Causes of grid cutoff, when using focused reciprocating grids, include which of the following?
1. Inadequate SID
2. X-ray tube off-center with the long axis of the lead strips
3. Angling the beam in the direction of the lead strips
   - ❏ A. 1 only
   - ❏ B. 1 and 2 only
   - ❏ C. 2 and 3 only
   - ❏ D. 1, 2, and 3

102. What are the effects of scattered radiation on a radiographic image?
1. It impairs visibility of details
2. It increases contrast
3. It increases grid cutoff
   - ❏ A. 1 only
   - ❏ B. 2 only
   - ❏ C. 1 and 2 only
   - ❏ D. 1, 2, and 3

103. Which of the following groups of exposure factors would be *most appropriate* to control involuntary motion?
   - ❏ A. 400 mA, 0.03 s
   - ❏ B. 200 mA, 0.06 s
   - ❏ C. 600 mA, 0.02 s
   - ❏ D. 100 mA, 0.12 s

104. Geometric blur can be evaluated using all the following devices, *except*
   - ❏ A. star pattern
   - ❏ B. slit camera
   - ❏ C. penetrometer
   - ❏ D. pinhole camera

105. Digital preprocessing functions include
1. rescaling
2. histogram analysis
3. equalization
   - ❏ A. 1 only
   - ❏ B. 1 and 2 only
   - ❏ C. 2 and 3 only
   - ❏ D. 1, 2, and 3

106. In digital imaging, milliampere seconds selection has an effect on
1. receptor exposure
2. patient dose
3. brightness
   - ❏ A. 1 only
   - ❏ B. 1 and 2 only
   - ❏ C. 2 and 3 only
   - ❏ D. 1, 2, and 3

107. What is the correct critique of the CR image shown in Figure 4-16?
   - ❏ A. Double exposure
   - ❏ B. Inverted IP
   - ❏ C. Incomplete erasure
   - ❏ D. Image fading

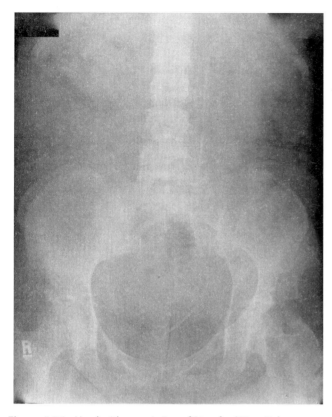

Figure 4-16. Used with permission of Stamford Hospital, Department of Radiology.

108. Which of the following affect(s) both the quantity and the quality of the primary beam?
1. Half-value layer (HVL)
2. Kilovoltage (kV)
3. Milliampere (mA)
   - ❏ A. 1 only
   - ❏ B. 2 only
   - ❏ C. 1 and 2 only
   - ❏ D. 1, 2, and 3

109. All of the following are related to spatial resolution, *except*
- ❏ A. milliamperage
- ❏ B. focal spot size
- ❏ C. SID
- ❏ D. OID

110. Which of the following would be useful for an examination of a patient suffering from Parkinson's disease?
1. Short exposure time
2. Decreased SID
3. Compensating filtration
   - ❏ A. 1 only
   - ❏ B. 1 and 2 only
   - ❏ C. 1 and 3 only
   - ❏ D. 1, 2, and 3

111. Reduction in x-ray photon intensity as it passes through numerous tissue densities is termed
- ❏ A. absorption
- ❏ B. scattering
- ❏ C. attenuation
- ❏ D. divergence

112. In digital imaging, as the size of the image matrix increases,
1. FOV increases
2. pixel size decreases
3. spatial resolution increases
   - ❏ A. 1 only
   - ❏ B. 1 and 2 only
   - ❏ C. 2 and 3 only
   - ❏ D. 1, 2, and 3

113. An anteroposterior (AP) projection of the femur was made using 300 mA, 0.03 s, 76 kV, 40-inch SID, and 1.2-mm focal spot. With all other factors remaining constant, which of the following exposure times would be required to maintain correct IR exposure at a 44-inch SID using 500 mA?
- ❏ A. 12 ms
- ❏ B. 22 ms
- ❏ C. 30 ms
- ❏ D. 36 ms

114. An AP radiograph of the femur was made using 300 mA, 0.03 s, 76 kV, 40-inch SID, and 1.2-mm focal spot. With all other factors remaining constant, which of the following exposure times would be required to maintain correct IR exposure using 87 kV and the addition of a 12:1 grid?
- ❏ A. 38 ms
- ❏ B. 60 ms
- ❏ C. 75 ms
- ❏ D. 150 ms

115. Scattered radiation can impact the image negatively, but has *no* effect on
- ❏ A. receptor exposure
- ❏ B. detail visibility
- ❏ C. spatial resolution
- ❏ D. occupational exposure

116. In a posteroanterior (PA) projection of the chest being used for cardiac evaluation, the heart measures 14.7 cm between its widest points. If the magnification factor (MF) is known to be 1.2, what is the actual diameter of the heart?
- ❏ A. 10.4 cm
- ❏ B. 12.25 cm
- ❏ C. 13.5 cm
- ❏ D. 17.64 cm

117. The material comprising the IP front must be
- ❏ A. homogenous/radiopaque
- ❏ B. heterogeneous/radiopaque
- ❏ C. homogeneous/radiolucent
- ❏ D. heterogeneous/radiolucent

118. OID is related to image sharpness/spatial resolution in which of the following ways?
- ❏ A. Sharpness/resolution is directly related to OID
- ❏ B. Sharpness/resolution is inversely related to OID
- ❏ C. As OID increases, so does sharpness/resolution
- ❏ D. OID is unrelated to sharpness/resolution

119. Which of the following statements are true with respect to the radiograph shown in Figure 4-17?
1. The image exhibits long-scale contrast
2. The image exhibits an exposure artifact
3. The image demonstrates motion blur
4. The image is a double exposure
- ❏ A. 1 and 2 only
- ❏ B. 1, 3, and 4 only
- ❏ C. 3 and 4 only
- ❏ D. 1, 2, and 3 only

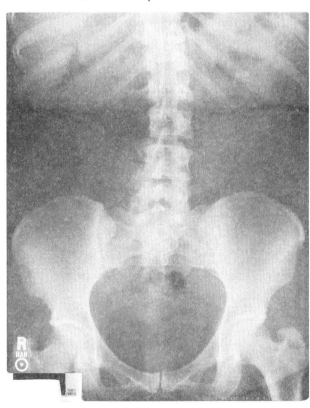

Figure 4-17. Used with permission of Stamford Hospital, Department of Radiology.

120. Which of the following grids would provide the best cleanup of scattered radiation using the following factors: 100 mA, 300 ms, 120 kVp?
- ❏ A. 8:1; 60 lines/inch
- ❏ B. 12:1; 103 lines/inch
- ❏ C. 16:1; 60 lines/inch
- ❏ D. 16:1; 103 lines/inch

121. All of the following statements are true, *except*
1. the relationship between SID and receptor exposure is inverse
2. the relationship between x-ray energy and wavelength is direct
3. maximum x-ray energy in an x-ray spectrum depends on the applied kilovoltage
4. the number of x-ray photons reaching the IR increases as field size increases
5. the purpose of x-ray tube filters is to produce a more polyenergetic beam
- ❏ A. 1 and 3
- ❏ B. 1 and 2
- ❏ C. 2 and 4
- ❏ D. 2 and 5
- ❏ E. 3 and 4
- ❏ F. 4 and 5

122. The purpose of the electroconductive layer of a CR-PSP plate is to
- ❏ A. provide support to the PSP layer
- ❏ B. provide mechanical strength
- ❏ C. facilitate transportation through the scanner/reader
- ❏ D. provide better resolution

123. Of the following groups of analog exposure factors, which is most likely to produce the shortest scale of image contrast?
- ❏ A. 500 mA, 0.040 s, 70 kV
- ❏ B. 100 mA, 0.100 s, 80 kV
- ❏ C. 200 mA, 0.025 s, 92 kV
- ❏ D. 700 mA, 0.014 s, 80 kV

124. What pixel size has a 2048 × 2048 matrix with a 60-cm FOV?
- ❏ A. 0.3 mm
- ❏ B. 0.5 mm
- ❏ C. 0.15 mm
- ❏ D. 0.03 mm

125. As window width increases
- ❏ A. contrast scale increases
- ❏ B. contrast scale decreases
- ❏ C. brightness increases
- ❏ D. brightness decreases

126. Which of the following matrix sizes is *most likely* to produce the best image resolution?
- ❏ A. 128 × 128
- ❏ B. 512 × 512
- ❏ C. 1024 × 1024
- ❏ D. 2048 × 2048

127. Ionizing radiation intensity decreases as
- ❏ A. distance from the source of radiation decreases
- ❏ B. distance from the source of radiation increases
- ❏ C. frequency increases
- ❏ D. wavelength decreases

128. Spatial resolution is inversely related to
1. SID
2. OID
3. part motion
   - ❏ A. 1 only
   - ❏ B. 1 and 2 only
   - ❏ C. 2 and 3 only
   - ❏ D. 1, 2, and 3

129. *Select the two correct completions.* When the FOV is reduced in size, while the matrix size remains the same,
1. spatial resolution is increased
2. pixel size is smaller
3. sampling frequency decreases
4. spatial resolution is decreased
5. pixel size is larger
6. sampling frequency increases
   - ❏ A. 1 and 2
   - ❏ B. 2 and 4
   - ❏ C. 5 and 6
   - ❏ D. 3 and 5
   - ❏ E. 4 and 6

130. The exposure factors of 400 mA, 17 ms, and 82 kV produce a milliampere seconds value of
   - ❏ A. 2.35
   - ❏ B. 6.8
   - ❏ C. 23.5
   - ❏ D. 68

131. The artifact(s) seen in Figure 4-18 include(s)
1. motion
2. jewelry artifacts
3. hair braid artifacts
4. denture artifact
   - ❏ A. 1 only
   - ❏ B. 1 and 2 only
   - ❏ C. 2 and 3 only
   - ❏ D. 1, 2, and 3

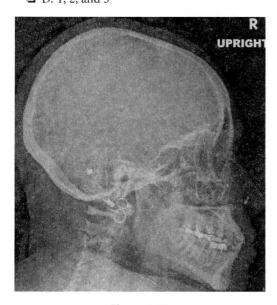

Figure 4-18

132. The radiographic accessory used to measure the thickness of body parts to determine optimal selection of exposure factors is the
   - ❏ A. fulcrum
   - ❏ B. caliper
   - ❏ C. densitometer
   - ❏ D. ruler

133. The x-ray image seen on the computer display monitor is a/an
   - ❏ A. analog image
   - ❏ B. digital image
   - ❏ C. phosphor image
   - ❏ D. emulsion image

134. Modifications to the degree of digital image brightness can be made by adjustments to
1. total IR exposure
2. monitor controls
3. window level postprocessing
   - ❏ A. 1 only
   - ❏ B. 1 and 2 only
   - ❏ C. 2 and 3 only
   - ❏ D. 1, 2, and 3

135. For which of the following examinations can the anode heel effect be an important consideration?
1. Lateral thoracic spine
2. AP femur
3. Right anterior oblique (RAO) sternum
   - ❏ A. 1 only
   - ❏ B. 1 and 2 only
   - ❏ C. 1 and 3 only
   - ❏ D. 1, 2, and 3

136. All of the following have an impact on receptor exposure, *except*
   - ❏ A. photon energy
   - ❏ B. grid ratio
   - ❏ C. OID
   - ❏ D. focal spot size

137. A radiograph made with a parallel grid demonstrates decreased receptor exposure on its lateral edges. This is *most likely* due to
   - ❏ A. static electrical discharge
   - ❏ B. the grid being off-centered
   - ❏ C. improper tube angle
   - ❏ D. decreased SID

138. What is the correct critique of the CR image shown in Figure 4-19?
- ❏ A. Double exposure
- ❏ B. Grid centering error
- ❏ C. Incorrect AEC photocell
- ❏ D. Inverted focused grid

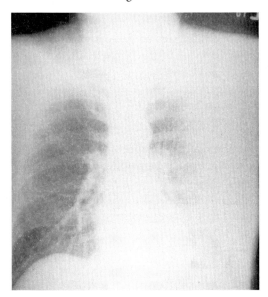

Figure 4-19. From the American College of Radiology Learning File. Used with permission of the ACR.

139. A particular milliampere seconds value, regardless of the combination of milliamperes and time, will reproduce the same receptor exposure. This is a statement of the
- ❏ A. line-focus principle
- ❏ B. inverse-square law
- ❏ C. reciprocity law
- ❏ D. law of conservation of energy

140. Differences between CR and DR include
1. DR images are displayed immediately
2. DR has higher DQE and lower patient dose
3. DR uses IPs
- ❏ A. 1 only
- ❏ B. 1 and 2 only
- ❏ C. 2 and 3 only
- ❏ D. 1, 2, and 3

141. If 300 mA has been selected for a particular exposure, what exposure time would be required to produce 6 mAs?
- ❏ A. 5 ms
- ❏ B. 10 ms
- ❏ C. 15 ms
- ❏ D. 20 ms

142. As digital detector element (DEL) size decreases
- ❏ A. brightness increases
- ❏ B. brightness decreases
- ❏ C. spatial resolution increases
- ❏ D. spatial resolution decreases

143. An increase in kilovoltage will serve to
- ❏ A. increase image brightness
- ❏ B. decrease image brightness
- ❏ C. increase photon energy
- ❏ D. decrease tissue penetration

144. The functions of automatic beam limitation devices include
1. reducing the production of scattered radiation
2. increasing the absorption of scattered radiation
3. changing the quality of the x-ray beam
- ❏ A. 1 only
- ❏ B. 2 only
- ❏ C. 1 and 2 only
- ❏ D. 1, 2, and 3

145. Factors that impact image sharpness/spatial resolution in digital imaging include
1. part motion
2. geometric factors
3. size of focal spot
- ❏ A. 1 only
- ❏ B. 1 and 2 only
- ❏ C. 2 and 3 only
- ❏ D. 1, 2, and 3

146. Which of the following combinations is most likely to be associated with quantum mottle noise?
- ❏ A. Decreased milliampere seconds, decreased SID
- ❏ B. Increased milliampere seconds, decreased kilovoltage
- ❏ C. Decreased milliampere seconds, increased kilovoltage
- ❏ D. Increased milliampere seconds, increased SID

147. The artifact seen in Figure 4-20 represents
- ❏ A. CR processing artifact
- ❏ B. static electrical discharge
- ❏ C. cleaning solution artifact
- ❏ D. secondary exposure artifact

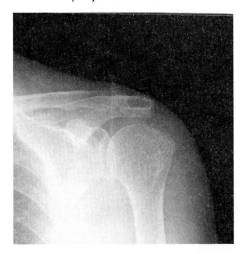

Figure 4-20. Reproduced with permission from Saia DA. *Radiography PREP Program Review and Exam Preparation.* 7th ed. New York, NY: McGraw Hill; 2012.

148. An exposure was made using 8 mAs and 60 kV. If the kilovoltage was changed to 70, what new milliampere seconds value is required to maintain receptor exposure?

❏ A. 2
❏ B. 4
❏ C. 16
❏ D. 32

149. Figure 4-21 is representative of

❏ A. the anode heel effect
❏ B. the line-focus principle
❏ C. the inverse-square law
❏ D. the reciprocity law

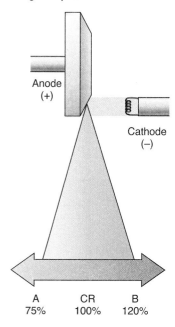

Figure 4-21

150. Of the following groups of technical factors, which will produce the greatest receptor exposure?

❏ A. 10 mAs, 74 kV, 44-inch SID
❏ B. 10 mAs, 74 kV, 36-inch SID
❏ C. 5 mAs, 85 kV, 48-inch SID
❏ D. 5 mAs, 85 kV, 40-inch SID

151. The maximum spatial resolution in digital imaging is equal to the

❏ A. DQE of the imaging system which should be at least 2 × the frequency of the ADC electrical signal
❏ B. wavelength of the detector systems ADCs electrical signal
❏ C. Nyquist frequency, which is 1/2 × the pixel pitch (mm)
❏ D. distance between the silver bromide grains in the IR

152. Which of the following is the *most* appropriate critique for the image seen in Figure 4-22?

❏ A. Double exposure
❏ B. Inverted IP
❏ C. Incomplete erasure
❏ D. Image fading

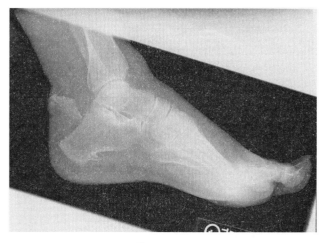

Figure 4-22

153. The *processing algorithm* represents the

❏ A. pixel value distribution
❏ B. anatomical part and projection
❏ C. image grayscale
❏ D. system speed

154. The relationship between the height of a grid's lead strips and the distance between them is called grid

❏ A. ratio
❏ B. radius
❏ C. frequency
❏ D. focusing distance

155. Advantage(s) of high-kilovoltage chest radiography include

1. it eliminates the need for a grid
2. it reduces patient dose
3. exposure time can be shorter
4. magnification distortion is reduced

❏ A. 1 only
❏ B. 2 and 3 only
❏ C. 1, 2 and 4 only
❏ D. 2, 3, and 4 only

156. Characteristics of high-ratio focused grids, compared with lower ratio grids, include which of the following?

1. They allow more positioning latitude
2. They are more efficient in collecting SR
3. They absorb more of the useful beam

❏ A. 1 only
❏ B. 1 and 2 only
❏ C. 2 and 3 only
❏ D. 1, 2, and 3

157. Factors that can affect histogram appearance include
1. beam restriction
2. centering errors
3. incorrect SID
   - ❑ A. 1 only
   - ❑ B. 1 and 2 only
   - ❑ C. 2 and 3 only
   - ❑ D. 1, 2, and 3

158. Which of the following statements provides the most accurate critique of the image seen in Figure 4-23?
   - ❑ A. Excessive scattered radiation fog
   - ❑ B. Part motion
   - ❑ C. Positioning aide artifact
   - ❑ D. Grid cutoff

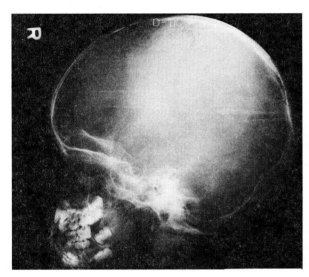

Figure 4-23. From the American College of Radiology Learning File. Used with permission of the ACR.

159. Changes in milliampere seconds can affect all of the following, *except*
   - ❑ A. quantity of x-ray photons produced
   - ❑ B. exposure rate
   - ❑ C. receptor exposure
   - ❑ D. spatial resolution

160. Lower kilovoltage exposure factors are often indicated for radiographic examinations using
1. water-soluble, iodinated media
2. a negative contrast agent
3. barium sulfate
   - ❑ A. 1 only
   - ❑ B. 1 and 2 only
   - ❑ C. 3 only
   - ❑ D. 1 and 3 only

161. Shape distortion is influenced by the relationship between the
1. x-ray tube and the part to be imaged
2. part to be imaged and the IR
3. IR and the x-ray tube
   - ❑ A. 1 only
   - ❑ B. 1 and 2 only
   - ❑ C. 1 and 3 only
   - ❑ D. 1, 2, and 3

162. The line-focus principle expresses the relationship between
   - ❑ A. the actual and the effective focal spot
   - ❑ B. exposure given to the IR and the resulting receptor exposure
   - ❑ C. SID used and the resulting receptor exposure
   - ❑ D. grid ratio and lines per inch

163. Each of the following can have an effect on image sharpness/spatial resolution, *except*
   - ❑ A. beam restriction
   - ❑ B. motion
   - ❑ C. OID
   - ❑ D. focal spot size

164. Subject/object unsharpness can result from all of the following, *except* when
   - ❑ A. object shape does not coincide with the shape of x-ray beam
   - ❑ B. object plane is not parallel with x-ray tube and/or IR
   - ❑ C. anatomic object(s) of interest is/are in the path of the CR
   - ❑ D. anatomic object(s) of interest is/are at a distance from the IR

165. Brightness and contrast resolution in digital imaging can be influenced by
1. window level (WL)
2. window width (WW)
3. lookup table (LUT)
   - ❑ A. 1 only
   - ❑ B. 1 and 2 only
   - ❑ C. 2 and 3 only
   - ❑ D. 1, 2, and 3

166. If a particular grid has lead strips 0.40-mm thick, 4.0-mm high, and 0.25-mm apart, what is its grid ratio?
   - ❑ A. 8:1
   - ❑ B. 10:1
   - ❑ C. 12:1
   - ❑ D. 16:1

167. A decrease from 200 to 100 mA will result in a decrease in which of the following?

1. Wavelength
2. Exposure rate
3. Beam intensity
   - ❏ A. 1 only
   - ❏ B. 1 and 2 only
   - ❏ C. 2 and 3 only
   - ❏ D. 1, 2, and 3

168. The radiograph shown in Figure 4-24 illustrates incorrect use of

- ❏ A. collimator
- ❏ B. grid
- ❏ C. photocell
- ❏ D. focal spot

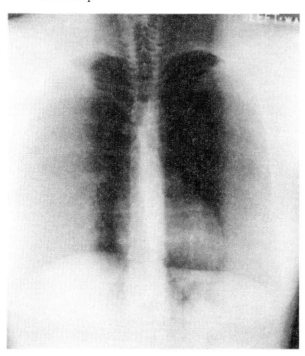

Figure 4-24

169. Factors that determine spatial resolution in direct digital imaging include

1. focal spot size
2. SID
3. DEL size
   - ❏ A. 1 only
   - ❏ B. 1 and 2 only
   - ❏ C. 2 and 3 only
   - ❏ D. 1, 2, and 3

170. A satisfactory radiograph of the abdomen was made at a 38-inch SID using 400 mA, 60-ms exposure, and 80 kV. If the distance is changed to 42 inches, what new exposure time would be required?

- ❏ A. 25 ms
- ❏ B. 50 ms
- ❏ C. 73 ms
- ❏ D. 93 ms

171. Which of the following is/are associated with differential attenuation?

1. Part thickness
2. Tissue density
3. Tissue Z number
   - ❏ A. 1 only
   - ❏ B. 1 and 2 only
   - ❏ C. 1 and 3 only
   - ❏ D. 1, 2, and 3

172. The interaction between x-ray photons and matter illustrated in Figure 4-25 is *most likely* to be associated with

1. high-energy photons
2. high tissue absorption
3. high Z number absorber
   - ❏ A. 1 only
   - ❏ B. 1 and 2 only
   - ❏ C. 2 and 3 only
   - ❏ D. 1, 2, and 3

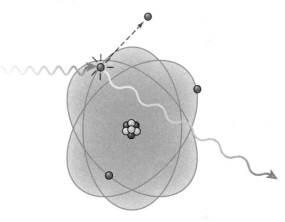

Figure 4-25

173. For which of the following examinations might the use of a grid *not* be necessary in an adult patient?

- ❏ A. Hip
- ❏ B. Knee
- ❏ C. Abdomen
- ❏ D. Lumbar spine

174. X-ray photon attenuation is not influenced by

1. pathology
2. structure atomic number
3. photon intensity
   - ❏ A. 1 only
   - ❏ B. 3 only
   - ❏ C. 2 and 3 only
   - ❏ D. 1, 2, and 3

175. Why is a very short exposure time essential in chest radiography?

- ❏ A. To avoid excessive focal spot blur
- ❏ B. To maintain short-scale contrast
- ❏ C. To minimize involuntary motion
- ❏ D. To minimize patient discomfort

176. Which of the following is the *most* appropriate critique for the image seen in Figure 4-26?

❏ A. Insufficient penetration
❏ B. Low ratio/no grid used
❏ C. Poor detail
❏ D. Excessive brightness

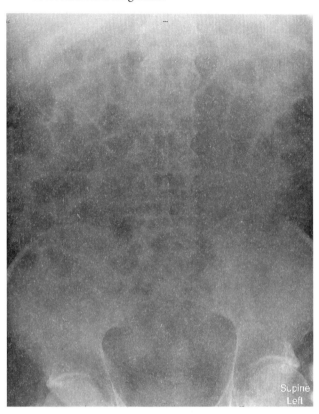

Figure 4-26

177. Image receptor spatial resolution in direct digital systems is

1. fixed
2. inversely related to the TFT and DEL size
3. always variable

❏ A. 1 only
❏ B. 1 and 2 only
❏ C. 2 and 3 only
❏ D. 1, 2, and 3

178. The term *windowing* describes the practice of

❏ A. varying the automatic brightness control
❏ B. changing the image brightness and/or contrast scale
❏ C. varying the FOV
❏ D. increasing resolution

179. The electronic term used to describe anything that interferes with visualization of the x-ray image is

❏ A. noise
❏ B. postprocessing
❏ C. modulation transfer function
❏ D. scintillation

180. How is SID related to exposure rate and image receptor exposure?

❏ A. As SID increases, exposure rate increases and receptor exposure increases
❏ B. As SID increases, exposure rate increases and receptor exposure decreases
❏ C. As SID increases, exposure rate decreases and receptor exposure increases
❏ D. As SID increases, exposure rate decreases and receptor exposure decreases

181. Which of the following is the *most* appropriate critique for the image seen in Figure 4-27?

❏ A. Underexposure
❏ B. Part motion
❏ C. Exposure artifact
❏ D. Grid cutoff

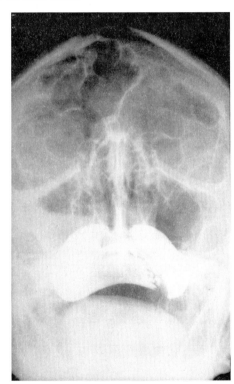

Figure 4-27

182. In digital imaging, thin film transistor (TFT) and detector element (DEL) size is related to

❏ A. contrast
❏ B. brightness
❏ C. spatial resolution
❏ D. plate size

183. Which of the following pathologic conditions would require an increase in exposure factors?

❏ A. Pneumoperitoneum
❏ B. Obstructed bowel
❏ C. Renal colic
❏ D. Ascites

184. The effect described as *differential absorption* is
1. a result of subject contrast
2. a result of attenuating characteristics of tissue
3. minimized by the use of a high kilovoltage
   - ❏ A. 1 only
   - ❏ B. 1 and 2 only
   - ❏ C. 1 and 3 only
   - ❏ D. 1, 2, and 3

185. A decrease in SNR can be the result of
1. excessive mA
2. incorrect part selection
3. grid cutoff
   - ❏ A. 1 only
   - ❏ B. 1 and 2 only
   - ❏ C. 2 and 3 only
   - ❏ D. 1, 2, and 3

186. The ratio of the pixel's sensing area to the area of the pixel itself refers to
- ❏ A. fill factor
- ❏ B. MTF
- ❏ C. Nyquist frequency
- ❏ D. SNR

187. One line pair is described as
- ❏ A. two black lines on a light background
- ❏ B. one black line on a light background and an interspace of the same width
- ❏ C. two black lines on a light background followed by two similar interspaces
- ❏ D. black lines that are 5, 8, 12, or 16 times taller than their adjacent interspaces

188. How is digital receptor exposure related to the square of the selected SID?
- ❏ A. Directly proportional
- ❏ B. Inversely proportional
- ❏ C. Directly, but not proportional
- ❏ D. Inversely, but not proportional

189. Foreshortening of an anatomic structure means that
- ❏ A. it is projected on the IR smaller than its actual size
- ❏ B. its image is more lengthened than its actual size
- ❏ C. it is accompanied by geometric blur
- ❏ D. it is significantly magnified

190. Digital radiographic imaging equipment provides a number of functions for optimization of image quality, including
1. exposure data recognition
2. automatic rescaling
3. narrow latitude
   - ❏ A. 1 only
   - ❏ B. 1 and 2 only
   - ❏ C. 2 and 3 only
   - ❏ D. 1, 2, and 3

191. The percentage of remnant/signal photons that are detected and absorbed by the receptor describes
- ❏ A. DEL
- ❏ B. FOV
- ❏ C. DQE
- ❏ D. TFT

192. The main difference between the *direct*-capture and *indirect*-capture DR is that
- ❏ A. direct capture/conversion has no scintillator
- ❏ B. direct capture/conversion uses a photostimulable phosphor
- ❏ C. in direct capture/conversion, light is detected by CCDs
- ❏ D. in direct capture/conversion, light is detected by TFTs

193. Which of the following may be used to reduce the effect of scattered radiation on the radiographic image?
1. Grids
2. Focal spot selection
3. Protective filtration
4. Collimators
5. Compression bands
   - ❏ A. 1 and 2 only
   - ❏ B. 2, 3, and 5 only
   - ❏ C. 1, 4, and 5 only
   - ❏ D. 3, 4, and 5 only

194. Figure 4-28 is representative of
- ❏ A. the anode heel effect
- ❏ B. the line-focus principle
- ❏ C. the inverse-square law
- ❏ D. the reciprocity law

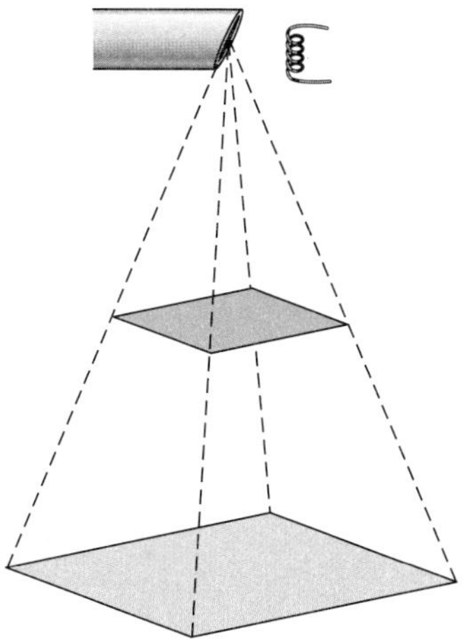

Figure 4-28

195. A compensating filter is used to
- ❏ A. absorb the harmful photons that contribute only to patient dose
- ❏ B. even out widely differing tissue densities
- ❏ C. eliminate much of the scattered radiation
- ❏ D. improve fluoroscopy

196. Digital image brightness is controlled by

1. IR exposure
2. monitor functions
3. postprocessing functions
   - ❏ A. 1 only
   - ❏ B. 1 and 2 only
   - ❏ C. 2 and 3 only
   - ❏ D. 1, 2, and 3

197. The changes seen among the images shown in Figure 4-29 represent changes made to

- ❏ A. pixel size
- ❏ B. matrix size
- ❏ C. window width
- ❏ D. window level

198. Which of the following statements about *histograms* is/are true?

1. A histogram illustrates pixel value distribution
2. There is a default histogram for each/different body parts
3. A histogram is representative of the image grayscale
   - ❏ A. 1 only
   - ❏ B. 1 and 2 only
   - ❏ C. 2 and 3 only
   - ❏ D. 1, 2, and 3

199. A change in the actual focal spot size will affect a change in

1. x-ray beam intensity
2. resolution/image sharpness
3. effective foal spot size
   - ❏ A. 1 only
   - ❏ B. 1 and 2 only
   - ❏ C. 2 and 3 only
   - ❏ D. 1, 2, and 3

200. What computer function corrects for exposure errors?

- ❏ A. Inversion
- ❏ B. Low-pass filtering
- ❏ C. Histogram analysis
- ❏ D. Rescaling

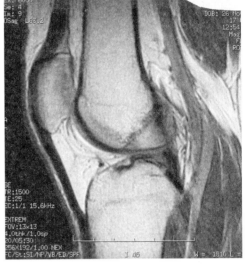

A

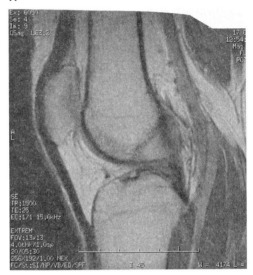

B

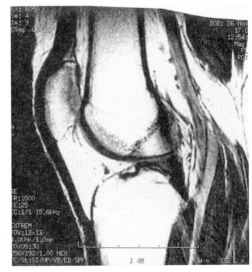

C

Figure 4-29. Used with permission of Stamford Hospital, Department of Radiology.

ANSWERS AND EXPLANATIONS

1. (A) Direct digital systems have a fixed spatial resolution that is determined by the size of the thin film transistor (TFT) and the detector element (DEL). The smaller the DEL, the greater the spatial resolution. Sampling frequency, laser scanner, and PSPs are all related to indirect digital systems.

2. (B) The digital image that we view is principally a result of computer functions rather than selection of technical factors. Technical factor selection does impact the *remnant x-ray photon signal*. The selection of kilovoltage determines the photon energy and therefore the *subject contrast* of the exit signal.

Rescaling, windowing, and especially LUT determine the image contrast of the digital image that we view.

3. (B) *Osteoporosis* is a condition, often seen in the elderly, marked by increased porosity and softening of bone. The bones are much less dense, and thus a decrease in exposure is required. *Osteomyelitis* and *osteochondritis* are inflammatory conditions that usually have no effect on bone density. *Osteosclerosis* is abnormal hardening of the bone, and an increase in exposure factors would be required.

4. (C) An *algorithm* is a series of computerized step-by-step instructions used to solve a problem. The instructions are flexible, that is, variable, and various options are checked to produce the best possible results from the range of available options. Radiographically speaking, the algorithm will test a range of variations to produce the best possible group of exposure factors for the anatomic particular part and circumstances.

5. (B) The image (Fig. 4-1) illustrates *aliasing artifact*, or Moiré effect. Aliasing, or Moiré, has the appearance of somewhat wavy linear lines and can occur in computed radiography when using *stationary grids*. If the grid's lead strip pattern (i.e., frequency) matches the scanning (sampling) pattern of the scanner/reader, the resulting interference can cause aliasing (also called Moiré) artifact. When sampling frequencies are decreased, aliasing/Moiré is less evident. As sampling frequencies increase, aliasing/Moiré is more obvious.

6. (A) The spatial resolution of direct digital systems is fixed and is related to the DEL size and its three component parts: the TFT, its fill factor, and the capacitor. Smaller DEL sizes provide better resolution. The fill factor/sensing area is the largest portion of the DEL and is generally made of amorphous selenium in direct digital systems. The greater the fill factor/sensing area, the higher the contrast resolution, spatial resolution, and SNR. A fill factor of 75%–80% is considered good. The capacitor stores electrical charges, and the TFT acts as the switch/gate to release charges for readout.

A CCD (charge coupled device) is typically coupled with an image intensifier; an ADC is an analog-to-digital converter.

7. (A) Geometric sharpness is affected by all three factors listed. As OID increases, magnification increases and therefore, geometric sharpness decreases. OID is *inversely* related to geometric sharpness. As SOD and SID increase, magnification decreases and geometric sharpness increases. SOD and SID are *directly* related to geometric sharpness.

8. (A) The spatial resolution of direct digital systems is fixed and is related to the DEL size and its three component parts: the TFT, its fill factor, and the capacitor. Smaller DEL sizes provide better resolution. The *fill factor/sensing area* is the largest portion of the DEL and is generally made of amorphous selenium in direct digital systems. The greater the fill factor, the better the spatial resolution. The *capacitor* stores electrical charges, and the *TFT* acts as the switch/gate to release charges for readout.

A *CCD* (charge coupled device) is typically coupled with an image intensifier; an ADC is an analog-to-digital converter.

9. (D) The radiograph shown in Figure 4-2 is that of an adult PA erect chest. The image is well positioned and exposed, but observe the *braids of hair* that extend past the neck and superimpose on the pulmonary apices. Braided hair should be pinned up or otherwise removed from superimposition on thoracic structures. The braided hair was imaged during the exposure of the PA chest and is, therefore, called an *exposure artifact*. Example of a scanner/reader artifact is laser jitter, which results in an image distortion. It is important to inquire about or examine patients for materials that will image radiographically and cast unwanted densities over essential anatomy.

10. (B) An increase in kilovoltage (photon energy) will result in a *greater number* (i.e., exposure rate) of scattered photons (Compton interaction) reaching the image receptor. These scattered photons carry no useful information and contribute to *image noise and decreased visibility of image details*. In *analog* (screen–film) imaging, this would result in decreased/lower radiographic contrast.

11. **(D)** A certain amount of object unsharpness is an inherent part of every radiographic image because of the position and shape of anatomic structures within the body. Anatomic structures are frequently not parallel to, and at some distance from, the IR. Consequently, some structures are imaged with more inherent distortion than others, and shapes of anatomic structures can be significantly misrepresented. As OID increases, structures *farther* from the IR will be distorted (magnified), resulting in decreased resolution/sharpness. *SID* is directly related to resolution/detail/sharpness and inversely related to magnification. As SID increases, magnification decreases and image sharpness increases.

    Photons emerging from various points on a measurable *focal spot* are responsible for producing anatomic details having *blurred, unsharp edges*. The extent or size of the unsharp area is *directly* related to focal spot size and OID and *inversely* related to the SID, that is, unsharpness increases as focal spot size and OID increase and as the SID decreases.

12. **(C)** Quantum *noise*, or *mottle*, is a grainy appearance; it has a spotted or freckled appearance. It looks very similar to a low-resolution photograph/image that has been enlarged. Low mAs and high kV factors are most likely to be the cause of quantum noise/mottle seen in Figure 4-3..

    Grid cutoff is absorption of the useful beam by the grid and usually results in loss of signal and visibility of grid lines. The anode heel effect is most pronounced using short SIDs, large IRs, small anode angles, and imaging parts having uneven tissue densities; it is represented by a noticeable IR exposure difference between the anode and cathode ends of the image.

13. **(B)** When an AEC is installed in an x-ray circuit, it is calibrated to produce brightness and contrast as required by the radiologist. Once the part being radiographed has been exposed to produce the correct receptor exposure, the AEC automatically terminates the exposure. The manual timer should be used as a backup timer; in case the AEC fails to terminate the exposure, the backup timer would protect the patient from overexposure and the x-ray tube from excessive heat load. The master receptor exposure override generally is set on normal to produce the required receptor exposure. In special cases, when this produces excessive or insufficient receptor exposure, the master receptor exposure override may be adjusted to plus or minus position.

14. **(C)** Milliampere seconds is the technical factor that regulates receptor exposure. Using the equation milliamperage × time = mAs, determine each mAs: (A) = 5 mAs, (B) = 8 mAs, (C) = 28 mAs, (D) = 18 mAs. Group C will produce the greatest exposure to the image receptor.

15. **(A)** Kilovoltage is the qualitative regulating factor; it has a *direct* effect on photon energy, that is, as kilovoltage is *increased*, photon energy *increases*. Photon energy is *inversely* related to wavelength, that is, as photon energy *increases*, wavelength *decreases*. Photon energy is unrelated to milliamperage.

16. **(D)** All the factor changes affect spatial resolution/sharpness, but focal spot size does not affect magnification. An increase in SID would *decrease* magnification. Although a decrease in SID will increase magnification, it does not have as significant an effect as an increase in OID. In general, it requires an increase of 7-inch SID to compensate for every inch of OID.

17. **(A)** Grids are composed of alternate strips of lead and interspace material and are used to trap scattered radiation after it emerges from the patient and before it reaches the IR. Accurate centering of the x-ray tube is required. If the x-ray tube is off-center but within the recommended focusing distance, there usually will be an overall loss of receptor exposure. Over- or underexposure under the anode is usually the result of exceeding the focusing distance limits in addition to being off-center.

18. **(B)** Image smoothing, or low-pass filtering, is a postprocessing spatial frequency filtering. Removal of high-frequency noise can be accomplished by averaging the frequency of each pixel with that of the surrounding pixels. This process is especially helpful when visualizing small/fine anatomic details. Windowing is also a postprocessing function used to adjust the brightness and contrast of the digital image. The edge (contrast) enhancement process averages fewer adjacent pixels, resulting in enhancement of the interface between adjacent structures.

19. **(B)** AEC backup time should be set to 150% of the expected exposure. *Backup time* protects the patient from overexposure and protects the x-ray tube from unnecessary heat production and wear and tear. *Minimum response time* is the shortest exposure time that particular AEC is capable of. If the selected mA is 500, and the minimum response time is 25 ms (0.025 s), then the exposure will be *at least* 12.5 mAs (500 mA × 0.025 s = 12.5). The *maximum* possible exposure would be 45 mAs (500 mA × 0.09 s/90 ms).

20. **(D)** The lateral projection of the coccyx seen in Figure 4-4 is markedly overexposed. Although a small focal spot would not be a practical selection for a lateral coccyx, focal spot size is unrelated to receptor exposure or contrast. If *insufficient* backup time had been selected, the image might be *under*exposed. The center photocell is the *appropriate* photocell to select because the part of interest, the coccyx, should be in the center of the image. Because the *coccyx was not centered* to the IR (but rather the thicker *hip* portion of the body was centered), the AEC correctly exposed the thicker portion—thus overexposing the less dense coccyx area. Accurate

positioning, centering, and photocell selection is essential when using AEC.

21. **(B)** *Resolution* describes how closely fine details may be associated and still be recognized as separate details before seeming to blend into each other and appear "as one." The degree of resolution transferred to the IR is a function of the resolving power of each of the system components and can be expressed in *line pairs per millimeter* (lp/mm), *line-spread function* (LSP), or *modulation transfer function* (MTF). Line pairs per millimeter can be measured using a resolution test pattern; a number of resolution test tools are available. LSP is measured using a 10-mm x-ray beam; MTF measures the amount of information lost between the object and the IR. The effective focal spot is the foreshortened size of the actual focal spot as it is projected down toward the IR, that is, as it would be seen looking up into the emerging x-ray beam. This is called the *line-focus principle* and is not a unit used to express resolution.

22. **(A)** That portion of the x-ray beam striking the IR and representing image anatomy is called the *signal*. Some of the initial x-ray beam is absorbed via photoelectric interaction; some is scattered via Compton scatter (creating *noise*). If the SID is above or below the recommended focusing distance, the useful beam will not coincide with the angled lead strips at the lateral edges. Consequently, there will be absorption of the useful beam, termed *grid cutoff*, and diminished signal to the IR. If the grid failed to move during the exposure, there would be grid lines throughout. Central ray angulation in the direction of the lead strips is appropriate and will not cause grid cutoff. If the central ray were off-center, there would be uniform loss of signal.

23. **(A)** Aligning the x-ray tube, anatomic part, and IR so that they are parallel reduces *shape distortion*. Angulation of the long axis of the part with respect to the IR results in *foreshortening* of the object. Tube angulation causes *elongation* of the part. Size distortion (magnification) is inversely proportional to SID and directly proportional to OID. Decreasing the SID and increasing the OID serve to increase size distortion.

24. **(D)** *The shortest possible exposure time should be used to minimize motion unsharpness*. Motion causes unsharpness that destroys detail. Careful and accurate patient *instruction* is essential for minimizing voluntary motion. *Suspended respiration* eliminates respiratory motion. Using the shortest possible *exposure time* is essential for decreasing involuntary motion. Immobilization is also very useful in eliminating motion unsharpness.

25. **(A)** When the variable-kilovoltage method is used, a particular milliampere seconds value is assigned to each body part. As part thickness increases, the kilovoltage (i.e., penetration) is also increased. The body part being radiographed must be measured carefully, and *for each*

centimeter of increase in thickness, 2 kV is added to the exposure.

26. **(B)** Using anatomically programmed radiography (APR), the radiographer uses console graphics or a touch screen to *select the anatomic part and its relative size* (S, M, L) to be imaged. The unit's microprocessor chooses the appropriate preprogrammed milliampere seconds and kilovoltage algorithm for that particular part and size—from the "internal technique chart" predetermined and stored upon installation.

APR is used in conjunction with AEC and is therefore still highly dependent on the skillfulness of its user. Accurate positioning, photocell selection, and control of scattered radiation is essential to the production of quality images using APR and AEC.

27. **(B)** The artifact shown in Figure 4-5 has *sharply delineated edges*, indicating that it is located adjacent to the PSP within the IP. The *farther* the object is from the IR, the more *blurred* its edges will be as a result of magnification distortion.

28. **(D)** The radiographic subject, the patient, is composed of many different tissue types of varying densities, resulting in varying degrees of photon attenuation. This *differential attenuation* impacts the exit radiation signal reaching the image receptor. Normal tissue density can be significantly altered in the presence of pathology. For example, destructive bone disease can cause a dramatic decrease in tissue density. Abnormal accumulation of fluid (as in ascites) will cause a significant increase in tissue density. Muscle atrophy, or highly developed muscles, will similarly decrease or increase tissue density. The most important way to limit the production of scattered radiation is by limiting the size of the irradiated field through *beam restriction*. As the size of the field is reduced, less tissue volume is irradiated; and less scattered radiation will be produced.

29. **(A)** As kilovoltage is increased, more high-energy photons are produced, and the overall energy of the primary beam is increased. Photon energy is *inversely* related to wavelength, that is, as photon energy increases, wavelength decreases. An increase in milliamperage serves to increase the *number* of photons produced at the target but is *unrelated* to their energy.

30. **(D)** The PA projection of the chest shown in Figure 4-6 demonstrates faint visualization of the thoracic vertebrae through the heart—characteristic of adequate penetration. Many shades of gray are seen, illustrating a long scale of contrast. The image is representative of having been exposed at the ideal milliampere seconds and kilovoltage factors. Ten pairs of posterior ribs are seen through the lung fields above the diaphragm; this illustrates adequate inspiration.

31. **(D)** A parallel-plate ionization chamber is a type of AEC. A radiolucent chamber is beneath the patient (between the patient and the IR). As photons emerge from the patient, they enter the chamber and ionize the air within it. Once a predetermined charge has been reached, the exposure is terminated automatically.

32. **(C)** *Grid ratio* is defined as the height of the lead strips to the width of the interspace material (Fig. 4-30). The higher the lead strips (or the smaller the distance between the strips), the higher the grid ratio, and the greater the percentage of scattered radiation absorbed. However, a grid does absorb some primary/useful radiation as well. The higher the lead strips, the *more* critical is the need for accurate centering because the lead strips will more readily trap photons whose direction does not parallel them.

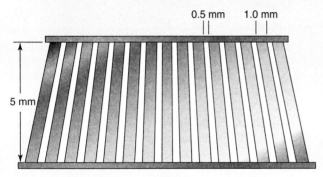

0.5 mm   1.0 mm

5 mm

Figure 4-30

33. **(C)** As kilovoltage is increased, *more* electrons are driven to the anode with greater speed and energy. More high-energy electrons will result in production of *more high-energy*, more penetrating *x-rays.* Thus, kilovoltage affects both quantity and quality (energy) of the x-ray beam. However, although kilovoltage and receptor exposure are directly *related*, they are not directly proportional—that is, twice the receptor exposure does not result from doubling the kilovoltage. With respect to the effect of kilovoltage on receptor exposure, if it is desired to double the exposure to the IR yet impossible to adjust the milliampere seconds, a similar effect can be achieved by *increasing the kilovoltage by 15%.* Conversely, the receptor exposure may be cut in half by decreasing the kilovoltage by 15%. Therefore, a decrease in kilovoltage will produce fewer x-ray photons, resulting in decreased exposure to the IR. Kilovoltage is unrelated to spatial resolution.

34. **(D)** The image shown in Figure 4-7 is a lateral soft tissue neck radiograph. The air-filled airway is well demonstrated. There is no loss of detail from motion unsharpness. The image lacks sufficient receptor exposure to demonstrate the bony anatomy of the cervical vertebra.

35. **(C)** It is our ethical responsibility to minimize radiation dose to our patients. X-rays produced at the target comprise a heterogeneous primary beam. There are many "soft" (low-energy) photons that only penetrate a small thickness of tissue and are absorbed. If not removed, they

contribute to greater patient dose. They have insufficient energy to penetrate the part and contribute to image formation. Filters, usually made of aluminum, are used in *radiography to reduce patient dose by removing these low-energy photons*, resulting in an x-ray beam of higher overall average energy. Total filtration is composed of inherent filtration plus added filtration.

36. **(B)** First, evaluate the change(s): The kilovoltage was increased by 15% (78 + 15% = 90). A 15% increase in kilovoltage will double the image receptor exposure; therefore, it is necessary to use *half* the original milliampere seconds value to maintain the original IR exposure. The original milliampere seconds value was 28 mAs (300 mA × 0.07 s [70 ms] 28 mAs), so we now need 14 mAs, using 500 mA. Because mA × s = mAs:

$$500x = 14$$
$$x = 0.028 \text{ s (28 ms)}$$

37. **(B)** A review of the problem reveals that three changes are being made: an increase in SID, a decrease in kilovoltage, and a change in exposure time (to be considered last). The original milliampere seconds value was 9. The decrease in kilovoltage requires us to double the milliampere seconds to 18 in order to maintain sufficient exposure. Now, we must deal with the distance change. Using the exposure-maintenance formula (and remembering that 18 is now the old milliampere seconds value), we find that the required new milliampere seconds value at 42 inches is 22.

$$\frac{(\text{Old mAs})18}{(\text{New mAs})x} = \frac{(\text{Old }D^2)36^2}{(\text{New }D^2)40^2}$$
$$1296x = 28,800$$

Thus, $x = 22.22$ mAs at 40-inch SID. Because milliamperage is unchanged, we must determine the exposure time that, when used with 300 mA, will yield 22 mAs.

$$300x = 22$$
$$x = 0.07 \text{ s exposure}$$

38. **(B)** The spatial resolution of direct digital systems is fixed and is related to the DEL size and its three component parts: the TFT, its fill factor, and the capacitor. Smaller DEL sizes provide better resolution. The *fill factor/sensing area* is the largest portion of the DEL and is generally made of amorphous selenium in direct digital systems. The greater the fill factor, the better the spatial resolution. The *capacitor* stores electrical charges, and the *TFT* acts as the switch/gate to release charges for readout.

A *CCD* (charge coupled device) is typically coupled with an image intensifier; an ADC is an analog-to-digital converter.

39. (C) Receptor exposure is directly proportional to milliampere seconds. If exposure time is *halved* from 40 ms (0.04 or 1/25 s) to 20 ms (0.02 or 1/50 s), IR exposure will be cut in half. Changing to 150 mA also will halve the milliampere seconds, effectively halving the IR exposure. If the kilovoltage is decreased by 15%, from 85 to 72 kV, receptor exposure will be halved according to the *15% rule*. To cut the receptor exposure in half, the milliampere seconds value must be reduced to 6 mAs (rather than 10 mAs).

40. (B) A 15-min oblique image of an IVU is pictured in Figure 4-8. IVU requires the use of iodinated contrast medium. Low kilovoltage was recommended in *analog* imaging to enhance the photoelectric effect and, in turn, better visualize the renal collecting system. Higher kilovoltage produced excessive SR and undermined the effect of the contrast agent. *Digital* imaging and its postprocessing of acquired data permit the use of higher kilovoltage while providing good contrast at reduced patient exposure.

A higher milliamperage with a shorter exposure time is preferred to decrease the possibility of motion.

41. (D) Exposure rate is regulated by milliamperage. Distance significantly affects the exposure rate according to the inverse-square law of radiation. Kilovoltage also has an effect on exposure rate because an increase in kilovoltage will increase the number of high-energy photons produced at the target. The size of the x-ray field determines the volume of tissue irradiated, the amount of scattered radiation generated, but is unrelated to the exposure *rate*.

42. (C) Receptor exposure is greatly affected by changes in the SID, as expressed by the inverse-square law of radiation. As distance from the radiation source increases, exposure rate decreases, and IR exposure decreases. Exposure rate is inversely proportional to the square of the SID. *Kilovoltage* and *scattered radiation* can have an effect on receptor exposure, but they are not controlling factors. Aluminum filtration functions to reduce patient skin dose and has little to no effect on receptor exposure.

43. (B) The *radiographic subject*, the patient, is composed of many different tissue types that have varying tissue densities, resulting in varying degrees of photon attenuation and absorption. The *atomic number* of the tissues under investigation is directly related to their *attenuation coefficient*. This *differential absorption* contributes to the energies of the exit photons. Normal tissue density may be altered significantly in the presence of *pathologic processes*. Subject contrast is unrelated to milliampere seconds.

44. (C) *Grid ratio* is defined as the height of the lead strips compared with (divided by) the width of the interspace

material. The width of the lead strips has no bearing on the grid ratio. The height of the lead strips is 5 mm; the width of the interspace material (same as the distance between the lead strips) is 0.5 mm. Therefore, the grid ratio is 5/0.5, or a 10:1 grid ratio.

45. (B) Magnification is part of every radiographic image. Anatomic parts within the body are at various distances from the IR and, therefore, have various degrees of magnification. The formula used to determine the amount of image magnification is

$$\frac{\text{Image size}}{\text{Object size}} = \frac{\text{SID}}{\text{SOD}}$$

Substituting known values:

$$\frac{x}{5\,\text{inches}} = \frac{44\,\text{inches (SID)}}{38\,\text{inches (SOD)}}$$
$$(\text{SOD} = \text{SID} - \text{OID})$$
$$38x = 220$$

Thus, $x = 5.78$-inch image width.

46. (C) Contrast is defined as the difference between adjacent brightness levels. The function of contrast is to make details visible. The number of brightness levels, or shades of gray, is often termed *grayscale*. The computer software's processing algorithms determine contrast. Many brightness levels/gray shades, with only slight difference between shades, is termed long-scale (or low) contrast. Few brightness levels/gray shades, with significant difference between shades, is termed short-scale (or high) contrast.

47. (D) Digital image storage is located in a *pixel*, which is a *two-dimensional "picture element"*, measured in the "XY" direction. The third dimension, "Z" direction, in the matrix of pixels is the *depth* that is called the *voxel* (volume element). The depth of the block is the number of bits required to describe the gray level that each pixel can take on—known as the bit depth.

Bit depth in CT is approximately 2^{12} with a dynamic range of almost 5000 gray shades, approximately 2^{14} in CR/DR with a dynamic range of more than 16,000 gray shades, and approximately 2^{16} in digital mammography with a dynamic range of more than 65,500 gray shades. The matrix is the number of pixels in the XY direction. As matrix size increases, for a fixed FOV, pixel size is smaller and better spatial resolution results. An electronic/digital image is formed by a matrix of pixels in rows and columns. A matrix having 512 pixels in each row and column is a 512×512 matrix (a typical CT image).

The term *FOV* is used to describe how much of the patient is included in the matrix. Either the matrix or the

FOV can be changed without one affecting the other, but changes in either will change pixel size. As FOV increases, for a fixed matrix size, the size of each pixel increases and spatial resolution decreases. Fewer and larger pixels result in a poor-resolution "pixely" or "mosaicked" image, that is, one in which you can actually see the individual pixel boxes.

48. **(C)** Each of these factors—SID, OID, and patient/part motion—can have an impact on special resolution/detail sharpness. As SID increases, resolution/sharpness increases (because magnification decreases). As OID increases, resolution/sharpness decreases (because magnification increases). As patient/part motion increases, resolution/shortness decreases. SID and resolution/sharpness are directly related. OID and patient/part motion are inversely related.

49. **(A)** A *compensating filter* is used when the part to be radiographed is of uneven thickness or density (in the chest, mediastinum vs. lungs). The filter (made of aluminum or lead acrylic) is constructed in such a way that it will *absorb* much of the x-ray photons that would have exposed the *low* tissue density area while allowing the remaining x-ray photons to *pass unaffected* to the high tissue density area. A *collimator* is used to decrease the production of scattered radiation by limiting the volume of tissue irradiated. The *grid* functions to trap scattered radiation before it reaches the IR, thus reducing scattered radiation fog. *Added filtration* addresses patient protection, decreasing patient dose.

50. **(C)** The tiny areas of increased brightness, termed *dropout artifacts*, seen in the proximal portion of the CR image of the radius shown in Figure 4-10 are representative of *dust/dirt particles* that have accumulated on the PSP. PSPs (as well as any other reflective surface) are susceptible to dust, and can appear as little clear pinholes. PSPs are sensitive to scattered radiation fog and backscatter, but these would give the image the typical overall gray appearance of fog. Phantom image artifacts are a result of incomplete erasure of a previous image on that PSP. Image fading occurs if an exposed PSP has been left several hours without processing and usually affects the entire image.

51. **(B)** Every radiographic image must include (1) the patient's name or identification number, (2) the correct left- or right-side marker, (3) the date of the examination, and (4) the identity of the institution or office. Additional information *may* be included (but is not required): the patient's birth date or age, the name of the attending physician, and the time of day the examination was performed. When multiple follow-up examinations are made on the same day, it becomes crucial that the time the radiographs were taken be included on the image. This allows the physician to track the patient's progress.

52. **(B)** The presence of pathology often modifies tissue composition. Changes/conditions that occur are generally spoken of as *additive* or *degenerative*. Additive pathology is that which increases tissue density, requiring an increase in technical factors (e.g., ascites, pulmonary edema, and skeletal sclerosis). Increased *BMI* (body mass index) increases thickness of body soft tissues. Degenerative pathology involves deterioration of the part (e.g., osteoporosis, osteomalacia, and emphysema) and requires a decrease in technical factors. Correct use of AEC will compensate for changes in tissue thickness, density, and/or pathologic conditions and will be reflected in appropriate EI range.

53. **(C)** Image storage is located in a *pixel*, which is a two-dimensional "picture element." Pixels are measured in the "XY" direction. The third dimension in the matrix of pixels is the depth that, together with the pixel, is called the *voxel*. The voxels are measured in the "Z" direction. The depth of the block is the number of bits required to describe the gray level that each pixel can take on. This is known as the *bit depth*. The *matrix* is the number of pixels in the XY direction. The larger the matrix size, the better the image resolution. The smaller the pixels and *pixel pitch* (i.e., distance between the center of one pixel to the center of adjacent pixel), the better the resolution.

54. **(C)** Because the anode's focal track is beveled (angled, facing the cathode), x-ray photons can freely diverge toward the cathode end of the x-ray tube. However, the "heel" of the focal track prevents x-ray photons from diverging toward the anode end of the tube. This results in varying intensity from anode to cathode, with fewer photons at the anode end and more photons at the cathode end. *The anode heel effect is most noticeable when using large IRs, short SIDs, and steep target angles.*

55. **(A)** *CR* uses traditional x-ray tables and *IPs* to enclose and protect the flexible PSP screen, whereas *DR* requires the use of significantly different equipment. DR does not use IPs or a traditional x-ray table—it is a direct-capture/conversion or indirect-capture/conversion system of x-ray imaging. Besides eliminating IPs and their handling, DR affords the advantage of *immediate display* of the image (compared with CR's slightly delayed image display), and DR *exposures can be lower* because of the detector's *higher DQE* (i.e., ability to perceive and interact with x-ray photons). DR, like CR, also offers the advantage of image preview and postprocessing.

56. **(C)** Digital image storage is located in a *pixel*, which is a two-dimensional "*picture element*," measured in the "XY" direction. The third dimension, "Z" direction, in the matrix of pixels is the *depth* that is called the *voxel* (volume element). The *depth* of the block is the number of bits required to describe the gray level that each pixel can take on—known as the bit depth.

Bit depth in CT is approximately 2^{12} with a dynamic range of almost 5000 gray shades, approximately 2^{14} in CR/DR with a dynamic range of more than 16,000 gray shades, and approximately 2^{16} in digital mammography with a dynamic range of more than 65,500 gray shades. The matrix is the number of pixels in the XY direction. As matrix size increases, for a fixed FOV, pixel size is smaller and better spatial resolution results. An electronic/digital image is formed by a matrix of pixels in rows and columns. A matrix having 512 pixels in each row and column is a 512×512 matrix (a typical CT image).

The term *FOV* is used to describe how much of the patient is included in the matrix. Either the matrix or the FOV can be changed without one affecting the other, but changes in either will change pixel size. As FOV increases, for a fixed matrix size, the size of each pixel increases and spatial resolution decreases. Fewer and larger pixels result in a poor-resolution "pixelly" or "mosaicked" image, that is, one in which you can actually see the individual pixel boxes.

57. (D) Magnification radiography may be used to delineate a suspected hairline fracture or to enlarge tiny, contrast-filled blood vessels. It also has application in mammography. To magnify an object to twice its actual size, the part must be placed midway between the focal spot and the IR. Magnification factor can be calculated with the formula: $MF = SID/SOD$.

58. (C) To change nongrid exposures to grid exposures, or to adjust exposure when changing from one grid ratio to another, you must remember the factor for each grid ratio:

$$No\ grid = 1 \times original\ mAs$$
$$5:1\ grid = 2 \times original\ mAs$$
$$6:1\ grid = 3 \times original\ mAs$$
$$8:1\ grid = 4 \times original\ mAs$$
$$12:1\ grid = 5 \times original\ mAs$$
$$16:1\ grid = 6 \times original\ mAs$$

To adjust exposure factors, you simply compare the old with the new:

$$\frac{12\,(Old\ mAs)}{x\,(New\ mAs)} = \frac{6\,(Old\ grid\ factor)}{4\,(New\ grid\ factor)}$$
$$6x = 48$$
$$x = 8\,mAs$$

Slightly different conversion factors are often recommended for digital equipment.

59. (D) Pathologic processes and abnormal conditions that alter tissue composition or thickness can have a significant effect on receptor exposure. The radiographer must be aware of these variants and processes to make an appropriate and accurate adjustment of technical factors.

Examples of *additive* pathologic conditions:

- Ascites
- Rheumatoid arthritis
- Paget's disease
- Pneumonia
- Atelectasis
- Congestive heart failure
- Edematous tissue

Examples of *destructive* pathologic conditions:

- Osteoporosis
- Osteomalacia
- Pneumoperitoneum
- Emphysema
- Degenerative arthritis
- Atrophic and necrotic conditions

60. (A) Digital imaging differs from analog imaging in its method of acquisition; in a one-step (*direct conversion*) or two-step (*indirect conversion*) process, remnant x-ray photons (which carry the *signal image*) are converted into an electric charge latent image. Computer hardware and software are required in both CR and DR. *Analog-to-digital conversion is required in CR*; that conversion is the second step in the two-step process. Screen-film (SF) is an analog system.

61. (D) The PSP plate within the CR image plate has several layers. Its uppermost layer is a *protective* coat for the phosphor layer below. This layer affords durability and must be translucent to allow passage of photostimulable luminescent light. The *phosphor layer* is the "active" layer that responds to the x-ray photons that reach it. Under the phosphor layer is the *electroconductive layer* that serves to facilitate transportation through the scanner/reader and prevent image artifacts resulting from static electricity. Below the electroconductive layer is the plate *support layer*. Below the support layer is a *light-shield layer* that serves to prevent light from erasing image plate data or from approaching through the rear protective layer. Behind the light-shield layer is the rear *protective* layer of the PSP plate.

62. (B) FOV refers to the area being viewed. The FOV can be increased or decreased. As the FOV is increased, the part being examined is magnified; as the FOV is decreased, the part returns closer to actual size. Pixel size is affected by changes in either the FOV or matrix size. For example, if the matrix size is increased from 256×256 to 512×512, the pixel size must decrease. If FOV increases, pixel size must increase. Pixel size is inversely related to *resolution*. As pixel size decreases, resolution increases.

63. (C) If a fairly large patient is turned *prone*, the abdominal measurement will be significantly different from the AP measurement as a result of the effect of *compression*. Thus, the part is essentially "thinner," and less scattered radiation will be produced. If the patient remains supine and a compression band is applied, a similar effect will be produced. *Beam restriction* is probably the single most effective means of reducing the production of scattered radiation. *Grid ratio* affects the *cleanup* of scattered radiation; it has *no effect* on the *production* of scattered radiation.

64. (C) Figure 4-11A is a *PA* erect chest taken at a distance of 6 feet and demonstrates an accurate representation of the heart shadow and various parenchymal and bony structures. Figure 4-11B is an *AP* erect chest performed at 50 inches on the same patient and taken within 24 h with no change in patient condition. The AP chest heart appears markedly larger (15.5 cm on PA and 20 cm on AP) for two reasons: (1) the heart is farther from the IR on the AP projection and (2) the SID is decreased; thus, the heart is magnified.

Both images demonstrate adequate inspiration and correct exposure.

65. (D) To change nongrid to grid exposure or to adjust exposure when changing from one grid ratio to another, it is necessary to recall the factor for each grid ratio:

$$\text{No grid} = 1 \times \text{original mAs}$$
$$5:1 \text{ grid} = 2 \times \text{original mAs}$$
$$6:1 \text{ grid} = 3 \times \text{original mAs}$$
$$8:1 \text{ grid} = 4 \times \text{original mAs}$$
$$12:1 \text{ (or } 10:1) \text{ grid} = 5 \times \text{original mAs}$$
$$16:1 \text{ grid} = 6 \times \text{original mAs}$$

Therefore, to change from nongrid to a 12:1 grid, multiply the original milliampere seconds value by a factor of 5. A new milliampere seconds value of 15 is required.

66. (A) Digital image storage is located in a *pixel*, a two-dimensional "picture element," measured in the "XY" direction. The third dimension, "Z" direction, in the matrix of pixels is the *depth*—called the *voxel* (volume element). The depth of the block is the number of bits required to describe the *gray level* that each pixel can take on—known as *bit depth*. Bit depth in *CT* is about 2^{12} with a dynamic range of almost 5000 gray shades, about 2^{14} in *CR/DR* with a dynamic range of more than 16,000 gray shades, and about 2^{16} in digital *mammography* with a dynamic range of more than 65,500 gray shades. The *matrix* is the number of pixels in the XY direction. *As matrix size increases, for a fixed FOV, pixel size is smaller and better image resolution results.* An electronic/digital image is formed by a *matrix* of pixels in *rows* and *columns*. A matrix having 512 pixels in each row and column is a 512 × 512 matrix (a typical CT image). The term FOV is used to describe how much of the patient is included in the matrix. Either the matrix or the FOV can be changed without one affecting the other, but changes in either will change pixel size. *As FOV increases, for a fixed matrix size, the size of each pixel increases and spatial resolution decreases.* Fewer and

larger pixels result in a poor-resolution "pixelly" (*mosaicked*) image, that is, one in which you can actually see the individual pixel boxes. In Figure 4-12, *image #1 is the most pixelly/mosaicked, having a matrix of 16 × 16, and demonstrates the poorest spatial resolution.* The images improve with image #2 having a matrix of 32 × 32, image #3 having a matrix 64 × 64, and *image #4 having a matrix of 128 × 128—and the best spatial resolution.* An image matrix of 256 × 256 would demonstrate even better resolution.

67. (C) *Size* distortion (magnification) is inversely proportional to SID and directly proportional to OID. Increasing the SID and decreasing the OID decrease size distortion. Aligning the tube, part, and IR so that they are parallel reduces *shape* distortion. There are two types of shape distortion—*elongation* and *foreshortening*. Angulation of the part with relation to the IR results in foreshortening of the object. Tube angulation causes elongation of the object.

68. (D) Digital image storage is located in a *pixel*, which is a two-dimensional "picture element," measured in the "XY" direction. The third dimension, "Z" direction, in the matrix of pixels is the depth that is called the *voxel* (volume element). The depth of the block is the number of bits required to describe the gray level that each pixel can take on—known as the bit depth.

The *matrix* is the number of pixels in the XY direction. As matrix size increases, for a fixed FOV, *pixel size is smaller and better spatial resolution results.* An electronic/digital image is formed by a matrix of pixels in rows and columns. A matrix having 512 pixels in each row and column is a 512 × 512 matrix (a typical CT image).

The term *FOV* is used to describe how much of the patient is included in the matrix. Either the matrix or the FOV can be changed without one affecting the other, but changes in either will change pixel size. As FOV increases, for a fixed matrix size, the size of each pixel increases and spatial resolution decreases. Fewer and larger pixels result in a poor-resolution "pixelly" or "mosaicked" image, that is, one in which you can actually see the individual pixel boxes.

69. (B) The formula for mAs is mA × s = mAs. Substituting known values:

$$0.05x = 30$$
$$x = 600 \text{ mA}$$

70. (A) As the distance from focal spot to IR (SID) increases, so does image detail sharpness. Because the part is being exposed by more perpendicular (less divergent) rays, less magnification and blur are produced. Although the best sharpness is obtained using a long SID, the necessary increase in exposure factors and resulting increased patient exposure become problematic. An optimal 40-inch

SID is used for most radiography, with the major exception being chest examinations.

71. **(B)** According to the exposure-maintenance formula, if the SID is changed to 42 inches, 16.33 mAs is required to maintain the original receptor exposure:

$$\frac{(\text{Old mAs})12}{(\text{New mAs})x} = \frac{(\text{Old }D^2)36^2}{(\text{New }D^2)42^2}$$

$$\frac{12}{x} = \frac{1296}{1764}$$

$$1296x = 21{,}168$$

Thus, $x = 16.33$ mAs at 42-inch SID. Then, to compensate for changing from a 12:1 grid to a 5:1 grid, the milliampere seconds value becomes 6.53 mAs:

$$\frac{(\text{Old mAs})16.33}{(\text{New mAs})x} = \frac{(\text{Old grid factor})5}{(\text{Old grid factor})2}$$

$$5x = 32.66$$

Thus, $x = 6.53$ mAs with 5:1 grid at 42-inch SID. Hence, 6.53 mAs is required to produce a receptor exposure similar to that of the original radiograph. The following are the factors used for milliampere seconds conversion from nongrid to grid:

No grid = 1 × original mAs

5:1 grid = 2 × original mAs

6:1 grid = 3 × original mAs

8:1 grid = 4 × original mAs

12:1 grid = 5 × original mAs

16:1 grid = 6 × original mAs

Slightly different conversion factors are often recommended for digital equipment.

72. **(C)** The formula mA × s = mAs is used to determine each milliampere second setting (remember to first change milliseconds to seconds). The *greatest* receptor exposure (a patient dose) will be produced by the combination of highest milliampere seconds value and shortest SID. The groups in choices (B) and (D) should produce *identical receptor exposure*, according to the inverse-square law, because group in choice (D) includes twice the distance and 4 times the milliampere seconds value of group in choice (B). The group in choice (A) has twice the distance of the group in choice (B) but only twice the milliampere seconds; therefore, it has the *least* receptor exposure. The group in choice (C) has the same distance as the group in choice (B) and twice the milliampere seconds, making group in choice (C) the group of technical factors that will produce the *greatest* receptor exposure. In digital imaging, predetermined algorithm selections control the required contrast and brightness requirements.

73. **(C)** The spatial resolution of direct digital systems is fixed and is related to the *detector element* (DEL) size of the TFT and its *fill factor*. The DEL is the sensing element of the TFT and its largest portion should be used for its sensing function to maintain/improve resolution. For example, if 25% of the DEL is used for other functions, the DEL is said to have a *fill factor* of 75%.

The smaller the TFT-DEL size, and the larger the fill factor, the better the spatial resolution. DEL size of 100 μ provides a spatial resolution of about 5 lp/mm (available only in some digital mammography systems). DEL size of 200 μ provides a spatial resolution of about 2.5 lp/mm (general radiography). A 100-speed intensifying screen system offers a spatial resolution of about 10 lp/mm—significantly greater than, and currently unachievable in, digital imaging.

74. **(B)** In digital imaging, brightness and contrast are determined by computer software and monitor controls; however, the principal factor in good digital image visibility and patient dose is still the result of proper IR exposure. Selection of kilovoltage and milliampere seconds in digital imaging is very similar to SF imaging, that is, kilovoltage still affects penetration, but not contrast; milliampere seconds still determines dose, but has no impact on brightness. Window level adjustments are associated with image brightness changes; window width adjustments are associated with changes in image contrast. The terms density and brightness do not mean the same thing and therefore are not used interchangeably.

75. **(B)** In *digital* imaging, brightness and contrast are determined by computer software and monitor controls; *however, the principal factor in good digital image visibility and patient dose is still the result of proper IR exposure.* Kilovoltage selection determines penetration but not contrast; milliampere seconds determines receptor exposure and dose but has no impact on brightness.

76. **(C)** Equipment must be properly calibrated to produce consistently predictable results; specifically, the equipment must have *linearity* and *reproducibility*. When adjacent mA stations are tested, for example 100 and 200 mA, and the exposure time is kept constant, the 200-mA station should produce twice exposure rate of the 100-mA station—this is *linearity*. *Reproducibility* refers to consistency in exposure output during repeated exposures at a particular setting.

77. **(B)** Milliampere seconds is directly related to x-ray intensity/quantity. Exposure to the IR will be *doubled* when the milliampere seconds is doubled. Although kilovoltage describes beam quality and penetration, it also influences beam intensity, thereby having effect on IR exposure. Receptor exposure will be doubled when the kilovoltage is increased by 15%.

78. **(D)** *Focal spot size* affects spatial resolution by its effect on focal spot blur: The larger the focal spot size, the

greater is the blur produced. Spatial resolution is affected significantly by distance changes because of their effect on magnification. As SID increases and as OID decreases, magnification decreases and spatial resolution increases. SOD is determined by subtracting OID from SID.

79. **(C)** Significant scattered radiation is generated within the part when imaging large or dense body parts and when using high kilovoltage. A radiographic grid is made of alternating lead strips and interspace material; it is placed between the patient and the IR to absorb energetic scatter emerging from the patient. Although a grid prevents much of the scattered radiation from reaching the radiograph, its use does necessitate a significant *increase* in patient exposure.

80. **(B)** The radiograph shown in Figure 4-13 demonstrates a 1.5-inch unexposed strip along the length of the IR. This occurred because, although the patient was centered correctly to the collimator light and x-ray field, the x-ray tube was not centered to the IR. If the patient was off-center, the entire image would be exposed, and the patient's spine would be off-center. Grid cutoff would not appear as such a sharply delineated line but rather as gradually decreasing loss of receptor exposure.

81. **(B)** The milliampere seconds value regulates the *number* of x-ray photons produced at the target and thus regulates *patient dose*. If the milliampere seconds is doubled, dose is doubled; therefore, milliampere seconds and patient dose are directly proportional.

82. **(B)** The image plate front material must not attenuate the remnant beam (which carries the *signal image*) yet must be sturdy enough to withstand daily use. Bakelite had long been used as the material for tabletops and IR fronts, but has been replaced largely by *magnesium* and *carbon fiber*. Lead would not be a suitable material because it would absorb the remnant beam, and no image would be formed.

83. **(C)** *Emphysema* is abnormal distension of the pulmonary alveoli (or tissue spaces) with air. The presence of abnormal amounts of air makes a decrease from normal exposure factors necessary to avoid excessive receptor exposure. *Congestive heart failure, pneumonia,* and *pleural effusion* all involve abnormal amounts of fluid in the chest and, therefore, would require an *increase* in exposure factors.

84. **(B)** In digital imaging, pixel size is determined by dividing the FOV by the matrix. In this case, the FOV is 20 cm; because the answer is expressed in millimeters, first change 20 cm to 200 mm. Then 200 divided by 512 equals 0.39 mm:

$$20\,\text{cm} = 200\,\text{mm}$$

$$\frac{200}{512} = 0.39\,\text{mm/pixel}$$

The FOV and matrix size are independent of one another, that is, either can be changed, and the other will remain

unaffected. However, pixel size is affected by changes in either the FOV or matrix size. For example, if the matrix size is increased, pixel size decreases. If FOV is increased, pixel size increases. Pixel size is inversely related to resolution. As pixel size increases, resolution decreases.

85. **(B)** If it is desired to reduce the exposure time for a particular radiograph, as it might be when radiographing patients who are unable to cooperate fully, the *milliamperage* must be *increased* sufficiently to maintain the original milliampere seconds value and thus correct IR exposure. A *higher kilovoltage* could be useful because it would allow further reduction of the milliampere seconds (exposure time) according to the 15% rule. Changing grid ratio is unrelated to desired changes in exposure time. Use of a higher ratio grid would only necessitate an increase in milliampere seconds and not likely a decrease in exposure time.

86. **(D)** As kilovoltage is increased, more electrons are driven to the anode with greater speed and energy. More high-energy electrons result in the production of *a greater number of high-energy x-rays*. Higher energy x-rays are associated with shorter wavelength, hence the relationship between kilovoltage and wavelength is inverse. Thus, kilovoltage affects both *quality* (energy/wavelength) and *quantity* (intensity/quantity) of the x-ray beam. However, although kilovoltage and receptor exposure are directly *related*, they are not directly proportional. The effect of kilovoltage on quantity is not proportional because an increase in kilovoltage produces an increase in photons of *all energies*.

With respect to the effect of kilovoltage on receptor exposure, the *15% rule* can be used. If it is desired to double the receptor exposure, without adjusting the milliampere seconds, a similar effect can be achieved by *increasing the kilovoltage by 15%*. Conversely, the receptor exposure may be reduced to half by decreasing the kilovoltage by 15%. Using the 15% rule to decrease milliampere seconds can play a significant role in *decreasing patient absorbed dose* because increased kilovoltage provides a *more penetrating* beam.

87. **(B)** Spatial resolution in *CR (indirect)* imaging improves with increased *sampling frequency* (pixels/mm or pixel density), smaller *pixel pitch*, smaller *pixel size*, and larger image matrix. The smaller the pixels and *pixel pitch* (i.e., distance between the center of one pixel to the center of adjacent pixel), the better the resolution.

DEL size of the TFT is related to direct and indirect digital imaging.

88. **(C)** One of the biggest advantages of digital over analog imaging is the *dynamic range/latitude* it offers. In CR/DR, there is a *linear* relationship between the exposure given the PSP and its resulting luminescence, as it is scanned by the laser, as illustrated in Figure 4-14. This affords much

greater dynamic range and latitude; technical inaccuracies can be effectively eliminated. Overexposure of greater than 200% and underexposure of up to 50% are reported as recoverable, thus eliminating most retakes. This possibly affords increased efficiency, but the professional radiographer has a responsibility to keep dose reduction to a minimum.

89. **(B)** Artifacts can be a result of *exposure, handling, and storage,* or *processing.* Exposure artifacts include *motion, double exposure,* and *patient clothing/jewelry*—the effects of these are seen as a result of the exposure. Handling and storage artifacts include fogged PSP, image fading, upside-down IP, damaged PSP—all these occur as a result of improper use or storage. Processing artifacts occur while the PSP is in the scanner/reader and include skipped scan lines, and laser jitter. Slightly different conversion factors are often recommended for digital equipment.

90. **(B)** As the kilovoltage is increased, a *greater number* of electrons are driven across to the anode with *greater force.* Therefore, as energy conversion takes place at the anode, *more high-energy* (short-wavelength) photons are produced. However, because they are higher energy photons, there will be less patient absorption.

91. **(D)** The term *distortion* refers to misrepresentation of the actual *size* (magnification) or *shape* (foreshortening or elongation) of the structures imaged, which may be partly or wholly caused by inherent object unsharpness. Foreshortening and elongation are a result of improper alignment of tube, part, and image receptor. *Foreshortening* results when the part or IR is not parallel. Elongation results from tube angulation. All of the geometric factors—OID, SID, focal spot size, distortion, structural position/shape, and motion—impact resolution/detail.

92. **(A)** Shape distortion (e.g., foreshortening or elongation) is caused by improper alignment of the tube, part, and IR. Size distortion, or magnification, is caused by too great an OID or too short an SID. Focal spot blur is caused by the use of a large focal spot.

93. **(B)** An *increase in SID* will help to decrease the effect of excessive OID. For example, in the lateral projection of the cervical spine, there is normally a significant OID that would result in obvious magnification at a 40-inch SID. This effect is decreased by the use of a 72-inch SID. However, especially with larger body parts, increased SID usually requires a significant increase in exposure factors. Focal spot size and grid ratio are unrelated to magnification.

94. **(B)** The addition of a grid will help to clean up the scattered radiation produced by higher kilovoltage, but the grid requires an *adjustment of milliampere seconds.* According to the grid conversion factors listed here, the addition of an 8:1 grid requires that the original milliampere seconds be multiplied by a factor of 4:

No grid = 1 × original mAs
5:1 grid = 2 × original mAs
6:1 grid = 3 × original mAs
8:1 grid = 4 × original mAs
12:1 (or 10:1) grid = 5 × original mAs
16:1 grid = 6 × original mAs

The original milliampere seconds value is 1.2. The ideal adjustment, therefore, requires a 4.8 mAs at 90 kV. Although 2.4 mAs with 100 kV (choice C), or 1.2 mAs with 110 kV (choice A), also might seem workable, an increase in kilovoltage would further compromise contrast, nullifying the effect of the grid. In addition, kilovoltage exceeding 100 should not be used with an 8:1 grid.

95. **(A)** Of the two radiographs illustrated, Figure 4-15A was made recumbent and Figure 4-15B was made in erect position; this may be discerned by the presence of clearly defined air–fluid levels in the lower abdomen. Abdominal viscera move to a lower position in the erect position, making the abdomen "thicker" and requiring an *increase* in exposure (usually the equivalent of about 10 kV).

96. **(A)** Exposure rate *decreases* with an increase in SID according to the inverse-square law of radiation. The *quantity* of x-ray photons produced at the focal spot is the function of milliampere seconds. The *quality* (i.e., wavelength, penetration, and energy) of x-ray photons produced at the target is the function of kilovoltage. The kilovoltage also has an effect on exposure rate because an increase in kilovoltage will increase the number of high-energy x-ray photons produced at the anode.

97. **(A)** Pixel depth is directly related to shades of gray—called *dynamic range*—and is measured in *bits.* The greater the number of bits, the more shades of gray. For example, a 1-bit (2^1) pixel will demonstrate 2 shades of gray, whereas a 6-bit (2^6) pixel can display 64 shades, and a 7-bit (2^7) pixel can display 128 shades. However, pixel depth is unrelated to resolution.

A digital image is formed by a *matrix of pixels* (picture elements) in rows and columns. A matrix that has 512 pixels in each row and column is a 512 × 512 matrix. The term *field of view* is used to describe how much of the patient (e.g., 150-mm diameter) is included in the matrix. The matrix and the field of view can be changed independently without one affecting the other, but changes in either will change pixel size. As in traditional radiography, *spatial resolution* is measured in line pairs per millimeter (lp/mm). As *matrix size is increased* (e.g., from 512 × 512 to 1024 × 1024) there are more and smaller pixels in the matrix and, therefore, *improved resolution.* Fewer and larger pixels result in poor resolution, a "pixelly" image, that is, one in which you can actually see the individual pixel boxes.

98. (D) Distortion is caused by *improper alignment of the tube, body part, and IR.* Anatomic structures within the body are rarely parallel to the IR in a simple recumbent position. In an attempt to overcome this distortion, we position the part to be parallel with the IR or angle the central ray to "open up" the part. Examples of this technique are obliquing the pelvis to place the ilium parallel to the IR or angling the central ray cephalad to "open up" the sigmoid colon.

99. (D) As OID is increased, spatial resolution is diminished as a result of magnification distortion. If the OID cannot be minimized, an increase in SID is required to reduce the effect of magnification distortion. However, the relationship between OID and SID is not an equal relationship. In fact, to compensate for every 1 inch of OID, an increase of 7 inches of SID is required. Therefore, an OID of 6 inches requires an SID increase of 42 inches. This is why a chest radiograph with a 6-inch air gap usually is performed at a 10-foot SID.

100. (A) Limiting the size of the radiographic field (irradiated area) serves to limit the amount of scattered radiation produced within the anatomic part. Therefore, as field size *decreases*, scattered radiation production *decreases*, and image quality increases. Limiting the size of the radiographic field is a very effective means of reducing the quantity of non–information-carrying scattered radiation (fog) produced, resulting in improved detail *visibility.* Limiting the size of the radiographic field is also the most effective means of patient radiation protection.

101. (A) If the SID is above or below the recommended focusing distance, the primary beam will not coincide with the angled lead strips at their lateral edges. Consequently, there will be *absorption of the primary beam* termed *grid cutoff.* If the central ray is off-center *longitudinally*, there will be no ill effects. If the central ray is off-center *side to side*, the lead strips are no longer parallel with the divergent x-ray beam, and there will be loss of receptor exposure owing to grid cutoff. Central ray angulation *in the direction of* the lead strips is appropriate and will not cause grid cutoff. Central ray angulation *against the direction of* the lead strips will cause grid cutoff.

102. (A) Scattered radiation is produced as x-ray photons travel through matter, interact with atoms, and are scattered (change direction). If these scattered rays are energetic enough to exit the body and contribute to the signal image, they will strike the IR from all different angles. They, therefore, do not carry useful information and produce fog over the image that impairs visibility of image details. Grid cutoff *increases* contrast and is caused by an improper relationship between the x-ray tube and the grid, resulting in absorption of some of the useful/primary beam.

103. (C) Control of motion, both voluntary and involuntary, is an important part of radiography. Patients are unable to control certain types of motion, such as heart action, peristalsis, and muscle spasm. In these circumstances, it is essential to use the shortest possible exposure time to have a "stop action" effect.

104. (C) *Motion*, voluntary or involuntary, is most detrimental to sharpness of detail/spatial resolution. Even if all other factors are adjusted to maximize sharpness, if motion occurs during exposure, detail sharpness is lost. The most important ways to reduce the possibility of motion are using the shortest possible exposure time, careful patient instruction (for suspended respiration), and adequate immobilization when necessary. Minimizing magnification through the use of *increased* SID and *decreased* OID functions to improve detail sharpness/spatial resolution.

105. (B) Flaws in "raw" digital images are corrected during preprocessing functions. These corrections are required as a result of *flaws in the image acquisition process* or as a result *processor flaws.* Preprocessing is also called acquisition processing. Examples of preprocessing corrections include flat-field corrections, correction for noise reduction as a result of DEL dropout, rescaling, exposure field recognition, segmentation recognition, and histogram analysis. Equalization refers to the dynamic range compression which is a postprocessing function.

106. (B) In *digital* imaging, brightness and contrast are determined by computer software and monitor controls; *however, the principal factor in good digital image visibility and patient dose is still the result of proper IR exposure.* Kilovoltage selection determines penetration but not contrast; milliampere seconds determines dose but has no impact on brightness.

107. (A) The image shown in Figure 4-16 is a double exposure. Note the ilia and lower pelvic structures. Two pelves are clearly identifiable. Particularly noteworthy is how CR will "correct" the exposure values. The image does not appear overexposed, but the superimposed abdominal images are unmistakably evident. An inverted IP would have imaged the rear panel of the IP—a large grid-like appearance. An incomplete erasure or image fading would show only a portion of the image—here we have the entire superimposed abdomen.

108. (C) *Kilovoltage* and the *HVL* affect both the quantity and the quality of the primary beam. The principal qualitative factor for the primary beam is kilovoltage, but an increase in kilovoltage will also create an increase in the *number* of photons produced at the target. *HVL* is defined as the amount of material necessary to decrease the intensity of the beam to one-half its original value, thereby effecting a change in both beam quality and quantity. The milliampere seconds value is adjusted to regulate the number of x-ray photons produced at the target. X-ray-beam quality is unaffected by changes in milliampere seconds.

109. (A) The *focal spot size* selected will determine the amount of focal spot, or geometric, blur produced in the image. OID and SID are responsible for image magnification and hence spatial resolution. The *milliamperage* is unrelated to spatial resolution; it affects only the quantity of x-ray photons produced and thus the receptor exposure.

110. (A) *The shortest possible exposure should be used as a matter of routine.* Parkinson's disease is characterized by uncontrollable tremors, and the resulting unsharpness can destroy image resolution/detail. A short exposure time is essential. That can be achieved by increasing the mA or the kilovoltage—AEC will react with a shorted exposure time. SID and compensating filtration are unrelated to the problem and are not indicated here.

111. (C) *Absorption* occurs when an x-ray photon interacts with matter and disappears, as in the photoelectric effect. *Scattering* occurs when there is partial transfer of energy to matter, as in the Compton effect. The *reduction in the intensity* of an x-ray beam as it passes through matter (in the form of absorption and scattering) is called *attenuation*.

112. (C) The FOV and matrix size are independent of one another, that is, either can be changed, and the other will remain unaffected. However, *pixel size is affected by changes in either the FOV or matrix size.* For example, if the matrix size is increased, pixel size decreases. If FOV increases, pixel size increases. Pixel size is inversely related to resolution. As pixel size decreases, resolution increases.

113. (B) The original milliampere seconds value was 9 (300 mA × 0.03 s). Using the *exposure-maintenance formula*, the new milliampere seconds value must be determined for the distance change from 40 to 44 inches of the SID:

$$\frac{(\text{Old mAs})\,9}{(\text{New mAs})\,x} = \frac{(\text{Old }D^2)\,40^2}{(\text{New }D^2)\,44^2}$$

$$1600x = 17{,}424$$

Thus, $x = 10.89$ (11) mAs at 44-inch SID. Then, if 500 is the new milliamperage, we must determine what exposure time is required to achieve 8.1 mAs:

$$500x = 11$$

Thus, $x = 0.022$ s (22 ms) at 500 mA and 44-inch SID.

114. (C) A 15% increase in kilovoltage was made, increasing the kilovoltage to 87 kV. Because the kilovoltage change effectively doubles the receptor exposure, the milliampere seconds value now must be cut in half (from 9 to 4.5 mAs) to compensate. Grids are used to absorb scattered radiation from the remnant beam before it can contribute to the x-ray image. Because the grid removes scattered radiation (and some useful photons as well) from the beam, an increase in exposure factors is required. The amount of increase depends on the grid ratio; the higher the grid ratio, the higher is the correction factor. The correction factor for a 12:1 grid is 5; therefore, the milliampere seconds value (4.5) is multiplied by 5 to arrive at the new required milliampere seconds value (22.5). Using the milliampere seconds equation mA × s = mAs, it is determined that 0.15 s will be required at 300 mA:

$$300x = 22.5$$

$$x = 0.075\,\text{s} = 75\,\text{ms}$$

115. (C) High kilovoltage is desirable in terms of patient dose and x-ray tube life, but excessive kilovoltage can contribute to scattered radiation that reaches the *IR* and can diminish *visibility* of image details. Scatter emerging from the patient also contributes to *occupational exposure.* The production of scattered radiation increases with an increase in kilovoltage, an increase in field size, and an increase in part thickness/density. *Spatial resolution* is affected by OID, SID, focal spot size, patient factors, and motion as well as pixel pitch, DEL size, and sampling frequency. Scattered radiation has no impact on spatial resolution.

116. (B) The formula for MF = image size/object size. In the stated problem, the anatomic measurement is 14.7 cm, and the magnification factor is known to be 1.2. Substituting the known factors in the appropriate equation:

$$\text{MF} = \frac{\text{image size}}{\text{object size}}$$

$$1.2 = \frac{14.7}{x}$$

$$x = \frac{14.7}{1.2}$$

$$x = 12.25\,\text{cm}$$

(actual anatomic size)

117. (C) IP front material must be radiolucent and homogeneous in nature, to avoid excessive absorption of x-ray photons and/or production of unwanted details/densities on the image receptor. The material must not absorb an excessive amount of the exit beam. It must be uniform in nature so as not to absorbed in an irregular fashion.

118. (B) As the distance from the object to the IR (OID) increases, so does magnification distortion, thereby decreasing sharpness/spatial resolution. Some magnification is inevitable in radiography because it is not possible to place anatomic structures directly on the IR. However, our understanding of how to minimize magnification distortion is an important part of our everyday work.

119. (D) The abdomen radiograph shown in Figure 4-17 demonstrates *motion* blur. This can be seen particularly in the upper abdomen and in the bowel gas patterns.

Motion obliterates detail. Patients who are in pain often are unable to cooperate as fully as patients who are not in pain. Careful positioning and patient instruction are helpful, but it remains useful to use the shortest exposure time possible. The radiograph also demonstrates good *long*-scale contrast that enables visualization of many tissue densities. The dark horizontal line across the abdomen is an exposure artifact resulting from a taut elastic underwear clothing waistband. There are no superimposed anatomical structures that would indicate double exposure.

120. **(C)** A *grid* is a device interposed between the part and IR that functions to absorb a large percentage of scattered radiation before it reaches the IR. It is composed of alternating strips of lead foil and radiolucent filler material. Two of a grid's physical characteristics that determine its degree of efficiency in the removal of SR are *grid ratio* and the *number of lead strips per inch.* As the lead strips are made taller, or the distance between them decreases, grid ratio increases and scattered radiation is more likely to be trapped before reaching the IR. A 12:1 ratio grid will absorb more SR radiation than an 8:1 ratio grid. The number of lead strips per inch is also called *grid frequency.* The advantage of many lead strips per inch is that there is less visibility of the lead strips. As the number of lead foil strips per inch increases, the lead foil strips must become thinner and therefore less visible. However, as lead strips get thinner, more energetic SR can pass through them and reach the IR and the grid becomes less efficient.

   SR absorption is improved using higher ratio grids having lower grid frequency. *Higher ratio grids* absorb more SR, *lower grid frequency* has thicker lead strips and absorbs more SR. To maintain the efficiency of grids having high-grid frequency/many lead strips per inch, grid ratio is increased as well, that is, the lead strips are made taller to increase the absorption of SR.

121. **(D)** The relationship between SID and RE is inverse, that is, as SID increases, RE decreases (1). The relationship between x-ray energy and wavelength is *inverse,* that is, as x-ray energy increases, wavelength decreases (2). The maximum x-ray energy in an x-ray spectrum depends on the applied kilovoltage, that is, as kilovoltage increases, x-ray photon energy increases (3).

   The number of x-ray photons reaching the IR increases as field size increases, that is, as field size increases, more SR is generated in a greater volume of tissue and reaches the IR (4). The purpose of x-ray tube filters is to absorb low-energy photons, thus producing a *less* polyenergetic beam (5).

122. **(C)** The PSP plate within the CR cassette/IP has several layers. Its uppermost layer is a *protective* coat for the phosphor layer below. This layer affords durability and must be translucent to allow passage of photostimulable

luminescent light. The *phosphor layer* is the "active" layer that responds to the x-ray photons that reach it. Under the phosphor layer is the *electroconductive layer* that serves to facilitate transportation through the scanner/reader and prevents image artifacts resulting from static electricity. Below the electroconductive layer is the plate support layer. Below the *support* layer is a *light-shield layer* that serves to prevent light from erasing image plate data or from approaching through the rear protective layer. Behind the light-shield layer is the rear protective layer of the PSP plate.

123. **(A)** Kilovoltage has been the exposure factor of choice for regulation of part penetration and image contrast. The lower the kilovoltage, the less part penetration and the shorter the scale of contrast. All the milliampere seconds values in this problem have been adjusted for kilovoltage changes to maintain receptor exposure, but just a glance at each of the kilovoltages is often a good indicator of which will produce the longest scale or shortest scale contrast. Systems using computerized rescaling of x-ray images effectively control image contrast.

124. **(A)** In digital imaging, pixel size is determined by dividing the FOV by the matrix. In this case, the FOV is 60 cm; because the answer is expressed in millimeters, first change 60 cm to 600 mm. Then 600 divided by 2048 equals 0.3 mm:

$$60\,cm = 600\,mm$$

$$\frac{600}{2048} = 0.29\,mm$$

   The FOV and matrix size are independent of one another, that is, either can be changed, and the other will remain unaffected. However, pixel size is affected by changes in either the FOV or matrix size. For example, if the matrix size is increased, pixel size decreases. If FOV increases, pixel size increases. Pixel size is inversely related to resolution. As pixel size increases, resolution decreases.

125. **(A)** In electronic/digital imaging, changes in window width affect changes in contrast scale, whereas changes in window level affect changes in brightness. As window width increases, the scale of contrast increases (i.e., contrast decreases). Window level adjustments are associated with image brightness changes. This can be easily illustrated as you postprocess/window your own digital photographs or scanned documents. As the brightness scale is moved in one direction or the other, images become more or less bright.

126. **(D)** The *matrix* is the number of pixels in the *xy* direction. *The larger the matrix size, the better is the image resolution.* Typical image matrix sizes used in radiography are

   • Nuclear medicine: 128 × 128

   • Digital subtraction angiography (DSA): 1024 × 1024

- CT: 512 × 512
- Chest radiography: 2048 × 2048

A digital image is formed by a *matrix* of pixels in rows and columns. A matrix having 512 pixels in each row and column is a 512 × 512 matrix. The term *field of view* is used to describe how much of the patient (e.g., 150-mm diameter) is included in the matrix. The matrix or field of view can be changed without affecting the other, but changes in either will change pixel size. As in traditional radiography, *spatial resolution* is measured in line pairs per millimeter (*lp/mm*). As matrix size is increased, there are more and smaller pixels in the matrix and, therefore, improved spatial resolution. Fewer and larger pixels result in a poor-resolution "pixely" image, that is, one in which you can actually see the individual pixel boxes.

127. (B) As distance from a light source increases, the light diverges and covers a larger area; the quantity of light available per unit area becomes less and less as distance increases. The intensity (quantity) of light decreases according to the *inverse-square law*, that is, the intensity of light at a particular distance from its source is inversely proportional to the square of the distance. For example, if you decreased the distance between a book you were reading and your illuminating lamp from 6 to 3 feet, you would have 4 times as much light available.

Similarly, SID has a significant impact on x-ray beam intensity. As the distance between the x-ray tube and IR increases, exposure rate decreases according to the inverse-square law.

128. (C) SID is *directly* related to spatial resolution because as SID increases, so does spatial resolution (because magnification is decreased). OID is *inversely* related to spatial resolution because as OID increases, spatial resolution decreases. Motion is also inversely related to spatial resolution because as motion increases, spatial resolution decreases—as a result of motion blur, the greatest enemy of resolution. Therefore, of the given choices, OID and motion are *inversely* related to spatial resolution. SID is *directly* related to spatial resolution.

129. (A) An FOV change will not affect matrix size and a change in matrix size will not affect FOV. However, a change in FOV and/or a change in matrix size will affect a change in pixel size.

If FOV is reduced (with matrix size unchanged), pixel size will become smaller and spatial resolution will increase. If FOV is increased (with matrix size unchanged), pixel size will become larger and spatial resolution will decrease.

Scanning frequency is related to the Nyquist theory as applied to converting an analog-to-digital image.

130. (B) To calculate milliampere seconds, multiply milliamperage by exposure time. In this case, 400 mA × 0.017 s (17 ms) = 6.8 mAs. Careful attention to proper decimal placement will help to avoid basic math errors.

131. (C) Before the radiologic examination begins, patients often need to change their clothing and/or remove radiopaque objects (e.g., jewelry, dentures, and braided hair) from superimposition on structures of interest. Figure 4-18 illustrates multiple *braids* of hair superimposed on skull structures, as well as nose and ear jewelry. Loose hair is radiolucent, whereas hair that is braided becomes more dense and is often imaged radiographically. Dental fillings, and so on, are seen, but there are no dentures. The ensuing artifacts can interfere with accurate diagnosis; otherwise, the bony detail is good and no motion is present.

132. (B) A technique chart identifies the standardized factors for a particular x-ray unit for various examinations/positions of anatomic parts of different sizes. To be used effectively, these technique charts require that the anatomic part in question be measured correctly with a *caliper*. A *fulcrum* is related to conventional tomography; a *densitometer* is used in analog/film sensitometry and QA.

133. (A) Remnant x-rays (which carry the *signal image*) emerging from the patient/part are converted to electrical signals. This is an analog image. These electrical signals are sent to the ADC (analog-to-digital converter) to be converted to digital data (in binary digits or bits). Then, the digital image data are transferred to a DAC (digital-to-analog converter) to be converted to a perceptible analog image on the display monitor. The initial processed/displayed image can be manipulated, postprocessed, stored, or transmitted.

134. (C) In digital imaging, brightness and contrast are determined by computer software and monitor controls; however, the principal factor in good digital image visibility and patient dose is still the result of proper IR exposure. Selection of kilovoltage and milliampere seconds in digital imaging is very similar to SF imaging, that is, kilovoltage still affects penetration, but not contrast; milliampere seconds value still determines dose, but has no impact on brightness. Window level adjustments are associated with image brightness changes; window width adjustments are associated with changes in image contrast. The terms density and brightness do not mean the same thing and therefore are not used interchangeably.

135. (B) The heel effect is characterized by a variation in beam intensity that *increases gradually from anode to cathode*. This can be effectively put to use when performing radiographic examinations of large body parts with uneven tissue density. For example, the AP thoracic spine is thicker caudally than cranially, so the thicker portion is best placed under the cathode. However, in the lateral projection of the thoracic spine, the upper portion is thicker because of superimposed shoulders, and therefore, that portion is best placed under the cathode end of the beam. The femur is also uneven in tissue density, particularly in the AP position, and can benefit from use of the heel effect. However, the sternum and its surrounding anatomy are fairly uniform in thickness and would not benefit from use of the anode heel effect. *The anode heel effect is most pronounced when using large IRs at short SIDs and with an anode having a steep (small) target angle.*

136. **(D)** As *photon energy* increases, more x-ray photons penetrate the parts and reach the image receptor. As *grid ratio* increases, more scattered radiation is absorbed, and fewer x-ray photons reach the image receptor. As OID increases, the distance between the part and the IR acts as a grid, and consequently, less scattered radiation reaches the IR. Focal spot size is related only to spatial resolution.

137. **(D)** The lead strips in a parallel grid are *parallel to one another* and, therefore, are *not parallel to the x-ray beam.* The more divergent the x-ray beam, the more likely there is to be cutoff/decreased receptor exposure at the *lateral edges* of the radiographic image. This problem becomes more pronounced at short SIDs. A centering or tube angle problem would more likely be a noticeable receptor exposure loss on *one side* or the other.

138. **(B)** The image shown in Figure 4-19 is an example of *both* off-focus and lateral decentering errors. Note the asymmetric cutoff from right to left. The individual grid errors, as well as the result of both errors together, are summarized as follows:

- *Off-focus errors:* Grid cutoff will occur if the SID is below the lower limits, or above the upper limits, of the specified focal range. This type of error is also called *focus–grid distance decentering.* Off-focus errors are usually characterized by loss of receptor exposure at the *periphery* of the image.
- *Off-center errors:* If the x-ray beam is not centered to the grid (i.e., if it is shifted laterally), grid cutoff will occur. This type of error is called lateral decentering and characterized by a *uniform receptor exposure loss* across the radiographic image.

If the x-ray beam is *both off-center and off-focus below the focusing distance,* the portion of the image below the focus will show *increased* receptor exposure; if the x-ray beam is *off-center and off-focus above the focusing distance,* the image below the focus will show *decreased* receptor exposure.

139. **(C)** The *reciprocity law* states that a particular milliampere seconds value, regardless of the milliamperage and exposure time used, will provide identical radiographic receptor exposure. This holds true with direct exposure techniques, but it does fail somewhat with the use of intensifying screens. However, the fault is so slight as to be unimportant in most radiographic procedures.

140. **(B)** *CR* uses traditional x-ray tables and *IPs* to enclose and protect the flexible PSP screen, whereas *DR* requires the use of significantly different equipment. DR does not use IPs or a traditional x-ray table—it is a direct-capture/conversion or indirect-capture/conversion system of x-ray imaging. Besides eliminating IPs and their handling, DR affords the advantage of *immediate display* of the image (compared with CR's slightly delayed image display), and DR *exposures can be lower* because of the detector's *higher DQE* (i.e., ability to perceive and interact with x-ray photons). DR, like CR, also offers the advantage of image preview and postprocessing.

141. **(D)** Milliampere seconds (mAs) is the exposure factor that regulates receptor exposure. The equation used to determine mAs is mA × s = mAs. Substituting the known factors:

$$300x = 6$$
$$x = 0.02\,\text{s}\,(20\,\text{ms})$$

142. **(C)** Factors influencing spatial resolution in digital imaging are very much the same as those factors affecting recorded detail in analog imaging, that is, *motion, geometric factors* (focal spot size, OID, and SID). The spatial resolution of direct digital systems, however, is *fixed* and is related to the *DEL* size of the thin film transistor (*TFT*). The smaller the TFT-DEL size, the better the spatial resolution. DEL size of 100 μ provides a spatial resolution of about 5 lp/mm (available only in some digital mammography systems). DEL size of 200 μ provides a spatial resolution of about 2.5 lp/mm (general radiography). Spatial resolution in digital imaging is fixed, but it is very important that radiographers are alert to the opportunity they have to utilize and control the remaining recorded detail factors (motion and geometric factors).

143. **(C)** An increase in kilovoltage increases the overall average *energy* of the x-ray photons produced at the target, thus giving them greater *penetrability.* This can also increase the incidence of Compton interaction and, therefore, the production of scattered radiation. Excessive scattered radiation reaching the IR will cause SR fog noise. In digital imaging, predetermined algorithm selections control the required contrast and *brightness* requirements.

144. **(A)** Beam restrictors function to limit the size of the irradiated field. In so doing, they limit the volume of tissue irradiated (thereby decreasing the percentage of scattered radiation generated in the part) and help to reduce patient dose. Beam restrictors do not affect the quality

(energy) of the x-ray beam—that is the function of kilovoltage and filtration. Beam restrictors do not absorb scattered radiation—that is a function of grids.

145. (D) Factors influencing image sharpness/spatial resolution in digital imaging are very much the same as those factors affecting recorded detail in analog imaging, that is, *motion* and *geometric factors* (focal spot size, OID, and SID). The spatial resolution of direct digital systems is fixed and is related to the detector element (*DEL*) size of the thin film transistor (*TFT*). The smaller the TFT-DEL size, the better the spatial resolution. DEL size of 100 μ provides a spatial resolution of about 5 lp/mm (available only in some digital mammography systems). DEL size of 200 μ provides a spatial resolution of about 2.5 lp/mm (general radiography). A 100-speed intensifying screen system offers a spatial resolution of about 10 lp/mm— significantly greater than, and currently unachievable in, digital imaging. Spatial resolution in digital imaging is fixed, but it is very important that radiographers are alert to the opportunity they have to utilize and control the remaining recorded detail factors (motion and geometric factors).

146. (C) Quantum *noise,* or *mottle,* is a grainy appearance; it has a spotted or freckled appearance. It looks very similar to a low-resolution photograph/image that has been enlarged. Low-milliampere seconds and high-kilovoltage factors are most likely to be the cause of quantum noise/mottle. SID is unrelated to quantum noise. Image *noise* is any negative/degrading input that interferes with visibility of image details. There are many types of image noise.

147. (A) The artifact seen in Figure 4-20 is a *vertical processing artifact* (a type of CR processing artifact) resulting from irregular movement as PSP is removed from the IP. A cleaning solution artifact usually appears as a splatter-like effect. Secondary exposure results in fogging of the very sensitive PSP.

148. (B) According to the *15% rule,* if the kilovoltage is increased by 15%, receptor exposure will be doubled. Therefore, to compensate for this change and to maintain IR exposure, the milliampere seconds value should be reduced to 4 mAs.

149. (A) Figure 4-21 represents the *anode heel effect.* Because the anode's focal track is beveled, x-ray photons can freely diverge toward the cathode end of the x-ray tube. However, the "heel" of the focal track prevents x-ray photons from diverging toward the anode end of the tube. This results in varying intensity with fewer photons at the anode end (A) and more photons at the cathode end (B).

The *line-focus principle* (Fig. 4-31) relates to the anode's focal spot, and x-ray tube targets are constructed according to the line-focus principle—the focal spot is angled to

the vertical. As the actual focal spot is projected downward, it is foreshortened; thus, the effective focal spot is always smaller than the actual focal spot.

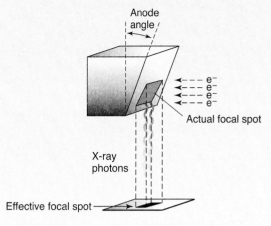

Figure 4-31

The inverse-square law deals with the changing x-ray intensity with changes in distance. This principle is important in image formation and in radiation protection.

150. (B) If (A) and (B) are reduced to 5 mAs for consistency, the kilovoltage will increase to 85 kV in both cases, thereby balancing radiographic receptor exposures. Thus, the greatest receptor exposure is determined by the shortest SID (greatest exposure rate).

151. (C) Spatial resolution is related to pixel pitch. The maximum spatial resolution is equal to the Nyquist frequency, 1/2 × the pixel pitch (mm). The wavelength of the electrical signal in the ADC is constant, and unaffected by the pixel pitch. DQE expresses the efficiency of digital system in detecting x-ray photons and convert them into an image signal, regardless of the size and pitch of the image matrix pixels. Digital imaging detectors do not use silver bromide grains.

152. (C) Once the PSP storage plate reading process is completed, any remaining data stored on the PSP are erased by exposing it to high-intensity light (called "erasure"); the PSP storage plate is then ready for reuse. If the erasure process is incomplete, remnants of the previous image remain and degrade the new image. The image shown in Figure 4-22 is an example of *incomplete erasure.* Residual image of ribs can be seen outside the collimated area, above the foot. The PSP undergoes three cycles: x-ray exposure, reading, and erasure.

153. (B) The radiographer selects a *processing algorithm* by selecting the anatomic part and particular projection on the computer/control panel. The CR unit then matches that information with a particular lookup table (LUT)—a characteristic curve that best matches the anatomic part being imaged. The observer is able to review the image and, if desired, change its appearance (through "windowing"); doing so changes the LUT. Hence, histogram analysis and use of the appropriate LUT together function to produce predictable image quality in CR.

154. **(A)** Grids are used in radiography to trap scattered radiation that otherwise would cause fog on the radiograph. *Grid ratio* is defined as the ratio of the height of the lead strips to the distance between them. *Grid frequency* refers to the number of lead strips per inch. *Focusing distance* and *grid radius* are terms denoting the distance range with which a focused grid may be used.

155. **(B)** The chest is composed of tissues with widely differing densities (bone and air), constituting high subject contrast. In an effort to "even out" these tissue densities and better visualize pulmonary vascular markings, high kilovoltage is generally used. This provides uniform penetration and permits visualization of the pulmonary vascular markings as well as bone and air tissue densities. The fact that the kilovoltage is increased means that the milliampere seconds value is reduced accordingly, and thus patient dose is reduced as well. Lower milliampere seconds value permits the use of sort of exposure time. A grid is usually used whenever high kilovoltage is required.

156. **(C)** Two of a grid's physical characteristics that determine its degree of efficiency in the removal of scattered radiation are *grid ratio* (the height of the lead strips compared with the distance between them) and the number of *lead strips per inch.* As the lead strips are made taller or the distance between them decreases, scattered radiation is more likely to be trapped before reaching the IR. A 12:1 ratio grid will absorb more scattered radiation than an 8:1 ratio grid. An undesirable but unavoidable characteristic of grids is that they do absorb some primary/useful photons as well as scattered photons. The higher the ratio grid, the more scatter radiation the grid will clean up, but more useful photons will be absorbed as well. The higher the primary to scattered photon transmission ratio, the more desirable is the grid. Higher ratio grids restrict positioning latitude more severely—grid centering must be more accurate (than with lower ratio grids) to avoid grid cutoff.

157. **(D)** In digital imaging, there are numerous *tonal values* that represent various *tissue densities* (i.e., x-ray attenuation properties), for example, bone, muscle, fat, blood-filled organs, air/gas, metal, contrast media, and pathologic processes. In CR, the CR scanner/reader recognizes these values and constructs a representative *grayscale* histogram of them, corresponding to the *anatomic characteristics of the imaged part.* Thus, all PA chest histograms are similar, all lateral chest histograms are similar, all pelvis histograms are similar, and so on.

A histogram is a *graphic representation* of *pixel value distribution.* The histogram is an analysis and graphic representation of all the densities from the PSP screen,

demonstrating the quantity of exposure, the number of pixels, and their value. Histograms are *unique to each body part* imaged.

Histogram appearance and *patient dose* can be affected by the radiographer's knowledge and skill using digital imaging, in addition to their degree of accuracy in *positioning* and *centering.* Collimation is exceedingly important to avoid *histogram analysis errors.* Lack of adequate collimation can result in signals outside the anatomic area being included in the exposure data recognition/histogram analysis. This can result in a variety of histogram analysis errors including excessively light, dark, or noisy images. Poor *collimation* can affect exposure level and exposure latitude; these changes are reflected in the images' informational numbers ("S number," "exposure index," etc.).

Other factors affecting histogram appearance, and therefore these informational numbers, include selection of the *correct processing algorithm* (e.g., chest vs. femur vs. cervical spine), changes in *scatter, source-to-image-receptor distance* (SID), *object-to-image-receptor distance* (OID), and *collimation*—in short, anything that affects scatter and/or dose.

158. **(C)** Tape used for immobilization is often imaged and can impair visualization of details. The *tape* used here (see Fig. 4-23) to assist with immobilization is a type of exposure *artifact.* Other examples of exposure artifacts include hairpins, dentures, and dressing gown snaps.

Excessive scattered radiation fog would produce a much more gray image; part motion would produce obvious blurriness; grid cutoff would be characterized by grid lines and/or loss of receptor exposure.

159. **(D)** Milliampere seconds (mAs) is the product of milliamperes (mA) and exposure time (s). Any combinations of milliamperes and time that will produce a given milliampere seconds value (i.e., a particular quantity of x-ray photons) will produce identical receptor exposure. This is known as the *reciprocity law.* The milliampere seconds value is directly proportional to x-ray beam *intensity, exposure rate, quantity,* or *number* of x-ray photons produced and greatly impacts patient dose. If the milliampere seconds value is doubled, the exposure rate, the patient dose, and the receptor exposure are doubled. If the milliampere seconds value is cut in half, the exposure rate, the patient dose, and receptor exposure are cut in half. The milliampere seconds value has no effect on spatial resolution.

160. **(B)** Positive contrast medium is *radiopaque;* negative contrast material is *radioparent.* Barium sulfate (radiopaque, positive contrast material) is used most frequently for examinations of the intestinal tract, and high-kilovoltage exposure factors are used to penetrate (to see through and behind) the barium. Water-based iodinated contrast media are also positive contrast agents. However, the K-edge binding energy of iodine *prohibits the use of much greater than 70 kV* with these materials. Higher kilovoltage values can obviate the effect of the contrast agent. Air is an example of a negative contrast agent, and high-kilovoltage factors are clearly not indicated.

161. (D) Shape distortion is caused by *misalignment of the x-ray tube, the part to be radiographed, and the image receptor/detector.* An object can be falsely imaged (*foreshortened* or *elongated*) by incorrect placement of the tube, the body part, or the IR. Only one of the three needs be misaligned for distortion to occur.

162. (A) The line-focus principle is a geometric principle illustrating that the *actual focal spot is larger than the effective (projected) focal spot.* The actual focal spot (target) is larger to accommodate heat over a larger area, and is angled so as to *project* a smaller focal spot, thus maintaining spatial resolution by reducing blur. The relationship between the exposure given to the IR and the resulting receptor exposure is expressed in the reciprocity law; the relationship between the SID and resulting IR exposure is expressed by the inverse-square law. Grid ratio and lines per inch are unrelated to the line-focus principle.

163. (A) Geometric factors affecting image sharpness/spatial resolution are focal spot size, source-to-image-receptor distance (SID), and object-to-image-receptor distance (OID). Motion is the single most important factor affecting sharpness/resolution. Even with all other factors being perfect, motion will destroy sharpness/resolution. Beam restriction/field size has a big impact on the production of scattered radiation and on patient dose/dose area product (DAP) but is unrelated to sharpness/spatial resolution.

164. (C) A certain amount of object unsharpness is an inherent part of every radiographic image because of the position and shape of anatomic structures within the body. Structures within the three-dimensional human body lie in different *planes*. In addition, the three-dimensional *shape* of solid anatomic structures rarely coincides with the shape of the divergent beam. Consequently, some structures are imaged with more inherent distortion than others, and shapes of anatomic structures can be entirely misrepresented. Structures *farther* from the IR will be distorted (i.e., *magnified*) more than those *closer* to the IR; structures *closer* to the x-ray source will be distorted (i.e., magnified) more than those *farther* from the x-ray source.

For the *shape* of anatomic structures to be accurately recorded, the structures must be parallel to the x-ray tube and the IR, and aligned with the central ray (CR). *The shape of anatomic structures lying at an angle within the body or placed away from the CR will be misrepresented on*

the IR. There are two types of shape distortion. If a linear structure is angled within the body, that is, not parallel with the long axis of the part/body and not parallel to the IR, that anatomic structure will appear *smaller—it will be foreshortened.* On the contrary, *elongation* occurs when the x-ray tube is angled.

Image details placed away from the path of the CR will be exposed by more divergent rays, resulting in *rotation distortion.* This is why the CR must be directed to the part of greatest interest.

Unless the edges of a three-dimensional *object* conform to the shape of the x-ray beam, blur or unsharpness will occur at the partially attenuating edge of the object. This can be accompanied by changes in receptor exposure, according to the thickness of areas traversed by the x-ray beam.

165. (D) The radiographer selects a *processing algorithm* by selecting the anatomic part and particular projection on the computer/control panel. The CR unit then matches that information with a particular LUT—a characteristic curve that best matches the anatomic part being imaged. The observer is able to review the image and, if desired, change its appearance (through "windowing"); doing so changes the LUT. Histogram analysis and use of the appropriate *LUT* together function to produce predictable image quality in CR. In addition, the radiographer can manipulate, that is, change and enhance, the digital image displayed on the display monitor through *postprocessing.* One way to alter image contrast and/or brightness is through *windowing.* The term *windowing* refers to some changes made to window width and/or window level, that is, a change in the LUT. Change in window *width* affects change in the number of gray shades, that is, *image contrast.* Change in window *level* affects change in the image *brightness.* Therefore, windowing and other postprocessing mechanisms permit the radiographer to affect changes in the image and produce "special effects," such as *contrast enhancement, edge enhancement, and image stitching.*

166. (D) *Grid ratio* is defined as the ratio between the height of the lead strips and the width of the distance between them (i.e., their height divided by the distance between them). If the height of the lead strips is 4.0 mm and the lead strips are 0.25 mm apart, the grid ratio must be 16:1 (4.0 divided by 0.25). The thickness of the lead strip is unrelated to grid ratio.

167. (C) Technical factors can be expressed in terms of milliampere seconds rather than milliamperes and time. The milliampere seconds value is a *quantitative* factor because it regulates x-ray beam *intensity, exposure rate, quantity,* or *number* of x-ray photons produced (the milliampere seconds value is the single most important technical factor associated with receptor exposure). *The milliampere seconds value is directly proportional to the intensity (i.e.,* exposure rate, number, and quantity) of x-ray photons produced and the resulting receptor exposure. If the milliampere seconds value is doubled, the exposure rate and the receptor exposure are doubled. If the milliampere seconds value is cut in half, the exposure rate and resulting receptor exposure are cut in half. Kilovoltage is the *qualitative* exposure factor—it determines beam quality by regulating photon energy (i.e., wavelength). Kilovoltage has an effect on receptor exposure, but it is not a proportional effect.

168. **(B)** An *upside-down focused grid* presents its lead strips in the opposite direction to that of the x-ray beam. This results in severe grid cutoff everywhere except in the central portion of the radiographic image (see Fig. 4-24). Severe grid cutoff of skull anatomy can be seen outside the central exposed area. A misaligned collimator would not show such symmetrical loss of receptor exposure, nor would an incorrectly selected AEC photocell. Focal spot is unrelated to image receptor exposure.

169. **(D)** Factors influencing spatial resolution in digital imaging are *motion* and *geometric factors* (focal spot size, OID, and SID). The spatial resolution of *direct* digital systems is fixed and is related to the detector element (*DEL*) size of the thin film transistor (*TFT*). The smaller the TFT-DEL size, the better the spatial resolution. DEL size of 100 μ provides a spatial resolution of about 5 lp/mm (available only in some digital mammography systems). DEL size of 200 μ provides a spatial resolution of about 2.5 lp/mm (general radiography). A 100-speed intensifying screen (analog) system offers a spatial resolution of about 10 lp/mm—significantly greater than, and currently unachievable in, digital imaging. Spatial resolution in digital imaging is fixed, but it is very important that radiographers are alert to the opportunity they have to utilize and control the remaining recorded detail factors (motion and geometric factors).

170. **(C)** According to the inverse-square law of radiation, as the distance between the radiation source and the IR decreases, the exposure rate increases. Therefore, a decrease in technical factors is indicated. The *exposure-maintenance formula* is used to determine new milliampere seconds values when changing distance:

$$\frac{(Old\ mAs)\,24}{(New\ mAs)\,x} = \frac{(Old\ D^2)\,38^2}{(New\ D^2)\,42^2}$$

$$\frac{24}{x} = \frac{1444}{1764}$$

$$1444x = 42{,}336$$

Thus, $x = 29.31$ mAs at 42-inch SID. Then, to determine the new exposure time (mA × s = mAs),

$$400x = 29.31$$

Thus, $x = 0.073$ s (73 ms) at 400 mA.

171. **(D)** The anatomic parts being imaged are composed of many different tissue types and have varying tissue densities, resulting in varying degrees of photon attenuation. This *differential attenuation* impacts the signal reaching the image receptor. Differential attenuation refers to differences in x-ray photon transmission through the part resulting in differences in signal (photons) reaching the digital image receptor. As tissue *thickness, density*, and *Z number* increase, attenuation increases via photoelectric and Compton processes.

172. **(A)** Diagnostic x-ray photons interact with tissue in a number of ways, but mostly they are involved in the photoelectric effect or the production of Compton scatter. *Compton scatter* is pictured in Figure 4-25; it occurs when a relatively *high-energy* (kilovoltage) photon uses *some* of its energy to eject an *outer*-shell electron. In so doing, the photon is deviated in direction and becomes a scattered photon. Compton scatter can cause objectionable scattered radiation fog in large structures such as the abdomen, but because its high energy is transmitted through the part, it is associated with less tissue absorption and patient dose than the photoelectric affect. Compton scatter poses a radiation hazard to personnel during procedures such as fluoroscopy. In the *photoelectric effect*, a relatively *low-energy* x-ray photon uses *all* its energy to eject an *inner*-shell electron, leaving a hole in the K shell. An L-shell electron then drops down to fill the K-shell vacancy and in so doing emits a characteristic ray whose energy is equal to the difference between the binding energies of the K and L shells. The photoelectric effect occurs with *high atomic number* absorbers such as bone and positive contrast media and is responsible for the production of radiographic contrast. It is helpful for the production of the radiographic image, but it contributes to the dose received by the patient (because it involves complete absorption of the incident photon).

173. **(B)** The abdomen is a thick structure that contains many structures of similar tissue density; thus, it requires increased exposure and a grid to absorb scattered radiation. The lumbar spine and hip are also dense structures requiring increased exposure and use of a grid. The knee, however, is frequently small enough to be radiographed without a grid. The general rule is that structures measuring more than 10 cm should be radiographed with a grid.

174. **(B)** *Attenuation* (decreased intensity/quantity through scattering or absorption) of the x-ray beam is a result of its *original energy and its interactions with different types and thicknesses of tissue*. The greater the original energy/quality (the higher the kilovoltage) of the incident beam, the less is the attenuation. The greater the effective *atomic number* of the tissues (tissue type and pathology determine absorbing properties), the greater is the beam attenuation. The greater the *volume of tissue* (subject density and thickness), the greater is the beam attenuation.

175. (C) Radiographers usually are able to stop voluntary motion using suspended respiration, careful instruction, and immobilization. However, *involuntary* motion also must be considered. To have a "stop action" effect on the heart when radiographing the chest, it is essential to use a short exposure time.

176. (B) The image shown in Figure 4-26 is an AP projection of the abdomen. The most obvious characteristic is its lack of contrast. The image is very gray because a grid was not used. The major function of a grid it is to improve image contrast. Remember that a grid is usually indicated for parts measuring greater than 10 cm. Image detail is related to image geometry, which is not impacted here. The lack of contrast impacts detail *visibility*.

177. (B) Spatial resolution is the term used to describe the IR's impact on image sharpness in digital imaging. Spatial resolution is receptor dependent. The IRs spatial resolution in direct digital systems is *fixed* and is inversely related to the detector element (*DEL*) size of the thin film transistor (*TFT*). The *smaller* the TFT-DEL size, the greater the spatial resolution. TFT-DEL sizes range from approximately 140 μ to 200 μ.

178. (B) The radiographer can manipulate the digital image displayed on the CRT through *postprocessing*. One way to alter image contrast and/or brightness is through *windowing*. This refers to some change made to *window width* and/or *window level*. Change in window width changes the number of gray shades, that is, *contrast scale/contrast resolution*. Change in window level changes the image brightness. Windowing and other postprocessing mechanisms permit the radiographer to produce "special effects" such as edge enhancement, image stitching, and image inversion, rotation, and reversal. A digital image is formed by a matrix of pixels in rows and columns. A matrix having 512 pixels in each row and column is a 512 × 512 matrix. The term *field of view* is used to describe how much of the patient (e.g., 150-mm diameter) is included in the matrix. The matrix or field of view can be changed without affecting the other, but changes in either will change pixel size. Automatic brightness control is associated with image intensification.

179. (A) *Noise* is an electronic term for anything that interferes with visualization of the image we wish to see. The signal-to-noise ratio (*SNR*) is important in image quality. The signal is directly related to the intensity/quantity of x-ray photons. An insufficient number of x-ray photons (milliampere seconds) can result in image noise. Digital images are subject to noise; it can appear as *graininess* called *quantum mottle*. There are several kinds of noise; noise cannot be removed in postprocessing.

As SNR increases, image quality increases but at the expense exposure dose. Intelligent selection of technical factors is still required and radiographers must be even more vigilant in minimizing patient exposure.

180. (D) According to the inverse-square law of radiation, the intensity or exposure rate of radiation is inversely proportional to the square of the distance from its source. Thus, as distance from the source of radiation increases, exposure rate decreases. Because exposure rate and image receptor exposure are directly proportional, if the exposure rate of a beam directed to an IR is decreased, the resulting image receptor exposure would be decreased proportionately.

181. (C) Radiopaque objects within the area of interest, such as buttons, snaps, zippers, hairpins, and dentures, should be removed before imaging whenever possible. Bulky or bunched clothing can produce undesirable radiographic artifacts and should therefore be removed whenever possible and replaced with a hospital dressing gown. Elastic waist garments can contribute to unnecessary and distracting exposure variations on abdominal images. Figure 4-27 demonstrates *dentures* artifact.

182. (C) Factors influencing sharpness/spatial resolution in digital imaging are very much the same as those factors affecting sharpness in analog imaging, that is, *motion* and *geometric factors* (focal spot size, OID, and SID). The spatial resolution of direct digital systems is *fixed* and is related to the *DEL* size of the *TFT*. The smaller the TFT-DEL size, the better the spatial resolution. DEL size of 100 μ provides a spatial resolution of about 5 lp/mm (available only in some digital mammography systems). DEL size of 200 μ provides a spatial resolution of about 2.5 lp/mm (general radiography). A 100-speed analog system offers a spatial resolution of about 10 lp/mm—significantly greater than, and currently unachievable in, digital imaging. Spatial resolution in digital imaging is fixed, but it is very important that radiographers are alert to the opportunity they have to utilize and control the remaining sharpness/detail factors (motion and geometric factors).

183. (D) Because *pneumoperitoneum* is an abnormal accumulation of *air or gas* in the peritoneal cavity, it would require a *decrease* in exposure factors. *Obstructed bowel* usually involves distended, air- or gas-filled bowel loops, again requiring a *decrease* in exposure factors. With *ascites*, there is an abnormal accumulation of *fluid* in the abdominal cavity, necessitating an *increase* in exposure factors. *Renal colic* is the pain associated with the passage of renal calculi; no change from the normal exposure factors is usually required.

184. (D) *Differential absorption* refers to the x-ray absorption characteristics of neighboring anatomic structures. The radiographic representation of these structures is called *radiographic contrast;* it may be enhanced with high-contrast technical factors, especially using low-kilovoltage levels. At low-kilovoltage levels, the photoelectric effect predominates.

185. **(C)** Software processing algorithms control digital image brightness. The *number* of x-ray photons produced, as determined by the programmed algorithm, is probably the most important aspect of the digital imaging process.

The total number of x-ray photons exiting the part is divided among all the pixels—and each pixel must have enough x-ray photons to provide a grayscale range. If there are *insufficient* x-ray photons for each pixel, noise (graininess) increases. Therefore, as SNR decreases, graininess increases. Digital image *graininess* can be caused by underexposure, incorrect processing, incorrect part algorithm selection (from the anatomic menu), inadequate collimation, and grid cutoff.

186. **(A)** *Fill factor* is described as the ratio of a pixel's *sensing area* to the area of the entire pixel. A pixel's sensing area receives data from the captured x-ray photons in the layer above, which are then converted to *light in indirect* flat-panel detectors or to *electrical charges and direct* flat-panel detectors. The Nyquist frequency is $1/2 \times$ the pixel pitch (mm) and describes the digital system spatial resolution. SNR refers to signal-to-noise ratio.

187. **(B)** Every x-ray image can be evaluated according to its spatial resolution and its contrast resolution. These qualities are closely related to the clarity, or detail, of the radiographic image. Spatial frequency can be used as an indication/measure of spatial resolution. Spatial frequency is measured in line pairs per millimeter. One line pair is defined as one black line on a light background having an interspace of the same width. Spatial resolution increases as spatial frequency increases, that is, they are directly related.

188. **(B)** As distance from the x-ray source increases, the x-ray beam diverges and covers a larger area and the quantity/intensity of x-ray available per unit area becomes less and less as distance increases. The intensity (quantity) of x-ray decreases according to the *inverse-square law,* that is, the intensity of x-ray at a particular distance from its source is *inversely proportional to the square of the distance.*

If the distance is *decreased,* the *intensity* of the x-ray beam *increases* according to the inverse-square law. The resulting *increase* in *receptor exposure* will require an adjustment of milliampere seconds (according to the exposure-maintenance formula) to reproduce the original receptor exposure.

189. **(A)** If a structure of a given length is not positioned parallel to the recording medium/detector, it will be projected smaller than its actual size (foreshortened). An example of this can be a lateral projection of the third digit. If the finger is positioned so as to be parallel to the IR, no distortion will occur. If, however, the finger is positioned so that its distal portion rests on the cassette while its proximal portion remains a distance from the IR, foreshortening will occur.

190. **(B)** Digital imaging *exposure data recognition* (EDR) and *automatic rescaling* offer *wide* latitude and automatic optimization of the values of interest (VOI) in the radiologic image. EDR, using the selected processing algorithm and its LUT, enables compensation for approximately 50% underexposure and 200% overexposure.

Although automatic/computerized optimization of the radiologic image is a wonderful tool, radiographers must be even more aware of their responsibility to keep patient dose to a minimum. Overexposure, though correctable via EDR, results in *increased patient dose*; underexposure results in decreased image quality because of increased image *noise*.

191. **(C)** Detective quantum efficiency (DQE) describes the percentage of incoming x-ray photons that are detected and absorbed by the receptor, for transformation to the x-ray image. Receptor systems having higher DQEs have the ability to produce high-quality images at lower doses. In CR, the receptor is the PSP. Digital receptors include TFTs and CCDs. DR can be either direct or indirect conversion. Systems without a scintillation/light conversion step generally have a higher DQE.

192. **(A)** One type of *indirect*-capture flat-panel detector uses cesium iodide or gadolinium oxysulfide as the *scintillator*, that is, which captures x-ray photons and emits light. That light is then transferred via a photodetector coupling agent—a CCD or TFT. In *direct*-capture flat-panel detector systems, x-ray energy is converted to an electrical signal in a single layer of material such as the semiconductor a-Se. Electric charges are applied to both surfaces of the a-Se, electron–hole pairs are created, and charges are read by TFT arrays located on the surfaces. The electrical signal is transferred directly to the ADC. The number of TFTs is equal to the number of image pixels.

Thus, the direct-capture system *eliminates the scintillator* step required in indirect DR. Because selenium has a relatively low Z number (compared with gadolinium [$Z = 64$] or cesium [$Z = 55$]), a-Se detectors are made thicker to improve detection, thus compensating for the low x-ray absorption of selenium. There is no diffusion of electrons, so spatial resolution is not affected in this manner.

193. **(C)** *Collimators* restrict the size of the irradiated field, thereby limiting the volume of irradiated tissue, and hence less scattered radiation is produced. Once radiation has scattered and emerged from the body, it can be trapped by the grid's lead strips. *Grids* effectively remove much of the scattered radiation in the remnant beam (which carry the *signal image*) before it reaches the IR where it forms the *latent* image, prior to digital processing. *Compression* can be applied to reduce the effect of excessive fatty tissue (e.g., in the abdomen)—in effect,

reducing the thickness of the part to be radiographed. Protective filtration impacts patient skin dose and is unrelated to exit x-ray photons; focal spot size impacts image sharpness/resolution and is unrelated to scattered radiation.

194. (C) Figure 4-28 illustrates that as distance from a light/x-ray source increases, the light/x-rays diverge and cover a larger area; the quantity of light/x-ray available per unit area becomes less and less as distance increases. The intensity (quantity) of light/x-ray decreases according to the *inverse-square law*, that is, the intensity at a particular distance from its source is inversely proportional to the square of the distance. *As the distance between the x-ray tube and image receptor increases, exposure rate (and IR exposure) decreases according to the inverse-square law.*

Because the anode's focal track is beveled, x-ray photons can freely diverge toward the cathode end of the x-ray tube. However, the "heel" of the focal track prevents x-ray photons from diverging toward the anode end of the tube. This results in varying intensity with fewer photons at the anode end and more photons at the cathode end.

X-ray tube targets are constructed according to the line-focus principle—the focal spot is angled to the vertical. As the actual focal spot is projected downward, it is foreshortened; thus, the effective focal spot is always smaller than the actual focal spot.

195. (B) A compensating filter is used to make up for widely differing tissue densities. For example, it is difficult to obtain a satisfactory image of the mediastinum and lungs simultaneously without the use of a compensating filter to "even out" the densities. With this device, the chest is radiographed using mediastinal factors, and a trough-shaped filter (thicker laterally) is used to absorb excess photons that would overexpose the lungs. The middle portion of the filter lets the photons pass to the mediastinum almost unimpeded. Filters that absorb the photons contributing to skin dose are inherent and added filters. Compensating filtration is unrelated to elimination of scattered radiation or fluoroscopy.

196. (C) In *digital* imaging, brightness and contrast are determined by computer software and monitor controls; *however, the principal factor in good digital image visibility and patient dose is still the result of proper IR exposure.* Kilovoltage selection determines penetration but not contrast; milliampere seconds determines dose but has no impact on brightness.

197. (C) The images shown in Figure 4-29 clearly demonstrate different scales of contrast. The radiographer can manipulate, that is, change or enhance, digital images displayed on the monitor through postprocessing. One way to alter image contrast and/or brightness is through windowing. The term windowing refers to some change made to window width and/or window level. Change in window width affects change in the number of gray shades, that is, image contrast—as demonstrated in the Figure 4-29. Change in window level affects change in the image brightness. Windowing and other postprocessing mechanisms permit the radiographer to affect changes in the image and produce special effects such as image enhancement, image stitching (useful in scoliosis examinations), image inversion, rotation, and reversal.

198. (D) In digital imaging, there are numerous *tonal values* that represent various *tissue densities* (i.e., x-ray attenuation properties), for example, bone, muscle, fat, blood-filled organs, air/gas, metal, contrast media, and pathologic processes. In CR, the CR scanner/reader recognizes all these values and constructs a representative *grayscale* histogram of them, corresponding to the *anatomic characteristics of the imaged part*. Thus, all PA chest histograms are similar, all lateral chest histograms are similar, all pelvis histograms are similar, and so on.

A histogram is a *graphic representation* of *pixel value distribution*. The histogram is an analysis and graphic representation of all the densities from the PSP screen, demonstrating the quantity of exposure, the number of pixels, and their value. Histograms are *unique to each body part* imaged.

Histogram appearance and *patient dose* can be affected by the radiographer's knowledge and skill using digital imaging, in addition to their degree of accuracy in *positioning* and *centering*. Collimation is exceedingly important to avoid *histogram analysis errors*. Lack of adequate collimation can result in signals outside the anatomic area being included in the exposure data recognition/histogram analysis. This can result in a variety of histogram analysis errors including excessively light, dark, or noisy images. Poor collimation can affect exposure level and exposure latitude; these changes are reflected in the images' informational numbers ("S number," "exposure index," etc.).

Other factors affecting histogram appearance, and therefore these informational numbers, include selection of the *correct processing algorithm* (e.g., chest vs. femur vs. cervical spine), changes in *scatter, source-to-image-receptor distance* (SID), *object-to-image-receptor distance* (OID), and *collimation*—in short, anything that affects scatter and/or dose.

199. (C) The actual focal spot is foreshortened as it projects down to the IR, becoming foreshortened and smaller in size. This is the line-focus principle. A smaller effective focal spot will produce better resolution/image sharpness. Focal spot has no effect on beam intensity (quantity).

200. (D) Slight-to-moderate over-/underexposure is corrected through the rescaling process. Input data are rearranged to match the desired pixel values. Low-pass filtering occurs during image reconstruction and removes high frequencies that can obscure low-frequency structures.

Question Number and Subspecialty correspond to subcategories in each of the four ARRT examination specification sections

1. Digital imaging characteristics
2. Selection of technical factors affecting radiographic quality
3. Technique charts
4. Digital imaging characteristics
5. Criteria for image evaluation of technical factors
6. Digital imaging characteristics
7. Selection of technical factors affecting radiographic quality
8. Digital imaging characteristics
9. Criteria for image evaluation of technical factors
10. Selection of technical factors affecting radiographic quality
11. Selection of technical factors affecting radiographic quality
12. Criteria for image evaluation of technical factors
13. Automatic exposure control
14. Technique charts
15. Selection of technical factors affecting radiographic quality
16. Criteria for image evaluation of technical factors
17. Criteria for image evaluation of technical factors
18. Digital imaging characteristics
19. Automatic exposure control
20. Criteria for image evaluation of technical factors
21. Digital imaging characteristics
22. Quality control of imaging equipment and accessories
23. Criteria for image evaluation of technical factors
24. Criteria for image evaluation of technical factors
25. Selection of technical factors affecting radiographic quality
26. Technique charts
27. Quality control of imaging equipment and accessories
28. Selection of technical factors affecting radiographic quality
29. Selection of technical factors affecting radiographic quality
30. Criteria for image evaluation of technical factors
31. Automatic exposure control
32. Quality control of imaging equipment and accessories
33. Selection of technical factors affecting radiographic quality
34. Criteria for image evaluation of technical factors
35. Selection of technical factors affecting radiographic quality
36. Selection of technical factors affecting radiographic quality
37. Selection of technical factors affecting radiographic quality
38. Digital imaging characteristics
39. Selection of technical factors affecting radiographic quality
40. Selection of technical factors affecting radiographic quality
41. Selection of technical factors affecting radiographic quality
42. Selection of technical factors affecting radiographic quality
43. Selection of technical factors affecting radiographic quality
44. Quality control of imaging equipment and accessories
45. Criteria for image evaluation of technical factors
46. Criteria for image evaluation of technical factors
47. Digital imaging characteristics
48. Selection of technical factors affecting radiographic quality
49. Quality control of imaging equipment and accessories
50. Quality control of imaging equipment and accessories
51. Image identification
52. Technique charts
53. Digital imaging characteristics
54. Quality control of imaging equipment and accessories
55. Digital imaging characteristics
56. Digital imaging characteristics
57. Criteria for image evaluation of technical factors
58. Selection of technical factors affecting radiographic quality
59. Technique charts
60. Digital imaging characteristics
61. Digital imaging characteristics
62. Digital imaging characteristics
63. Selection of technical factors affecting radiographic quality
64. Criteria for image evaluation of technical factors
65. Selection of technical factors affecting radiographic quality
66. Digital imaging characteristics
67. Criteria for image evaluation of technical factors
68. Digital imaging characteristics

69. Digital imaging characteristics
70. Selection of technical factors affecting radiographic quality
71. Selection of technical factors affecting radiographic quality
72. Selection of technical factors affecting radiographic quality
73. Selection of technical factors affecting radiographic quality
74. Digital imaging characteristics
75. Digital imaging characteristics
76. Quality control of imaging equipment and accessories
77. Selection of technical factors affecting radiographic quality
78. Selection of technical factors affecting radiographic quality
79. Criteria for image evaluation of technical factors
80. Criteria for image evaluation of technical factors
81. Selection of technical factors affecting radiographic quality
82. Quality control of imaging equipment and accessories
83. Technique charts
84. Digital imaging characteristics
85. Selection of technical factors affecting radiographic quality
86. Selection of technical factors affecting radiographic quality
87. Digital imaging characteristics
88. Digital imaging characteristics
89. Quality control of imaging equipment and accessories
90. Selection of technical factors affecting radiographic quality
91. Selection of technical factors affecting radiographic quality
92. Selection of technical factors affecting radiographic quality
93. Criteria for image evaluation of technical factors
94. Technique charts
95. Criteria for image evaluation of technical factors
96. Selection of technical factors affecting radiographic quality
97. Digital imaging characteristics
98. Criteria for image evaluation of technical factors
99. lection of technical factors affecting radiographic quality
100. Quality control of imaging equipment and accessories
101. Criteria for image evaluation of technical factors
102. Criteria for image evaluation of technical factors
103. Selection of technical factors affecting radiographic quality
104. Quality control of imaging equipment and accessories
105. Digital imaging characteristics
106. Digital imaging characteristics
107. Criteria for image evaluation of technical factors
108. Selection of technical factors affecting radiographic quality
109. Digital imaging characteristics
110. Technique charts
111. Selection of technical factors affecting radiographic quality
112. Selection of technical factors affecting radiographic quality
113. Selection of technical factors affecting radiographic quality
114. Selection of technical factors affecting radiographic quality
115. Digital imaging characteristics
116. Criteria for image evaluation of technical factors
117. Quality control of imaging equipment and accessories
118. Selection of technical factors affecting radiographic quality
119. Criteria for image evaluation of technical factors
120. Quality control of imaging equipment and accessories
121. Selection of technical factors affecting radiographic quality
122. Quality control of imaging equipment and accessories
123. Selection of technical factors affecting radiographic quality
124. Digital imaging characteristics
125. Digital imaging characteristics
126. Digital imaging characteristics
127. Selection of technical factors affecting radiographic quality
128. Digital imaging characteristics
129. Digital imaging characteristics
130. Selection of technical factors affecting radiographic quality
131. Criteria for image evaluation of technical factors
132. Technique charts
133. Digital imaging characteristics
134. Digital imaging characteristics
135. Selection of technical factors affecting radiographic quality
136. Selection of technical factors affecting radiographic quality
137. Quality control of imaging equipment and accessories
138. Criteria for image evaluation of technical factors
139. Selection of technical factors affecting radiographic quality
140. Digital imaging characteristics
141. Selection of technical factors affecting radiographic quality
142. Digital imaging characteristics
143. Selection of technical factors affecting radiographic quality

144. Automatic exposure control
145. Digital imaging characteristics
146. Digital imaging characteristics
147. Quality control of imaging equipment and accessories
148. Selection of technical factors affecting radiographic quality
149. Quality control of imaging equipment and accessories
150. Selection of technical factors affecting radiographic quality
151. Digital imaging characteristics
152. Criteria for image evaluation of technical factors
153. Digital imaging characteristics
154. Selection of technical factors affecting radiographic quality
155. Selection of technical factors affecting radiographic quality
156. Selection of technical factors affecting radiographic quality
157. Digital imaging characteristics
158. Criteria for image evaluation of technical factors
159. Selection of technical factors affecting radiographic quality
160. Technique charts
161. Criteria for image evaluation of technical factors
162. Selection of technical factors affecting radiographic quality
163. Selection of technical factors affecting radiographic quality
164. Criteria for image evaluation of technical factors
165. Digital imaging characteristics
166. Criteria for image evaluation of technical factors
167. Selection of technical factors affecting radiographic quality
168. Criteria for image evaluation of technical factors
169. Digital imaging characteristics
170. Selection of technical factors affecting radiographic quality

171. Technique charts
172. Technique charts
173. Technique charts
174. Technique charts
175. Selection of technical factors affecting radiographic quality
176. Criteria for image evaluation of technical factors
177. Digital imaging characteristics
178. Digital imaging characteristics
179. Digital imaging characteristics
180. Selection of technical factors affecting radiographic quality
181. Criteria for image evaluation of technical factors
182. Digital imaging characteristics
183. Technique charts
184. Selection of technical factors affecting radiographic quality
185. Digital imaging characteristics
186. Digital imaging characteristics
187. Quality control of imaging equipment and accessories
188. Selection of technical factors affecting radiographic quality
189. Criteria for image evaluation of technical factors
190. Digital imaging characteristics
191. Digital imaging characteristics
192. Digital imaging characteristics
193. Criteria for image evaluation of technical factors
194. Selection of technical factors affecting radiographic quality
195. Quality control of imaging equipment and accessories
196. Digital imaging characteristics
197. Digital imaging characteristics
198. Digital imaging characteristics
199. Selection of technical factors affecting radiographic quality
200. Digital imaging characteristics

TARGETED READING

Bushong SC. *Radiologic Science for Technologists.* 11th ed. St Louis, MO: Mosby; 2017.

Carlton RR, Adler AM, Balas V. *Principles of Radiographic Imaging.* 6th ed. Albany, NY: Delmar; 2020.

Carroll QB. *Radiography in the Digital Age.* 3rd ed. Springfield, IL: Charles C Thomas; 2018.

Carter C, Vealé B. *Digital Radiography and PACS.* 3rd ed. St Louis, MO: Mosby Elsevier; 2019.

Johnston JN, Fauber TL. *Essentials of Radiographic Physics and Imaging.* 3rd ed. St Louis, MO: Mosby Elsevier; 2020.

Orth D, *Essentials of Radiologic Science.* 2nd ed. Baltimore, MD: Lippincott Williams & Wilkins; 2017.

Saia DA. *Radiography PREP.* 9th ed. New York, NY: McGraw Hill; 2018.

Shephard CT. *Radiographic Image Production and Manipulation.* New York, NY: McGraw Hill; 2003.

Wolbarst AB. *Physics of Radiology.* 2nd ed. Madison, WI: Medical Physics Publishing; 2005.

Image Production: Equipment Operation and Quality Assurance

QUESTIONS

DIRECTIONS: Each of the numbered items or incomplete statements in this section is followed by answers or by completions of the statement. Select the *one* letter answer or completion that is *best* in each case.

1. Compared with the image on the input phosphor, the image on the output phosphor of the image intensifier is (select three)
- ❑ A. magnified
- ❑ B. distorted
- ❑ C. brighter
- ❑ D. dimmer
- ❑ E. inverted
- ❑ F. minified

2. Which of the following is/are components of the primary or low-voltage side of the x-ray circuit?
1. mA meter
2. Autotransformer
3. kV meter
- ❑ A. 1 only
- ❑ B. 1 and 2 only
- ❑ C. 2 and 3 only
- ❑ D. 1, 2, and 3

3. Which of the following is/are true statements regarding viewing conditions for digital images?
1. Excessive light causes dilation of the pupils of the eyes
2. Low-light level is desirable
3. Too much light causes images to appear dark
- ❑ A. 1 only
- ❑ B. 1 and 2 only
- ❑ C. 2 and 3 only
- ❑ D. 1, 2, and 3

4. As FOV decreases in image intensification (select three)
- ❑ A. output screen image is magnified
- ❑ B. output screen image has more noise
- ❑ C. mA increases
- ❑ D. output screen image has improved resolution
- ❑ E. the focal point is closer to the output phosphor
- ❑ F. voltage to the focusing lenses is decreased

5. Design characteristics of x-ray tube targets that determine heat capacity include the
1. rotation of the anode
2. diameter of the anode
3. size of the focal spot
- ❑ A. 1 only
- ❑ B. 1 and 2 only
- ❑ C. 1 and 3 only
- ❑ D. 1, 2, and 3

6. If exposure factors of 85 kV, 400 mA, and 12 ms yield an output exposure of 1.3 mGy, what is the value of milligray per milliampere seconds (mGy/mAs)?
- ❑ A. 36.9
- ❑ B. 17.2
- ❑ C. 3.69
- ❑ D. 0.27

7. The digital imaging processing function known as equalization (select three)
- ❑ A. is a preprocessing function
- ❑ B. is a computer software operation
- ❑ C. removes high-frequency noise
- ❑ D. removes densities that veil image details
- ❑ E. compresses the contrast scale

8. Which of the following waveforms shown in Figure 5-1 is illustrative of three-phase 12-pulse current?

❏ A. Diagram D
❏ B. Diagram E
❏ C. Diagram F
❏ D. Diagram G

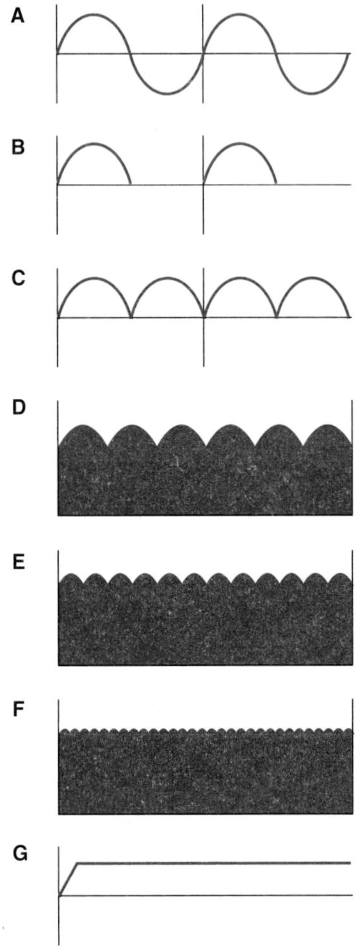

Figure 5-1

9. Advantages of flat-panel fluoroscopy over image-intensified fluoroscopy include (select four) which of the following?

❏ A. Greater maneuverability
❏ B. Improved contrast resolution
❏ C. Reduced DQE
❏ D. Eliminates need for ADC
❏ E. Considerably smaller size and weight
❏ F. Images require smaller data files

10. Which of the following terms is used to describe unsharp edges of tiny radiographic details?

❏ A. Diffusion
❏ B. Mottle
❏ C. Blur
❏ D. Umbra

11. How often are radiographic equipment collimators required to be evaluated?

❏ A. Annually
❏ B. Biannually
❏ C. Semiannually
❏ D. Quarterly

12. Which of the following will improve the spatial resolution of image-intensified images?

1. A very thin input phosphor layer
2. A larger diameter input screen
3. Increased total brightness gain
   ❏ A. 1 only
   ❏ B. 1 and 2 only
   ❏ C. 1 and 3 only
   ❏ D. 1, 2, and 3

13. X-ray tube characteristics/qualities include which of the following?

1. The target material should have a high atomic number and a high-melting point
2. The useful beam emerges from the port window
3. The cathode assembly receives both low and high voltages
   ❏ A. 1 only
   ❏ B. 2 only
   ❏ C. 1 and 2 only
   ❏ D. 1, 2, and 3

14. A parallel-plate ionization chamber receives a particular charge as x-ray photons travel through it. This is the operating principle of which of the following devices?

❏ A. AEC
❏ B. Image intensifier
❏ C. Video recorder
❏ D. Photospot camera

15. The total number of x-ray photons produced at the target is contingent on the

1. tube current
2. target material
3. square of the kilovoltage
   ❏ A. 1 only
   ❏ B. 1 and 2 only
   ❏ C. 2 and 3 only
   ❏ D. 1, 2, and 3

16. Which of the following combinations would pose the greatest heat hazard to a particular single-phase anode?

❏ A. 1.2-mm focal spot, 92 kV, 1.5 mAs
❏ B. 0.6-mm focal spot, 80 kV, 3 mAs
❏ C. 1.2-mm focal spot, 70 kV, 6 mAs
❏ D. 0.6-mm focal spot, 60 kV, 12 mAs

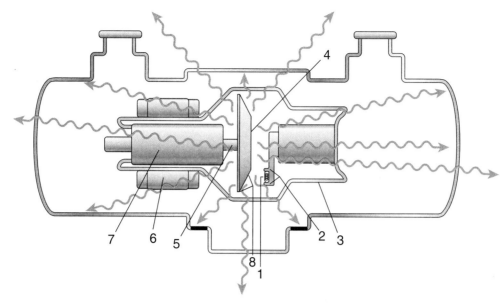

Figure 5-2

17. Of what material is number 1 in Figure 5-2 made?
- ❏ A. Nickel
- ❏ B. Molybdenum
- ❏ C. Tungsten
- ❏ D. Copper

18. Which of the following systems functions to compensate for changes in patient/part thicknesses, FOV, and OID during flat-panel detector (FPD) fluoroscopic procedures?
- ❏ A. Automatic exposure rate control
- ❏ B. Electronic magnification
- ❏ C. Automatic resolution control
- ❏ D. Flux gain

19. Delivery of large exposures to a cold anode or the use of exposures exceeding tube limitation can result in
1. increased tube output
2. cracking of the anode
3. rotor-bearing damage
- ❏ A. 1 only
- ❏ B. 1 and 2 only
- ❏ C. 2 and 3 only
- ❏ D. 1, 2, and 3

20. Deposition of vaporized tungsten on the inner surface of the x-ray tube glass window
1. acts as additional filtration
2. results in increased tube output
3. results in anode pitting
- ❏ A. 1 only
- ❏ B. 1 and 2 only
- ❏ C. 2 and 3 only
- ❏ D. 1, 2, and 3

21. What is the relationship between kilovoltage and HVL?
- ❏ A. As kilovoltage increases, the HVL increases
- ❏ B. As kilovoltage decreases, the HVL increases
- ❏ C. If the kilovoltage is doubled, the HVL doubles
- ❏ D. If the kilovoltage is doubled, the HVL is squared

22. As window width decreases
- ❏ A. contrast scale increases
- ❏ B. contrast scale decreases
- ❏ C. brightness increases
- ❏ D. brightness decreases

23. Circuit devices that permit electrons to flow in only one direction are
- ❏ A. solid-state diode rectifiers
- ❏ B. resistors
- ❏ C. transformers
- ❏ D. autotransformers

24. Scintillation is associated with all the following, *except*
- ❏ A. amorphous silicon
- ❏ B. amorphous selenium
- ❏ C. cesium iodide
- ❏ D. gadolinium oxysulfide

25. The AEC backup timer functions to
1. protect the patient from overexposure
2. protect the x-ray tube from excessive heat
3. increase or decrease programmed receptor exposure
- ❏ A. 1 only
- ❏ B. 1 and 2 only
- ❏ C. 2 and 3 only
- ❏ D. 1, 2, and 3

26. Which of the following devices converts mechanical energy to electrical energy?
- ❑ A. Motor
- ❑ B. Generator
- ❑ C. Stator
- ❑ D. Rotor

27. The filtering effect of the x-ray tube's glass envelope and its oil coolant are collectively called
- ❑ A. inherent filtration
- ❑ B. added filtration
- ❑ C. compensating filtration
- ❑ D. port filtration

28. A slit camera is used to measure
1. focal spot size
2. spatial resolution
3. dynamic range
- ❑ A. 1 only
- ❑ B. 1 and 2 only
- ❑ C. 1 and 3 only
- ❑ D. 1, 2, and 3

29. All of the following statements regarding mobile radiographic equipment are true, *except*
- ❑ A. exposure switches must be the "dead-man" type
- ❑ B. the radiographer must alert individuals in the area before making the exposure
- ❑ C. the exposure cord must permit the operator to stand at least 4 feet from the patient, x-ray tube, and useful beam
- ❑ D. a lead apron should be carried with the unit and worn by the radiographer during exposure

30. Which of the following causes pitting, or many small surfaces melt, of the anode's focal track?
- ❑ A. Vaporized tungsten on the glass envelope
- ❑ B. Loss of anode rotation
- ❑ C. A large amount of heat to a cold anode
- ❑ D. Repeated, frequent overloading

31. The advantages of collimators over aperture diaphragms and flare cones include which of the following?
1. The variety of field sizes available
2. More efficient beam restriction
3. Better cleanup of scattered radiation
- ❑ A. 1 only
- ❑ B. 1 and 2 only
- ❑ C. 1 and 3 only
- ❑ D. 2 and 3 only

32. Which of the following evaluates focal spot accuracy as a function of geometric blur?
- ❑ A. Pinhole camera
- ❑ B. Slit camera
- ❑ C. Star pattern
- ❑ D. Focus pattern

33. Which of the following are the characteristics of the metallic element tungsten?
1. Ready dissipation of heat
2. High-melting point
3. High atomic number
- ❑ A. 1 only
- ❑ B. 1 and 2 only
- ❑ C. 2 and 3 only
- ❑ D. 1, 2, and 3

34. What grid ratio is represented in the illustration shown in Figure 5-3?
- ❑ A. 5:1
- ❑ B. 8:1
- ❑ C. 12:1
- ❑ D. 16:1

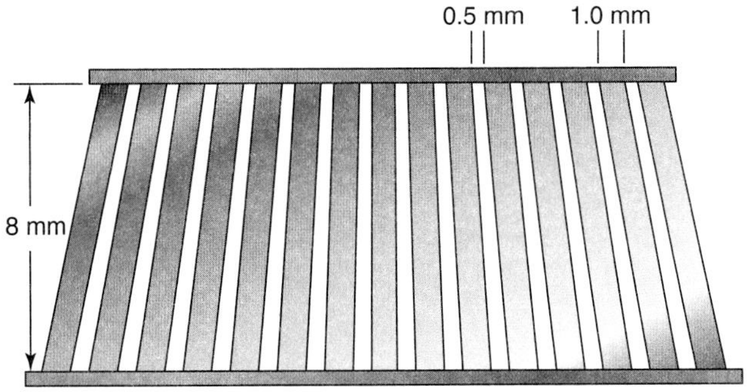

Figure 5-3

35. The voltage ripple associated with a three-phase, six-pulse rectified generator is about
- ❑ A. 4%
- ❑ B. 13%
- ❑ C. 32%
- ❑ D. 100%

36. Which of the following modes of a triple-field image intensifier will result in the highest patient dose?
- ❑ A. Its 25-inch mode
- ❑ B. Its 17-inch mode
- ❑ C. Its 12-inch mode
- ❑ D. Diameter does not affect patient dose

37. A high-speed electron is decelerated as it is attracted to a tungsten atom nucleus. This results in
- ❑ A. Bremsstrahlung radiation
- ❑ B. characteristic radiation
- ❑ C. Compton scatter
- ❑ D. a photoelectric effect

38. All of the following are components of the image intensifier, *except*
- ❑ A. the photocathode
- ❑ B. the focusing lenses
- ❑ C. the TV monitor
- ❑ D. the accelerating anode

39. Which of the following are components of digital imaging?
1. Computer manipulation of the image
2. Formation of an electronic image on the radiation detector
3. Formation of an x-ray image directly on the IR
   - ❏ A. 1 only
   - ❏ B. 1 and 2 only
   - ❏ C. 2 and 3 only
   - ❏ D. 1, 2, and 3

40. Which of the following is used in digital fluoroscopy (DF), replacing the image intensifier's television camera tube?
- ❏ A. Solid-state diode
- ❏ B. Charge coupled device
- ❏ C. Photostimulable phosphor
- ❏ D. Vidicon

41. With what frequency must radiographic equipment be checked for linearity and reproducibility?
- ❏ A. Annually
- ❏ B. Biannually
- ❏ C. Semiannually
- ❏ D. Quarterly

42. The regular measurement and evaluation of radiographic equipment components and their performance is most accurately termed as
- ❏ A. postprocessing
- ❏ B. quality assurance
- ❏ C. quality control
- ❏ D. quality congruence

43. Which of the following are typical examples of digital imaging?
1. MRI
2. CT
3. CR
   - ❏ A. 1 only
   - ❏ B. 1 and 2 only
   - ❏ C. 1 and 3 only
   - ❏ D. 1, 2, and 3

44. In fluoroscopy, the automatic brightness control is used to adjust the
- ❏ A. kilovoltage (kV) and milliamperage (mA)
- ❏ B. backup timer
- ❏ C. milliamperage (mA) and time
- ❏ D. kilovoltage (kV) and time

45. Which of the following terms describes the amount of electric charge flowing per second?
- ❏ A. Voltage
- ❏ B. Current
- ❏ C. Resistance
- ❏ D. Capacitance

46. How often are radiographic equipment kilovoltage settings required to be evaluated?
- ❏ A. Annually
- ❏ B. Biannually
- ❏ C. Semiannually
- ❏ D. Quarterly

47. What is the device that directs the light emitted from the image intensifier to various viewing and imaging apparatus?
- ❏ A. Output phosphor
- ❏ B. Beam splitter
- ❏ C. Spot image device
- ❏ D. Automatic brightness control

48. The image-intensifier tube's input phosphor functions to convert
- ❏ A. kinetic energy to light
- ❏ B. x-rays to light
- ❏ C. electrons to light
- ❏ D. fluorescent light to electrons

49. Which of the following contribute(s) to inherent filtration?
1. X-ray tube glass envelope
2. X-ray tube port window
3. Aluminum between the tube housing and the collimator
   - ❏ A. 1 only
   - ❏ B. 1 and 2 only
   - ❏ C. 1 and 3 only
   - ❏ D. 1, 2, and 3

50. Digital imaging subject contrast is the result of
- ❏ A. x-ray beam quantity and quality
- ❏ B. varying intensities of the primary beam
- ❏ C. signal differences within the remnant beam
- ❏ D. grid ratio and alignment

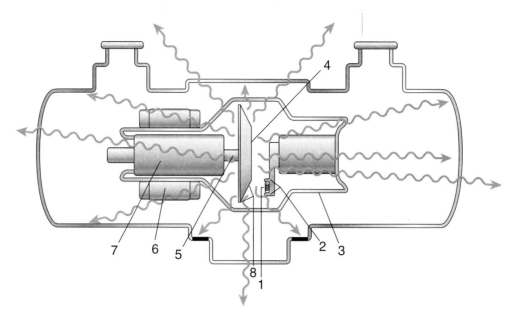

Figure 5-4

51. Which x-ray tube component does the number 7 in Figure 5-4 indicate?

❑ A. Anode stem
❑ B. Rotor
❑ C. Stator
❑ D. Focal track

52. Select the three correct statements regarding the structures identified as numbers 6 and 7 in Figure 5-4?

❑ A. They operate on the principle of electromagnetic induction
❑ B. Number 6 is the stator
❑ C. They function to produce thermionic emission
❑ D. They function to rotate the anode
❑ E. They operate on the principle of self-induction
❑ F. Number 6 is the rotor

53. The total brightness gain of an image intensifier is the product of

1. flux gain
2. minification gain
3. focusing gain
    ❑ A. 1 only
    ❑ B. 2 only
    ❑ C. 1 and 2 only
    ❑ D. 1 and 3 only

54. The advantages of CMOS (complementary metal oxide semiconductors) over CCDs (charge coupled devices) include which of the following?

1. Less expensive
2. Much greater speed
3. Better image quality
    ❑ A. 1 only
    ❑ B. 1 and 2 only
    ❑ C. 2 and 3 only
    ❑ D. 1, 2, and 3

55. Which of the following occurs during Bremsstrahlung (Brems) radiation production?

❑ A. An electron makes a transition from an outer to an inner electron shell
❑ B. An electron approaching a positive nuclear charge changes direction and loses energy
❑ C. A high-energy photon ejects an outer-shell electron
❑ D. A low-energy photon ejects an inner-shell electron

56. Which of the following are the functions of a picture archiving and communication system (PACS)?

1. Processing of digital images
2. Reception of digital images
3. Storage of digital images
    ❑ A. 1 only
    ❑ B. 1 and 2 only
    ❑ C. 2 and 3 only
    ❑ D. 1, 2, and 3

57. How many half-value layers will it take to reduce an x-ray beam whose intensity is 88 mGy/min to an intensity of less than 12 mGy/min?
- ❏ A. 2
- ❏ B. 3
- ❏ C. 4
- ❏ D. 8

58. Which of the following functions to increase the milliamperage?
- ❏ A. Increase in charge of anode
- ❏ B. Increase in heat of the filament
- ❏ C. Increase in kilovoltage
- ❏ D. Increase in focal spot size

59. As a general rule, a grid is usually used when
1. less patient dose is required
2. using high kV
3. radiographing a large or dense body part
- ❏ A. 1 only
- ❏ B. 1 and 2 only
- ❏ C. 2 and 3 only
- ❏ D. 1, 2, and 3

60. Which of the following combinations will offer the greatest detail sharpness?
- ❏ A. 17° target angle, 1.2-mm actual focal spot
- ❏ B. 10° target angle, 1.2-mm actual focal spot
- ❏ C. 17° target angle, 0.6-mm actual focal spot
- ❏ D. 10° target angle, 0.6-mm actual focal spot

61. Which number in the Figure 5-5 represents magnification mode?
- ❏ A. Number 1
- ❏ B. Number 2
- ❏ C. Number 7
- ❏ D. Number 8

62. Which number in the Figure 5-5 represents electrostatic focusing lens?
- ❏ A. Number 5
- ❏ B. Number 6
- ❏ C. Number 4
- ❏ D. Number 2

63. Advantages of CCDs over the use of television cameras in image intensification include which of the following?
1. Compact size
2. Improved resolution
3. Higher DQE
- ❏ A. 1 only
- ❏ B. 1 and 2 only
- ❏ C. 2 and 3 only
- ❏ D. 1, 2, and 3

64. Which of the following information is necessary to determine the maximum safe kilovoltage using the appropriate x-ray tube rating chart?
1. Milliamperage and exposure time
2. Focal spot size
3. Imaging system speed
- ❏ A. 1 only
- ❏ B. 1 and 2 only
- ❏ C. 2 and 3 only
- ❏ D. 1, 2, and 3

65. Spatial resolution in computed radiography increases as
1. monitor matrix size decreases
2. PSP crystal size decreases
3. laser beam size decreases
- ❏ A. 1 only
- ❏ B. 1 and 2 only
- ❏ C. 2 and 3 only
- ❏ D. 1, 2, and 3

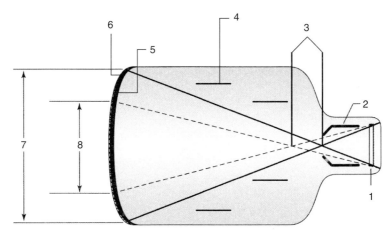

Figure 5-5

66. The voltage across the x-ray tube in three-phase equipment
1. drops to zero every 180°
2. is 87%–96% of the maximum value
3. is at nearly constant potential
   - ❏ A. 1 only
   - ❏ B. 2 only
   - ❏ C. 1 and 2 only
   - ❏ D. 2 and 3 only

67. Which of the following would be appropriate IP front material(s)?
1. Tungsten
2. Magnesium
3. Bakelite
   - ❏ A. 1 only
   - ❏ B. 1 and 2 only
   - ❏ C. 2 and 3 only
   - ❏ D. 1, 2, and 3

68. If the distance from the focal spot to the center of the collimator's mirror is 6 inches, what distance should the illuminator's light bulb be from the center of the mirror?
   - ❏ A. 3 inches
   - ❏ B. 6 inches
   - ❏ C. 9 inches
   - ❏ D. 12 inches

69. The image intensifier's input phosphor generally is composed of
   - ❏ A. cesium iodide
   - ❏ B. zinc cadmium sulfide
   - ❏ C. gadolinium oxysulfide
   - ❏ D. calcium tungstate

70. The essential function of an AEC is to
   - ❏ A. provide a brighter fluoroscopic image
   - ❏ B. automatically restrict the field size
   - ❏ C. terminate the x-ray exposure once the IR is correctly exposed
   - ❏ D. automatically increase or decrease incoming line voltages

71. Grid interspace material can be made of
1. carbon fiber
2. aluminum
3. plastic fiber
   - ❏ A. 1 only
   - ❏ B. 1 and 2 only
   - ❏ C. 2 and 3 only
   - ❏ D. 1, 2, and 3

72. If the primary coil of a high-voltage transformer is supplied by 220 V and has 400 turns and the secondary coil has 100,000 turns, what is the voltage induced in the secondary coil?
   - ❏ A. 80 kV
   - ❏ B. 55 kV
   - ❏ C. 80 V
   - ❏ D. 55 V

73. Which of the following circuit devices operate(s) on the principle of self-induction?
1. Autotransformer
2. Rectifiers
3. High-voltage transformer
   - ❏ A. 1 only
   - ❏ B. 1 and 2 only
   - ❏ C. 2 and 3 only
   - ❏ D. 1, 2, and 3

74. When the radiographer selects kilovoltage on the control panel, which device is adjusted?
   - ❏ A. Step-up transformer
   - ❏ B. Autotransformer
   - ❏ C. Filament circuit
   - ❏ D. Rectifier circuit

75. The brightness level of the fluoroscopic image can vary with
1. milliamperage
2. kilovoltage
3. patient thickness
   - ❏ A. 1 only
   - ❏ B. 1 and 2 only
   - ❏ C. 1 and 3 only
   - ❏ D. 1, 2, and 3

76. Which of the following does Figure 5-6 represent?
   - ❏ A. Compton scatter
   - ❏ B. Bremsstrahlung radiation
   - ❏ C. Photoelectric effect
   - ❏ D. Characteristic radiation

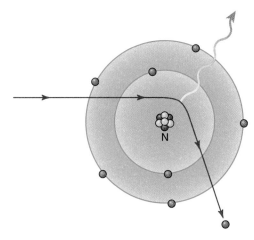

Figure 5-6

77. Guidelines regarding the use, care, and maintenance of protective lead aprons include (select three) which of the following?

❏ A. They should be hung on a rack or draped over a bar when not in use

❏ B. Federal law requires a minimum Pb equivalent of 0.25 mm

❏ C. They should be folded carefully and stored safely when not in use

❏ D. They should be x-rayed semiannually to detect any cracks

❏ E. They protect from scatter and leakage radiation

78. A change in the size of the actual focal spot will cause a change in (select three)

❏ A. detail sharpness

❏ B. image contrast

❏ C. effective focal spot size

❏ D. spatial resolution

❏ E. image brightness

79. All of the following are associated with the anode, *except*

❏ A. the line-focus principle

❏ B. the heel effect

❏ C. the focal track

❏ D. thermionic emission

80. Which part of an induction motor is located within the x-ray tube glass envelope?

❏ A. Filament

❏ B. Focusing cup

❏ C. Stator

❏ D. Rotor

81. Regulations governing quality control of imaging equipment include (select three) which of the following?

❏ A. The variation in x-ray intensity for a given exposure must not exceed 10%

❏ B. Beam alignment must be accurate to within 2% of the SID

❏ C. The control panel must indicate when the x-ray tube is energized

❏ D. Linearity variation must not exceed 20% when testing mA stations

❏ E. Total filtration must be at least 2.5-mm Al equivalent for 70 kV and above

82. As electrons impinge on the anode surface, less than 1% of their kinetic energy is changed to

❏ A. x-rays

❏ B. heat

❏ C. gamma rays

❏ D. recoil electrons

83. Moving the image intensifier closer to the patient during fluoroscopy

1. decreases the SID
2. decreases patient dose
3. improves image quality

❏ A. 1 only

❏ B. 1 and 2 only

❏ C. 1 and 3 only

❏ D. 1, 2, and 3

84. Figure 5-7 illustrates the

❏ A. inverse-square law

❏ B. line-focus principle

❏ C. reciprocity law

❏ D. anode heel effect

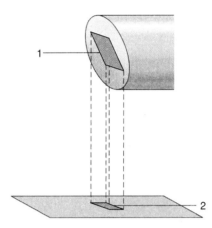

Figure 5-7

85. Although the stated focal spot size is measured directly under the actual focal spot, focal spot size actually varies along the length of the x-ray beam. At which portion of the x-ray beam is the effective focal spot the smallest?

❏ A. At its outer edge

❏ B. Along the path of the central ray

❏ C. At the cathode end

❏ D. At the anode end

86. Which of the following x-ray circuit devices is located in the secondary/high-voltage portion of the x-ray circuit?

❏ A. The timer

❏ B. The kilovoltage meter

❏ C. The milliamperage meter

❏ D. The autotransformer

87. Which of the following is/are associated with magnification fluoroscopy?

1. Higher patient dose than nonmagnification fluoroscopy
2. Higher voltage to the focusing lenses
3. Image intensifier focal point closer to the input phosphor
   - ❏ A. 1 only
   - ❏ B. 1 and 2 only
   - ❏ C. 2 and 3 only
   - ❏ D. 1, 2, and 3

88. Advantages of battery-powered mobile x-ray units include their

1. ability to store a large quantity of energy
2. ability to store energy for extended periods of time
3. ease of maneuverability
   - ❏ A. 1 only
   - ❏ B. 1 and 2 only
   - ❏ C. 2 and 3 only
   - ❏ D. 1, 2, and 3

89. The device that receives the remnant beam, converts it into light, and then increases the brightness of that light is the

- ❏ A. charge coupled device (CCD)
- ❏ B. spot image device
- ❏ C. image intensifier
- ❏ D. television monitor

90. Off-focus, or extrafocal, radiation is minimized by

- ❏ A. avoiding the use of very high kilovoltages
- ❏ B. restricting the x-ray beam as close to its source as possible
- ❏ C. using compression devices to reduce tissue thickness
- ❏ D. avoiding extreme collimation

91. Which of the following factors contribute(s) to the efficient performance of a grid?

1. Grid ratio
2. Number of lead strips per inch
3. Amount of scatter transmitted through the grid
   - ❏ A. 1 only
   - ❏ B. 2 only
   - ❏ C. 1 and 2 only
   - ❏ D. 1, 2, and 3

92. The AEC device operates on which of the following principles?

1. Delivery of the required exposure time
2. A parallel-plate ionization chamber charged by x-ray photons
3. Motion of magnetic fields inducing current in a conductor
   - ❏ A. 1 only
   - ❏ B. 2 only
   - ❏ C. 1 and 2 only
   - ❏ D. 1, 2, and 3

93. The kilovoltage settings on radiographic equipment must be tested annually and must be accurate to within

- ❏ A. ± 2 kV
- ❏ B. ± 4 kV
- ❏ C. ± 6 kV
- ❏ D. ± 8 kV

94. If 92 kV and 15 mAs were used for a particular abdominal exposure with single-phase equipment, what milliampere seconds value would be required to produce a similar radiograph with three-phase, 12-pulse equipment?

- ❏ A. 36
- ❏ B. 24
- ❏ C. 10
- ❏ D. 7.5

95. Bone densitometry is often performed to

1. measure degree of bone (de)mineralization
2. evaluate the results of osteoporosis treatment/therapy
3. evaluate the condition of soft tissue adjacent to bone
   - ❏ A. 1 only
   - ❏ B. 1 and 2 only
   - ❏ C. 2 and 3 only
   - ❏ D. 1, 2, and 3

96. Required corrections made to "raw" digital image data that occur as a result of inherent flaws in the image acquisition system is called

- ❏ A. preprocessing
- ❏ B. postprocessing
- ❏ C. windowing
- ❏ D. leveling

97. When using the smaller field in a dual-field image intensifier

1. the image is magnified
2. the image is brighter
3. a larger anatomic area is viewed
   - ❏ A. 1 only
   - ❏ B. 1 and 3 only
   - ❏ C. 2 and 3 only
   - ❏ D. 1, 2, and 3

98. In Figure 5-8, what is the maximum safe milliamperage that may be used with a 0.05-s exposure and 120 kV, using the three-phase, 2.0-mm focal spot x-ray tube?

❏ A. 300 mA
❏ B. 400 mA
❏ C. 500 mA
❏ D. 600 mA

99. Referring to the anode cooling chart in Figure 5-9, if the anode is saturated with 300,000 heat units (HU), how long will the anode need to cool before another 100,000 HU can be safely applied?

❏ A. 1 min
❏ B. 2 min
❏ C. 3 min
❏ D. 4 min

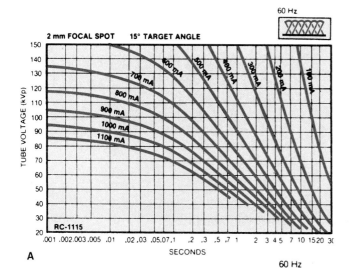

A

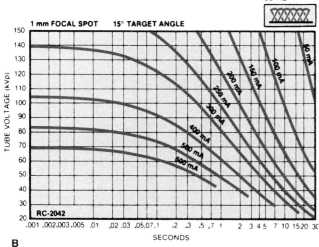

B

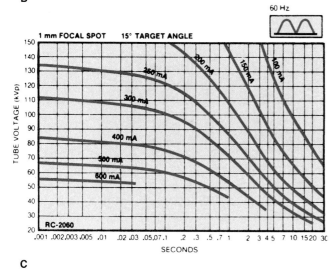

C

Figure 5-8. Reproduced, with permission, from Dunlee Tech Data Publication 50014.

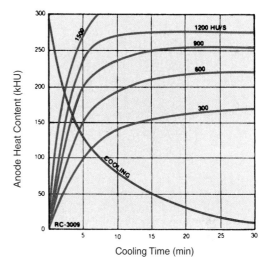

Figure 5-9. Reproduced, with permission, from Dunlee Tech Data Publication 50014.

100. Which digital postprocessing operation removes image noise?

❏ A. Edge enhancement
❏ B. Smoothing
❏ C. Aliasing
❏ D. Windowing

101. Anode angle will have an effect on the
1. severity of the heel effect
2. focal spot size
3. heat-load capacity

❏ A. 1 only
❏ B. 2 only
❏ C. 1 and 2 only
❏ D. 1, 2, and 3

102. The minimum response time of an automatic exposure control (AEC)

❏ A. is the time required to energize the intensifying phosphors
❏ B. is its shortest possible exposure time
❏ C. functions to protect the patient from overexposure
❏ D. functions to protect the tube from excessive heat

103. In which of the following examinations would an IP front with very low absorption properties be especially important?

❏ A. Abdominal radiography
❏ B. Extremity radiography
❏ C. Angiography
❏ D. Mammography

104. Which of the following is most closely related to Figure 5-10?

❏ A. Low kV
❏ B. High kV
❏ C. Low mA
❏ D. High mA

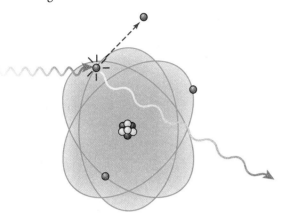

Figure 5-10

105. Which of the following formulas would the radiographer use to determine the total number of heat units (HU) produced with a given exposure using three-phase, six-pulse equipment?

❏ A. mA × time × kV
❏ B. mA × time × kV × 0.6
❏ C. mA × time × kV × 1.2
❏ D. mA × time × kV × 1.4

106. A device used to ensure reproducible radiographs, regardless of tissue density variations, is the

❏ A. automatic exposure control
❏ B. penetrometer
❏ C. grid device
❏ D. induction motor

107. The number of details visibly represented on the digital image is increased by

1. increased dynamic range
2. longer grayscale
3. increased bit depth

❏ A. 1 only
❏ B. 1 and 2 only
❏ C. 2 and 3 only
❏ D. 1, 2, and 3

108. Advantages of smaller diameter input screens in image intensification include which of the following?

1. Improved resolution
2. Availability of large FOV
3. Image magnification

❏ A. 1 and 2 only
❏ B. 2 and 3 only
❏ C. 1 and 3 only
❏ D. 1, 2, and 3

109. The device used to change alternating current to unidirectional current is

❏ A. a capacitor
❏ B. a solid-state diode
❏ C. a transformer
❏ D. a generator

110. Star and wye configurations are related to

❏ A. autotransformers
❏ B. three-phase transformers
❏ C. rectification systems
❏ D. AECs

111. Which x-ray tube component does the number 5 in Figure 5-11 indicate?

❏ A. Anode stem
❏ B. Rotor
❏ C. Stator
❏ D. Focal track

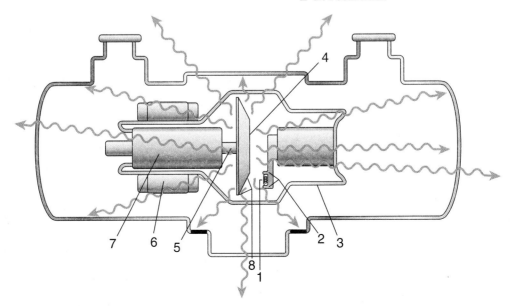

Figure 5-11

112. Which part of an induction motor is located outside the x-ray tube glass envelope?

❏ A. Filament
❏ B. Focusing cup
❏ C. Stator
❏ D. Rotor

113. Which of the following factors determine AEC exposure termination?

1. Tissue thickness and density
2. Positioning of the object with respect to the photocell
3. Beam restriction

❏ A. 1 only
❏ B. 1 and 2 only
❏ C. 2 and 3 only
❏ D. 1, 2, and 3

114. To maintain image clarity in an image-intensifier system, the path of electron flow from the photocathode to the output phosphor is controlled by

❏ A. the accelerating anode
❏ B. electrostatic lenses
❏ C. the vacuum glass envelope
❏ D. the input phosphor

115. Which of the following will serve to increase the effective energy of the x-ray beam?

1. Increase in added filtration
2. Increase in kilovoltage
3. Increase in milliamperage

❏ A. 1 only
❏ B. 2 only
❏ C. 1 and 2 only
❏ D. 1, 2, and 3

116. A photostimulable phosphor (PSP) is used with

❏ A. CR
❏ B. DR
❏ C. FOV
❏ D. ROI

117. The angle of transmitted scattered radiation is smaller with

❏ A. high-ratio grids
❏ B. low-ratio grids
❏ C. high mAs factors
❏ D. low mAs factors

118. An incorrect relationship between the primary beam and the center of a focused grid results in

1. an increase in scattered radiation production
2. grid cutoff
3. insufficient receptor exposure

❏ A. 1 only
❏ B. 1 and 2 only
❏ C. 2 and 3 only
❏ D. 1, 2, and 3

119. A quality control (QC) program includes checks on which of the following radiographic equipment conditions?

1. Reproducibility
2. Linearity
3. Positive beam limitation/automatic collimation

❏ A. 1 only
❏ B. 1 and 2 only
❏ C. 1 and 3 only
❏ D. 1, 2, and 3

120. Which of the following will most likely produce the highest quality radiographic image?

❏ A. High SNR
❏ B. Low SNR
❏ C. Low-contrast resolution
❏ D. Moderate noise

121. The absorption of useful radiation by a grid is called

❏ A. grid selectivity
❏ B. grid cleanup
❏ C. grid cutoff
❏ D. latitude

122. The number of exposures per second in pulsed fluoroscopy is called

❏ A. automatic exposure rate control
❏ B. FPD rate
❏ C. pulse rate
❏ D. pulse width

123. Image plate front material can be made of which of the following?

1. Carbon fiber
2. Magnesium
3. Lead

❏ A. 1 only
❏ B. 1 and 2 only
❏ C. 1 and 3 only
❏ D. 1, 2, and 3

124. An increase in the kilovoltage applied to the x-ray tube increases the

1. x-ray wavelength
2. exposure rate
3. patient absorption

❏ A. 1 only
❏ B. 2 only
❏ C. 2 and 3 only
❏ D. 1, 2, and 3

125. Diagnostic x-rays are generally associated with

❏ A. high frequency and long wavelength
❏ B. high frequency and short wavelength
❏ C. low frequency and long wavelength
❏ D. low frequency and short wavelength

126. Which of the following devices is used to overcome severe variation in patient anatomy or tissue density, providing more uniform receptor exposure?

❏ A. Compensating filter
❏ B. Grid
❏ C. Collimator
❏ D. Added filtration

127. Which of the following are desirable conditions for viewing digital images?

1. Increased ambient light
2. Reduced monitor glare
3. Well-lit area
   ❏ A. 1 only
   ❏ B. 2 only
   ❏ C. 2 and 3 only
   ❏ D. 1, 2, and 3

128. What is the purpose of the thin layer of lead that is often located in the rear portion of an IP (cassette)?

❏ A. To prevent crossover
❏ B. To increase speed
❏ C. To diffuse light photons
❏ D. To reduce backscatter

129. HVL can increase as a result of

1. an increase in kV
2. vaporized tungsten on inner surface of glass envelope
3. a decrease in kV
   ❏ A. 1 only
   ❏ B. 1 and 2 only
   ❏ C. 2 and 3 only
   ❏ D. 1, 2, and 3

130. Magnification fluoroscopy is accomplished by

1. moving the image intensifier focal point further from the output phosphor
2. selecting a smaller portion of the input phosphor
3. decreasing the voltage to the electrostatic lenses
   ❏ A. 1 only
   ❏ B. 1 and 2 only
   ❏ C. 2 and 3 only
   ❏ D. 1, 2, and 3

131. Minimizing the dose to patient and personnel during fluoroscopic procedures can be achieved in which of the following ways (select four)?

❏ A. Tabletop intensity should not exceed 88 mGy/min
❏ B. At least 0.25-mm Pb equivalent protective curtain
❏ C. QC inspection at least every 12 months
❏ D. Maximum use of magnification
❏ E. At least 0.25-mm Pb equivalent Bucky slot cover
❏ F. SSD at least 38 cm for stationary/fixed equipment

132. Advantages of direct-capture flat-panel fluoroscopy over image-intensified fluoroscopy include (select four) which of the following?

❏ A. Wider dynamic range
❏ B. Uses several kinds of recording devices
❏ C. Ability to record static images
❏ D. Higher spatial resolution
❏ E. Reduced patient dose
❏ F. Uses high-quality camera tube

133. Which interaction is responsible for producing the most x-ray photons at the x-ray tube target?

❏ A. Bremsstrahlung
❏ B. Characteristic
❏ C. Photoelectric
❏ D. Compton

134. The polyenergetic nature of the x-ray beam can be accounted for by which of the following?

1. Incident electrons interacting with several layers of tungsten target atoms
2. Electrons moving to fill different shell vacancies
3. Its nuclear origin
   ❏ A. 1 only
   ❏ B. 1 and 2 only
   ❏ C. 1 and 3 only
   ❏ D. 1, 2, and 3

135. The line-focus principle expresses the relationship between

❏ A. the actual and the effective focal spot
❏ B. exposure given to the IR and resulting receptor exposure
❏ C. SID used and resulting receptor exposure
❏ D. grid ratio and lines per inch

136. How would the shape/object shown in Figure 5-12 most likely appear when imaged using a perpendicular central ray?

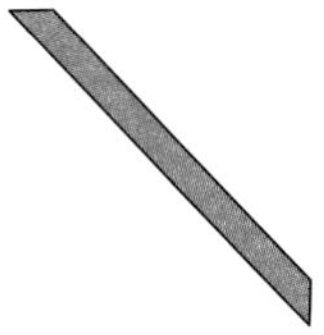

Figure 5-12

❏ A. 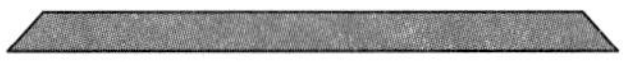
❏ B. 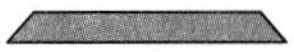
❏ C. 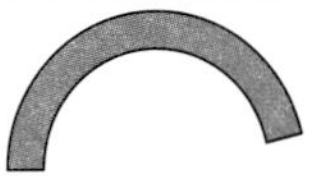
❏ D.

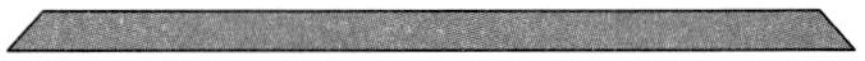

137. If an unused PSP has been stored for 48 h or more, it should be erased prior to use to avoid
- ❏ A. phantom image formation
- ❏ B. aliasing artifact
- ❏ C. image distortion
- ❏ D. image fog

138. The term *interrogation time* refers to
- ❏ A. the shortest possible exposure time permitted by a particular x-ray tube
- ❏ B. the amount of time required for x-ray tube morning warming
- ❏ C. the time required for the x-ray tube to turn off
- ❏ D. the time it takes the x-ray tube to reach the required technical factors

139. The difference in x-ray photon attenuation between various adjacent tissues and structures within the body is called
- ❏ A. remnant radiation
- ❏ B. differential absorption
- ❏ C. SNR
- ❏ D. scattering

140. The system that allows multiple users to view the same image at the same time at different locations is
- ❏ A. PACS
- ❏ B. RIS
- ❏ C. HIS
- ❏ D. LET

141. The focal spot size should be evaluated
1. upon installation
2. annually
3. monthly
- ❏ A. 1 only
- ❏ B. 1 and 2 only
- ❏ C. 1 and 3 only
- ❏ D. 1, 2, and 3

142. The type of x-ray tube designed to turn on and off rapidly, providing multiple short, precise exposures, is
- ❏ A. high speed
- ❏ B. grid-controlled
- ❏ C. diode
- ❏ D. electrode

143. The electron cloud within the x-ray tube is the product of a process called
- ❏ A. electrolysis
- ❏ B. thermionic emission
- ❏ C. rectification
- ❏ D. induction

144. Which of the following conditions contribute to x-ray tube damage?
1. Lengthy anode rotation
2. Exposures to a cold anode
3. Low-milliampere seconds/high-kilovoltage exposure factors
- ❏ A. 1 only
- ❏ B. 1 and 2 only
- ❏ C. 1 and 3 only
- ❏ D. 1, 2, and 3

145. If a high-voltage transformer has 100 primary turns and 50,000 secondary turns and is supplied by 220 V and 100 A, what are the secondary voltage and current?
- ❏ A. 200 A and 110 V
- ❏ B. 200 mA and 110 kV
- ❏ C. 20 A and 100 V
- ❏ D. 20 mA and 100 kV

1. **(C, E, and F)** Light photons from the input phosphor strike the photocathode which emits electrons. These electrons are focused toward the output phosphor/screen by negatively charged electrostatic focusing lenses. They then pass through the neck of the image-intensifier tube where they are accelerated and strike the small 1.27–2.54 cm (1/2–1 inch) output screen, resulting in a *minified* image. Image minification and electron acceleration both account for increased *brightness* of the output image. For undistorted focusing of electrons onto the output screen, each electron must travel the same distance. This is accomplished by a slight curvature of the input screen, which is responsible for *inverting* the image on the output screen. The image on the input screen is reproduced as a minified image on the output screen. The output screen being much smaller than the input screen, the amount of fluorescent light emitted from it per unit area is significantly greater than the quantity of light emitted from the input screen.

2. **(C)** All circuit devices located *before* the primary coil of the high-voltage transformer are said to be on the *primary or low-voltage* side of the x-ray circuit. The timer, autotransformer, and (prereading) kilovoltage meter are all located in the *low*-voltage circuit.

   The *secondary/high-voltage* side of the circuit begins with the *secondary coil* of the high-voltage transformer. The *milliamperage meter* is connected at the midpoint of the secondary coil of the high-voltage transformer. Following the secondary coil is the *rectification system* and the *x-ray tube.*

   Transformers are used to change the value of alternating current (AC). They operate on the principle of mutual induction. The secondary coil of the step-up transformer is located on the high-voltage (secondary) side of the x-ray circuit. The step-down transformer, or filament transformer, is located in the filament circuit and serves to regulate the voltage and current provided to heat the x-ray tube filament. The rectification system is also located on the high-voltage, or secondary side of the x-ray circuit.

3. **(C)** Digital images are best viewed in areas with low-lighting levels that will avoid undesirable monitor screen glare. Digital images usually have a black "mask" covering the white unexposed areas, further reducing objectionable ambient light and glare. If the radiographer views images in a brightly lit area, the image can appear excessively dark. The same image, when reviewed by the radiologist, might look most adequate. As light level increases, the pupils of the eye contract and admit less light causing images to appear dark. It is an effect similar to walking from a sunny day into a darkened theater.

4. **(A, C, and D)** Image-intensifier output phosphor/screen diameters of 5–12 inches are available. Although smaller diameter input screens improve *resolution,* they do not permit a large fluoroscopic *FOV.*

   Dual- and triple-field image intensifiers are available that permit *magnified* viewing of fluoroscopic images. To achieve magnification, the voltage to the focusing lenses is increased and a smaller portion of the input phosphor is used, thereby resulting in a smaller FOV (and subsequent loss of brightness). The milliamperage is automatically increased to compensate for the loss in brightness when the image intensifier is switched to the magnification mode. When voltage applied to the focusing lenses

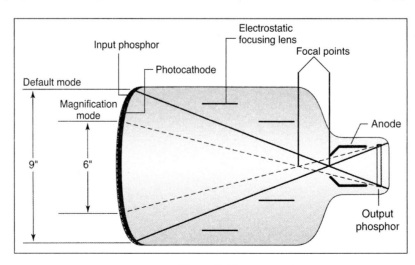

Figure 5-13

increases, the *focal point* is further away from the output phosphor, and the output image is magnified.

ESE can increase dramatically as the FOV decreases (i.e., as magnification increases).

As FOV decreases, *magnification* of the output screen image increases, there is less noise because increased milliamperage provides a greater number of x-ray photons, and contrast and resolution improve. The focal point in the magnification mode is further away from the output phosphor (as a result of increased voltage applying to the focusing lenses) and therefore the output images magnified.

5. **(D)** Each time an x-ray exposure is made, less than 1% of the total energy is converted to x-rays, and the remainder (>99%) of the energy is converted to heat. Thus, it is important to use target material with a high atomic number and high-melting point. The larger the actual focal spot size is, the larger is the area over which the generated heat is spread, and the more heat tolerant the x-ray tube is. Heat is particularly damaging to the target if it is concentrated or limited to a small area. A target that rotates during the exposure is spreading the heat over a large area, the entire surface of the focal track. If the diameter of the anode is greater, the focal track will be longer and heat will be spread over an even larger area.

6. **(D)** Determining milligray per milliampere seconds output is often done to determine linearity among x-ray machines. However, all the equipment being compared must be of the same type (e.g., all single-phase or all three-phase, six-pulse). If there is linearity among these machines, then identical technique charts can be used. In the example given, 400 mA and 12 ms were used, equaling 4.8 mAs. If the output for 4.8 mAs was 1.3 mGy, then 1 mAs is equal to 0.27 mGy/4.8 mAs = 0.27 mGy/mAs).

7. **(B, D, and E)** Equalization, or dynamic range control (DRC), is a *post*processing function of the computer software that actually compresses the contrast scale. It serves to remove densities that veil/obscure image details. If many very dark densities are removed, it permits visualization of previously hidden anatomic details. Removal of high-frequency noise is a function of the postprocessing function called smoothing or low-pass filtering.

8. **(B)** Seven waveforms are illustrated in Figure 5-1. Figure 5-1A represents alternating current. Figure 5-1B illustrates half-wave rectification; each useful pulse (of x-ray) is followed by a pause of equal length. Figure 5-1C illustrates full-wave rectification. Note the 100% voltage ripple as each pulse starts at 0 potential, makes its way to 100%, and returns to 0 potential. Figure 5-1D represents three-phase, six-pulse current exhibiting a 13% voltage drop between peak potentials. Figure 5-1E represents three-phase, 12-pulse current having only about a 4%

voltage drop between peak potentials. A big advantage of three-phase current is the very small drop in voltage between pulses. Figure 5-1F illustrates high-frequency current, which is most efficient and produces less than 1% voltage ripple. Here, 60-Hz full-wave-rectified current is converted to higher frequency (500–25,000 Hz). Mobile x-ray units first used this technology, because one of its greatest advantages is its small size. High-frequency generators are also used in mammography units and helical CT. More and more traditional x-ray equipment is using high-frequency technology because of its compact size, lower cost, and greater efficiency. Figure 5-1G illustrates direct current (DC).

9. **(A, B, D, and E)** Flat-panel detectors (FPDs) used in fluoroscopy replace the large and bulky image intensifier. *Smaller size and weight of FPDs permit greater maneuverability.* The amorphous selenium direct-capture detector produces a digital signal so there is no need for a camera tube or ADC. The system is capable of recording both static images and dynamic images; however, *these systems produce very large data files.* The system produces higher spatial resolution, wider dynamic range, *improved contrast resolution,* and *improved DQE*—as compared with image-intensified fluoroscopy. In addition, patient dose decreases approximately 50% compared with image-intensified systems.

10. **(C)** Spatial resolution is evaluated by how sharply tiny anatomic details are imaged on the radiograph. The area of blurriness that may be associated with small image details is termed *geometric blur.* The blurriness can be produced by using a large focal spot or by diffused fluorescent light from intensifying screens. The image proper (i.e., without blur) is termed the *umbra. Mottle* is a grainy appearance caused by fast imaging systems.

11. **(C)** Quality control refers to our equipment and its safe and accurate operation. Various components must be tested at specified intervals, and test results must be within specified parameters. Any deviation from those parameters must be corrected. Examples of equipment components that are tested annually are the focal spot size, linearity, reproducibility, filtration, kilovoltage, and exposure time. Congruence is a term used to describe the relationship between the collimator light field and the actual x-ray field—they must be congruent (i.e., match) to within 2% of the SID. Radiographic equipment collimators should be inspected and verified as accurate semiannually, that is, twice a year. Kilovoltage settings can most effectively be tested using an electronic kilovoltage meter; to meet required standards, the kilovoltage should be accurate to within ±4 kV. Reproducibility testing should specify that radiation output be consistent to within ±5%.

12. **(A)** An image's *spatial resolution* refers to its recorded detail/sharpness. As the input phosphor layer (usually cesium iodide) is made *thinner,* detail sharpness (resolution) increases. Also, the *smaller* the input phosphor

diameter, the greater is the spatial resolution. A brighter image is easier to see but, like mottle, does not affect image sharpness/resolution. Using magnification mode in image intensification does impact (and improve) spatial resolution (but does increase dose).

13. (D) Anode target material with a *high atomic number* produces higher energy x-rays more efficiently. Because a great deal of heat is produced at the target, the material should have a *high-melting point* so as to avoid damage to the target surface. X-rays produced at the target are emitted isotropically; those passing through the *port window* are the most useful diagnostically. The cathode filament receives *low-voltage* current to heat it to the point of thermionic emission. Then, *high voltage* is applied to drive the electrons across to the focal track.

14. (A) A parallel-plate ionization chamber is a type of AEC. A radiolucent chamber is beneath the patient (between the patient and the IR). As photons emerge from the patient, they enter the chamber and ionize the air within it. Once a predetermined charge has been reached, the exposure is terminated automatically.

15. (D) The greater the number of electrons making up the electron stream and bombarding the target, the greater is the number of x-ray photons produced. Although kilovoltage usually is associated with the energy of the x-ray photons, because a greater number of more energetic electrons will produce more x-ray photons, an increase in kilovoltage also will increase the number of photons produced. Specifically, the quantity of radiation produced increases as the square of the kilovoltage. The material composition of the tube target also plays an important role in the number of x-ray photons produced. The higher the atomic number of this material, the denser and more closely packed are the atoms making up the material, and therefore, the greater is the chance of an interaction between a high-speed electron and the target material.

16. (D) Radiographic rating charts enable the radiographer to determine the maximum safe milliamperage, exposure time, and kilovoltage for a particular exposure using a particular x-ray tube. Focal spot size also plays an important role in determining heat-load capacity. An exposure that can be made safely with the *large* focal spot may not be safe for use with the *small* focal spot of the same x-ray tube. The total number of *heat units* that an exposure generates also influences the amount of stress (in the form of heat) imparted to the anode. The product of milliampere seconds and kilovoltage determines heat units. Group (A) produces 138 HU, group (B) produces 240 HU, group (C) produces 420 HU, and group (D) produces 720 HU. The *most hazardous* group of technical factors is, therefore, group (D). The larger the focal spot and smaller the milliampere seconds value, the greater the heat-load capacity.

17. (C) Figure 5-2 illustrates the component parts of a rotating-anode x-ray tube enclosed within a glass envelope (number 3) that preserves the vacuum necessary for efficient x-ray production. Number 4 is the *rotating anode,* consisting of a light-weight molybdenum disk with beveled focal track at the periphery (number 8) and *stem* (number 5). The focal track is made of a tungsten–rhenium alloy. Numbers 6 and 7 are the *stator* and *rotor,* respectively—the two components of an induction motor—whose function is to rotate the anode. Number 1 is the filament of the cathode assembly, which is made of thoriated tungsten and functions to liberate electrons (thermionic emission) when heated to white hot (incandescence). Number 2 is the nickel focusing cup, which functions to direct the liberated filament electrons to the focal spot.

18. (A) Parts being examined during fluoroscopic procedures change in thickness and tissue density as the patient is required to change positions and as the fluoroscope is moved to examine different regions of the body. Changes in tissue attenuation characteristics, beam restriction, OID, and FOV can also necessitate an increase or decrease in exposure. The *automatic exposure rate control* (AERC) functions to vary the required changes in milliamperage, kilovoltage, pulse width, and even filtration as necessary. With AERC, beam intensity varies, and image quality is maintained. Electronic magnification is related to FOV selection. Flux gain is related to brightness gain.

19. (C) A large quantity of heat applied to a cold anode can cause enough surface heat to crack the anode. Excessive heat to the target can cause pitting or localized melting of the focal track. Localized melts can result in vaporized tungsten deposits on the glass envelope, which can cause a filtering effect, decreasing tube output. Excessive heat also can be conducted to the rotor bearings, causing increased friction and tube failure.

20. (A) Through the action of thermionic emission, as the tungsten filament continually gives up electrons, it gradually becomes thinner with age. This evaporated tungsten frequently is deposited on the inner surface of the glass envelope at the tube window. When this happens, *it acts as an additional filter* to the x-ray beam, thereby *reducing tube output.* Also, the tungsten deposit actually may attract electrons from the filament, creating a tube current, and causing *puncture of the glass envelope.*

21. (A) The HVL of a particular beam is defined as that thickness of a material that will reduce the exposure rate to one-half of its original value. The more energetic the beam (the higher the kilovoltage), the greater is the HVL thickness required to cut its intensity in half. *Therefore, it may be stated that kilovoltage and HVL have a direct relationship: as kilovoltage increases, HVL increases.*

22. (B) In electronic/digital imaging, changes in window width affect changes in contrast scale, whereas changes in window level affect changes in brightness. As window width increases, the scale of contrast increases (i.e., contrast decreases). Window level adjustments are associated with image brightness changes. This process can also be illustrated while postprocessing/windowing personal digital photographs or scanned documents.

23. (A) *Rectifiers change AC into unidirectional current* by allowing current to flow through them in only one direction. Valve tubes are vacuum rectifier tubes found in older equipment. *Solid-state diodes* are the types of rectifiers used in x-ray equipment these days. Rectification systems are found between the secondary coil of the high-voltage transformer and the x-ray tube. *Resistors,* such as rheostats or choke coils, are circuit devices used to vary voltage or current. *Transformers,* operating on the principle of mutual induction, change the voltage (and current) to useful levels. *Autotransformers,* operating on the principle of self-induction, enable us to select the required kilovoltage.

24. (B) Phosphors that fluoresce are said to *scintillate.* Fluorescent/scintillating phosphors used in indirect-conversion systems include amorphous silicon, cesium iodide, and gadolinium oxysulfide. Amorphous selenium is used in direct-conversion systems and functions to convert to x-ray photon energy into electrical charges.

25. (B) When an AEC is installed in an x-ray circuit, it is calibrated to produce radiographic densities as required by the radiologist. Once the part being radiographed has been exposed to produce the correct receptor exposure, the AEC automatically terminates the exposure. The manual timer should be used as a backup timer; in case the AEC fails to terminate the exposure, the backup timer would protect the patient from overexposure and the x-ray tube from excessive heat load. The master receptor exposure override generally is set on normal to produce the required receptor exposure. In special cases, when this produces excessive or insufficient receptor exposure, the master receptor exposure override may be adjusted to plus or minus position.

26. (B) A *generator* converts mechanical energy into electrical energy—as alternating or direct current. A *motor* is a device used to convert electrical energy to mechanical energy. The stator and rotor are the two principal parts of an induction motor.

27. (A) The x-ray photons emitted from the anode focus are heterogeneous in nature. The low-energy photons must be removed because they are not penetrating enough to contribute to the image and because they *do* contribute to the patient's skin dose. The glass envelope and oil coolant provide approximately 0.5- to 1.0-mm Al equivalent filtration, which is called *inherent* because it is a built-in, permanent part of the tube head.

28. (B) A quality assurance (QA) program requires the use of a number of devices to test the efficiency of various parts of the imaging system. Spatial resolution is significantly affected by focal spot size. A *slit camera*, as well as a *star pattern* (Fig. 5-14), or pinhole camera, is used to test focal spot size. The slit camera is considered the standard for (annual) measurement of the effective focal spot size. Dynamic range is the range of exposures that can be captured by a detector, and is unrelated to measurement of focal spot.

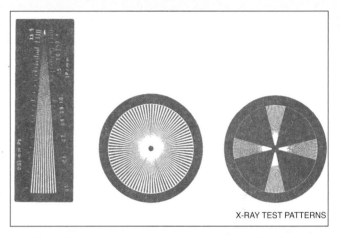

Figure 5-14. Used with permission of Nuclear Associates.

29. (C) NCRP Report No. 102 states that the exposure switch on mobile radiographic units shall be so arranged that the operator can stand at least 2 m (*6 feet*) from the patient, the x-ray tube, and the useful beam. An appropriately long exposure cord accomplishes this requirement. The fluoroscopic and/or radiographic exposure switch or switches must be of the "dead-man" type, that is, the exposure will terminate should the switch be released. At least one lead apron should be carried with every mobile x-ray unit for the operator to wear during the exposure. Finally, the radiographer must be certain to alert individuals in the area, enabling unnecessary occupants to move away, before making the exposure. Many facilities require a second lead apron to be available for family/staff/patient who are unable to leave.

30. (D) As the filament ages, vaporized tungsten may be deposited on the port window and act as an additional filter. Tungsten may also vaporize as a result of anode abuse. Exposures in excess of safe values deliver sufficient heat to cause surface melts, or pits, on the focal track. This results in roughening of the anode surface and decreased tube output. Delivery of a large amount of heat to a cold anode can cause cracking if the anode does not have sufficient time to disperse the heat. Loss of anode rotation would cause one large melt on the focal track because the electrons would bombard only one small area. If the anode is not heard to be rotating, the radiographer should not make an exposure.

31. **(B)** There are three types of beam restrictors—aperture diaphragms, cones and cylinders, and collimators. The most practical and efficient type is the collimator. Its design makes available an infinite number of field-size variations that are not available with the other types of beam restrictors. Because aperture diaphragms and flare cones have a fixed aperture size and shape, their beam restriction is not as efficient as that of the variable size collimator. Aperture diaphragms, cones, and cylinders may be placed on a collimator track so that the illuminated crosshairs are visualized. Although the collimator assembly contributes approximately 1.0-mm Al equivalent to the added filtration of the x-ray tube (because of the plastic exit portal and silver-coated reflective mirror), its functions are unrelated to the cleanup of scattered radiation. This is so because the *patient* is the principal scatterer, and grids function to clean up scattered radiation generated by the patient.

32. **(C)** Focal spot size accuracy is related to the degree of *geometric blur*, that is, edge gradient or penumbra. Manufacturer tolerance for new focal spots is 50%, that is, a 0.3-mm focal spot actually may be 0.45 mm. In addition, the focal spot can increase in size as the x-ray tube ages; hence, the importance of *testing* newly arrived focal spots and periodic testing to monitor focal spot changes. Focal spot size can be measured with a *pinhole camera*, *slit camera*, or *star-pattern-type resolution device*. The pinhole camera is rather difficult to use accurately and requires the use of excessive tube (heat) loading. With a *slit camera*, two exposures are made; one measures the length of the focal spot, and the other measures the width. The *star pattern*, or similar resolution device, such as the *bar pattern*, can measure focal spot size *as a function of geometric blur* and is readily adaptable in a QA program to monitor focal spot changes over a period of time. It is recommended that focal spot size be checked on installation of a new x-ray tube and annually thereafter.

33. **(D)** The x-ray anode may be a molybdenum disk coated with a tungsten–rhenium alloy. Because tungsten has a *high atomic number* (74), it produces high-energy x-rays more efficiently. Because a great deal of heat is produced at the target, tungsten's *high-melting point* (3410°C) helps to avoid damage to the target surface. Heat produced at the target should be dissipated readily, and tungsten's *conductivity is similar to that of copper.* Therefore, as heat is applied to the focus, it can be conducted throughout the disk to equalize the temperature and thus avoid pitting, or localized melting, of the focal track.

34. **(D)** *Grid ratio* is defined as the height of the lead strips compared to (divided by) the width of the interspace material. The width of the lead strips has no bearing on the grid ratio. The height of these lead strips is 8 mm; the width of the interspace material (that is the same as the *distance between* the lead strips) is 0.5 mm.

    Therefore, the grid ratio is 8/0.5, or a 16:1 grid.

35. **(B)** *Voltage ripple* refers to the percentage drop from maximum voltage each pulse of current experiences. In single-phase rectified equipment, the entire pulse (half-cycle) is used; therefore, there is first an increase to the maximum (peak) voltage value and then a decrease to zero potential (90° past peak potential). The entire waveform is used; at 100 kV, the actual average kilovoltage output would be approximately 70 kV. Three-phase rectification produces almost constant potential, with small ripples (drops) in maximum potential between pulses. Approximately a 13% voltage ripple (drop from maximum value) characterizes the operation of three-phase, six-pulse generators. Three-phase, 12-pulse generators have about a 4% voltage ripple. High-frequency current is most efficient and produces less than 1% voltage ripple. The high-frequency generator is small in size and produces an almost constant potential waveform.

36. **(C)** Most image-intensifier tubes are either dual-field or triple-field, indicating the diameter of the input phosphor. When a change to a smaller diameter mode is made, the voltage on the electrostatic focusing lenses is increased, and the result is a *magnified but dimmer* image. The milliamperage will be increased automatically to compensate for the loss in brightness with a magnified image, resulting in *higher patient dose in the smaller diameter modes.*

37. **(A)** The incident electron has a certain amount of energy as it approaches the tungsten target. If the positive nucleus of a tungsten atom attracts the electron, changing its course, a certain amount of energy is released during the "braking" action. This energy is given up in the form of an x-ray photon called *Bremsstrahlung* (braking) *radiation. Characteristic radiation* is also produced at the target (less frequently) when an incident electron ejects a K-shell electron, and an L-shell electron drops into its place. Energy is liberated in the form of a characteristic ray, and its energy is representative of the difference in energy levels. *Compton scatter* and the *photoelectric effect* are interactions between x-ray photons and tissue atoms.

38. **(C)** The *input phosphor* of an image intensifier receives remnant radiation emerging from the patient and converts it to a fluorescent light image. Directly adjacent to the input phosphor is the *photocathode*, which is made of a photoemissive alloy (usually, a cesium and antimony compound). The fluorescent light image strikes the photocathode and is converted to an electron image. The electrons are focused carefully, to maintain image resolution, by the *electrostatic focusing lenses*, through the *accelerating anode* and to the *output phosphor* for conversion back to light. The *TV monitor* is not part of the image intensifier but serves to display the image that is transmitted to it from the output phosphor.

39. (B) In digital imaging, x-rays form an electronic image on a special radiation detector. This electronic image can be manipulated by a computer and stored in the computer memory or displayed as a matrix of intensities. This final digital image can be viewed on a computer monitor and the computer has the capability of postprocessing and image enhancement.

40. (B) In DF, the image-intensifier output screen image is coupled via a *charge coupled device* (CCD) for viewing on a display monitor. A CCD converts visible light to an electrical charge that is then sent to the analog-to-digital converter (ADC) for processing. When output screen light strikes the CCD cathode, a proportional number of electrons are released by the cathode and stored as digital values by the CCD. The CCD's rapid discharge time virtually eliminates image lag and is useful in high-speed imaging procedures, such as cardiac catheterizations. CCD cameras have replaced analog cameras (e.g., the Vidicon and Plumbicon) in fluoroscopic equipment. CCDs are more sensitive to the light emitted by the output phosphor (than the analog cameras) and are associated with less "noise." DF photospot images are simply still-frame images requiring less patient dose, and offering postprocessing capability. DF also offers "road-mapping" capability, a technique useful in procedures involving guidewire/catheter placement. During the fluoroscopic examination, the most recent fluoroscopic image is stored on the monitor, thereby reducing the need for continuous x-ray exposure. This technique can offer significant reductions in radiation exposure to the patient and personnel.

41. (A) Quality control refers to our equipment and its safe and accurate operation. Various components must be tested at specified intervals and test results must be within specified parameters. Any deviation from those parameters must be corrected. Examples of equipment components that are tested annually are the focal spot size, linearity, reproducibility, filtration, kilovoltage, and exposure time. Reproducibility specifies that radiation output must be consistent to within ±5%. Linearity tests x-ray output with increasing milliampere seconds value; mR/mAs should be accurate to within 10%. Kilovoltage settings can most effectively be tested using an electronic kilovoltage meter; to meet required standards, the kilovoltage should be accurate to within ±4 kV. Congruence is a term used to describe the relationship between the collimator light field and the actual x-ray field—they must be congruent to within 2% of the SID. Radiographic equipment collimators should be inspected and verified as accurate semiannually.

42. (C) Quality control refers to our equipment and its safe and accurate operation. Various components must be tested at specified intervals and test results must be within specified parameters. Any deviation from those parameters must be corrected. Examples of equipment components that are tested annually are the focal spot

size, linearity, reproducibility, collimation, filtration, kilovoltage, and exposure time. Quality assurance is associated with patients and staff, and their interactions and relationships. Congruence is a term used to describe the relationship between the collimator light field and the actual x-ray field—they must be congruent (i.e., match) to within 2% of the SID. Postprocessing refers to the windowing or other manipulation of a digital image.

43. (D) CT (computed tomography), MRI (magnetic resonance imaging), and CR (computed radiography) are three common examples of *digital imaging*. Special equipment is also available for direct digital radiography (DR)—images produced by either a fan-shaped x-ray beam received by linearly arrayed radiation detectors or a traditional fan-shaped x-ray beam received by a light-stimulated phosphor plate. Digital images can also be obtained in digital subtraction angiography (DSA), nuclear medicine, and diagnostic sonography.

44. (A) As body areas of different thicknesses and densities are scanned with the image intensifier, image brightness and contrast require adjustment. The ABC functions to maintain constant brightness and contrast of the output screen image, correcting for fluctuations in x-ray beam attenuation with adjustments in kilovoltage and/or milliamperage. There are also brightness and contrast controls on the monitor that the radiographer can regulate.

45. (B) *Current* is defined as the amount of electric charge flowing per second. *Voltage* is the potential difference existing between two points. *Resistance* is the property of a circuit that opposes current flow. *Capacitance* describes a quantity of stored electricity.

46. (A) Quality control refers to our equipment and its safe and accurate operation. Various components must be tested at specified intervals and test results must be within specified parameters. Any deviation from those parameters must be corrected. Examples of equipment components that are tested annually are the focal spot size, linearity, reproducibility, filtration, kilovoltage, and exposure time. Kilovoltage settings can most effectively be tested using an electronic kilovoltage meter; to meet required standards, the kilovoltage should be accurate to within ±4 kV. Congruence is a term used to describe the relationship between the collimator light field and the actual x-ray field—they must be congruent (i.e., match) to within 2% of the SID. Collimators should be inspected and verified as accurate semiannually. Reproducibility testing should specify that radiation output be consistent to within ±5%.

47. (B) The light image emitted from the output phosphor of the image intensifier is directed to the TV monitor for viewing and sometimes to recording devices, such as a spot image or cine device. The light is directed to these places by a *beam splitter* or objective lens located between the output phosphor and the CCD. The majority of the light will go to the recording device, whereas a small portion goes to the monitor so that the procedure may continue to be observed during imaging.

48. **(B)** The image intensifier's input phosphor receives the remnant radiation emerging from the patient and converts it into a fluorescent light image. Very close to the input phosphor, separated by a thin, transparent layer, is the photocathode. The photocathode is made of a photoemissive alloy, usually an antimony and cesium compound. The fluorescent light image strikes the photocathode and is converted to an electron image that is focused by the electrostatic lenses to the output phosphor.

49. **(B)** *Inherent* filtration is that which is "built into" the construction of the x-ray tube. Before exiting the x-ray tube, x-ray photons must pass through the tube's glass envelope and port window; the photons are filtered somewhat as they do so. This inherent filtration is usually the equivalent of 0.5 mm Al. Aluminum filtration *placed* between the x-ray tube housing and the collimator is added to contribute to the total necessary requirement of 2.5-mm Al equivalent. The collimator itself is considered part of the *added filtration* (1.0-mm Al equivalent) because of the silver surface of the mirror within. It is important to remember that as aluminum filtration is added to the x-ray tube, the HVL increases.

50. **(C)** Normal tissue variants and pathologic processes that alter tissue thickness and composition can have a significant effect on degree of alteration of the applied x-ray beam—and, ultimately, on the characteristics of the remnant beam. The degree to which the x-ray beam is weakened/diminished by varying tissues is termed differential absorption. These tissue variants affect differential absorption, the amount of SR generated, and the number of photons reaching the IR. Subject contrast refers to the various body tissue densities and thicknesses, which results in *differential absorption* of the x-ray beam and the resulting *signal differences* within the remnant beam.

51. **(B)** Figure 5-4 illustrates the component parts of a rotating-anode x-ray tube enclosed within a glass envelope (number 3) to preserve the *vacuum* necessary for x-ray production. Number 4 is the *rotating anode* with its beveled focal track at the periphery (number 8) and its *stem* (at number 5). Numbers 6 and 7 are the *stator* and *rotor*, respectively—the two components of an induction motor—whose function is to rotate the anode. Number 1 is the filament of the cathode assembly, which is made of thoriated tungsten and functions to liberate electrons (thermionic emission) when heated to white hot (incandescence). Number 2 is the nickel focusing cup, which functions to direct the liberated filament electrons to the focal spot. Aliasing, or moiré, has the appearance of somewhat wavy linear lines and can occur in computed radiography when using *stationary* grids.

52. **(A, B, and D)** Figure 5-4 illustrates the component parts of a rotating-anode x-ray tube enclosed within a glass envelope (number 3) that preserves the vacuum necessary for x-ray production. Number 4 is the rotating anode, consisting of a light-weight molybdenum disk with beveled focal track at the periphery (number 8) and *stem* (number 5). The focal track is made of a tungsten–rhenium alloy. Numbers 6 and 7 are the *stator* and *rotor*, respectively—the two components of an induction motor. The induction motor's function is to *rotate the anode* via *electromagnetic induction*. Number 1 is the filament of the cathode assembly, which is made of thoriated tungsten and functions to liberate electrons (thermionic emission) when heated to white hot (incandescence). Number 2 is the nickel focusing cup, which functions to direct the liberated filament electrons to the anode's focal track.

53. **(C)** The brightness gain of image intensifiers is 5000–20,000. This increase is accounted for in two ways. As the electron image is focused to the output phosphor, it is accelerated by high voltage (about 25 kV). The output phosphor is only a fraction of the size of the input phosphor, and this decrease in image size represents brightness gain, termed *minification gain*. The *ratio* of the number of x-ray photons at the input phosphor compared with the number of light photons at the output phosphor is termed *flux gain*. *Total brightness gain is equal to the product of minification gain and flux gain.*

54. **(B)** CCDs have been used to replace the television camera associated with image intensification. They are much more compact than a television camera and can efficiently capture the fluoroscopic image. In comparison to television cameras, CCDs provide better resolution and contrast and have a higher DQE (detective quantum efficiency) and SNR (signal-to-noise ratio). CMOS efficiency has improved greatly over the past decade. Advantages of CMOS over CCDs include significantly less cost, greater speed, and much more energy efficiency (less power consumption). The CCD still provides somewhat better image quality.

55. **(B)** Two types of interactions between high-speed incident electrons and the tungsten-target atoms account for the production of x-rays within the x-ray tube. (1) In the production of Brems (braking) radiation, a high-speed electron is attracted to the positive nuclear charge of a tungsten atom. In doing so, it is "braked" and gives up energy in the form of an x-ray photon. Most of the primary beam is made up of Brems radiation. (2) If the incident electron were to eject a K-shell electron, an L-shell electron would move in to fill the vacancy. It releases a photon (K-characteristic ray) whose energy equals the difference between the K- and L-shell energy levels. This is characteristic radiation; it is responsible for only a small portion of the primary beam.

56. (C) PACS refers to a *picture archiving and communication system*. PACS systems *receive* digital images and *display* them on monitors for interpretation. These systems also *store* images and allow their retrieval at a later time. Computer software is responsible for digital image processing.

57. (B) HVL may be used to express the quality of an x-ray beam. The HVL of a particular beam is that thickness of an absorber that will decrease the intensity of the beam to one-half of its original value. If the original intensity of the beam was 88 mGy/min, the first HVL will reduce the intensity to 44 mGy/min, the second HVL will reduce it to 22 mGy/min, and the third HVL will reduce it to 11 mGy/min, and so on.

58. (B) The x-ray tube filament is made of thoriated tungsten. When heated to incandescence (white hot), the filament liberates electrons—a process called *thermionic emission*. It is these electrons that will become the tube current (mA). As heat is increased, more electrons are released, and milliamperage increases.

59. (C) Significant scattered radiation is produced when radiographing large dense body parts and when using high kilovoltage. A grid is a radiographic accessory made of alternating lead strips and interspace material; it is placed between the patient and the image receptor to absorb energetic scattered photons emerging from the patient. Although the grid prevents much scattered radiation (fog) from reaching the image receptor, its use necessitates a significant increase in exposure and patient dose.

60. (D) The smaller the focal spot, the more limited the anode is with respect to the quantity of heat it can safely accept, but the better the detail sharpness because there is less focal spot blur. As the target angle decreases, the effective focal spot size decreases. Therefore, group (D) offers the best combination for good detail sharpness/resolution. It must be remembered, however, *that a steep target angle increases the heel effect*, and IR coverage may be compromised.

61. (D) The image intensifier's input phosphor (number 6) receives the remnant radiation emerging from the patient and converts it into a fluorescent light image. Very close to the input phosphor, separated by a thin, transparent layer, is the photocathode (number 5). The photocathode is made of a photoemissive alloy, usually an antimony and cesium compound. The fluorescent light image strikes the photocathode and is converted to an electron image that is focused by the electrostatic lenses (number 4) to the output phosphor (number 1).

Dual- and triple-field image intensifiers are available that permit *magnified* viewing of fluoroscopic images. To achieve magnification, the *voltage* to the focusing lenses is increased and a *smaller portion of the input phosphor is used* (number 8), thereby resulting in a smaller FOV.

Because minification gain is now decreased, the image is not as bright. The milliamperage is automatically increased to compensate for the loss in brightness when the image intensifier is switched to magnification mode. Entrance skin exposure (ESE) can increase dramatically as the FOV decreases (i.e., as magnification increases). The magnified output screen image has better resolution because there is less *noise*; increased milliamperage provides a greater number of x-ray photons, and *contrast* and *resolution* improve. The *focal point* (number 3) in the magnification mode is *further away from* the output phosphor (as a result of increased voltage applied to the focusing lenses) and therefore the output image is magnified.

62. (C) The image intensifier's input phosphor (number 6), usually made of cesium iodide, receives the remnant radiation emerging from the patient and converts it into a fluorescent light image. Very close to the input phosphor and separated by a thin transparent layer is the photocathode (number 5). The photocathode is made of a photoemissive alloy, usually an antimony and cesium compound. The fluorescent light image strikes the photocathode and is converted to an electron image that is focused by the electrostatic lenses (number 4), through the accelerating anode, to the output phosphor (number 1).

63. (D) CCDs have been used to replace the television camera associated with image intensification. They are much more compact than a television camera and can efficiently capture the fluoroscopic image. In comparison to television cameras, CCDs provide better resolution and contrast and have a higher DQE (detective quantum efficiency) and SNR (signal-to-noise ratio). CMOS efficiency has improved greatly over the past decade. Advantages of CMOS over CCDs include significantly less cost, greater speed, and much more energy efficiency (less power consumption). The CCD still provides somewhat better image quality.

64. (B) Given the milliamperage and exposure time, a radiographic rating chart enables the radiographer to determine the maximum safe kilovoltage for a particular exposure. Because the heat load an anode will safely accept varies with the size of the focal spot and the type of rectification, these variables must be identified. Each x-ray tube has its own radiographic rating chart. The speed of the imaging system has no impact on the use of a radiographic rating chart.

65. (C) Spatial resolution in CR is impacted by the size of the PSP, the size of the scanning laser beam, and monitor matrix size. *High-resolution monitors* (2–4 megapixels) are required for high-quality, high-resolution image display. *The larger the matrix size, the better is the image resolution.* Typical image matrix size (rows and columns) used in chest radiography is 2048 × 2048. *Spatial resolution* is measured in line pairs per millimeter (lp/mm). As matrix size is increased, there are more and smaller pixels in the matrix and, therefore, improved spatial resolution. Other factors contributing to image resolution are the *size of the laser beam* and the *size of the PSP phosphors.* Smaller phosphor size improves resolution—anything that causes an increase in light diffusion will result in a decrease in resolution. Smaller PSP phosphors permit less light diffusion. In addition, the scanning laser light must be of the correct intensity and size. A narrow laser beam is required for optimal resolution.

66. **(D)** With *single-phase*, full-wave-rectified equipment, the voltage is constantly changing from 0% to 100% of its maximum value. It drops to 0 every 180° (of the AC waveform), that is, there is 100% voltage ripple. With *three-phase* equipment, the voltage ripple is significantly smaller. Three-phase, six-pulse equipment has a 13% voltage ripple, and three-phase, 12-pulse equipment has a 3.5% ripple. Therefore, *the voltage never falls below 87%–96.5% of its maximum value with three-phase equipment*, and it closely approaches constant potential (direct current [DC]).

67. **(C)** The IP is used to house, support, and protect the PSP *within* the IP (cassette). The IP front should be made of a sturdy material with a low atomic number because attenuation of the remnant beam is undesirable. Bakelite (the forerunner of plastics these days) and magnesium (the lightest structural metal) are the materials used most commonly for cassette fronts. The high atomic number of tungsten makes it inappropriate as an IP front material.

68. **(B)** The collimator assembly includes a series of lead shutters, a mirror, and a light bulb (Fig. 5-15). The mirror and light bulb function to project the size, location, and center of the irradiated field. The bulb's emitted beam of light is deflected by a mirror placed at an angle of 45° in the path of the light beam. *In order for the projected light beam to be the same size as the x-ray beam, the focal spot and the light bulb must be exactly the same distance from the center of the mirror.*

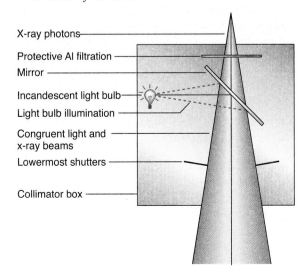

X-ray photons

Protective Al filtration

Mirror

Incandescent light bulb

Light bulb illumination

Congruent light and x-ray beams

Lowermost shutters

Collimator box

Figure 5-15

69. **(A)** The image intensifier's input phosphor receives the remnant beam from the patient and converts it to a fluorescent light image. To maintain resolution, the input phosphor is made of cesium iodide crystals. Cesium iodide is much more efficient in this conversion process than was the phosphor used previously, zinc cadmium sulfide. Calcium tungstate was one of the earliest phosphors used many years prior to the development of rare earth phosphors, such as gadolinium oxysulfide.

70. **(C)** AEC devices are used in equipment these days and serve to produce consistent and comparable radiographic results. In the most common type of AEC, an *ionization chamber* is located just beneath the tabletop above the IR. The part to be examined is centered to the AEC's sensor and imaged. When a predetermined quantity of ionization has occurred (equal to the correct receptor exposure), the x-ray exposure terminates automatically. *The manual timer should always be used as a backup timer.* In case of AEC malfunction, it would terminate the exposure, thus avoiding patient overexposure and x-ray tube overload. An image intensifier functions to provide a brighter fluoroscopic image, and positive beam limitation (PBL), or automatic collimation, serves to restrict the field size to the size of the cassette/IR used in the Bucky tray. The line-voltage compensator automatically adjusts the incoming line voltage to the x-ray machine to correct for any voltage drops or surges.

71. **(C)** Grids are composed of alternating strips of lead and radiolucent interspace material. The interspace material is either aluminum or plastic fiber. Aluminum resists moisture, is sturdier, provides a "smoother" appearance with less visible grid lines, but requires a higher milliampere seconds value and therefore increases patient dose. Plastic fiber interspace material can be affected by moisture, resulting in warping. Carbon fiber is often used as image plate front material because of its durability and homogeneity.

72. **(B)** The high-voltage, or step-up, transformer functions to *increase voltage* to the necessary kilovoltage. It *decreases the amperage* to milliamperage. The amount of increase or decrease *depends on the transformer ratio*, that is, the ratio of the number of turns in the primary coil to the number of turns in the secondary coil. The transformer law is as follows:

To determine secondary V,

$$\frac{V_s}{V_p} = \frac{N_s}{N_p}$$

To determine secondary I,

$$\frac{N_s}{N_p} = \frac{I_p}{I_s}$$

Substituting known values:

$$\frac{x}{220} = \frac{100,000}{400}$$
$$400x = 22,000,000$$

Thus, $x = 55,000$ V (55 kV).

73. **(A)** The principle of self-induction is an example of the second law of electromagnetics (Lenz's law), which states that an induced current within a conductive coil will oppose the direction of the current that induced it. It is important to note that self-induction is a characteristic of AC only. The fact that AC is constantly changing direction accounts for the opposing current set up in the coil. The autotransformer operates on the principle of self-induction and enables the radiographer to vary the kilovoltage. The high-voltage transformer operates on the principle of mutual induction. Rectifiers function to change alternating current to the unidirectional pulsating current required for efficient x-ray tube operation.

74. **(B)** Because the high-voltage transformer has a fixed ratio, there must be a means of changing the voltage sent to its primary coil; otherwise, there would be a fixed kilovoltage. The autotransformer makes these changes possible. When kilovoltage is selected on the control panel, the radiographer actually is adjusting the autotransformer and selecting the amount of voltage to send to the high-voltage transformer to be stepped up (to kilovoltage). The filament circuit supplies the proper current and voltage to the x-ray tube filament for proper thermionic emission. The rectifier circuit is responsible for changing AC to unidirectional current.

75. **(D)** The thicker and denser the anatomic part being studied, the less bright will be the fluoroscopic image. Both milliamperage and kilovoltage affect the fluoroscopic image in a way similar to the way in which they affect the radiographic image. For optimal contrast, especially taking patient dose into consideration, higher kilovoltage and lower milliamperage are generally preferred.

76. **(B)** In Bremsstrahlung (Brems) or "braking" x-ray production, a high-speed electron, accelerated toward a tungsten atom, is attracted (and "braked," i.e., slowed down) by the positively charged nucleus and therefore is deflected from its original course with a resulting loss of kinetic energy. This energy loss re-emerges in the form of an x-ray photon. The electron might not give up all its kinetic energy in one such interaction; it might go on to have several more interactions deeper in the target, each time giving up an x-ray photon having less and less energy. This is one reason the x-ray beam is heterogeneous (i.e., has a spectrum of energies). *Brems radiation comprises 70%–90% of the x-ray beam.* The other type of x-ray production that occurs in the tungsten anode is *characteristic* radiation. In this case, a high-speed

electron encounters the tungsten atom and ejects a K-shell electron, leaving a vacancy in the K shell. An electron from a shell above (e.g., the L shell) fills the vacancy and in doing so emits a K-characteristic ray. The energy of the characteristic ray is equal to the difference in energy between the K and L shells. K-characteristic x-rays from a tungsten-target x-ray tube have 69 keV of energy. Characteristic radiation comprises very little of the x-ray beam (15%–20%).

77. **(A, B, and E)** Lead aprons protect the radiation worker from leakage and scatter radiation; they do not protect from the primary beam. Federal law requires that lead aprons must have at least 0.25-mm lead equivalent protection. When not in use, they should be hung on a rack or draped over a bar. Folding lead aprons can cause creases and cracks in the protective material. Lead aprons must be x-rayed, either fluoroscoped or radiographed, annually to detect any cracks or other flaws.

78. **(A, C, and D)** According to the line-focus principle, the effective focal spot size is always smaller than the actual focal spot size. If the large focal spot is selected, the effective focal spot size will be larger than if the small focal spot were selected. The smaller the focal spot size, the better the sharpness of image details and spatial resolution. Focal spot side has no effect on image contrast or brightness.

79. **(D)** The rotating *anode* has a target (or focal spot) on its beveled edge that forms the target angle. As the anode rotates, it constantly turns a new face to the incoming electrons; this is the *focal track*. The portion of the focal track that is bombarded by electrons is the actual focal spot, and because of the target's angle, the effective or projected focal spot is always smaller (line-focus principle). The *anode heel effect* refers to decreased beam intensity at the anode end of the x-ray beam. The electrons impinging on the target have "boiled off" the cathode filament as a result of thermionic emission.

80. **(D)** The anode is made to rotate through the use of an *induction motor*. An induction motor has two main parts, a *stator* and a *rotor*. The stator is the part located *outside the glass envelope* and consists of a series of electromagnets occupying positions around the stem of the anode. The stator's electromagnets are supplied with current, and the associated magnetic fields function to exert a drag or pull on the *rotor within the glass envelope*. The anode is a 2- to 5-inch diameter molybdenum or graphite disk with a beveled edge. The beveled surface has a *focal track* of tungsten–rhenium alloy. The anode rotates at about 3600 rpm (high-speed anode rotation is about 10,000 rpm) so that heat generated during x-ray production is evenly distributed over the entire track. *Rotating anodes* can withstand delivery of a greater amount of heat for a longer period of time than *stationary anodes*.

81. **(B, C, and E)** Quality control concerns the regular testing for accuracy of equipment and accessories. Safe and accurate equipment, and its use, helps to ensure patient safety. These guidelines state that beam alignment must be accurate to within 2% of the SID, the control panel must indicate when the x-ray tube is energized, total filtration must be at least 2.5-mm Al equivalent for 70 kV and above, the variation in x-ray intensity for a given exposure must not exceed 5%, and linearity variation must not exceed 10% when testing milliamperage stations.

82. **(A)** The vast majority of target interactions involve the incident electrons and outer-shell tungsten electrons. No ionization occurs, and the energy loss is reflected in heat generation. The production of x-rays is an amazingly inefficient process: *More than 99% of the electrons' kinetic energy is changed to heat energy and less than 1% into x-ray photon energy.* This presents a serious heat-buildup problem in the anode because heat production is directly proportional to tube current.

83. **(D)** Moving the image intensifier *closer to the patient* during fluoroscopy *reduces* the distance between the x-ray tube (source) and the image intensifier (which is the image receptor in this case), that is, the SID. It follows that the distance between the part being imaged (object) and the image intensifier (IR), that is, the object-to-image-receptor distance (OID), is also reduced. The shorter OID produces *less magnification* and *better image quality.* As the SID is reduced, the intensity of the x-ray photons at the image intensifier's input phosphor increases, stimulating the automatic brightness control (ABC) to decrease the milliamperage and thereby *decreasing patient dose* (Fig. 5-16).

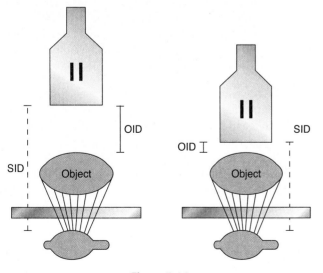

Figure 5-16

84. **(B)** X-ray tube focal spots/targets are constructed according to the *line-focus principle*—the focal spot is angled (usually, 12°–17°) to the vertical. As the actual focal spot is projected downward, it is foreshortened;

thus, the effective focal spot is always smaller than the actual focal spot. As it is projected toward the *cathode* end of the x-ray beam, the effective focal spot becomes *larger* and approaches its actual size. As it is projected toward the anode end, and foreshortening becomes more pronounced, the effective focal spot becomes smaller. Anode heel effect refers to the variation in x-ray beam intensity between the anode and cathode. Because of the anode angle, x-ray beam intensity is greater at the cathode end of the beam and less at the anode into the beam—as the x-ray beam attempts to diverge, it is absorbed by the "heel" of the anode at that end of the x-ray tube.

85. **(D)** X-ray tube targets are constructed according to the *line-focus principle*—the focal spot is angled (usually, 12°–17°) to the vertical. As the actual focal spot is projected downward, it is foreshortened; thus, the effective focal spot is always smaller than the actual focal spot. As it is projected toward the *cathode* end of the x-ray beam, the effective focal spot becomes *larger* and approaches its actual size. As it is projected toward the anode end, and foreshortening becomes more pronounced, the effective focal spot becomes smaller.

86. **(C)** All circuit devices located before the primary coil of the high-voltage transformer are said to be on the primary or low-voltage side of the x-ray circuit. The timer, autotransformer, and (prereading) kilovoltage meter are all located in the low-voltage circuit. The milliampere meter, however, is connected at the midpoint of the secondary coil of the high-voltage transformer. When studying a diagram of the x-ray circuit, it will be noted that the milliampere meter is grounded at the midpoint of the secondary coil (where it is at zero potential). Therefore, it may be placed in the control panel safely.

87. **(D)** The input phosphor of image intensifiers is usually made of cesium iodide. For each x-ray photon absorbed by cesium iodide, approximately 5000 light photons are emitted. As the light photons strike a photoemissive *photocathode*, a number of electrons are released from the photocathode and focused toward the output side of the image tube by voltage applied to the negatively charged *electrostatic focusing lenses*. The electrons are then accelerated through the neck of the tube, where they strike the small (0.5–1 inch) *output phosphor* that is mounted on a flat glass support. The entire assembly is enclosed within a 2- to 4-mm thick vacuum glass envelope. Remember that the image on the output phosphor is *minified, brighter,* and *inverted* (electron focusing causes image inversion).

Input screen diameters of 5–12 inches are available. Although smaller diameter input screens improve resolution, they do not permit a large FOV, that is, viewing of large patient areas.

Dual- and triple-field image intensifiers are available that permit *magnified* viewing of fluoroscopic images. To achieve magnification, the *voltage* to the focusing lenses is increased and a *smaller* portion of the input phosphor is used, thereby resulting in a smaller FOV. Because minification gain is now decreased, the image is not as bright. The milliamperage is automatically increased to compensate for the loss in brightness when the image intensifier is switched to magnification mode. Entrance skin exposure (ESE) can increase dramatically as the FOV decreases (i.e., as magnification increases).

As FOV decreases, *magnification* of the output screen image increases, there is less *noise* because increased milliamperage provides a greater number of x-ray photons, and *contrast* and *resolution* improve. The *focal point* in the magnification mode is *further away from* the output phosphor (as a result of increased voltage applied to the focusing lenses) and therefore the output image is magnified.

88. **(D)** There are two main types of mobile x-ray equipment—capacitor-discharge and battery-powered. Capacitor-discharge units are light, and therefore fairly easy to maneuver. Battery-powered mobile units, with their heavy-duty power sources, have become much lighter in weight and they have the advantage of being capable of storing a large milliampere seconds capacity for extended periods of time. These units frequently have a capacity of 10,000 mAs, with 12 h required for a full charge.

89. **(C)** The visual apparatus that is responsible for visual acuity and contrast perception is the *cones* within the retina. Cones are also used for daylight vision. Therefore, the most desirable condition for fluoroscopic viewing is to have a bright enough image to permit cone (daylight) vision for better detail perception. The image intensifier accomplishes this. The intensified image is then transferred to a TV monitor for viewing. Cine and spot image devices can be used to record fluoroscopic events.

90. **(B)** Off-focus, or extrafocal, radiation is produced as electrons strike metal surfaces other than the focal track and produce x-rays that emerge with the primary beam at a variety of angles. This radiation is responsible for indistinct images outside the collimated field. Mounting a pair of shutters as close to the source as possible minimizes off-focus radiation.

91. **(D)** *Grid ratio* is defined as *the ratio of the height of the lead strips to the width of the interspace material*; the higher the lead strips, the more scattered radiation they will trap and the greater is the grid's efficiency. The greater the *number of lead strips per inch*, the thinner and less visible they will be on the finished radiograph. The function of a grid is to absorb scattered radiation to improve radiographic contrast. The *selectivity* of a grid is

determined by the amount of primary radiation *transmitted* through the grid divided by the amount of scattered radiation *transmitted* through the grid.

92. **(C)** A parallel-plate *ionization chamber* is the most commonly used AEC. A radiolucent chamber of air is located beneath the patient (between the patient and the IR). As photons emerge from the patient, they enter the chamber and ionize the air within it. Once a predetermined charge has been reached, the exposure is terminated automatically. AEC determines exposure time; the radiographer must determine optimum kilovoltage and milliamperage. Motion of magnetic fields inducing current in a conductor refers to the *principle of mutual induction*.

93. **(B)** Quality control refers to our equipment and its safe and accurate operation. Various components must be tested at specified intervals and test results must be within specified parameters. Any deviation from those parameters must be corrected. Examples of equipment components that are tested annually are the focal spot size, linearity, reproducibility, filtration, kilovoltage, and exposure time. Kilovoltage settings can most effectively be tested using an electronic kilovoltage meter; to meet required standards, the kilovoltage should be accurate to within ±4 kV.

Congruence is a term used to describe the relationship between the collimator light field and the actual x-ray field—they must be congruent (i.e., match) to within 2% of the SID. Collimators should be inspected and verified as accurate semiannually, that is, twice a year. Reproducibility testing should specify that radiation output be consistent to within ±5%.

94. **(D)** Single-phase radiographic equipment is less efficient than three-phase equipment because it has a 100% voltage ripple. *With three-phase equipment, voltage never drops to zero*, and x-ray intensity is significantly greater. To produce similar receptor exposure, only *two-thirds* of the original milliampere seconds value would be used for three-phase, six-pulse equipment. With three-phase, 12-pulse equipment, the original milliampere seconds value would be cut in *half* (one-half of 15 mAs = 7.5).

95. **(B)** DXA imaging is used to evaluate bone mineral density (BMD). Bone densitometry (i.e., DXA) can be used to evaluate bone mineral content of the body, or part of it, to diagnose osteoporosis or to evaluate the effectiveness of treatments for osteoporosis. It is the most widely used method of bone densitometry—it is low-dose, precise, and uncomplicated to use/perform. DXA uses two photon energies—one for soft tissue and one for bone. Because bone is denser and attenuates x-ray photons more readily, their attenuation is calculated to represent the degree of bone density. Soft-tissue attenuation information is not used to measure bone density.

96. **(A)** Digital image acquisition has inherent system flaws. Corrections made to the "raw" digital images to repair these flaws is termed *preprocessing* (or acquisition processing). The inherent flaws are attributable to image receptor system elements and processor circuitry. Any later adjustments made by the operator or by equipment default settings are called *postprocessing*.

97. **(A)** When a dual-field image intensifier is switched to the smaller field, the electrostatic focusing lenses are given a greater charge to focus the electron image more tightly. The focal point, then, moves further from the output phosphor (the diameter of the electron image is, therefore, smaller as it reaches the output phosphor), and the brightness gain is somewhat diminished. Hence, the patient area viewed is somewhat *smaller* and is *magnified*. However, the minification gain has been reduced, and the image is somewhat *less bright*.

98. **(D)** A radiographic rating chart enables the radiographer to determine the maximum safe milliamperage, exposure time, and kilovoltage for a given exposure using a particular x-ray tube. Because the heat load that an anode will safely accept varies with the size of the focal spot, type of rectification, and anode rotation, these variables must also be identified. Each x-ray tube has its own characteristics and its own rating chart. Find the correct chart for the three-phase, 2.0-mm focal spot x-ray tube. Locate 0.05 s on the horizontal (seconds) axis and follow it up to where it intersects with the 120-kV line on the vertical (kV) axis. They intersect just above the 700-mA curve, at approximately 680 mA. Thus, 600 mA is the maximum safe milliamperage for this particular group of exposure factors and x-ray tube.

99. **(B)** Each x-ray exposure made by the radiographer produces hundreds or thousands of heat units at the target. If the examination requires several consecutive exposures, the potential for extreme heat load is increased. Just as each x-ray tube has its own radiographic rating chart, each tube also has its own anode cooling curve to describe its unique heating and cooling characteristics. An x-ray tube generally cools most rapidly during the first 2 min of nonuse. First, note that the tube is saturated with heat at 300,000 HU. In order for another 100,000 HU to be safely applied, the x-ray tube must first release 100,000 HU, which means that it has to cool down at least to 200,000 HU. Find the 200,000 HU point on the vertical axis and follow across to where it intersects with the cooling curve. It intersects at about the 2-min point.

100. **(B)** Image *smoothing* (also called low-pass filtering) is used in digital image postprocessing to remove high-frequency noise, having a blurring effect. The reduction in noise also results in a reduction in contrast. Smoothing must not be used to remedy severe mottle, which represents underexposure.

Edge enhancement (also called high-pass filtering) removes low spatial frequencies and produces higher contrast and is particularly useful in digital vascular imaging.

Aliasing is a wraparound artifact that occurs when the spatial frequency is greater than the Nyquist frequency and the sampling occurs less than twice per cycle. This causes loss of information and a wraparound image, appearing as superimposed images out of alignment, and a moiré effect. The Nyquist theorem states that the sampling frequency must be greater than twice the bandwidth of the input signal in order for the image to be properly displayed.

Windowing is a postprocessing method of adjusting brightness and/or contrast. Window level adjusts the overall image brightness, whereas window width adjusts image contrast. Narrow window width provides higher contrast (short-scale contrast), whereas wide window width provides lower contrast (long-scale contrast).

101. **(D)** As the anode angle is decreased (made steeper), a larger actual focal spot may be used while still maintaining the same small effective focal spot. Because the actual focal spot is larger, it can accommodate a greater heat load. However, with steeper (smaller) anode angles, the anode heel effect is accentuated and can compromise IR coverage.

102. **(B)** The *minimum response time*, or *minimum reaction time*, is the length of the shortest exposure possible with a particular AEC. If less than the minimum response time is required for a particular exposure, the radiograph will exhibit excessive receptor exposure. The problem may become apparent when using fast imaging systems (e.g., high milliamperage) or when imaging small or easily penetrated body parts. The backup timer functions to protect the patient from overexposure and the x-ray tube from overload.

103. **(D)** Because mammography uses such low-kilovoltage levels, IR front material becomes especially important. Any attenuation of the beam by the IR front would be most undesirable. Low-attenuating carbon fibers or special plastics that resist impact and heat softening (e.g., polystyrene and polycarbonate) are used frequently as IR front material.

104. **(B)** In *Compton scatter*, a *high-energy* (high kilovoltage) x-ray photon ejects an *outer-shell* electron in tissue or other absorber. The ejected electron is called a *recoil electron*. Although the x-ray photon is deflected with somewhat reduced energy (modified *scatter*), it *retains most* of its original energy and exits the body as an energetic scattered photon. Because the scattered photon exits the body, it does not pose a radiation hazard to the patient. It can, however, contribute to *image fog* and pose a *radiation hazard to personnel* (as in fluoroscopic procedures). In the *photoelectric effect*, a relatively *low-energy* (low kilovoltage) x-ray photon uses *all* its energy (true/total absorption) to eject an *inner-shell* electron, leaving an

orbital vacancy. An electron from the shell above drops down to fill the vacancy and in doing so gives up energy in the form of a *characteristic ray.* The photoelectric effect is more likely to occur in absorbers having *high atomic number* (e.g., bone or positive contrast media) and contributes significantly to patient dose because all the photon energy is absorbed by the patient (and, therefore, is responsible for the production of short-scale contrast). Brems and characteristic x-rays are produced at the focal spot as high-speed electrons are rapidly decelerated.

105. **(D)** Each time an x-ray exposure is made, *heat* is produced in the x-ray tube. Of all the energy used to make an exposure, 99.8% is converted to heat, and only 0.2% is converted to x-ray photon energy. Because greater heat production leads to increased wear and tear on the x-ray tube, decreasing its useful life, the radiographer should be able to calculate heat units and to understand the means of keeping heat production to a minimum. Heat units for a *single-phase* x-ray unit are determined by using the formula HU = mA × kV × time. Heat units for three-phase and high-frequency x-ray equipment are determined by using the formula HU = mA × kV × time × 1.4. High-milliampere seconds technical factors produce far more heat units than low-milliampere seconds technical factors.

106. **(A)** Radiographic reproducibility is an important concept in producing high-quality diagnostic images. Radiographic results should be consistent and predictable not only in terms of positioning accuracy but also with respect to exposure factors. AEC devices (ionization chambers and phototimers) automatically terminate the x-ray exposure once a predetermined quantity of x-rays has penetrated the patient, thus ensuring consistent results. A penetrometer can be used to demonstrate effects of kilovoltage on contrast. An induction motor has two parts, a stator and a rotor, and is used to rotate the anode.

107. **(D)** The function of contrast is to make details visible. Bit depth describes the number of gray shades stored in an image; the higher the bit depth, the greater is the dynamic range and the longer the grayscale. The greater the number of gray shades, the greater is the number of visible anatomic details. Dynamic range describes grayscale; as dynamic range and grayscale increase, so does the number of visible details.

108. **(C)** Image-intensifier output screen diameters of 5–12 inches are available. Although smaller diameter input phosphors/screens improve *resolution,* they do not permit a large fluoroscopic *FOV.*

Dual- and triple-field image intensifiers are available that permit *magnified* viewing of fluoroscopic images. To achieve magnification, the voltage to the focusing lenses is increased and a smaller portion of the input phosphor is used, thereby resulting in a smaller FOV (and

subsequent loss of brightness). The milliamperage is automatically increased to compensate for the loss in brightness when the image intensifier is switched to the magnification mode. When voltage applied to the focusing lenses increases, the *focal point* is further away from the output phosphor, and the output image is magnified.

ESE can increase dramatically as the FOV decreases (i.e., as magnification increases).

As FOV decreases, *magnification* of the output screen image increases, there is less noise because increased milliamperage provides a greater number of x-ray photons, and contrast and resolution improve. The focal point in the magnification mode is further away from the output phosphor (as a result of increased voltage applying to the focusing lenses) and therefore the output images magnified.

109. **(B)** Some x-ray circuit devices, such as the transformer and autotransformer, will operate only on AC. The efficient operation of the x-ray tube, however, requires the use of unidirectional current, so current must be *rectified* before it gets to the x-ray tube. The process of full-wave *rectification* changes the negative half-cycle to a useful positive half-cycle. An x-ray circuit rectification system is located between the secondary coil of the high-voltage transformer and the x-ray tube. Rectifiers are solid-state diodes made of *semiconductive materials,* such as silicon, selenium, or germanium that conduct electricity *in only one direction.* Thus, a series of rectifiers placed between the transformer and x-ray tube function to change AC to a more useful unidirectional current.

110. **(B)** The terms *star* and *wye* (or *delta*) refer to the configuration of transformer windings in three-phase equipment. Instead of having a single primary coil and a single secondary coil, the high-voltage transformer has three primary and three secondary windings—one winding for each phase (Fig. 5-17). Autotransformers operate on the principle of self-induction and have only one winding. Three-phase x-ray equipment often has three autotransformers.

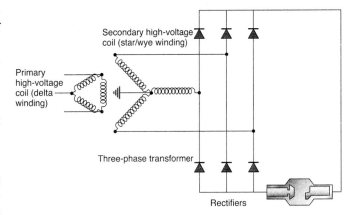

Figure 5-17

111. (A) Figure 5-11 illustrates the component parts of a rotating-anode x-ray tube enclosed within a glass envelope (number 3) to preserve the *vacuum* necessary for x-ray production. Number 4 is the *rotating anode* with its beveled focal track at the periphery (number 8) and its *stem* (at number 5). Numbers 6 and 7 are the *stator* and *rotor*, respectively—the two components of an induction motor—whose function is to rotate the anode. Number 1 is the filament of the cathode assembly, which is made of tho-riated tungsten and functions to liberate electrons (thermi-onic emission) when heated to white hot (incandescence). Number 2 is the nickel focusing cup, which functions to direct the liberated filament electrons to the focal spot.

112. (C) The anode is made to rotate through the use of an *induction motor*. An induction motor has two main parts, a *stator* and a *rotor*. The stator is the part located *outside the glass envelope* and consists of a series of electromag-nets occupying positions around the stem of the anode. The stator's electromagnets are supplied with current and the associated magnetic fields function to exert a drag or pull on the *rotor within the glass envelope*. The anode is a 2- to 5-inch diameter molybdenum or graphite disk with a beveled edge. The beveled surface has a *focal track* of tungsten–rhenium alloy. The anode rotates at about 3600 rpm (high-speed anode rotation is about 10,000 rpm), so that heat generated during x-ray produc-tion is evenly distributed over the entire track. *Rotating anodes* can withstand delivery of a greater amount of heat for a longer period of time than *stationary anodes*.

113. (D) The AEC automatically terminates the exposure when the proper receptor exposure has been reached. The important advantage of the AEC, then, is that it can accurately duplicate receptor exposures. It is very useful in providing accurate comparison in follow-up examina-tions and in decreasing patient exposure dose by reduc-ing the number of "retakes" needed because of improper exposure. The AEC automatically adjusts the exposure required for body parts with different thicknesses and densities. However, proper functioning of the AEC depends on accurate positioning by the radiographer. The correct photocell(s) must be selected, and the ana-tomic part of interest must completely cover the photo-cell to achieve the desired receptor exposure. If collimation is inadequate and a field size larger than the part is used, excessive scattered radiation from the body or tabletop can cause the AEC to terminate the exposure prematurely, resulting in an underexposed image.

114. (B) The *input phosphor* of an image intensifier receives remnant radiation emerging from the patient and con-verts it to a fluorescent light image. Directly adjacent to the input phosphor is the *photocathode*, which is made of a photoemissive alloy (usually, a cesium and antimony compound). The fluorescent light image strikes the pho-tocathode and is converted to an electron image. The electrons are carefully focused to maintain image resolu-tion by the *electrostatic focusing lenses* through the

accelerating anode and to the *output phosphor* for conver-sion back to light.

115. (C) As *filtration* is added to the x-ray beam, the lower energy photons are removed, and the overall energy or wavelength of the beam is greater. As *kilovoltage* is increased, more high-energy photons are produced, and again, the overall, or average, energy of the beam is greater. An increase in *milliamperage* serves to increase the number of photons produced at the target but is unrelated to their energy.

116. (A) A *photostimulable* (light-stimulated) *phosphor*, or simply *PSP*, is used in CR. The CR image plate (IP) con-tains a photostimulable phosphor that functions as the IR. On x-ray exposure, the PSP stores information. During processing the PSP is exposed to a monochro-matic laser light source. The phosphors emit polychro-matic light, termed photostimulated luminescence (PSL). The PSL signal represents varying tissue densities and the latent image. The PMT or photodiode (PD) detects the PSL and converts it to electrical signals, which is then transferred to an analog-to-digital converter (ADC)—converting the analog electrical signal to digital data. These digital data are then transferred to a digi-tal-to-analog converter (DAC) to be converted to a per-ceptible analog image on the display monitor. Direct digital imaging, DR, involves no scintillation. The abbre-viation FOV refers to field of view; the abbreviation ROI refers to region of interest.

117. (A) Lower ratio grids have shorter lead strips and diver-gent scattered photons are much more likely to pass between the lead strips and reach the image receptor. High-ratio grids have taller lead strips and so the diverg-ing scattered photons are much more likely to be absorbed by the lead strip. Scattered radiation is not impacted by milliampere seconds selection.

Comparison of Scatter Absorption

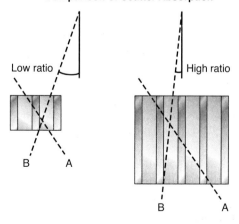

Figure 5-18

118. (C) The lead strips of a focused grid are angled to corre-spond to the configuration of the divergent x-ray beam. Thus, any radiation that is changing direction, as is typi-cal of scattered radiation, will be trapped by the lead foil strips. However, if the central ray and the grid center do not correspond, the lead strips will absorb the useful radiation. The absorption of primary radiation is termed *cutoff* and results in diminished receptor exposure.

119. **(D)** The accuracy of all three is important to ensure adequate patient protection. *Reproducibility* means that repeated exposures using given technical factors must provide consistent intensity. *Linearity* means that a given milliampere seconds value, using different milliamperage stations with appropriate exposure time adjustments, will provide consistent intensity. PBL is automatic collimation and must be accurate to 2% of the SID. Light-localized collimators must be available and must be accurate to within 2%.

120. **(A)** That portion of the x-ray beam striking the IR and representing image anatomy is called the *signal*. Some of the initial x-ray beam is absorbed via photoelectric interaction; some is scattered via Compton scatter (creating *noise*). Signal-to-noise ratio (SNR) is an important factor in all of medical imaging. Noise impairs image resolution; a high SNR is desirable (more signal, less noise). Noise impairs contrast resolution. Generally speaking, SNR increases as the milliampere seconds value increases; however, this is at the expense of patient dose. It is the responsibility of the radiographer to select technical factors and techniques that will provide a quality diagnostic image while keeping the ALARA concept in mind and minimizing patient dose.

121. **(C)** Grids are used in radiography to *absorb scattered radiation* before it reaches the IR (grid "cleanup"), thus improving radiographic contrast. Contrast obtained with a grid compared with contrast without a grid is termed *contrast-improvement factor*. The greater the percentage of scattered radiation absorbed compared with absorbed primary radiation, the greater is the "selectivity" of the grid. If a grid absorbs an abnormally large amount of useful radiation as a result of improper centering, tube angle, or tube distance, *grid cutoff* occurs.

122. **(C)** Pulsed fluoroscopy is rapid on/off of the x-ray beam. They are typically quite short (pulsed) exposures. The *length* of each pulse is called pulse width, whereas the *number* of pulsed exposures per second is called pulse rate.

Automatic exposure rate control (AERC) automatically modifies the exposure rate to that required by varying milliamperage, kilovoltage, pulse width.

123. **(B)** The image plate front material must not attenuate the remnant beam yet must be sturdy enough to withstand daily use. Bakelite has long been used as the material for tabletops and IR fronts, but now it has been replaced largely by *magnesium* and *carbon fibers*. Lead would not be a suitable material because it would absorb the remnant beam, and no image would be formed.

124. **(B)** As the kilovoltage is increased, a *greater number* of electrons are driven across to the anode with *greater force*. Therefore, as energy conversion takes place at the anode, *more high-energy* (short-wavelength) photons are produced. However, because they are higher energy photons, there will be less patient absorption.

125. **(B)** Electromagnetic radiation can be described as wave-like fluctuations of electric and magnetic fields. There are many kinds of electromagnetic radiation; visible light, microwaves, and radio waves, as well as x-ray and gamma rays, are all part of the electromagnetic spectrum. All the electromagnetic radiations have the same velocity, that is, 3×10^8 m/s (186,000 miles/s); however, they differ greatly in wavelength and frequency. Wavelength refers to the distance between two consecutive wave crests. Frequency refers to the number of cycles per second; its unit of measurement is hertz (Hz), which is equal to 1 cycle per second. Frequency and wavelength are closely associated with the relative energy of electromagnetic radiations. More energetic radiations have *shorter wavelength and higher frequency*. The relationship among frequency, wavelength, and energy is graphically illustrated in the electromagnetic spectrum.

Some radiations are energetic enough to rearrange atoms in materials through which they pass, and they can therefore be hazardous to living tissue. These radiations are called *ionizing radiation* because they have the energetic potential to break apart electrically neutral atoms, resulting in the production of negative and/or positive ions.

126. **(A)** A *compensating filter* is used when the part to be radiographed is of uneven thickness or tissue density (in the chest, mediastinum vs. lungs). The filter (made of aluminum or lead acrylic) is constructed in such a way that it will *absorb* much of the x-ray photons that would have exposed the *low*-tissue density area while allowing the remaining x-ray photons to *pass unaffected* to the high-tissue density area. A *collimator* is used to decrease the production of scattered radiation by limiting the volume of tissue irradiated. The *grid* functions to trap scattered radiation before it reaches the IR, thus reducing scattered radiation fog. *Added filtration* addresses patient protection, decreasing patient dose.

127. **(B)** Digital images are best viewed in areas with low-lighting levels that will avoid undesirable monitor screen glare. Digital images usually have a black "mask" covering the white unexposed areas, further reducing objectionable ambient light and glare. If the radiographer views images in a brightly lit area, the image can appear excessively dark. The same image, when reviewed by the radiologist, might look most adequate. As light level increases, the pupils of the eye contract and admit less light, causing images to appear dark. It is an effect similar to walking from a sunny day into a darkened theater.

128. (D) The purpose of the thin layer of lead that is often located in the rear portion of an IP is to absorb x-ray photons that strike the rear of the IP and bounce back toward the PSP, resulting in scattered radiation fog. The thin layer of lead absorbs these x-ray photons and thus improves the radiographic image.

129. (B) HVL testing provides beam quality information that is different from that obtained from kilovoltage testing. HVL is defined as the thickness of any absorber that will reduce x-ray beam intensity (kerma rate) to one-half of its original value. It is determined by measuring the beam intensity/kerma without an absorber and then recording the intensity as successive millimeters of Al are added. It is influenced by the type of rectification, total filtration, and kilovoltage. The x-ray tube HVL should remain almost constant. If HVL decreases, it is an indication of a decrease in the actual kilovoltage. If the HVL increases, it indicates the deposition of vaporized tungsten on the inner surface of the glass envelope (as a result of tube aging) or an increase in the actual kilovoltage.

130. (B) The input phosphor of image intensifiers is usually made of cesium iodide. For each x-ray photon absorbed by cesium iodide, approximately 5000 light photons are emitted. As the light photons strike a photoemissive *photocathode*, a number of electrons are released from the photocathode and focused toward the output side of the image tube by voltage applied to the negatively charged *electrostatic focusing lenses*. The electrons are then accelerated through the neck of the tube where they strike the small (0.5–1 inch) *output phosphor* that is mounted on a flat glass support. The entire assembly is enclosed within a 2- to 4-mm thick vacuum glass envelope. Remember that the image on the output phosphor is *minified*, *brighter*, and *inverted* (electron focusing causes image inversion).

Input screen diameters of 5–12 inches are available. Although smaller diameter input screens improve resolution, they do not permit a large FOV, that is, viewing of large patient areas.

Dual- and triple-field image intensifiers are available that permit *magnified* viewing of fluoroscopic images. To achieve magnification, the *voltage* to the focusing lenses is increased and a *smaller* portion of the input phosphor is used, thereby resulting in a smaller FOV. Because minification gain is now decreased, the image is not as bright. The milliamperage is automatically increased to compensate for the loss in brightness when the image intensifier is switched to magnification mode. Entrance skin exposure (ESE) can increase dramatically as the FOV decreases (i.e., as magnification increases).

As FOV decreases, *magnification* of the output screen image increases, there is less *noise* because increased milliamperage provides a greater number of x-ray photons, and *contrast* and *resolution* improve. The *focal* point in the magnification mode is *further away from* the output phosphor (as a result of increased voltage applied to the focusing lenses) and therefore the output image is magnified.

131. (A, B, E, and F) Regulating agencies identify quality control guidelines for fluoroscopic procedures. These quality control inspections must occur at least once every *6 months*. Fluoroscopic tabletop intensity must not exceed 88 mGy/min. The *Bucky slot cover* and the *protective curtain* each have 0.25-mm lead equivalent. The SSD for *stationary/fixed* equipment must be at least 38 cm, and at least 30 cm for mobile C-arm units. Magnification mode increases dose, so *minimum* use of magnification is encouraged.

132. (A, C, D, and E) Flat-panel detectors (FPDs) used in fluoroscopy replace the large and bulky image intensifier. Smaller size and weight of FPDs permit greater maneuverability. The amorphous selenium direct-capture detector produces a digital signal so there is *no need for a camera tube* or ADC. The system is capable of *recording both static images and dynamic* images; however, these systems produce very large data files. The system produces *higher spatial resolution, wider dynamic range*, improved contrast resolution, and improved DQE—as compared with image-intensified fluoroscopy. In addition, patient *dose decreases approximately 50%* compared with image-intensified systems.

133. (A) Diagnostic x-rays are produced within the x-ray tube when high-speed electrons are rapidly decelerated upon encountering the tungsten atoms of the anode/target. The *source of electrons* is the heated cathode filament; they are driven across to the anode focal spot when thousands of volts (kV) are applied. When the high-speed electrons are suddenly decelerated at the focal spot, their kinetic energy is converted to x-ray photon energy. This happens in two ways.

Bremsstrahlung (Brems) or "braking" *radiation*: A high-speed electron, passing near or through a tungsten atom, is attracted and "braked" (i.e., slowed down) by the positively charged nucleus and deflected from its course with a loss of energy. *This energy loss is given up in the form of an x-ray photon*. The electron might not give up all its kinetic energy in one interaction; it can go on to have several more interactions deeper in the anode, each time producing an x-ray photon having less and less energy. This is one reason the x-ray beam is *polyenergetic*, that is, has a spectrum of energies. *Brems radiation comprises at least 80% of the x-ray beam.*

Characteristic radiation: In this case, a high-speed electron encounters a tungsten atom within the anode and *ejects* a K-shell electron, leaving a vacancy in that shell. An electron from the adjacent L shell moves to the K shell to fill its vacancy and in doing so *emits a K-characteristic ray*. The energy of the characteristic ray is equal to the difference in energy between the K- and L-shell energy levels. *Characteristic radiation comprises up to 20% of the x-ray beam.*

Photoelectric effect and Compton scatter are interactions that occur between x-ray photons and matter.

134. (B) The x-ray photons produced at the tungsten target comprise a heterogeneous beam, that is, a spectrum of photon energies. This is accounted for by the fact that the incident electrons have different energies. Also, the incident electrons travel through several layers of tungsten target material, lose energy with each interaction, and therefore produce increasingly weaker x-ray photons. During characteristic x-ray production, vacancies may be filled in the K, L, or M shells, differing with each other in binding energies, and therefore, a variety of energy photons are emitted.

135. (A) The line-focus principle is a geometric principle illustrating that the *actual focal spot is larger than the effective (projected) focal spot*. The actual focal spot (target) is larger, to accommodate heat over a larger area, and is angled so as to *project* a smaller focal spot, thus maintaining spatial resolution by reducing blur. The relationship between the exposure given the IR and the resulting receptor exposure is expressed in the reciprocity law; the relationship between the SID and resulting IR exposure is expressed by the inverse square law. Grid ratio and lines per inch are unrelated to the line-focus principle.

136. (B) If the object/structure forms an angle with the image receptor, the resulting image will appear shorter/smaller than the actual part because of *foreshortening*. Think about the scaphoid and femoral neck and the imaging requirements because of their position in the body and relationship with the IR. Elongation can occur as a result of tube angulation.

137. (D) PSP storage plates are very sensitive to not only x-rays but also ultraviolet, gamma, and particulate radiations. Building materials such as concrete, marble, and others constantly emit natural radiation; bedrock in some geographic areas contributes significantly to background radiation. If PSPs are stored for extended periods of time, the possibility of artifacts must be considered. These artifacts typically appear as randomly placed small black spots. If an IP and its PSP storage plate has been stored, unused, for 48 h or more, the PSP should be erased prior to use.

Aliasing artifact can occur if a grid's lead strip pattern (i.e., frequency) matches the scanning (sampling) pattern of the scanner/reader. Phantom image artifacts are a result of incomplete erasure of a previous image on that PSP. Image fading occurs if an exposed PSP has been left several hours without processing and usually affects the entire image.

138. (D) The use of a fluoroscopic flat-panel detector can offer the benefit of reduction in patient dose because of increased DQE and pulsed x-ray beam. *The x-ray tube must be able to turn on and off very quickly.* The term *interrogation time* refers to the time it takes the tube to reach the required technical factors. The term *extinction time* refers to the time it takes the tube to turn off. The required time is less than 1 ms.

139. (B) Normal tissue variants and pathologic processes that alter tissue thickness and composition can have a significant effect on degree of alteration of the applied x-ray beam. The degree to which the x-ray beam is weakened/diminished by varying tissues is termed *differential absorption*. These tissue variants affect differential absorption, the amount of SR generated, and the number of photons reaching the IR. Subject contrast refers to the various body tissue densities and thicknesses, which results in *differential absorption* of the x-ray beam and *signal differences* within the remnant beam.

140. (A) Health care information technology, or health *informatics*, has ever-increasing application and use in the imaging sciences. PACS (picture archiving and communication systems) is used by health care facilities to economically store, archive, exchange, and transmit digital images from multiple imaging modalities. *PACS allows viewing of different modality images at one monitor and allows multiple users to view the same image at the same time at different locations.*

RIS (radiology information system) and HIS (hospital information system) can be integrated with PACS for electronic health information storage. The purpose of HIS is to manage health care information and documents electronically, and to ensure data security and availability. RIS is a system for tracking radiological and imaging procedures. RIS is used for patient registration and scheduling, radiology workflow management, reporting and printout, manipulation and distribution and tracking of patient data, and billing. RIS complements HIS and is critical to competent workflow to radiologic facilities.

141. (B) Focal spot size accuracy is related to the degree of *geometric blur*. Manufacturer tolerance for new focal spots is quite large. In addition, the focal spot can increase in size as the x-ray tube ages; hence, the importance of *testing newly arrived* focal spots and *annual* testing to monitor focal spots changes.

142. **(B)** X-ray tubes are diode tubes, that is, they have two electrodes—a positive electrode called the *anode* and a negative electrode called the *cathode.* The cathode filament is heated to incandescence and releases electrons—a process called *thermionic emission.* During the exposure, these electrons are driven by thousands of volts toward the anode, where they are suddenly decelerated. That deceleration is what produces x-rays. Some x-ray tubes, such as those used in fluoroscopy, digital radiography, and DSA are required to make short, precise—sometimes multiple–exposures. This need is met by using a grid-controlled tube. A grid-controlled tube uses the molybdenum focusing cup as the switch, permitting very precise control of the tube current (flow of electrons between cathode and anode).

143. **(B)** The thoriated tungsten filament of the cathode is heated by its own filament circuit. The x-ray tube filament is made of thoriated tungsten and is part of the cathode assembly. Its circuit provides current and voltage to heat it to incandescence, at which time it undergoes *thermionic emission*—the liberation of valence electrons from the filament atoms. *Electrolysis* describes the chemical ionization effects of an electric current. *Rectification* is the process of changing alternating current to unidirectional current.

144. **(B)** X-ray tube life may be extended by using exposure factors that produce a *minimum of heat*, that is, a lower milliampere seconds and higher kilovoltage combination, whenever possible. When the rotor is activated, the filament current is increased to produce the required electron source (thermionic emission). *Prolonged rotor time*, then, can lead to shortened filament life as a result of early vaporization. Large exposures to a cold anode will heat the anode surface, and the big temperature difference can cause cracking of the anode. This can be avoided by proper warming of the anode prior to use, thereby allowing sufficient dispersion of heat through the anode.

145. **(B)** The high-voltage, or step-up, transformer functions to increase voltage to the necessary kilovoltage. It decreases the amperage to milliamperage. The amount of increase or decrease depends on the transformer ratio—the ratio of the number of turns in the primary coil to the number of turns in the secondary coil. The transformer law is as follows:

To determine secondary V,

$$\frac{V_s}{V_p} = \frac{N_s}{N_p}$$

To determine secondary I,

$$\frac{N_s}{N_p} = \frac{I_p}{I_s}$$

Substituting known factors to determine voltage:

$$\frac{x}{220} = \frac{50,000}{100}$$
$$100x = 11,000,000$$
$$x = 110,000\,\text{V}\,(110\,\text{kV})$$

Substituting known factors to determine current:

$$\frac{50,000}{100} = \frac{100}{x}$$
$$50,000x = 10,000$$
$$x = 0.2\,\text{A}\,(200\,\text{mA})$$

SUBSPECIALTY LIST

Question Number and Subspecialty correspond to subcategories in each of the four ARRT examination specification sections

1. Imaging equipment
2. Imaging equipment
3. Image processing and display
4. Criteria for image evaluation of technical factors
5. Imaging equipment
6. Imaging equipment
7. Image processing and display
8. Imaging equipment
9. Imaging equipment
10. Criteria for image evaluation of technical factors
11. Quality control of imaging equipment and accessories
12. Imaging equipment
13. Imaging equipment
14. Imaging equipment
15. Imaging equipment
16. Quality control of imaging equipment and accessories
17. Imaging equipment
18. Imaging equipment
19. Quality control of imaging equipment and accessories
20. Quality control of imaging equipment and accessories
21. Imaging equipment
22. Image processing and display
23. Imaging equipment
24. Image processing and display
25. Imaging equipment
26. Imaging equipment
27. Imaging equipment
28. Quality control of imaging equipment and accessories
29. Quality control of imaging equipment and accessories
30. Imaging equipment
31. Criteria for image evaluation of technical factors
32. Quality control of imaging equipment and accessories
33. Imaging equipment
34. Imaging equipment
35. Imaging equipment
36. Image processing and display
37. Imaging equipment
38. Imaging equipment
39. Imaging equipment
40. Imaging equipment
41. Quality control of imaging equipment and accessories
42. Quality control of imaging equipment and accessories
43. Imaging equipment
44. Criteria for image evaluation of technical factors
45. Imaging equipment
46. Quality control of imaging equipment and accessories
47. Image processing and display
48. Imaging equipment
49. Imaging equipment
50. Criteria for image evaluation of technical factors
51. Imaging equipment
52. Imaging equipment
53. Imaging equipment
54. Imaging equipment
55. Imaging equipment
56. Image processing and display
57. Imaging equipment
58. Imaging equipment
59. Criteria for image evaluation of technical factors
60. Quality control of imaging equipment and accessories
61. Imaging equipment
62. Imaging equipment
63. Imaging equipment
64. Quality control of imaging equipment and accessories
65. Criteria for image evaluation of technical factors
66. Imaging equipment
67. Quality control of imaging equipment and accessories
68. Criteria for image evaluation of technical factors
69. Imaging equipment
70. Imaging equipment
71. Imaging equipment
72. Imaging equipment
73. Imaging equipment
74. Imaging equipment
75. Imaging equipment
76. Imaging equipment
77. Quality control of imaging equipment and accessories
78. Criteria for image evaluation of technical factors
79. Imaging equipment
80. Imaging equipment
81. Quality control of imaging equipment and accessories
82. Imaging equipment
83. Imaging equipment
84. Imaging equipment
85. Imaging equipment
86. Imaging equipment

87. Imaging equipment
88. Quality control of imaging equipment and accessories
89. Image processing and display
90. Criteria for image evaluation of technical factors
91. Imaging equipment
92. Imaging equipment
93. Quality control of imaging equipment and accessories
94. Imaging equipment
95. Imaging equipment
96. Image processing and display
97. Image processing and display
98. Imaging equipment
99. Imaging equipment
100. Image processing and display
101. Criteria for image evaluation of technical factors
102. Imaging equipment
103. Quality control of imaging equipment and accessories
104. Imaging equipment
105. Quality control of imaging equipment and accessories
106. Quality control of imaging equipment and accessories
107. Image processing and display
108. Image processing and display
109. Imaging equipment
110. Imaging equipment
111. Imaging equipment
112. Imaging equipment
113. Imaging equipment
114. Image processing and display
115. Imaging equipment
116. Imaging equipment

117. Imaging equipment
118. Criteria for image evaluation of technical factors
119. Quality control of imaging equipment and accessories
120. Criteria for image evaluation of technical factors
121. Imaging equipment
122. Imaging equipment
123. Quality control of imaging equipment and accessories
124. Imaging equipment
125. Imaging equipment
126. Criteria for image evaluation of technical factors
127. Image processing and display
128. Quality control of imaging equipment and accessories
129. Imaging equipment
130. Image processing and display
131. Quality control of imaging equipment and accessories
132. Image processing and display
133. Imaging equipment
134. Imaging equipment
135. Imaging equipment
136. Criteria for image evaluation of technical factors
137. Quality control of imaging equipment and accessories
138. Image processing and display
139. Imaging equipment
140. Image processing and display
141. Quality control of imaging equipment and accessories
142. Imaging equipment
143. Imaging equipment
144. Quality control of imaging equipment and accessories
145. Imaging equipment

TARGETED READING

Bushong SC. *Radiologic Science for Technologists.* 11th ed. St Louis, MO: Mosby; 2017.

Carlton RR, Adler AM, Balas V. *Principles of Radiographic Imaging.* 6th ed. Albany, NY: Delmar; 2020.

Carroll QB. *Radiography in the Digital Age.* 3rd ed. Springfield, IL: Charles C Thomas; 2018.

Carter C, Vealé B. *Digital Radiography and PACS.* 3rd ed. St Louis, MO: Mosby Elsevier; 2019.

Fuji Computed Radiography. Minato-Ku, Japan; 2002.

Johnston JN, Fauber TL. *Essentials of Radiographic Physics and Imaging.* 3rd ed. St Louis, MO: Mosby Elsevier; 2020.

Practice Test 1

QUESTIONS

DIRECTIONS: Each of the numbered items or incomplete statements in this section is followed by answers or by completions of the statement. Select the *one* letter answer or completion that is *best* in each case.

1. The portion of the remnant x-ray beam representing anatomical details having desirable quality is called
   - ❏ A. photoelectric
   - ❏ B. Compton
   - ❏ C. signal
   - ❏ D. noise

2. Which type of error results in grid cutoff at the periphery of the radiographic image?
   - ❏ A. Off-focus
   - ❏ B. Off-center
   - ❏ C. Off-level
   - ❏ D. Off-angle

3. In which of the following projections was the image in Figure 6-1 made?
   - ❏ A. AP
   - ❏ B. Medial/internal oblique
   - ❏ C. Lateral/external oblique
   - ❏ D. Acute flexion

4. During measurement of blood pressure, which of the following occurs as the radiographer controls arterial tension with the sphygmomanometer?
   - ❏ A. The brachial vein is collapsed
   - ❏ B. The brachial artery is temporarily collapsed
   - ❏ C. The antecubital vein is monitored
   - ❏ D. Oxygen saturation of arterial blood is monitored

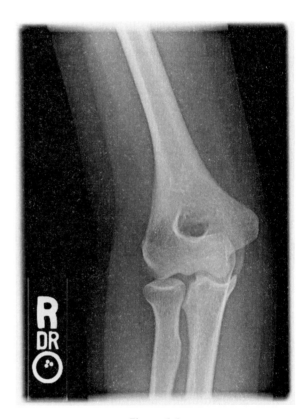

Figure 6-1

5. As the CR laser scanner/reader recognizes the phosphostimulated luminescence (PSL) released by the PSP storage plate, it constructs a graphic representation of pixel value distribution, called a/an
   - ❏ A. processing algorithm
   - ❏ B. histogram
   - ❏ C. lookup table
   - ❏ D. exposure index

6. An accurately positioned oblique projection of the first through fourth lumbar vertebrae will demonstrate the classic "Scotty dog." What bony structure does the Scotty dog's "eye" represent?

- ❏ A. Superior articular process
- ❏ B. Pedicle
- ❏ C. Transverse process
- ❏ D. Pars interarticularis

7. The term used to describe the gradual decrease in exposure rate as an x-ray beam passes through the matter is

- ❏ A. attenuation
- ❏ B. absorption
- ❏ C. scattered radiation
- ❏ D. secondary radiation

8. Which three of the following elements *must* be included on an x-ray image for it to be considered as legitimate legal evidence?

1. Name of facility where examination performed
2. Examination date
3. Date of birth
4. Referring physician
5. Patient identification
6. Radiographer initials
   - ❏ A. 1, 4, and 5
   - ❏ B. 1, 2, and 5
   - ❏ C. 4, 5, and 6
   - ❏ D. 2, 3, and 4

9. Referring to Figure 6-2, the pulmonary veins empty blood into which chamber of the heart?

- ❏ A. 2
- ❏ B. 4
- ❏ C. 5
- ❏ D. 6
- ❏ E. 8

10. Late effects of radiation include late tissue reactions. Examples of late tissue reactions include

1. organ atrophy
2. genetic effects
3. malignant disease
4. cataract formation
5. reduced fertility
   - ❏ A. 1, 3, and 4 only
   - ❏ B. 2, 3, and 5 only
   - ❏ C. 1, 4, and 5 only
   - ❏ D. 1, 2, and 3

11. Which of the following procedures requires that contrast medium is injected into the ureters?

- ❏ A. Cystogram
- ❏ B. Urethrogram
- ❏ C. Retrograde pyelogram
- ❏ D. Intravenous urogram

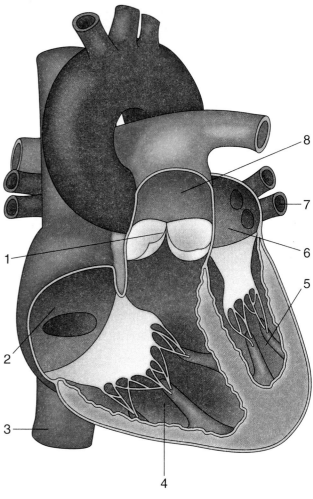

Figure 6-2

12. The unit for *kerma* is

- ❏ A. R
- ❏ B. rad
- ❏ C. gray
- ❏ D. coulomb

13. Which of the following combinations would pose the *greatest* hazard to a particular anode?

- ❏ A. 0.6-mm focal spot, 75 kVp, 30 mAs
- ❏ B. 0.6-mm focal spot, 85 kVp, 15 mAs
- ❏ C. 1.2-mm focal spot, 75 kVp, 30 mAs
- ❏ D. 1.2-mm focal spot, 85 kVp, 15 mAs

14. What is the structure indicated by the letter A in Figure 6-3?

- ❏ A. Greater tubercle
- ❏ B. Coronoid process
- ❏ C. Coracoid process
- ❏ D. Acromion process

15. Which of the following indicates the glenoid cavity seen in Figure 6-3?

- ❏ A. B
- ❏ B. C
- ❏ C. H
- ❏ D. M

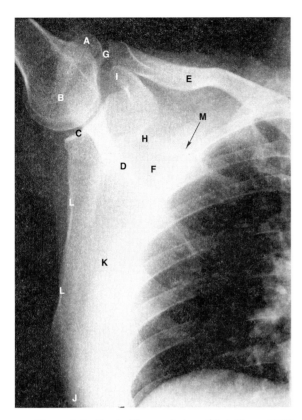

Figure 6-3. Used with permission of Bob Wong, RT(R).

16. The CR should be directed to the center of the part of greatest interest to avoid
- ❏ A. shape distortion
- ❏ B. magnification
- ❏ C. foreshortening
- ❏ D. elongation

17. Federal regulations regarding infection control in the workplace, as amended by the Occupational Safety and Health Administration (OSHA), make which of the following requirements?
1. Hepatitis B immunizations must be made available to all hospital employees
2. Puncture-proof containers must be provided for all used needles
3. Follow-up care must be provided to any staff accidentally exposed to blood splash/needlestick
- ❏ A. 1 only
- ❏ B. 1 and 2 only
- ❏ C. 2 and 3 only
- ❏ D. 1, 2, and 3

18. Methods of decreasing patient dose during fluoroscopic examinations include
1. use of last-image hold
2. using the lowest practical pulse rate
3. keeping the patient/part as close to the image intensifier as possible
- ❏ A. 1 only
- ❏ B. 1 and 2 only
- ❏ C. 2 and 3 only
- ❏ D. 1, 2, and 3

19. Which of the following radiologic examinations requires preparation consisting of a low-residue diet, cathartics, and enemas?
- ❏ A. Upper GI series
- ❏ B. Small bowel series
- ❏ C. Barium enema (BE)
- ❏ D. Intravenous (IV) cystogram

20. The exposure timer settings on three-phase radiographic equipment must be tested annually and must be accurate to within
- ❏ A. ±2%
- ❏ B. ±5%
- ❏ C. ±10%
- ❏ D. ±20%

21. Fluoroscopic equipment features designed to eliminate unnecessary radiation exposure to patients and/or personnel include
1. protective Pb curtain
2. primary beam filtration
3. collimation
- ❏ A. 1 only
- ❏ B. 1 and 2 only
- ❏ C. 1 and 3 only
- ❏ D. 1, 2, and 3

22. Verbal disclosure of confidential information that is detrimental to the patient is called
- ❏ A. invasion of privacy
- ❏ B. slander
- ❏ C. libel
- ❏ D. assault

23. If 300 mA has been selected for a particular exposure, what exposure time should be selected to produce 18 mAs?
- ❏ A. 40 ms
- ❏ B. 60 ms
- ❏ C. 400 ms
- ❏ D. 600 ms

24. During endoscopic retrograde cholangiopancreatography (ERCP) examination, contrast medium is injected into the
- ❏ A. hepatic duct
- ❏ B. cystic duct
- ❏ C. pancreatic duct
- ❏ D. common bile duct

25. Which of the following should be well demonstrated in the oblique position of the cervical vertebrae?
1. Pedicles
2. Disk spaces
3. Zygapophyseal joints
- ❏ A. 1 only
- ❏ B. 1 and 2 only
- ❏ C. 1 and 3 only
- ❏ D. 1, 2, and 3

CHAPTER 6 · PRACTICE TEST 1

26. Which of the following is most likely to produce a high-quality image?
- ❏ A. Small image matrix
- ❏ B. High signal-to-noise ratio (SNR)
- ❏ C. Large pixel size
- ❏ D. Low resolution

27. Select from the following the type(s) of x-ray beam filtration whose function is to decrease patient's skin dose.
1. Inherent
2. Added
3. Compensating
4. Collimation
- ❏ A. 1 only
- ❏ B. 1 and 2 only
- ❏ C. 1 and 3 only
- ❏ D. 2 and 3 only
- ❏ E. 1, 2, and 3

28. The image shown in Figure 6-4 was made in which of the following recumbent positions?
- ❏ A. RAO
- ❏ B. Lateral
- ❏ C. LPO
- ❏ D. PA

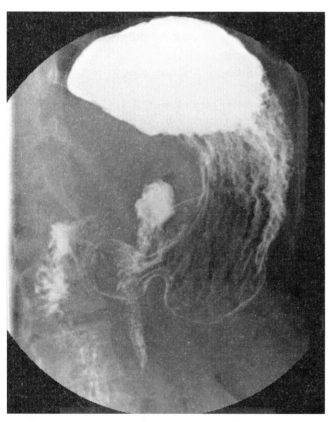

Figure 6-4. Used with permission of Stamford Hospital, Department of Radiology.

29. Terms that refer to size distortion include
1. magnification
2. attenuation
3. elongation
- ❏ A. 1 only
- ❏ B. 1 and 2 only
- ❏ C. 1 and 3 only
- ❏ D. 1, 2, and 3

30. Advantages of high-frequency generators include
1. small size
2. decreased patient dose
3. nearly constant potential
- ❏ A. 1 only
- ❏ B. 1 and 2 only
- ❏ C. 2 and 3 only
- ❏ D. 1, 2, and 3

31. The source-to-table distance in fixed/stationary fluoroscopy must
- ❏ A. be at least 38 cm (15 inches)
- ❏ B. not exceed 38 cm (15 inches)
- ❏ C. be at least 30 cm (12 inches)
- ❏ D. not exceed 30 cm (12 inches)

32. Which of the following is the *preferred* scheduling sequence?
- ❏ A. Lower GI series, abdomen ultrasound, upper GI series
- ❏ B. Abdomen ultrasound, lower GI series, upper GI series
- ❏ C. Abdomen ultrasound, upper GI series, lower GI series
- ❏ D. Upper GI series, lower GI series, abdomen ultrasound

33. Which of the following is/are demonstrated in the lateral projection of the thoracic spine?
1. Intervertebral spaces
2. Zygapophyseal joints
3. Intervertebral foramina
- ❏ A. 1 only
- ❏ B. 2 only
- ❏ C. 1 and 3 only
- ❏ D. 1, 2, and 3

34. As window width increases
- ❏ A. contrast scale increases
- ❏ B. contrast scale decreases
- ❏ C. brightness increases
- ❏ D. brightness decreases

35. The AP axial projection of the chest for pulmonary apices
1. projects the apices above the clavicles
2. requires 15°–20° of cephalad angulation
3. should demonstrate the medial ends of the clavicles equidistant from the vertebral column
    ❏ A. 1 only
    ❏ B. 1 and 2 only
    ❏ C. 2 and 3 only
    ❏ D. 1, 2, and 3

36. Rapid onset of severe respiratory or cardiovascular symptoms after ingestion or injection of a drug, vaccine, contrast agent, or food or after an insect bite describes
    ❏ A. asthma
    ❏ B. anaphylaxis
    ❏ C. myocardial infarction
    ❏ D. rhinitis

37. Select the statements from the following that correctly describe lines A and B in Figure 6-5.
1. Line A illustrates wider exposure latitude than line B
2. Line B is typical of digital imaging systems
3. Line A is typical of PSP response
4. Lines A and B are representative of analog imaging
    ❏ A. 1 and 4
    ❏ B. 1 and 3
    ❏ C. 2 and 3
    ❏ D. 3 and 4

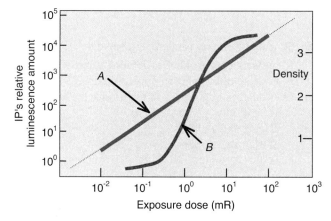

Figure 6-5. Used with permission of FUJIFILM Medical Systems USA, Inc.

38. Which of the following is/are used to indicate the appropriateness of radiation intensity reaching the IR?
1. Exposure index
2. Sensitivity (S) number
3. Field of view (FOV)
    ❏ A. 1 only
    ❏ B. 1 and 2 only
    ❏ C. 2 and 3 only
    ❏ D. 1, 2, and 3

39. Which of the following is the *most useful* for bone age evaluation?
    ❏ A. Lateral skull
    ❏ B. PA chest
    ❏ C. AP pelvis
    ❏ D. PA hand

40. The uppermost/first set of collimator shutters closest to the x-ray tube port window functions
    ❏ A. as a variable aperture beam restrictor
    ❏ B. to absorb scattered radiation
    ❏ C. to reduce off-focus radiation
    ❏ D. as positive beam limitation

41. Body substances and fluids that are considered infectious or potentially infectious include
1. sputum
2. synovial fluid
3. cerebrospinal fluid
    ❏ A. 1 only
    ❏ B. 1 and 2 only
    ❏ C. 2 and 3 only
    ❏ D. 1, 2, and 3

42. The National Council on Radiation Protection and Measurements (NCRP) has recommended what total equivalent dose limit to the embryo/fetus?
    ❏ A. 0.5 mSv
    ❏ B. 5.0 mSv
    ❏ C. 50 mSv
    ❏ D. 500 mSv

43. Fluids and medications are administered via the intravenous route for which of the following reason(s)?
1. To achieve a local effect
2. To administer parenteral nutrition
3. To promote rapid response
    ❏ A. 1 only
    ❏ B. 1 and 2 only
    ❏ C. 2 and 3 only
    ❏ D. 1, 2, and 3

44. Which of the following is/are tested as part of a QC program?
1. Beam alignment
2. Reproducibility
3. Linearity
    ❏ A. 1 only
    ❏ B. 1 and 2 only
    ❏ C. 1 and 3 only
    ❏ D. 1, 2, and 3

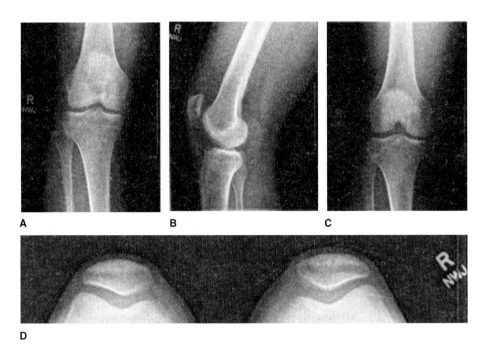

Figure 6-6. Used with permission of Orthopedic + Fracture Specialists, Portland, OR.

45. The line-focus principle refers to the fact that
- ❏ A. x-rays cannot be focused
- ❏ B. x-rays travel in straight lines
- ❏ C. the effective focal spot is larger than the actual focal spot
- ❏ D. the actual focal spot is larger than the effective focal spot

46. Which of the images shown in Figure 6-6 best demonstrates the intercondylar fossa?
- ❏ A. Figure 6-6A
- ❏ B. Figure 6-6B
- ❏ C. Figure 6-6C
- ❏ D. Figure 6-6D

47. Which of the following effects does an analgesic have on the body?
- ❏ A. Decreases pain
- ❏ B. Helps delay clotting
- ❏ C. Increases urine output
- ❏ D. Combats bacterial growth

48. Which of the following is/are associated with magnification fluoroscopy?
1. Less noise
2. Improved contrast resolution
3. Improved spatial resolution
- ❏ A. 1 only
- ❏ B. 1 and 2 only
- ❏ C. 2 and 3 only
- ❏ D. 1, 2, and 3

49. Histogram appearance can be skewed if there is inaccuracy in
1. part centering
2. part positioning
3. processing algorithm selection
- ❏ A. 1 only
- ❏ B. 1 and 2 only
- ❏ C. 2 and 3 only
- ❏ D. 1, 2, and 3

50. Bone densitometry is often performed to
1. measure degree of bone (de)mineralization
2. evaluate results of osteoporosis treatment/therapy
3. evaluate condition of soft tissue adjacent to bone
- ❏ A. 1 only
- ❏ B. 1 and 2 only
- ❏ C. 2 and 3 only
- ❏ D. 1, 2, and 3

51. Deficiency of blood to a body tissue describes
- ❏ A. necrosis
- ❏ B. ischemia
- ❏ C. dyspnea
- ❏ D. thrombus

52. If a part received 0.8 Gy during a 4-min fluoroscopic examination, what was the dose rate?
- ❏ A. 2 mGy/min
- ❏ B. 20 mGy/min
- ❏ C. 200 mGy/min
- ❏ D. 2000 mGy/min

53. The radiation barriers in a controlled area must keep worker exposure to less than
- ❏ A. 1 mSv/month
- ❏ B. 5 mSv/month
- ❏ C. 1 mSv/week
- ❏ D. 5 mSv/week

54. In the 45° medial oblique projection of the ankle, the
1. talotibial joint is visualized
2. tibiofibular joint is visualized
3. plantar surface is approximately perpendicular to the lower leg/IR
- ❏ A. 1 only
- ❏ B. 1 and 2 only
- ❏ C. 2 and 3 only
- ❏ D. 1, 2, and 3

55. Major effect(s) of irradiation of macromolecules include(s)
1. point lesions
2. cross-linking
3. main-chain scission
- ❏ A. 1 only
- ❏ B. 1 and 2 only
- ❏ C. 1 and 3 only
- ❏ D. 1, 2, and 3

56. Cells described as somatic include
1. neuron
2. muscle
3. oocytes
4. spermatozoa
5. osteoblasts
- ❏ A. 1, 2, and 3
- ❏ B. 2, 3, and 5
- ❏ C. 1, 2, and 5
- ❏ D. 3, 4, and 5

57. An animal host of an infectious organism that transmits the infection via a bite or sting is a
- ❏ A. vector
- ❏ B. fomite
- ❏ C. host
- ❏ D. reservoir

58. If the exposure rate at 2.0 m from a source of radiation is 18 mGy$_a$/min, what will be the exposure rate at 5 m from the source?
- ❏ A. 2.88 mGy$_a$/min
- ❏ B. 7.10 mGy$_a$/min
- ❏ C. 28.8 mGy$_a$/min
- ❏ D. 71.0 mGy$_a$/min

59. Imperfect expansion of the lung(s), often accompanied by dyspnea, is called
- ❏ A. COPD
- ❏ B. pneumonia
- ❏ C. pneumothorax
- ❏ D. atelectasis

60. An axial projection of the clavicle is often helpful in demonstrating a fracture that is not visualized using a perpendicular CR. When examining the clavicle in the PA position, how is the CR directed for the axial projection?
- ❏ A. Cephalad
- ❏ B. Caudad
- ❏ C. Medially
- ❏ D. Laterally

61. The x-ray tube's inherent filtration includes
1. glass envelope
2. insulating oil
3. collimator shutters
4. collimator mirror
5. glass window of tube housing
- ❏ A. 1, 2, and 3
- ❏ B. 1, 4, and 5
- ❏ C. 2, 3, and 5
- ❏ D. 1, 2, and 5
- ❏ E. 1, 3, and 4

62. All of the following are rules of good body mechanics, *except*
- ❏ A. keep the back straight, avoid twisting
- ❏ B. keep the load away from the body
- ❏ C. push, do not pull, the load
- ❏ D. keep a wide base of support

63. Which of the following is/are accurate positioning or evaluation criteria for an AP projection of the normal knee?
1. Femorotibial interspaces equal bilaterally
2. Patella superimposed on distal tibia
3. CR enters 1/2 inch distal to base of patella
- ❏ A. 1 only
- ❏ B. 1 and 2 only
- ❏ C. 1 and 3 only
- ❏ D. 1, 2, and 3

64. Biologic material is most sensitive to radiation exposure under which of the following conditions?
- ❏ A. Deoxygenated
- ❏ B. Oxygenated
- ❏ C. Hypoxic
- ❏ D. Anoxic

65. Each of the following statements regarding respiratory structures is true, *except*

❏ A. the left lung has two lobes
❏ B. the lower portion of the lung is the base
❏ C. each lung is enclosed in peritoneum
❏ D. the main stem bronchus enters the lung hilum

66. Ionizing radiation passing through tissue and depositing energy through ionization processes is known as

❏ A. the characteristic effect
❏ B. Compton scatter
❏ C. linear energy transfer
❏ D. the photoelectric effect

67. Images useful in demonstrating postspinal fusion degree of motion include

1. AP flexion and extension
2. lateral flexion and extension
3. AP right and left bending
   ❏ A. 1 only
   ❏ B. 1 and 2 only
   ❏ C. 2 and 3 only
   ❏ D. 1, 2, and 3

68. A blowout fracture usually occurs in which aspect of the orbital wall?

❏ A. Superior
❏ B. Inferior
❏ C. Medial
❏ D. Lateral

69. What is the name of the structure indicated as number 5 in Figure 6-7?

❏ A. Coracoid fossa
❏ B. Radial notch
❏ C. Olecranon fossa
❏ D. Coronoid fossa

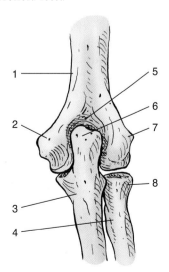

Figure 6-7

70. Which of the following projections/positions would best demonstrate structure number 8 seen in Figure 6-7?

❏ A. PA projection
❏ B. Lateral projection
❏ C. AP external oblique
❏ D. AP internal oblique

71. From the following, select the group identifying the correct blood path through the heart from systemic, to pulmonary, and back to systemic circulation.

❏ A. Left atrium, tricuspid valve, left ventricle, pulmonary semilunar valve, right atrium, mitral valve, right ventricle, aortic semilunar valve
❏ B. Right atrium, mitral valve, right ventricle, pulmonary semilunar valve, left atrium, tricuspid valve, left ventricle, aortic semilunar valve
❏ C. Right atrium, tricuspid valve, right ventricle, pulmonary semilunar valve, left atrium, mitral valve, left ventricle, aortic semilunar valve
❏ D. Left atrium, pulmonary semilunar valve, right atrium, tricuspid valve, left ventricle, aortic semilunar valve, right ventricle, mitral valve

72. Tungsten alloy is the usual choice of target material for radiographic equipment because it

1. has a high atomic number
2. has a high-melting point
3. can readily dissipate heat
   ❏ A. 1 only
   ❏ B. 1 and 2 only
   ❏ C. 2 and 3 only
   ❏ D. 1, 2, and 3

73. The portion of a hypodermic needle that attaches to the syringe is termed its

❏ A. hub
❏ B. gauge
❏ C. length
❏ D. bevel

74. X-ray tube life may be extended by

1. using high-mAs with low-kV technical factors
2. avoiding lengthy anode rotation
3. avoiding exposures to a cold anode
   ❏ A. 1 only
   ❏ B. 1 and 2 only
   ❏ C. 2 and 3 only
   ❏ D. 1, 2, and 3

75. Technical factors of 400 mA, 20 ms, 68 kVp at 40-inch SID were used to produce a satisfactory x-ray image. A change to 4 mAs can be *best* compensated for by which of the following?

❏ A. Increasing the SID to 60 inches
❏ B. Decreasing the SID to 20 inches
❏ C. Decreasing the kilovoltage to 60 kVp
❏ D. Increasing the kilovoltage to 78 kVp

76. A parallel-plate ionization chamber receiving a charge from x-ray photons is a/an
  ❏ A. photomultiplier tube
  ❏ B. induction motor
  ❏ C. autotransformer
  ❏ D. AEC

77. The position seen in Figure 6-8 is used to demonstrate
  ❏ A. distal humerus
  ❏ B. proximal forearm
  ❏ C. proximal humerus
  ❏ D. distal forearm

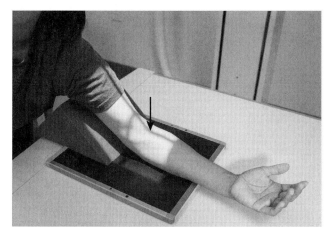

Figure 6-8. Reproduced with permission from Peart O. *Lange Radiographic Positioning Flashcards*. New York, NY: McGraw Hill; 2014.

78. Which of the following statements is/are true with respect to the differences between the male and female bony pelves?
  1. The female pelvic outlet is wider
  2. The pubic angle is 90° or less in the male
  3. The male pelvis is shallower
  ❏ A. 1 only
  ❏ B. 1 and 2 only
  ❏ C. 2 and 3 only
  ❏ D. 1, 2, and 3

79. Which interaction between x-ray photons and matter involves partial transfer of the incident photon energy to the involved atom?
  ❏ A. Photoelectric effect
  ❏ B. Compton scattering
  ❏ C. Coherent scattering
  ❏ D. Pair production

80. Improved visualization of interphalangeal joint spaces, seen in Figure 6-9, can be achieved by
  1. increasing obliquity of hand
  2. using a 45° foam wedge
  3. placing fingers parallel to IR
  ❏ A. 1 only
  ❏ B. 1 and 2 only
  ❏ C. 2 and 3 only
  ❏ D. 1, 2, and 3

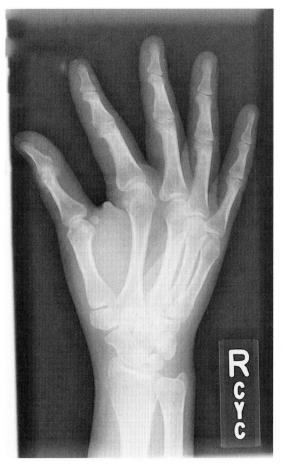

Figure 6-9

81. It is essential to question female patients of childbearing age regarding the
  1. date of their last menstrual period
  2. possibility of their being pregnant
  3. number of x-ray examinations they have had in the past 12 months
  ❏ A. 1 only
  ❏ B. 1 and 2 only
  ❏ C. 1 and 3 only
  ❏ D. 1, 2, and 3

82. Geometric unsharpness is influenced by which of the following?
  1. Distance from object to image
  2. Distance from source to object
  3. Distance from source to image
  ❏ A. 1 only
  ❏ B. 1 and 2 only
  ❏ C. 1 and 3 only
  ❏ D. 1, 2, and 3

83. A lesion with a stalk projecting from the intestinal mucosa into the lumen is a/an
  ❏ A. fistula
  ❏ B. polyp
  ❏ C. diverticulum
  ❏ D. abscess

84. Which of the following radiologic examinations would deliver the greatest ESE?
   - ❏ A. Chest
   - ❏ B. Skull
   - ❏ C. Abdomen
   - ❏ D. Thoracic spine

85. The medical term used to describe the vomiting of blood is
   - ❏ A. hematemesis
   - ❏ B. hemoptysis
   - ❏ C. hematuria
   - ❏ D. epistaxis

86. Select from the following the three types of motion permitted by saddle/sellar joints.
   1. Flexion
   2. Gliding
   3. Abduction
   4. Circumduction
   5. Medial/lateral rotation
      - ❏ A. 1, 2, and 4
      - ❏ B. 2, 3, and 5
      - ❏ C. 2, 3, and 4
      - ❏ D. 1, 3, and 4
      - ❏ E. 3, 4, and 5

87. How can OID be reduced for a PA projection of the wrist?
   - ❏ A. Extend the fingers
   - ❏ B. Flex the metacarpophalangeal joints
   - ❏ C. Extend the forearm
   - ❏ D. Oblique the metacarpals 45°

88. The positive electrode of the x-ray tube is the
   - ❏ A. capacitor
   - ❏ B. grid
   - ❏ C. cathode
   - ❏ D. anode

89. What is the most superior structure of the scapula?
   - ❏ A. Apex
   - ❏ B. Acromion process
   - ❏ C. Coracoid process
   - ❏ D. Superior angle

90. Impingement on the wrist's median nerve causing pain and disability of the affected hand and wrist is known as
   - ❏ A. carpal boss syndrome
   - ❏ B. carpal tunnel syndrome
   - ❏ C. carpopedal syndrome
   - ❏ D. radioulnar syndrome

91. Select from the following the three correct statements regarding characteristics of x-ray photons/the x-ray beam.
   - ❏ A. Fluorescent effect on certain phosphors
   - ❏ B. Travel at the speed of sound
   - ❏ C. Physiological effect on living tissue
   - ❏ D. Negative electrical charge
   - ❏ E. Collimators focus the x-ray beam
   - ❏ F. Travel in straight lines

92. A term that is often used to describe a particular control panel software selection in medical imaging is
   - ❏ A. hardware
   - ❏ B. algorithm
   - ❏ C. histogram
   - ❏ D. modem

93. The legal doctrine *res ipsa loquitur* relates to which of the following?
   - ❏ A. Let the master answer
   - ❏ B. The thing speaks for itself
   - ❏ C. A thing or matter settled by justice
   - ❏ D. A matter settled by precedent

94. Select from the following the two radiation monitoring devices that contain air chambers for radiation measurement.
   - ❏ A. Optically stimulated luminescence dosimeter
   - ❏ B. Thermoluminescent dosimeter
   - ❏ C. Film badge
   - ❏ D. Direct ion storage dosimeter
   - ❏ E. Pocket dosimeter

95. In the AP knee projection of an asthenic patient who measures 17 cm from the anterosuperior iliac spine (ASIS) to tabletop, the CR should be directed
   - ❏ A. perpendicularly
   - ❏ B. 5° medially
   - ❏ C. 5° cephalad
   - ❏ D. 5° caudad

96. Which of the following statements is/are true regarding Figure 6-10?
   1. There is inadequate inspiration
   2. Good collimation is evident
   3. Centering is not exact
      - ❏ A. 1 only
      - ❏ B. 1 and 2 only
      - ❏ C. 2 and 3 only
      - ❏ D. 1, 2, and 3

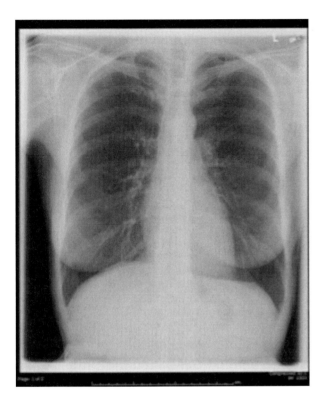

Figure 6-10

97. Hypochlorite bleach (Clorox) and Lysol are examples of
- ❏ A. antiseptics
- ❏ B. bacteriostatics
- ❏ C. antifungal agents
- ❏ D. disinfectants

98. Which of the following affect(s) both the quantity and quality of the primary beam?
1. kV
2. mA
3. Half-value layer (HVL)
4. Distance (SID)
- ❏ A. 3 and 4
- ❏ B. 2, 3, and 4
- ❏ C. 1 and 3
- ❏ D. 1, 2, and 4

99. Which of the following groups of organs/structures are located in the left upper quadrant?
- ❏ A. Left kidney, left suprarenal gland, and gastric fundus
- ❏ B. Left suprarenal gland, pylorus, and duodenal bulb
- ❏ C. Hepatic flexure, cecum, and pancreas
- ❏ D. Gastric fundus, liver, and cecum

100. For which of the following can a radiographer be found liable for a negligent tort?
1. Radiographer images the wrong forearm
2. Patient is injured while being positioned on the x-ray table
3. Radiographer fails to question patient about possible pregnancy before performing x-ray examination
- ❏ A. 1 only
- ❏ B. 1 and 2 only
- ❏ C. 2 and 3 only
- ❏ D. 1, 2, and 3

101. Technical factors of 100 kVp and 6 mAs are used with a 6:1 grid for a particular exposure. What should be the new milliampere seconds value if a 12:1 grid is substituted?
- ❏ A. 7.5 mAs
- ❏ B. 10 mAs
- ❏ C. 13 mAs
- ❏ D. 18 mAs

102. A diabetic patient who has not taken insulin while preparing for a fasting radiologic examination is susceptible to a hypoglycemic reaction. This is characterized by
1. fatigue
2. cyanosis
3. restlessness
- ❏ A. 1 only
- ❏ B. 1 and 2 only
- ❏ C. 1 and 3 only
- ❏ D. 1, 2, and 3

103. Which of the following structures are located on the distal anterior humerus?
1. Olecranon fossa
2. Capitulum
3. Medial epicondyle
4. Intertubercular groove
5. Coronoid fossa
- ❏ A. 1, 2, and 4
- ❏ B. 2, 3, and 5
- ❏ C. 1, 3, and 4
- ❏ D. 2, 4, and 5
- ❏ E. 3, 4, and 5

104. If the lumbar zygapophyseal articulation is not well visualized in the posterior oblique position, and the pedicle is seen on the posterior aspect of the vertebral body, what should be done to correct the position?
- ❏ A. Increase the degree of patient rotation
- ❏ B. Decrease the degree of patient rotation
- ❏ C. Flex knees to decrease lordotic curve
- ❏ D. Angle 5°–7° cephalad

105. Which of the following is the approximate dose for 2 min of fluoroscopy at 3 mA and 80 kV?

❏ A. 6 mGy$_a$
❏ B. 12 mGy$_a$
❏ C. 63 mGy$_a$
❏ D. 126 mGy$_a$

106. A *controlled area* is one that is

❏ A. restricted to access by nonradiation workers only
❏ B. monitored by survey meters
❏ C. occupied by radiation workers
❏ D. occupied by the general population

107. Gonadal shielding should be provided for male patients in which of the following examinations?

1. Femur
2. Abdomen
3. Pelvis

❏ A. 1 only
❏ B. 1 and 2 only
❏ C. 2 and 3 only
❏ D. 1, 2, and 3

108. Which of the following statements referring to Figure 6-11 is correct?

❏ A. Figure 6-11A was performed AP
❏ B. Figure 6-11B was performed AP
❏ C. Both images were obtained in the AP position
❏ D. Neither image was obtained in the AP position

109. Which of the following artifacts is occasionally associated with the use of grids in digital imaging?

❏ A. Incomplete erasure
❏ B. Aliasing
❏ C. Image fading
❏ D. Vignetting

110. The radiograph shown in Figure 6-12 can be produced with the

1. long axis of the plantar surface perpendicular to the IR
2. CR 40° cephalad to the base of the third metatarsal
3. CR 20° cephalad to the talotibial joint

❏ A. 1 only
❏ B. 2 only
❏ C. 1 and 2 only
❏ D. 1 and 3 only

111. Which of the following interactions between x-ray photons and matter is *most responsible* for patient dose?

❏ A. The photoelectric effect
❏ B. Compton scatter
❏ C. Classic scatter
❏ D. Thompson scatter

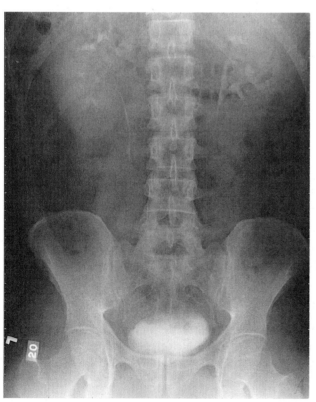

A

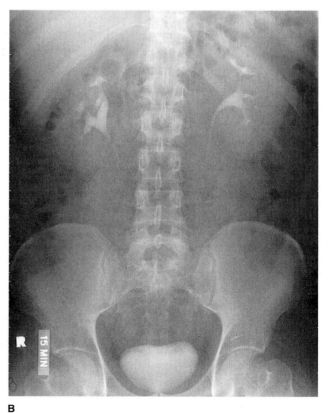

B

Figure 6-11. Used with permission of Stamford Hospital, Department of Radiology.

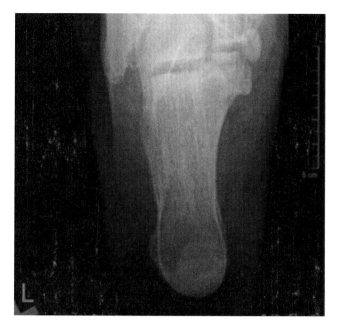

Figure 6-12. Used with permission of Orthopedic + Fracture Specialists, Portland, OR.

112. Select from the following the four bony features that are associated with the tibia.

1. Condyle
2. Plateau
3. Patellar surface
4. Malleolus
5. Styloid process
6. Intercondylar eminence
7. Head

❏ A. 1, 3, 5, and 7
❏ B. 1, 2, 4, and 6
❏ C. 2, 3, 4, and 7
❏ D. 3, 4, 5, and 6
❏ E. 2, 4, 5, and 7

113. The brightness level of the fluoroscopic image can vary with changes in

1. milliamperage
2. kilovoltage
3. patient thickness

❏ A. 1 only
❏ B. 1 and 2 only
❏ C. 1 and 3 only
❏ D. 1, 2, and 3

114. Which of the following methods can be used to decrease the effect of differential absorption?

1. Using high kV and low mAs
2. Using compensating filtration
3. Using factors that increase the photoelectric effect

❏ A. 1 only
❏ B. 1 and 2 only
❏ C. 2 and 3 only
❏ D. 1, 2, and 3

115. Select from the following the three correct completions: Scattered radiation exposure to personnel during C-arm fluoroscopic procedures can be reduced by positioning

❏ A. the fluoroscopy tube under the patient
❏ B. the image intensifier under the patient
❏ C. staff at the head of the x-ray table
❏ D. staff at right angles to the center of the x-ray beam
❏ E. staff at the foot of the x-ray table
❏ F. the image intensifier over the patient

116. Compared with that of the hypersthenic and sthenic body types, the stomach of an asthenic patient is most likely to be located

❏ A. higher and more medial
❏ B. lower and more medial
❏ C. higher and more lateral
❏ D. lower and more lateral

117. Which of the following correctly identifies the letter *T* in the radiograph shown in Figure 6-13?

❏ A. Plane joint
❏ B. Spheroid joint
❏ C. Sellar joint
❏ D. Ellipsoid joint

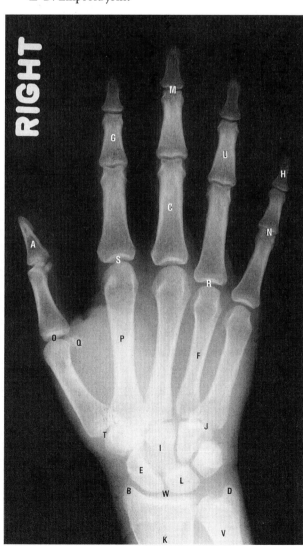

Figure 6-13. Used with permission of Bob Wong, RT(R).

118. Which of the following correctly identifies the letter *S* in the radiograph shown in Figure 6-13?

❏ A. Plane joint
❏ B. Spheroid joint
❏ C. Sellar joint
❏ D. Ellipsoid joint

119. The LAO position of the cervical spine requires which of the following combinations of tube angle and direction?

❏ A. 25°–30° cephalad
❏ B. 25°–30° caudad
❏ C. 15°–20° cephalad
❏ D. 15°–20° caudad

120. As x-ray field size increases,

1. amount of tissue exposure increases
2. DAP increases
3. beam intensity decreases

❏ A. 1 only
❏ B. 1 and 2 only
❏ C. 2 and 3 only
❏ D. 1, 2, and 3

121. Which of the following projection(s) require(s) that the shoulder be placed in external rotation?

1. AP humerus
2. Lateral forearm
3. Lateral humerus

❏ A. 1 only
❏ B. 1 and 2 only
❏ C. 2 and 3 only
❏ D. 1, 2, and 3

122. If the center ionization chamber was selected for a lateral projection of the lumbar spine that was positioned with the spinous processes centered to the IR, the result would be

❏ A. the image would be underexposed
❏ B. the image would be overexposed
❏ C. the image would be correctly exposed
❏ D. an exposure could not be made

123. What type of shock results from bodily invasion of infection?

❏ A. Septic
❏ B. Neurogenic
❏ C. Cardiogenic
❏ D. Hypovolemic

124. Which of the following statements are correct with respect to excretory system structures in the recumbent RPO position?

1. The right ureter is free of vertebral superposition
2. The left kidney is parallel to the IR
3. The right kidney is perpendicular to the IR
4. The left ureter is free of vertebral superposition
5. The right kidney is parallel to the IR

❏ A. 1, 2, and 3
❏ B. 1, 3, and 5
❏ C. 2, 4, and 5
❏ D. 2, 3, and 4

125. Occupational effective dose is assumed to be what percentage of the personal monitor dose?

❏ A. 5%
❏ B. 10%
❏ C. 20%
❏ D. 30%

126. Which of the following are examples of primary radiation barriers?

1. Radiographic room walls
2. Radiographic room floor
3. Lead aprons
4. Radiographic room ceiling
5. Lead gloves
6. Radiographic room control booth

❏ A. 1 and 2
❏ B. 2 and 5
❏ C. 1, 2, and 5
❏ D. 3, 4, and 6

127. How is source-to-image-receptor distance (SID) related to exposure rate and receptor exposure?

❏ A. As SID increases, exposure rate increases and receptor exposure increases
❏ B. As SID increases, exposure rate increases and receptor exposure decreases
❏ C. As SID increases, exposure rate decreases and receptor exposure increases
❏ D. As SID increases, exposure rate decreases and receptor exposure decreases

128. Which of the following cell types has the *lowest* radiosensitivity?

❏ A. Nerve cells
❏ B. Muscle cells
❏ C. Spermatids
❏ D. Lymphocytes

129. The substance used to induce vomiting is

❏ A. an emetic
❏ B. a cathartic
❏ C. a diuretic
❏ D. an antitussive

130. Although the stated focal spot size is measured directly under the actual focal spot, focal spot size in fact varies along the length of the x-ray beam. At which portion of the x-ray beam is the projected focal spot the largest?
- ❏ A. At its outer edge
- ❏ B. Along the path of the CR
- ❏ C. At the cathode end
- ❏ D. At the anode end

131. Extravasation occurs when
- ❏ A. there is an absence of collateral circulation
- ❏ B. there is a multitude of vessels supplying one area
- ❏ C. excessive contrast medium is injected
- ❏ D. contrast medium is injected into surrounding tissue

132. What is the *best* position/projection to demonstrate the longitudinal arch of the foot?
- ❏ A. Mediolateral
- ❏ B. Lateromedial
- ❏ C. Mediolateral weight-bearing lateral
- ❏ D. Lateromedial weight-bearing lateral

133. What anatomic structure is indicated by the letter B in Figure 6-14?
- ❏ A. Ischial tuberosity
- ❏ B. Iliac crest
- ❏ C. Anterior inferior iliac spine
- ❏ D. Obturator foramen

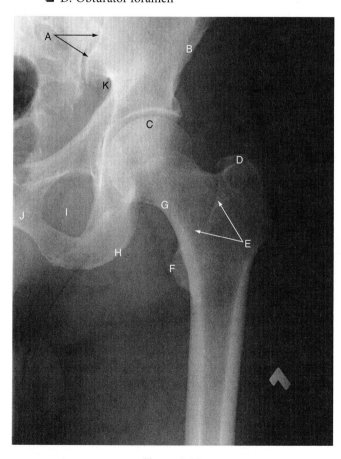

Figure 6-14

134. What is the minimum requirement for lead aprons used in general radiography, according to CFR 20?
- ❏ A. 0.05 mm Pb
- ❏ B. 0.50 mm Pb
- ❏ C. 0.25 mm Pb
- ❏ D. 1.0 mm Pb

135. Which of the following are associated with disease transmission via droplet route?
1. Influenza
2. Tuberculosis
3. Pertussis
4. SARS
5. Most pneumonias
   - ❏ A. 1, 3, and 5
   - ❏ B. 1, 2, and 4
   - ❏ C. 2, 3, and 4
   - ❏ D. 2, 4, and 5

136. Stochastic effects of radiation include
- ❏ A. blood changes
- ❏ B. genetic alterations
- ❏ C. epilation
- ❏ D. reduced fertility

137. In what way(s) is MRSA transmitted?
1. Contact with infected surfaces
2. Contact with infected objects
3. Direct contact
   - ❏ A. 1 only
   - ❏ B. 3 only
   - ❏ C. 1 and 2 only
   - ❏ D. 2 and 3 only
   - ❏ E. 1, 2, and 3

138. Which of the following conditions will require an increase in x-ray photon energy/penetration?
- ❏ A. Fibrosarcoma
- ❏ B. Osteomalacia
- ❏ C. Paralytic ileus
- ❏ D. Ascites

139. Combinations of milliamperage and exposure time that produce a particular milliampere seconds value will produce identical receptor exposures. This statement is an expression of the
- ❏ A. inverse-square law
- ❏ B. line-focus principle
- ❏ C. reciprocity law
- ❏ D. *D* log *E* curve

140. The position/projection most likely to offer the best visualization of the pulmonary apices is the
- ❏ A. lateral decubitus
- ❏ B. dorsal decubitus
- ❏ C. erect lateral
- ❏ D. AP axial lordotic

141. Which of the following is used to obtain a lateral projection of the upper humerus on patients who are unable to abduct their arm?

- ❏ A. Bicipital groove projection
- ❏ B. Superoinferior lateral
- ❏ C. Inferosuperior axial
- ❏ D. Transthoracic lateral

142. The term *differential absorption* is related to

1. beam intensity
2. subject contrast
3. pathology
   - ❏ A. 1 only
   - ❏ B. 1 and 2 only
   - ❏ C. 2 and 3 only
   - ❏ D. 1, 2, and 3

143. The RAO position is used to project the sternum to the left of the thoracic vertebrae to take advantage of the

- ❏ A. pulmonary markings
- ❏ B. heart shadow
- ❏ C. posterior ribs
- ❏ D. costal cartilages

144. Which of the following positions would demonstrate the right lumbar zygapophyseal articulations closest to the IR?

- ❏ A. LAO
- ❏ B. RAO
- ❏ C. LPO
- ❏ D. RPO

145. Which of the following features of digital fluoroscopy (DF) contribute to patient dose reduction?

1. Last-image hold
2. Pulsed exposure
3. Longer procedure times
   - ❏ A. 1 only
   - ❏ B. 1 and 2 only
   - ❏ C. 2 and 3 only
   - ❏ D. 1, 2, and 3

146. Grid interspace material can be made of

1. plastic
2. lead
3. aluminum
   - ❏ A. 1 only
   - ❏ B. 1 and 2 only
   - ❏ C. 1 and 3 only
   - ❏ D. 1, 2, and 3

147. What is the annual TEDE limit for radiation workers?

- ❏ A. 5 mSv
- ❏ B. 500 mSv
- ❏ C. 5000 mSv
- ❏ D. 50 mSv

148. All of the following statements regarding beam restriction are true, *except*

- ❏ A. beam restriction improves contrast resolution
- ❏ B. beam restriction improves spatial resolution
- ❏ C. field size should never exceed IR dimensions
- ❏ D. beam restriction reduces patient dose

149. An increase in technical factors usually is required in which of the following circumstances?

1. Edema
2. Ascites
3. Acromegaly
   - ❏ A. 1 only
   - ❏ B. 1 and 2 only
   - ❏ C. 1 and 3 only
   - ❏ D. 1, 2, and 3

150. Which of the following will *best* demonstrate the lumbosacral articulation in the AP position?

- ❏ A. CR perpendicular to L3
- ❏ B. CR perpendicular to L5–S1
- ❏ C. CR caudad 30°–35°
- ❏ D. CR cephalad 30°–35°

151. Which of the following medications commonly found on emergency carts functions to raise blood pressure?

- ❏ A. Heparin
- ❏ B. Norepinephrine
- ❏ C. Nitroglycerin
- ❏ D. Lidocaine

152. Focal spot blur is greatest

- ❏ A. toward the anode end of the x-ray beam
- ❏ B. toward the cathode end of the x-ray beam
- ❏ C. directly along the course of the CR
- ❏ D. as the SID is increased

153. Which of the following statements describe accurate comparisons between CCD (charge coupled device) and CMOS (complementary metal-oxide semiconductor) devices used for recording images?

1. The CCD has a higher DQE than the CMOS
2. CMOS has higher speed than CCD
3. CCD uses less power
4. CMOS is less expensive than CCD
   - ❏ A. 1, 3, and 4
   - ❏ B. 1, 2, and 4
   - ❏ C. 2, 3, and 4
   - ❏ D. 1, 2, and 3

154. Occupational exposure received by the radiographer is *mostly* from

- ❏ A. Compton scatter
- ❏ B. the photoelectric effect
- ❏ C. coherent scatter
- ❏ D. pair production

155. The bone labeled number 3 in Figure 6-15 is
- ❏ A. cuboid
- ❏ B. sesamoid
- ❏ C. tuberosity
- ❏ D. lateral cuneiform

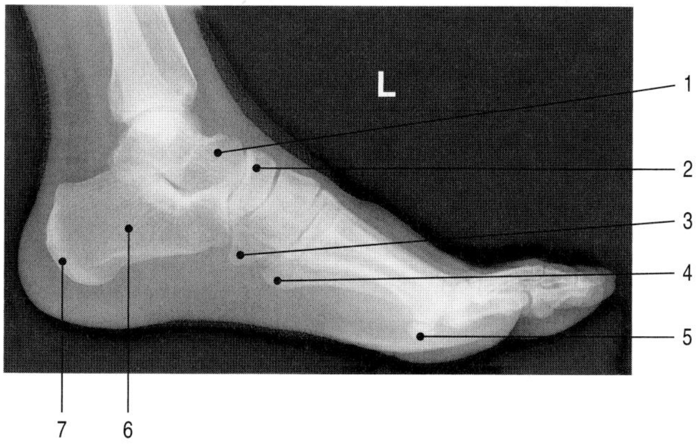

Figure 6-15

156. Sternal compressions during CPR are made with the heels of the hands located about
- ❏ A. 1½ inches superior to the xiphoid tip
- ❏ B. 1½ inches inferior to the xiphoid tip
- ❏ C. 3 inches superior to the xiphoid tip
- ❏ D. 3 inches inferior to the xiphoid tip

157. How is the introduction of a 6-inch OID likely to affect receptor exposure?
- ❏ A. Receptor exposure would increase
- ❏ B. Receptor exposure would decrease
- ❏ C. Receptor exposure would be unchanged
- ❏ D. Receptor exposure and OID are unrelated

158. Which of the following may be used as landmark(s) for an AP projection of the hip?
1. 2 inches medial to the ASIS
2. Prominence of the greater trochanter
3. Midway between the iliac crest and the pubic symphysis
- ❏ A. 1 only
- ❏ B. 1 and 2 only
- ❏ C. 1 and 3 only
- ❏ D. 1, 2, and 3

159. If an individual receives 3 mGy_a at a distance of 4 m from the source, what dose will that individual receive at a distance of 1 m from the source?
- ❏ A. 12 mGy_a
- ❏ B. 24 mGy_a
- ❏ C. 36 mGy_a
- ❏ D. 48 mGy_a
- ❏ E. 60 mGy_a

160. Recommended method(s) of minimizing motion unsharpness include(s)
1. suspended respiration
2. short exposure time
3. patient instruction
- ❏ A. 1 only
- ❏ B. 1 and 2 only
- ❏ C. 1 and 3 only
- ❏ D. 1, 2, and 3

161. Oral administration of barium sulfate suspension is usually required to demonstrate which of the following structures?
1. Descending duodenum
2. Ilium
3. Splenic flexure
- ❏ A. 1 only
- ❏ B. 1 and 3 only
- ❏ C. 2 and 3 only
- ❏ D. 3 only

162. Potential consequences of irradiation of DNA include
1. genetic effects
2. cell death
3. malignant disease
- ❏ A. 1 only
- ❏ B. 1 and 2 only
- ❏ C. 2 and 3 only
- ❏ D. 1, 2, and 3

163. The image intensifier's input phosphor differs from the output phosphor in that the input phosphor
- ❏ A. is much larger than the output phosphor
- ❏ B. emits electrons, whereas the output phosphor emits light photons
- ❏ C. absorbs electrons, whereas the output phosphor absorbs light photons
- ❏ D. is of a fixed size, and the size of the output phosphor can vary

164. Minor reactions to IV administration of a contrast agent can include
1. a few hives
2. nausea
3. a flushed face
- ❏ A. 1 only
- ❏ B. 1 and 2 only
- ❏ C. 1 and 3 only
- ❏ D. 1, 2, and 3

165. In an AP abdomen radiograph taken at 105-cm SID, one renal shadow measures 9 cm in width. If the OID is 18 cm, what is the actual width of the kidney?
- ❏ A. 5 cm
- ❏ B. 7.5 cm
- ❏ C. 11 cm
- ❏ D. 18 cm

166. An acute reaction caused by ingestion or injection of a sensitizing agent describes

- ❏ A. asthma
- ❏ B. anaphylaxis
- ❏ C. myocardial infarction
- ❏ D. rhinitis

167. A minimum total amount of aluminum filtration (inherent plus added) of 2.5 mm is required in stationary radiographic equipment operated

- ❏ A. above 50 kVp
- ❏ B. above 60 kVp
- ❏ C. above 70 kVp
- ❏ D. above 80 kVp

168. Which of the x-ray circuit devices shown in Figure 6-16 operates on the principle of self-induction?

1. Number 1
2. Number 2
3. Number 3
   - ❏ A. 1 only
   - ❏ B. 1 and 2 only
   - ❏ C. 2 and 3 only
   - ❏ D. 1, 2, and 3

169. Referring to the simplified x-ray circuit shown in Figure 6-16, what is indicated by the number 1?

- ❏ A. Primary coil of step-up transformer
- ❏ B. Secondary coil of filament transformer
- ❏ C. Autotransformer
- ❏ D. Secondary coil of step-up transformer

170. Which of the following pathologic conditions are considered *additive* conditions with respect to technical factor selection?

1. Atrophy
2. Bronchiectasis
3. Pneumonia
4. Emphysema
5. Pneumonectomy
6. Bowel obstruction
   - ❏ A. 1, 2, and 3
   - ❏ B. 2, 3, and 6
   - ❏ C. 4, 5, and 6
   - ❏ D. 2, 3, and 5
   - ❏ E. 3, 4, and 5

171. Which of the following would be *most likely* to cause the greatest skin dose (ESE)?

- ❏ A. Short SID
- ❏ B. High kilovoltage
- ❏ C. Increased filtration
- ❏ D. Increased milliamperage

172. Which of the following is/are essential to high-quality mammographic examinations?

1. Small focal spot x-ray tube
2. Short-scale contrast
3. Use of a compression device
   - ❏ A. 1 only
   - ❏ B. 1 and 2 only
   - ❏ C. 1 and 3 only
   - ❏ D. 1, 2, and 3

173. When medications are administered *parenterally,* they are given

- ❏ A. orally
- ❏ B. orally or intravenously
- ❏ C. intravenously or intramuscularly
- ❏ D. by any route other than oral

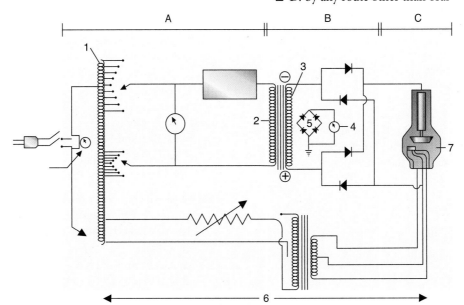

Figure 6-16

174. Which organization has the authority to impose professional sanction on a radiographer?
- ❏ A. ARRT
- ❏ B. ASRT
- ❏ C. JRCERT
- ❏ D. TJC

175. Patient factors such as size and pathology can have an impact on
1. receptor exposure
2. spatial resolution
3. distortion
- ❏ A. 1 only
- ❏ B. 1 and 2 only
- ❏ C. 2 and 3 only
- ❏ D. 1, 2, and 3

176. Advantages of CMOS (complementary metal oxide semiconductors) over CCDs (charge coupled devices) include
1. less expensive
2. better image quality
3. much greater speed
- ❏ A. 1 only
- ❏ B. 2 only
- ❏ C. 1 and 3 only
- ❏ D. 1, 2, and 3

177. The image seen in Figure 6-17 was obtained using which of the following positions?
- ❏ A. AP
- ❏ B. Unilateral frog-leg/modified Cleaves
- ❏ C. Axiolateral inferosuperior/Danelius-Miller
- ❏ D. Posterior oblique/Judet
- ❏ E. PA axial oblique/Teufel

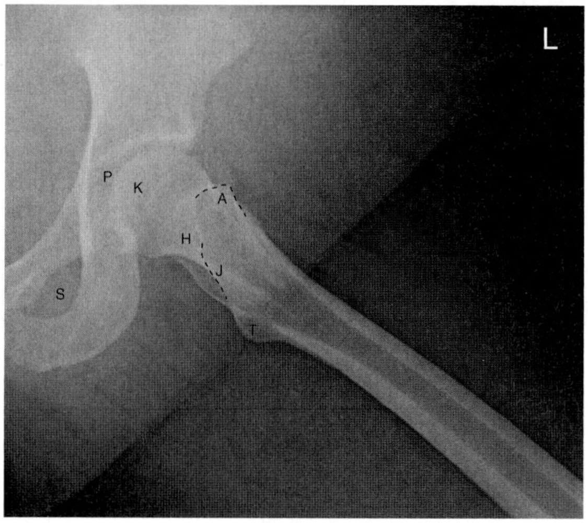

Figure 6-17

178. Referring to the image seen in Figure 6-17, the J identifies the
- ❏ A. greater tuberosity
- ❏ B. intercondylar line
- ❏ C. lesser trochanter
- ❏ D. intertrochanteric crest

179. The functions of x-ray beam filtration include which three of the following?
- ❏ A. Reduces patient skin exposure
- ❏ B. Absorbs low-energy photons
- ❏ C. Absorbs short-wavelength photons
- ❏ D. Decreases beam quality
- ❏ E. "Hardens" the x-ray beam

180. The effects of radiation on biologic material depend on several factors. If a quantity of radiation is delivered to a body over a long period of time, the effect
- ❏ A. will be greater than if it is delivered all at one time
- ❏ B. will be less than if it is delivered all at one time
- ❏ C. has no relation to how it is delivered in time
- ❏ D. solely depends on the radiation quality

181. The x-ray beam and collimator light field must coincide to within
- ❏ A. 10% of the OID
- ❏ B. 2% of the OID
- ❏ C. 10% of the SID
- ❏ D. 2% of the SID

182. When an injured patient requires assistance with dressing or undressing, the radiographer must remember to
1. place clothing on the injured side first
2. remove clothing from the injured side first
3. always start with the injured side
- ❏ A. 1 only
- ❏ B. 1 and 2 only
- ❏ C. 3 only
- ❏ D. 1, 2, and 3

183. Which of the following shoulder projections can be used to evaluate the lesser tubercle in profile?
- ❏ A. External rotation
- ❏ B. Internal rotation
- ❏ C. Neutral rotation
- ❏ D. Inferosuperior axial

184. The threat of bodily harm, with apparent ability to do so, is termed
- ❏ A. assault
- ❏ B. battery
- ❏ C. false imprisonment
- ❏ D. invasion of privacy

185. Which of the following structures will be filled with barium in the AP recumbent position of a sthenic patient during an upper GI examination?
- ❏ A. Duodenal bulb
- ❏ B. Descending duodenum
- ❏ C. Pyloric vestibule
- ❏ D. Gastric fundus

186. How often are radiographic equipment collimators required to be evaluated?

❏ A. Annually
❏ B. Biannually
❏ C. Semiannually
❏ D. Quarterly

187. Which of the following techniques might have been used in the production of Figure 6-18?

1. Motion
2. Anode heel effect
3. Compression
  ❏ A. 1 only
  ❏ B. 1 and 2 only
  ❏ C. 1 and 3 only
  ❏ D. 1, 2, and 3

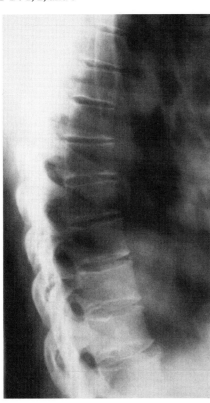

Figure 6-18. Reproduced, with permission, from Shephard C.T. *Radiographic Image Production and Manipulation*. New York: McGraw Hill; 2003.

188. Which of the following pathologic conditions require(s) a decrease in technical factors?

1. Pneumothorax
2. Emphysema
3. Multiple myeloma
  ❏ A. 1 only
  ❏ B. 1 and 2 only
  ❏ C. 2 and 3 only
  ❏ D. 1, 2, and 3

189. A diuretic is used to

❏ A. induce vomiting
❏ B. stimulate defecation
❏ C. increase urine output
❏ D. inhibit coughing

190. An exposed CR image plate's PSP will retain its image for about

❏ A. 2 h
❏ B. 8 h
❏ C. 24 h
❏ D. 48 h

191. The total number of x-ray photons produced at the target is contingent on the

1. tube current
2. target material
3. square of the kilovoltage
  ❏ A. 1 only
  ❏ B. 1 and 2 only
  ❏ C. 2 and 3 only
  ❏ D. 1, 2, and 3

192. Which of the following formulas is used to determine the total number of heat units (HU) produced with a given exposure using three-phase and high-frequency equipment?

❏ A. mA × kVp × s
❏ B. mA × kVp × s × 1.4
❏ C. mA × kVp × s × 1.7
❏ D. mA × kVp × s × 2.3

193. Figure 6-19 illustrates a sectional image of the abdomen. Which of the following is represented by the number 3?

❏ A. Left colic flexure
❏ B. Pancreas
❏ C. Left kidney
❏ D. Spleen

194. Select from the following the three correct statements regarding radiation monitoring control monitors.

1. The control monitor is stored in a radiation-free area
2. Control monitor reading is subtracted from the remaining personnel monitors
3. Control monitor can replace an employee's lost or misplaced monitor
4. A control monitor is supplied with each batch of dosimeters
5. Control monitor is stored in central area of radiology department
6. A control monitor is designated for each personnel monitor
  ❏ A. 1, 3, and 6
  ❏ B. 1, 2, and 4
  ❏ C. 3, 4, and 5
  ❏ D. 2, 5, and 6

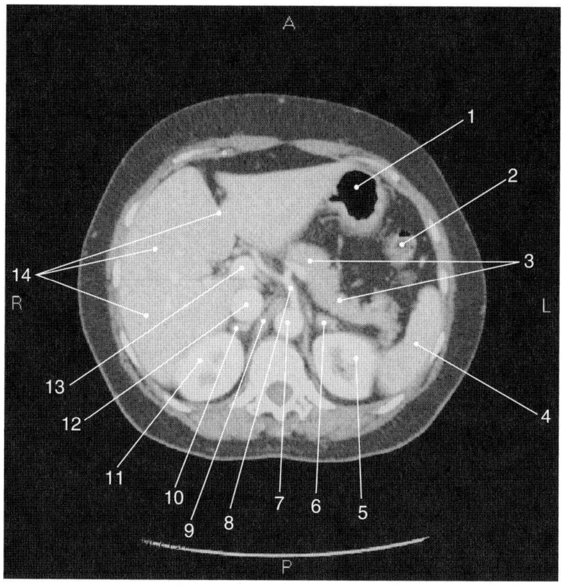

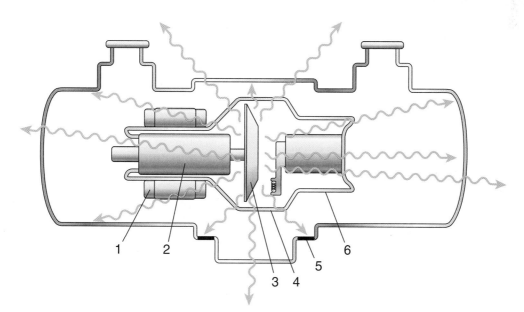

Figure 6-19. Used with permission of Stamford Hospital, Department of Radiology.

195. What is the *appropriate* action if a patient has signed consent for a procedure but, once on the radiographic table, refuses the procedure?
- ❏ A. Proceed—the consent form is signed
- ❏ B. Send the patient back to his or her room
- ❏ C. Honor the patient's request and proceed with the next patient
- ❏ D. Immediately stop the procedure and inform the radiologist and the referring physician of the patient's request

196. To maintain image clarity, the path of electron flow from photocathode to output phosphor is controlled by
- ❏ A. the accelerating anode
- ❏ B. electrostatic lenses
- ❏ C. the vacuum glass envelope
- ❏ D. the input phosphor

197. Which of the following terms is used to express resolution?
- ❏ A. Kiloelectronvolts (keV)
- ❏ B. Modulation transfer function (MTF)
- ❏ C. Relative speed
- ❏ D. Latitude

198. What is the function of the x-ray tube component numbered 2 in Figure 6-20?
- ❏ A. To release electrons when heated
- ❏ B. To rotate the anode
- ❏ C. To direct electrons to the focal track
- ❏ D. To heat the filament

199. Of what material is the x-ray tube component numbered 3 in Figure 6-20 made?
- ❏ A. Cesium
- ❏ B. Copper
- ❏ C. Nickel
- ❏ D. Tungsten

200. What is the structure labeled number 5 in Figure 6-20?
- ❏ A. Glass envelope
- ❏ B. Lead-lined tube housing
- ❏ C. Uppermost collimator shutter
- ❏ D. Added aluminum filtration

Figure 6-20

ANSWERS AND EXPLANATIONS

1. **(C)** The portion of the x-ray beam striking the IR and representing image anatomy is called the *signal*. Some of the initial x-ray beam is absorbed via photoelectric interaction; some is scattered via Compton scatter (creating *noise*). Signal-to-noise ratio (SNR) is an important factor in all of medical imaging. Noise impairs image resolution; a high SNR is desirable (more signal, less noise). Generally speaking, SNR increases as milliampere seconds value increases; however, this is at the expense of patient dose. It is the responsibility of the radiographer to select technical factors and techniques that will provide a quality diagnostic image while keeping the ALARA concept in mind and minimizing patient dose.

2. **(A)** The lead strips in a focused grid are angled so as to parallel the x-ray beam. Therefore, scattered radiation, which radiates in directions other than that of the primary beam, will be absorbed by the grid. When the x-ray beam does not parallel the lead strips, some type of grid cutoff occurs. If the x-ray beam is not centered to the grid (off-center error), or if the x-ray tube and grid surface are not parallel (off-level error), there will be a fairly *uniform decrease* in receptor exposure across the entire image. However, if the grid is not used within its recommended SID (focus) range (i.e., if the SID is too great or too little), there will be a decrease in density *at the periphery* of the image.

3. **(C)** Figure 6-1 illustrates an oblique view of the proximal radius and ulna and distal humerus with epicondyles 45° to the IR—the external oblique (lateral rotation) projection is shown demonstrating the radial head free of superimposition as well as the radial neck, tuberosity, and the humeral capitulum.

   The *medial oblique (internal rotation)* projection of the elbow is particularly useful to demonstrate the *coronoid process* in profile, the *trochlea,* and the *medial epicondyle.*

   The acute flexion projection (Jones method) of the elbow is a two-projection method demonstrating the elbow anatomy when the part cannot be extended for an AP projection.

4. **(B)** A stethoscope and a sphygmomanometer are used together to measure blood pressure. The sphygmomanometer's cuff is placed around the midportion of the upper arm. The cuff is inflated to a value higher than the patient's systolic pressure to temporarily collapse the brachial artery. As the inflation is gradually released, the first sound heard is the systolic pressure; the normal range is 110–140 mm Hg. When no more sound is heard, the diastolic pressure is recorded. The normal diastolic range is 60–90 mm Hg. Elevated blood pressure is called *hypertension. Hypotension,* low blood pressure, is not of concern unless it is caused by injury or disease; in that case, it can result in shock.

5. **(B)** As the CR laser scanner/reader recognizes the phosphostimulated luminescence (PSL) released by the PSP storage plate, it constructs a graphic representation of pixel value distribution called a *histogram.*

   The photostimulable storage phosphor (PSP) is the image receptor (IR) and is a europium-doped barium fluorohalide-coated storage plate. When exposed by x-ray photons, the PSP crystals emit a small amount of visible light, *but most of the x-ray energy is stored* (hence, the term *storage plate*). This stored energy represents the latent image.

   In the CR scanner/reader, a helium–neon, or solid-state, laser beam scans the PSP and its stored energy is released as blue-violet light (phosphostimulated luminescence [PSL]). This light signal represents varying tissue densities and the latent image that is then transferred to an *analog-to-digital converter (ADC).* The PSL values result in numerous image *brightness values* representing various *tissue densities* (i.e., x-ray attenuation properties). The CR scanner/reader recognizes these values and constructs a representative grayscale *histogram* of them corresponding to the anatomical characteristics of the imaged part. Thus, all PA chest histograms will be similar, all lateral chest histograms will be similar, all pelvis histograms will be similar, and so on.

   A histogram of the *actual* imaged part is compared with the programmed representative histogram for that part. Over time, if required diagnostic image characteristics change, a histogram can be updated to reflect the latest required characteristics.

6. **(B)** The 45° oblique position of the lumbar spine generally is performed for demonstration of the *zygapophyseal joints.* In a correctly positioned oblique lumbar spine, "Scotty dog" images are demonstrated. The Scotty's *ear* corresponds to the superior articular process, its *nose* to the transverse process, its *eye* to the pedicle, its *neck* to the pars interarticularis, its *body* to the lamina, and its *front foot* to the inferior articular process.

7. **(A)** The gradual decrease in exposure rate as radiation passes through matter is called *attenuation*. Attenuation is attributed to the two major types of interactions that occur in tissue between x-ray photons and matter in the

diagnostic x-ray range. In the photoelectric effect, absorption and secondary radiation occur. In the Compton effect, scattered radiation is produced. With each of these occurrences, there is a decrease in the exposure rate that is called *attenuation*.

8. (B) X-ray images are often subpoenaed as court evidence in cases of medical litigation. To be considered as a legitimate legal evidence, each x-ray image must contain certain essential and specific patient information. Essential information that must be included on each image is patient identification, the identity of the facility where the x-ray study was performed, the date when the study was performed, and a right- or left-side marker.

Other useful information that may be included, but that is not considered essential, is additional patient demographics such as date of birth, the identity of the referring physician, the time of day that the study was performed, and the identity/initials of the radiographer performing the examination.

9. (D) Figure 6-2 illustrates the component parts of cardiopulmonary circulation. Deoxygenated blood enters the RA (2) from the superior and inferior (3) venae cavae and coronary sinus. Blood flows from RA through the right atrioventricular/tricuspid valve into the RV (4). RV contraction opens the pulmonary semilunar valve (1) and blood flows into the pulmonary artery (8) to the lungs and undergoes oxygenation. Newly oxygenated blood enters LA (6) via four pulmonary veins (7).

Blood flows from the LA through left atrioventricular/mitral valve into the LV (5). LV contraction opens the aortic semilunar valve and blood flows into the ascending aorta. Aorta and its branches distribute oxygenated blood to all body tissues. CO_2 is collected by the venous system, and deoxygenated blood is returned via the superior and inferior (3) venae cavae to the RA (2).

10. (C) Late somatic effects of radiation can occur in tissues as a result of chronic exposure or tissues that have survived a previous irradiation months or years earlier. Late somatic effects can be either *stochastic* effects or *tissue reactions*. *Stochastic* effects, such as cancer, are usually determined at the time of radiation exposure and generally require years to manifest themselves. Stochastic effects such as cancer do not have a threshold dose, that is, any dose, however small, can cause an effect (thus, the importance of radiation protection). Increasing that dose will increase the *likelihood* of the occurrence but will not affect its severity; these effects are termed *stochastic*. Examples of *tissue reactions* include organ atrophy, reduced fertility, stability, fibrosis, and cataract formation.

11. (C) Contrast-medium injection into the ureters can be achieved only by first catheterizing the bladder, locating the ureteral orifices, and then injecting the contrast agent into the ureters. This procedure is called a *retrograde*

(because contrast is being introduced against the normal direction of flow) *pyelogram*. A *cystogram* is an examination of the bladder. A *cystourethrogram* is an examination of the bladder and urethra. An intravenous urogram requires that the contrast agent be injected intravenously. Intravenous urograms demonstrate function, whereas retrograde urograms demonstrate structure/anatomy.

12. (C) The term *kerma* is used to express *k*inetic *e*nergy *r*eleased in *ma*tter. For our purposes, that matter can be *air* or *tissue*. X-rays expend kinetic energy as they ionize the air or matter. Joule/kilogram is the metric unit used to express the release of kinetic energy in air or tissue. *Gray* is the unit for kerma, in both air and tissue. Gy_a describes gray in air and Gy_t describes gray in tissue.

13. (A) Radiographic rating charts enable the radiographer to determine the maximum safe milliamperage, exposure time, and peak kilovoltage for a particular exposure using a particular x-ray tube. An exposure that can be made safely with the large focal spot may not be safe for use with the small focal spot of the same x-ray tube. The total number of heat units that an exposure generates also influences the amount of stress (in the form of heat) imparted to the anode. The product of milliampere seconds and peak kilovolts determines HU. Groups (A) and (C) produce 2250 HU; groups (B) and (D) produce 1275 HU. Groups (B) and (D) deliver less heat load, but group (D) delivers it to a larger area (actual focal spot), making this the *least* hazardous group of technical factors. Groups (A) and (C) produce more heat, but group (A) delivers it to a smaller focal spot, making it the *most* hazardous group of technical factors for the anode.

14–15. (14, D; 15, B) The radiograph in Figure 6-3 illustrates an AP projection of the scapula; abduction of the arm moves the scapula away from the rib cage, revealing a greater portion of the scapula than would be visualized with the arm at the side. A number of bony structures are identified: the acromion process (A), the humeral head (B), glenoid fossa (C), scapular spine (D), clavicle (E), supraspinatus fossa (F), acromioclavicular joint (G), scapular notch (H), coracoid process (I), inferior angle/apex (J), body/costal surface (K), lateral/axillary border (L), and base of the scapula (M).

16. (A) Image details placed away from the path of the CR will be exposed by more divergent rays, resulting in *shape distortion*. This occurs to some degree in every radiograph—any structure not along the path of the central ray will be distorted. The further away from the central ray, the greater the divergence, and the greater the degree of distortion. The effect is similar to that of angling tube angulation, resulting in elongation.

Magnification occurs when an OID is introduced, or with a decrease in SID. Foreshortening and elongation are the two types of shape distortion—caused by non-alignment of the x-ray tube, part/subject, and IR.

17. **(C)** Federal regulations regarding infection control in the workplace, as amended by OSHA, require development of policies conforming to OSHA guidelines and instruction in their application/use. These regulations also require provision of hepatitis B immunization (free of charge) for all staff *who might be exposed to blood*/body substances, follow-up care for any staff accidentally exposed to blood/body fluids and/or needlestick injuries, and readily accessible personal protective equipment (PPE) and impermeable puncture-proof containers for used needles/syringes. It also requires that all health care workers and their employers follow/enforce standard precautions, transmission-based precautions, and these OSHA guidelines under penalty of law.

18. **(D)** Fluoroscopy is a potentially higher patient dose procedure. The principal reason for this is that the source of x-ray photons is in closer proximity to the patient than in overhead imaging. There are NCRP recommendations that provide guidelines for minimum source-to-skin distance (SSD), maximum tube output, collimation, timer and exposure switch specifications, and so on. An advantage of *digital* fluoroscopy (DF) is reduced patient dose. The principal reason for lower patient dose in DF is that DF x-ray beams are *pulsed,* rather than continuous.

Ways to Decrease Patient Fluoroscopic Dose

- Decrease length of fluoroscopic exposure/procedure
- Use last-image-hold feature
  - Keep patient as close to the image intensifier (II) as possible
  - Use automatic brightness control (ABC) setting with highest kV/lowest mA combination
- Minimize use of "boost" and "magnification" modes
- Collimation; use smallest field of view (FOV)
- Use lowest practical pulse rate
  - Change tube angle or patient position to spread dose over larger area

---

19. **(C)** To have high diagnostic quality, a barium enema (BE) examination requires rigorous and complete patient preparation. This usually consists of a modified low-residue diet for a few days before the examination, cathartics the day before, and cleansing enemas the morning of the examination. Instructions for an upper GI series, small bowel series, and IV cystogram are usually to be NPO after midnight.

20. **(B)** Quality control refers to our equipment and its safe and accurate operation. Various components must be tested at specified intervals and test results must be within specified parameters. Any deviation from those parameters must be corrected. Examples of equipment components that are tested annually are the focal spot size, linearity, reproducibility, filtration, kilovoltage, and exposure time. Three-phase x-ray generators should be able to time exposures to ±5% accuracy. Radiographic equipment collimators should be inspected and verified as accurate semiannually (twice a year); the relationship

between the collimator light field and the actual x-ray field must be congruent to within 2% of the SID. Kilovoltage settings can most effectively be tested using an electronic kilovoltage meter; to meet the required standards, the kilovoltage should be accurate to within ±4 kV. Reproducibility testing should specify that radiation output be consistent to within ±5%.

21. **(D)** The *protective curtain,* usually made of leaded vinyl with at least 0.25-mm Pb equivalent, must be positioned between the patient and the fluoroscopist to greatly reduce exposure of the fluoroscopist to energetic scatter from the patient. As with overhead equipment, fluoroscopic x-ray tube total *filtration* must be at least 2.5-mm Al equivalent to reduce excessive exposure to low-energy scatter radiation. Collimator/beam alignment must be accurate to within 2%.

22. **(B)** A radiographer who discloses confidential information to unauthorized individuals may be found guilty of invasion of privacy. If the disclosure is in some way detrimental or otherwise harmful to the patient, the radiographer may be accused of defamation. Spoken defamation is slander; written defamation is libel. Assault is to threaten harm; battery is to carry out the threat.

23. **(B)** The technical factor that regulates receptor exposure is milliampere seconds (mAs). The equation used to determine mAs is mA × s = mAs. Substituting known factors:

$$300x = 18 \text{ mAs}$$
$$x = 0.06 \text{ s} (60 \text{ ms})$$

24. **(D)** ERCP is performed to diagnose disease of the biliary and/or pancreatic organs. Fluoroscopic control is used to introduce the fiberoptic endoscope through the mouth and into the duodenum. The hepatopancreatic ampulla (of Vater) then is located and cannulated, and contrast medium is injected into the common bile duct.

25. **(A)** The cervical intervertebral foramina (and the pedicles that form them) form a 45° angle with the MSP and, therefore, are well visualized in a 45° *oblique* position. Zygapophyseal joints are formed by articulating surfaces of the inferior articular facet of one vertebra with the superior articular facet of the vertebra below; they are well demonstrated in the lateral position of the cervical spine. The intervertebral disk spaces are best demonstrated in the lateral position.

26. **(B)** SNR can refer to home television images, magnetic resonance images (MRIs), ultrasound images, x-ray images, and so on. Noise interferes with visualization of image details, for example, scattered radiation fog, and graininess from quantum mottle. The actual signal can be from x-rays, sound waves, and so on. The signal is desirable, the noise is not; therefore, a higher SNR produces a higher quality image. Low SNR severely impairs contrast resolution.

27. (B) X-ray equipment operated above 70 kV requires total filtration of 2.5-mm Al equivalent. Filtration reduces patient skin exposure by removing the low-energy, long-wavelength x-ray photons—thus increasing beam quality and "hardening" the x-ray beam. Total filtration is composed of *inherent* filtration plus *added* filtration.

Inherent (built-in) filtration includes the components of the x-ray tube structure: the x-ray tube glass envelope, oil insulation surrounding the glass tube, and the glass window of the tube housing. Inherent filtration is usually about 0.5-mm Al equivalent. Added filtration is mostly a result of the variable aperture light localizing collimator device which provides an additional 1.0-mm Al equivalent filtration; most of this is owing to the light localizing mirror. Additional aluminum is added to meet the required 2.5-mm total Al equivalent.

Compensating filtration is designed to even out the tissue density of uneven anatomy, and collimation is designed to limit the size of the exposed field.

28. (C) The stomach is generally not parallel with the long axis of the body—its fundus/superior portion lies more posterior, and the pylorus/inferior portion lies more anterior. Consequently, in the recumbent position, barium will gravitate to the fundus when the patient is supine and to the pylorus when the patient is prone. Because Figure 6-4 shows a barium-filled fundus, it must have been made in the AP projection or LPO position. A look at the vertebrae indicates that the body is somewhat obliqued, indicating an LPO position. Note the double-contrast demonstration of rugal folds in the body of the stomach and double-contrast delineation of the pylorus and duodenal bulb.

29. (A) *Distortion* is misrepresentation of the actual size or shape of the object being imaged. Size distortion is magnification. Shape distortion is a result of improper alignment of the x-ray tube, the part being radiographed, and the IR; the two types of shape distortion are foreshortening and elongation. The shapes of various structures can be misrepresented radiographically as a result of their position in the body, when the part is out of the central axis of the x-ray beam, or when the CR is angled (Fig. 6-21). Parts sometimes are elongated intentionally for better visualization (e.g., sigmoid colon). Some body parts, because of their position in the body, are foreshortened, such as the carpal scaphoid. *Attenuation* refers to decreasing beam intensity and is unrelated to distortion.

30. (D) Conventional 60-Hz full-wave rectified power is converted to a higher frequency of 500–25,000 Hz in the most recent generator design—the *high-frequency generator*. The high-frequency generator is small in size, in addition to producing an almost constant potential waveform. High-frequency generators first appeared in mobile x-ray units and were then adopted by mammography and CT equipment. Nowadays, more and more radiographic equipment uses high-frequency generators. Their compact size makes them popular, and the fact that they produce nearly constant potential voltage helps to improve image quality and decrease patient dose (fewer low-energy photons to contribute to skin dose).

31. (A) Lead and distance are the two most important ways to protect from radiation exposure. Fluoroscopy can be particularly hazardous because the SID is much shorter than in overhead radiography. Therefore, it has been established that mobile fluoroscopic equipment must provide at least 30 cm (12 inches) source-to-tabletop/skin distance for the protection of the patient, and fixed or stationary fluoroscopic equipment must provide at least 38 cm (15 inches) source-to-tabletop/skin distance.

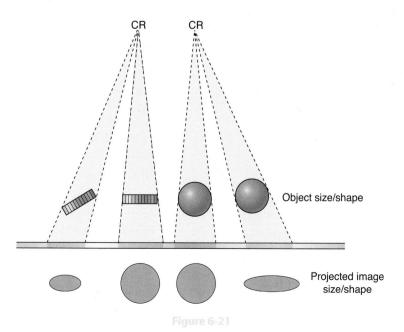

Figure 6-21

32. (B) Diagnostic imaging examinations must be scheduled appropriately. Retained barium sulfate contrast medium can obscure necessary anatomic details in x-ray or ultrasound studies that are scheduled later. Therefore, the ultrasound examination should come first, followed by the lower GI series (BE), and finally the upper GI series. Retained barium from the lower GI series probably will not obscure upper GI structures.

33. (C) The thoracic intervertebral (disk) spaces are demonstrated in the AP and lateral projections, although they are probably best demonstrated in the lateral projection. The thoracic zygapophyseal joints are 70° to the MSP and are demonstrated in a steep (70°) oblique position. The thoracic intervertebral foramina, formed by the vertebral notches of the pedicles, are 90° to the MSP. They are, therefore, well demonstrated in the lateral position.

34. (A) In digital imaging, changes in window width affect changes in contrast scale. As window width increases, the scale of contrast increases (i.e., contrast decreases). Window level adjustments are associated with image brightness changes. Brightness is measured in units of candela per square meter and describes the degree of luminance of areas on a radiographic image viewed on a monitor. Brightness changes can be illustrated while postprocessing/windowing personal digital photographs or scanned documents.

35. (C) The AP axial projection is used to avoid clavicle superimposition on the pulmonary apices. A 15°–20° cephalad angle projects the clavicles above the apices. The radiograph is evaluated for rotation by checking the distance between the medial ends of the clavicles and the lateral border of the vertebral column.

36. (B) *Anaphylaxis* is an acute reaction characterized by sudden onset of urticaria, respiratory distress, vascular collapse, or systemic shock; it sometimes leads to death. It is caused by ingestion or injection of a sensitizing agent such as a drug, vaccine, contrast agent, or food or by an insect bite. Asthma and rhinitis are examples of allergic reactions. Myocardial infarction results from a blocked coronary artery.

37. (B) One of the biggest advantages of CR and DR is the *latitude* it offers. The characteristic curve of film emulsion (line A) has a limited "range of correct exposure." In CR, there is a *linear* relationship between the exposure given to the PSP and its resulting luminescence as it is scanned by the laser, as illustrated in Figure 6-5. This affords much greater exposure latitude; technical inaccuracies can be effectively eliminated. Overexposure of up to 300% and underexposure of up to 80% are reported as recoverable, thus eliminating most retakes. *This surely affords increased efficiency; however, this does not mean that images can be exposed arbitrarily.* The professional radiographer has a responsibility to use anatomically appropriate technical factors in order to keep dose to a minimum.

38. (B) Digital imaging offers wide latitude and automatic optimization of the radiologic image. When AEC is not used, digital imaging can compensate for about 80% underexposure and 300% overexposure. This can be an important advantage in trauma and mobile radiography. The radiographer still must be vigilant with patient dose considerations—overexposure, though correctable, results in increased patient dose. Underexposure results in decreased image quality owing to increased image noise. CR systems provide an exposure indicator: an *S* (sensitivity) number, exposure index *EI,* or other relative exposure index depending on the manufacturer used. The manufacturer usually provides a chart identifying the acceptable range the exposure indicator should be within for various examination types. For example, a high *S* number often is related to underexposure, whereas a high *EI* number is related to overexposure. *Field of view* (FOV) refers to the anatomic area being visualized.

39. (D) A PA projection of the left hand and wrist is obtained most often to evaluate skeletal maturation. These images are compared with standard normal images for the age and sex of the child. Additional supplemental images may be requested.

40. (C) As high-speed electrons encounter the focal spot, as many as 25% of them can interact with other surfaces, for example, the glass envelope and the anode stem. This produces low-energy Brems photons that contribute to patient dose or are evidenced as exposed areas outside the collimated field. This *off-focus radiation* can be significantly reduced by the fixed diaphragm/uppermost collimator shutters located just outside the x-ray tube's port window. The tube housing, whose function is to reduce leakage radiation, also assists with reducing off-focus radiation.

The lower collimator shutters comprise the variable aperture beam restrictor. Scattered radiation is produced within the irradiated part and is absorbed with the use of a grid. Positive beam limitation is automatic collimation and functions to restrict the field size to the size of the IR.

41. (D) Body substance precaution procedures identify various body fluids as infectious or potentially infectious. These body substances include pleural, pericardial, peritoneal, and amniotic fluids; synovial fluid; CSF; breast milk; and vaginal secretions, as well as semen, nasal secretions, tears, saliva, sputum, feces, urine, and wound drainage.

42. (B) The NCRP recommends a total equivalent dose limit of 5 mSv (500 mrem, 0.5 rem) to the embryo/fetus. This dose limit is the total for the entire gestational period. The dose limit for 1 month during pregnancy is 0.5 mSv (50 mrem, 0.05 rem).

43. (C) Fluids and medications are administered to patients intravenously to achieve a more rapid response to the medication than if it were delivered orally or intramuscularly. The IV route is also often used to deliver parenteral nutrition to patients who cannot take their meals by mouth. Medications that are administered topically, such as calamine lotion, achieve a local effect.

44. (D) Each of the three is included in a good QC program. Beam alignment must be accurate to 2% of the SID. *Reproducibility* means that repeated exposures at a given technique must provide consistent intensity. *Linearity* means that a given milliampere seconds value, using different milliamperage stations with appropriate exposure-time adjustments, will provide consistent intensity.

45. (D) A distinction is made between the actual focal spot and the effective, or projected, focal spot. The *actual focal spot* is the finite area on the tungsten target that is actually bombarded by electrons from the filament. The *effective focal spot* is the foreshortened size of the focus as it is projected down toward the image receptor. This is called line focusing or the *line-focus principle*. The quoted focal spot size is the effective focal spot size.

46. (C) A four-view examination of the knee is shown in Figure 6-6. Figure 6-6A illustrates the AP projection. Figure 6-6B is the lateral projection. Figure 6-6C is the axial projection demonstrating the intercondylar fossa and tibial plateaus in profile. Figure 6-6D is the axial projection of the patellas demonstrating the patellofemoral joint spaces.

47. (A) An *analgesic* is any drug, such as aspirin, which functions to relieve pain. An *anticoagulant* (e.g., heparin) is used to prevent clotting of blood. A *diuretic* is used to increase urine output. An *antibiotic* (e.g., penicillin) fights the growth of bacterial microorganisms.

48. (D) The input phosphor of image intensifiers is usually made of cesium iodide. For each x-ray photon absorbed by cesium iodide, approximately 5000 light photons are emitted. As the light photons strike a photoemissive *photocathode,* a number of electrons are released from the photocathode and focused toward the output side of the image tube by voltage applied to the negatively charged *electrostatic focusing lenses.* The electrons are then accelerated through the neck of the tube, where they strike the small (0.5–1 inch) *output phosphor* that is mounted on a flat glass support. The entire assembly is enclosed within a 2- to 4-mm thick vacuum glass envelope. Remember that the image on the output phosphor is *minified, brighter,* and *inverted* (electron focusing causes image inversion).

Input phosphor diameters of 5–12 inches are available. Although smaller diameter input phosphors improve resolution, they do not permit a large FOV, that is, viewing of large patient areas.

Dual- and triple-field image intensifiers are available that permit *magnified* viewing of fluoroscopic images. To achieve magnification, the *voltage* to the focusing lenses is increased and a *smaller* portion of the input phosphor is used, thereby resulting in a smaller FOV. Because minification gain is now decreased, the image is not as bright. The milliamperage is automatically increased to compensate for the loss in brightness when the image intensifier is switched to magnification mode. Entrance skin exposure (ESE) can increase dramatically as the FOV decreases (i.e., as magnification increases).

As FOV decreases, *magnification* of the output phosphor image increases, there is less *noise* because increased mA provides a greater number of x-ray photons, and *contrast* and *resolution* improve. The *focal point* in the magnification mode is *further away from* the output phosphor (as a result of increased voltage applied to the focusing lenses) and therefore the output image is magnified.

49. (D) The computed radiography (CR) laser scanner recognizes the various tissue-density values and constructs a representative grayscale histogram. A *histogram* is a graphic representation showing the distribution of pixel values. Histogram analysis and use of the appropriate LUT together function to produce predictable image quality in CR. Histogram appearance can be affected by a number of things. Degree of accuracy in positioning and centering can have a significant effect on histogram appearance (as well as patient dose). Change is affected in average exposure level and exposure latitude; these changes will be reflected in the image's informational numbers (i.e., S number and exposure index). Other factors affecting histogram appearance, and therefore these informational numbers, include selection of the correct processing algorithm (e.g., chest vs. femur vs. cervical spine) and changes in scatter, SID, OID, and collimation. Figure 6-22 illustrates the effect of incorrect collimation on histogram appearance—in short, anything that affects scatter and/or dose.

Example A

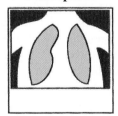

Properly collimated

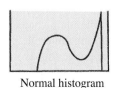

Normal histogram

Example B

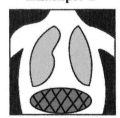

Noncollimated beam

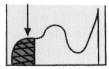

Wider histogram

Figure 6-22. Used with permission of FUJIFILM Medical Systems USA, Inc.

50. **(B)** Dual x-ray absorptiometry (DXA) imaging is used to evaluate bone mineral density (BMD). Bone densitometry/DXA can be used to evaluate bone mineral content of the body, or part of it, to diagnose osteoporosis, or to evaluate the effectiveness of treatments for osteoporosis. It is the most widely used method of bone densitometry—it is low dose, precise, and uncomplicated to use/perform. DXA uses two photon energies—one for soft tissue and one for bone. Because bone is denser and attenuates x-ray photons more readily, the attenuation is calculated to represent the degree of bone density. Soft-tissue attenuation information is not used to measure bone density.

51. **(B)** Insufficient oxygenated blood supply to a tissue is termed ischemia. It can be caused by construction or blockage of the vessel. Necrosis refers to the death of tissue resulting from lack of sufficient blood supply. A thrombus, or blood clot, can enter circulation and cause vessel obstruction. Dyspnea refers to difficulty breathing.

52. **(C)** If 0.8 Gy were delivered in 4 min, the dose rate would be 0.8/4, or 0.2 Gy/min. Thus, 0.2 Gy is equal to 200 mGy.

53. **(C)** A *controlled area* is occupied by radiology personnel and patients. The radiation barriers in a controlled area must keep the weekly dose to less than 1 mSv/week (100 mrem) to radiation workers. That limit is based on the annual occupational dose limit of 50 mSv/year.

    An uncontrolled area is one that is occupied by anyone; the maximum exposure permitted in an uncontrolled area is 20 µSv (2 mrem)/week. That limit is based on the recommended annual dose limit to the general population of 1 mSv (100 mrem)/year.

54. **(C)** The medial oblique projection of the ankle can be performed either as a 15°–20° oblique or as a 45° oblique. The 15°–20° oblique projection demonstrates the tibiofibular articulation and the entire ankle mortise, that is, the articulations between the talus, tibia, and fibula. The 45° oblique opens the distal tibiofibular joint. In addition, as degree of rotation increases, the space between the tibia and fibula increases. In all three cases, although the MSP/rotation can change, the plantar surface should be approximately perpendicular to the lower leg/IR.

55. **(D)** A *point lesion* is a disturbance of a single chemical bond that can result in malfunction within the affected cell. Following irradiation, a small extension-type molecule can develop, extending from the main chain. This molecule can attach to a neighboring molecule or to another portion of the same molecule; this is called *cross-linking. Main-chain scission* is breakage of the molecule's principal connection so that the molecule is broken into smaller molecules. Each of these radiation effects on macromolecules is repairable.

56. **(C)** The human body is composed of approximately 80% water; the remaining 20% is a combination of substances such as proteins, carbohydrates, and lipids. The smallest functional unit of the body is the cell; the structure/content of a cell often determines its function. Cells form tissues and organs that also have functional characteristics. The two basic types of cells are *somatic* and *genetic.* Somatic cells are all the body's cells (bone, muscle, nerve, etc.), except those concerned with reproduction (spermatozoa, oocytes)—those cells are termed as genetic.

57. **(A)** A *vector* is an animal host of an infectious organism that transmits the infection via a bite or sting, such as the mosquito (malaria) and the deer tick (Lyme disease). A *fomite* is an inanimate object that has been in contact with an infectious microorganism. A *reservoir* is a site where an infectious organism can remain alive and from which transmission can occur. Although an inanimate object can be a reservoir for infection, living objects (such as humans) can also be reservoirs. For infection to spread, there must be a *host* environment. Although an inanimate object may serve as a temporary host for microbes to grow, microbes flourish on and in the human host, where plenty of body fluids and tissue nourish and feed the microbes.

58. **(A)** The relationship between x-ray intensity and distance from the source is expressed in the inverse-square law of radiation. The formula is

$$\frac{I_1}{I_2} = \frac{D_2^2}{D_1^2}$$

Substituting known values:

$$\frac{18}{x} = \frac{25}{4}$$
$$25x = 72$$

Thus, $x = 2.88$ mGy$_a$/min at 5 m. Distance has a profound effect on dose received and, therefore, is one of the cardinal factors considered in radiation protection. As distance from the source increases, dose received decreases.

59. **(D)** *Atelectasis* is partial or complete collapse (i.e., imperfect expansion) of a lung or lobe of a lung. *Pneumonia* is an acute infection of the lung parenchyma characterized by productive cough, chest pain, fever, and chills and frequently accompanied by rales. *Pneumothorax* is the condition of air or gas in the pleural space. *Chronic obstructive pulmonary disease* (COPD) is the name given to a number of disease processes that decrease the lung's ability to perform its function of ventilation.

60. **(B)** With the patient in the AP position, the CR is directed cephalad 25°–30°. This serves to project the clavicle away from the pulmonary apices and ribs, projecting most of the clavicle above the thorax. The reverse

is true when the patient is examined in the PA position. The PA projection can be useful to obtain better recorded detail because of reduced OID.

61. **(D)** X-ray equipment operated above 70 kV requires total filtration of 2.5-mm Al equivalent. Filtration reduces patient skin exposure by removing the low-energy, long-wavelength x-ray photons—thus increasing beam quality and "hardening" the x-ray beam. Total filtration is composed of *inherent* filtration plus *added* filtration.

Inherent (built-in) filtration includes the components of the x-ray tube structure: the x-ray tube glass envelope, oil insulation surrounding the glass tube, and the glass window of the tube housing. Inherent filtration is usually about 0.5-mm Al equivalent. Added filtration is mostly a result of the variable aperture light localizing collimator device which provides an additional 1.0-mm Al equivalent filtration; most of this is owing to the light localizing mirror. Additional aluminum is added to meet the required 2.5-mm total Al equivalent.

62. **(B)** Proper body mechanics can help to prevent painful back injuries by making proficient use of the muscles in the arms and legs. Proper body mechanics includes a wide base of support. The *base of support* is the part of the body in touch with the floor or other horizontal plane. The back should always be kept *straight;* twisting increases the chance of injury. When lifting a load, keep it as *close* to the body as possible to avoid back strain. Always *push* a load (such as a mobile x-ray machine) rather than pull it.

63. **(A)** In the AP projection of the normal knee, the space between the tibial plateau and the femoral condyles is equal bilaterally. It is, therefore, important that there be no pelvic rotation that could change the appearance of an otherwise normal relationship. The AP projection of the knee superimposes the patella and femur. The CR should enter at the knee joint, located 1/2 inch distal to the patellar apex.

64. **(B)** Tissue is most sensitive to radiation exposure when it is in an oxygenated condition. *Anoxic* refers to a general lack of oxygen in tissue; *hypoxic* refers to tissue with little oxygen. Anoxic and hypoxic tumors typically are avascular (with little or no blood supply) and, therefore, more radioresistant.

65. **(C)** The trachea (windpipe) bifurcates into left and right main stem bronchi, each of which enters its respective lung hilum. The left bronchus divides into two portions—one for each lobe of the left lung. The right bronchus divides into three portions—one for each lobe of the right lung. The lungs are conical in shape, consisting of upper pointed portions, termed as the *apices* (plural of apex), and broad lower portions (or *bases*). The lungs are enclosed in a double-walled serous membrane called the *pleura*.

66. **(C)** As radiation passes through tissue, different types of ionization processes can take place depending on the photon energy and the type of material being irradiated. The photoelectric effect (whose end products include a characteristic ray) and Compton scatter are the two major interactions that take place in the diagnostic x-ray peak kilovoltage range. The rate at which energy is deposited in (or transferred to) tissue during these interactions is termed as *linear energy transfer* (LET). The greater the LET, the greater is the potential biologic effect. Diagnostic x-ray is considered low-LET radiation.

67. **(C)** Arthrodesis, or spinal fusion, is a surgical procedure that might be used in cases of certain fractures, degenerative disk disease, spinal stenosis, degenerative spondylolisthesis, and other vertebral conditions. It is most often seen in the lumbar region. Implants might be used to hold vertebrae in position/alignment. After approximately 6 months, postsurgery imaging is often helpful in demonstrating the degree of motion permitted at the site(s) of fusion. The images can include AP left and right bending to demonstrate degree of lateral motion, and lateral in flexion and extension to demonstrate degree of AP motion.

68. **(B)** The bony walls of the orbit are thin, fragile, and subject to fracture. A direct blow to the eye results in a pressure that can cause fracture. That fracture is usually to the orbital floor (the inferior aspect of the bony orbit). Because the fracture results from increased pressure within the eye, it is called a *blowout fracture*.

69–70. **(69, C; 70, C)** Figure 6-7 shows a posterior view of the elbow. The distal posterior humerus (number 1) is seen, as well as the proximal posterior radius (number 4) and ulna (number 3). Additional structures identified are the medial epicondyle (number 2), the olecranon fossa (number 5), olecranon process (number 6), lateral epicondyle (number 7), and radial head (number 8). The olecranon process (number 6) can be best demonstrated in the lateral projection; it can also be demonstrated in the acute flexion position. The AP internal oblique will demonstrate the coronoid process; the AP external oblique will demonstrate the radial head free of superimposition.

71. **(C)** *Pulmonary circulation* refers to deoxygenated blood flowing from the right ventricle (through the pulmonary semilunar valve) to the lungs for exchange of oxygen and carbon dioxide then through the pulmonary veins to the left atrium. *Systemic circulation* refers to oxygenated blood flowing from the left atrium, through the mitral/bicuspid valve, into the left ventricle (through the aortic semilunar valve) through the aorta, all the arterial branches, to tissue capillaries, then it returns to the heart through veins and ultimately to the superior and inferior venae cavae into the right atrium.

The sequence that identifies blood flow from systemic to pulmonary and back to systemic is (C) right atrium, tricuspid valve, right ventricle, pulmonary semilunar valve, left atrium, mitral valve, left ventricle, aortic semilunar valve.

72. **(D)** The x-ray anode may be a molybdenum disk coated with a tungsten–rhenium alloy. Tungsten, with a high atomic number ($Z = 74$), produces high-energy x-rays quite efficiently. Because a great deal of heat is produced at the target, its high-melting point (3410°C) helps to avoid damage to the target surface. Heat produced at the target should be dissipated readily, and tungsten's conductivity is similar to that of copper. Therefore, as heat is applied to the focus, it can be conducted throughout the disk to equalize the temperature and thus avoids pitting, or localized melting, of the focal track.

73. **(A)** The diameter of a needle is the needle's *gauge*. The higher the gauge number, the thinner is the diameter. For example, a very tiny gauge needle such as 25-gauge needle may be used on a pediatric patient for IV injection, whereas a large-gauge needle such as 16-gauge needle may be used for donating blood. The *hub* of the needle is the portion of the needle that attaches to a syringe. The *length* of the needle varies depending on its use. A longer needle is needed for intramuscular injections; a shorter needle, for a subcutaneous injection. The *bevel* of the needle is the slanted tip of the needle. For IV injections, the bevel should always face up.

74. **(C)** X-ray tube life may be extended by using technical factors that produce a minimum of heat, that is, a *lower* milliampere seconds and higher kilovoltage combination, whenever possible. When the rotor is activated, the filament current is increased to produce the required electron source (thermionic emission). Prolonged rotor time, then, can lead to shortened filament life as a result of early vaporization. Large exposures to a cold anode will heat the anode surface, and the big temperature difference can cause cracking of the anode. This can be avoided by proper warming of the anode prior to use, thereby allowing sufficient dispersion of heat through the anode.

75. **(D)** The milliampere seconds value used was 8 (400 mA $\times$ 0.02 s); the new milliampere seconds value is half, that is, 4 mAs, which will result in half the original receptor exposure. An increase in SID, as suggested by choice (A), would further decrease receptor exposure. The decrease in the milliampere seconds value could be compensated for by a decrease in SID—but according to the exposure-maintenance formula, that distance should be 28 inches. Decreasing the kilovoltage to 60 would also decrease the receptor exposure by another half. Increasing the kilovoltage by 15%, as suggested by choice (D), will best simulate the original receptor exposure.

76. **(D)** A parallel-plate *ionization chamber* is a type of automatic exposure control (AEC). A radiolucent chamber is beneath the patient (between the part and the IR). As photons emerge from the part, they enter the chamber and ionize the air within it. Once a predetermined charge has been reached, the exposure is terminated automatically. A *phototimer* is another type of AEC that actually measures light. As x-ray photons penetrate and emerge from a part, a fluorescent screen beneath the IR glows, and the fluorescent light charges a photomultiplier tube. Once a predetermined charge has been reached, the exposure terminates automatically. An induction motor is used to rotate the anode of the x-ray tube. An autotransformer operates on the principle of self-induction and is useful in kilovoltage selection.

77. **(B)** When the patient is unable to fully extend his or her elbow as a result of injury, an AP projection of the bony structures is still required. In this situation, two projections are necessary—one for the distal humerus and one for the proximal forearm. The *proximal forearm* elbow structures are demonstrated with the forearm parallel to the IR and a perpendicular CR as seen in Figure 6-8. The *distal humerus* elbow structures are demonstrated with the humerus parallel to the IR and a perpendicular CR. If the elbow is flexed to a greater degree, the CR can be directed 10°–15° into the joint space.

78. **(B)** The female pelvis differs from the male pelvis in that it is shallower and its bones generally are lighter and more delicate (Fig. 6-23). The pelvic outlet is wider and more circular in females, and the ischial tuberosities and acetabula are farther apart; the angle formed by the pubic arch is also greater (more than 100°) in females. All these bony characteristics facilitate childbearing and birth.

79. **(B)** The photoelectric effect and Compton scattering are the two predominant interactions between x-ray photons and matter in diagnostic x-ray. In *Compton scatter,* the high-energy incident photon uses only *part* of its energy to eject an outer-shell electron. It retains most of its original energy in the form of a scattered x-ray. The outer-shell electron leaves the atom and is called a *recoil electron*. Compton scatter is the interaction between x-ray photons and matter that occurs most frequently in diagnostic x-ray and is also the major contributor of scattered radiation fog. In the *photoelectric effect,* the low-energy incident photon uses all its energy to eject an atom's inner-shell electron. When photon ceases to exist, it means it has used all its energy to ionize the atom. The part has absorbed the x-ray photon. This interaction contributes to patient dose and produces short-scale contrast.

80. **(C)** The oblique projection of the hand is shown in Figure 6-9. The degree of obliquity is correct. Shape distortion exists because fingers are not parallel with x-ray

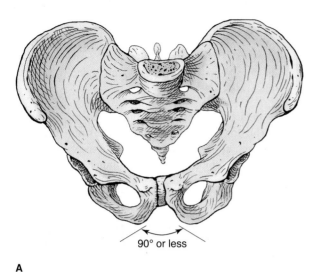
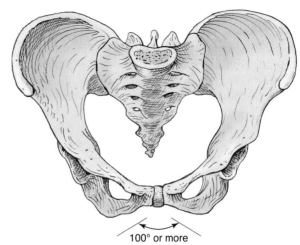

90° or less

A

100° or more

B

Figure 6-23

tube and IR. Consequently, interphalangeal joint spaces appear "closed." Using a 45° foam wedge/"finger sponge" to place the fingers parallel with the IR will eliminate shape distortion and will permit visualization of interphalangeal joints.

81. **(B)** It is the radiographer's responsibility to keep radiation exposure to patients and to himself or herself to a minimum. The embryo/fetus is particularly radiosensitive. One way to avoid irradiating a newly fertilized ovum is to inquire about the possibility of a female patient being pregnant or to ask her for the date of her last menstrual period. The safest time for a woman of childbearing age to have elective radiographic examinations is during the first 10 days following the onset of menstruation.

82. **(D)** Geometric unsharpness is affected by all three factors listed. As OID increases, so does magnification. As focal object distance and SID decrease, so does magnification. OID may be said to be directly proportional to magnification. Focal object distance and SID are inversely proportional to magnification.

83. **(B)** A *polyp* is a tumor with a pedicle (stalk) that is found commonly in vascular organs projecting inward from its mucosal wall. Polyps usually are removed surgically because, although usually benign, they can become malignant. A *diverticulum* is an outpouching from the wall of an organ, such as the colon. A *fistula* is an abnormal tube-like passageway between organs or between an organ and the surface. An *abscess* is a localized collection of pus as a result of inflammation.

84. **(C)** The quantity of radiation absorbed by the skin from the primary beam is called the ESE. Although the primary x-ray beam is filtered, it is still quite heterogeneous/polyenergetic, containing x-ray photons of low energy

that do not contribute to image formation but do contribute to patient skin dose. Thus, the greater the intensity of the initial primary beam, the greater the ESE will be. Therefore, the chest delivers the lowest ESE (0.1–0.22 mGy); the next is the skull (0.9–2.1 mGy), then the thoracic spine (2.5–4.2 mGy), and the examination delivering the greatest ESE is the abdomen (3.3–6.1 mGy).

85. **(A)** *Hematemesis* refers to vomiting blood. If the blood is dark in color, it is probably gastric in origin; if it is bright red, it is most likely pharyngeal in origin. Expectoration (coughing or spitting up) of blood is called *hemoptysis.* Blood is originating from the mouth, larynx, or respiratory structure. *Hematuria* is the condition of blood in the urine. *Epistaxis* is the medical term for nosebleed.

86. **(D)** The articulating bones that form saddle/sellar joints have a convex–concave-shaped relationship. The most common example is the first carpometacarpal joint, the thumb. The convex base of the first metacarpal fits into the concave surface of the trapezium. The ankle joint is now classified as a saddle joint as well; it was previously classified as ellipsoid/condylar. *Saddle* joints and ellipsoid joints permit the same types of motion: flexion, extension, abduction, abduction, and circumduction. Medial and lateral rotation is permitted by ball and socket/spheroidal joints. Gliding/sliding motion is permitted by plane/gliding joints such as intercarpal and carpometacarpal joint.

87. **(B)** When the hand is pronated and the fingers are extended for a PA projection of the wrist, the wrist arches, and an OID is introduced between the wrist and the cassette. To reduce this OID, the metacarpophalangeal joints should be flexed slightly. This maneuver will bring the anterior surface of the wrist into contact with the cassette.

88. **(D)** X-ray tubes are diode tubes, that is, they have two electrodes—a positive electrode called the *anode* and a negative electrode called the *cathode*. The cathode filament is heated to incandescence and releases electrons, a process called *thermionic emission*. During the exposure, these electrons are driven by thousands of volts toward the anode, where they are suddenly decelerated. This deceleration is what produces x-rays. Some x-ray tubes, such as those used in fluoroscopy and in capacitor-discharge mobile units, are required to make short, precise—sometimes, multiple—exposures. This need is met by using a grid-controlled tube. A grid-controlled tube uses the nickel focusing cup as the switch, permitting very precise control of the tube current (flow of electrons between cathode and anode).

89. **(B)** It is easy to determine the highest point of the scapula when it is viewed laterally. The coracoid process projects anteriorly and is quite superior. However, the acromion process, which is an anterior extension of the scapular spine, projects considerably more superior than the coracoid.

90. **(B)** *Carpal tunnel syndrome* involves pain and numbness to some parts of the median nerve distribution (i.e., palmar surface of the thumb, index finger, and radial half of the fourth finger and palm). Carpal tunnel syndrome occurs frequently in those who continually use vibrating tools or machinery. *Carpopedal spasm* is spasm of the hands and feet, commonly encountered during hyperventilation. *Carpal boss* is a bony growth on the dorsal surface of the third metacarpophalangeal joint.

91. **(A, C, and F)** X-rays are energetic enough to rearrange atoms in materials through which they pass, and they can, therefore, be hazardous to living tissue. X-rays are called *ionizing* radiation because they have the energetic potential to break apart electrically neutral atoms, resulting in the production of negative and/or positive *ions*. X-rays are infinitesimal bundles of energy called *photons* that deposit some of their energy into matter as they travel through it. This deposition of energy and subsequent *ionization* has the potential to cause chemical and biologic damage. Several of the outstanding properties of X-ray photons are as follows:

- X-rays are not perceptible by the senses
- X-rays travel in straight lines
- X-rays travel at the speed of light
- X-rays are electrically neutral
- X-rays have a penetrating effect on all matter
- X-rays have a physiological effect on living tissue
- X-rays have an ionizing effect on air
- X-rays have a photographic effect on film emulsion
- X-rays produce fluorescence in certain phosphors
- X-rays cannot be focused
- X-rays have a spectrum of energies
- X-rays are unaffected by a magnetic field

92. **(B)** Computer *hardware* describes the actual computer equipment (CPU, keyboard, memory chips, etc.). The *software* are the computer programs—*algorithms,* or programmed instructions, that are needed to perform specific tasks.

A *modem* converts a computer's outgoing digital signal to an analog signal, which is then transmitted via telephone line to another computer where it must first be changed back to a digital signal for computer processing.

A *histogram* is a graphic representation of pixel value distribution. The histogram is an analysis and graphic representation of all the values from the PSP, demonstrating the quantity of exposure, the number of pixels, and their value.

93. **(B)** The legal doctrine *res ipsa loquitur* relates to "a matter that speaks for itself." For instance, if a patient were admitted to the hospital to have a kidney stone removed and incorrectly was given an appendectomy, "that speaks for itself," and negligence could be proven. *Respondeat superior* is the phrase meaning "let the master answer" or "the one ruling is responsible." If a radiographer is negligent, there may be an attempt to prove that the radiologist was responsible because the radiologist oversees the radiographer. *Res judicata* means "a thing or matter settled by justice." *Stare decisis* refers to "a matter settled by precedent."

94. **(D and E)** The newest type of personnel monitoring device is the direct ion storage dosimeter (DIS); it is a digital ionization dosimeter. The DIS eliminates the need to collect and send dosimeters for monthly or quarterly processing. The user wears the DIS, which looks like a small flash drive, in the same way as other monitors such as an OSL (optically stimulated luminescence dosimeter). The DIS has a gas-filled ionization chamber within and uses Bluetooth technology to relate its raw data via mobile device or any computer with Internet access and a USB connection. Occupational exposure can be read, and reread, at any time without loss of information.

The pocket dosimeter, or pocket ionization chamber, resembles a penlight and has a thimble ionization chamber within. Ions are counted and radiation quantity is registered in milliroentgens (mR). The use of the pocket dosimeter is indicated when working with high exposures or large quantities of radiation for short periods of time, so that an immediate reading is available to the user. The pocket dosimeter is sensitive and accurate but has limited application in diagnostic radiography.

95. **(D)** In the AP projection of the knee, the position of the joint space is significantly affected by the patient's overall body habitus and the distance between the ASIS and tabletop. When the patient is of sthenic habitus with a distance of 19–24 cm between the ASIS and tabletop, the CR is directed perpendicularly. When the patient is of asthenic habitus with a distance of less than 19 cm

between the ASIS and tabletop, the CR is directed 5° caudad. For a patient with a hypersthenic habitus and an ASIS-to-table measurement of greater than 24 cm, the CR is directed 5° cephalad.

96. **(C)** A PA projection of the chest is shown in Figure 6-10. Adequate *inspiration* is evidenced by visualization of 10 pairs of posterior ribs. Costophrenic angles and pulmonary apices are well demonstrated. There is an excellent evidence of *beam restriction;* collimation is evident on all four sides of the image. Patient is somewhat *off-centered to the left.*

97. **(D)** Hypochlorite bleach (Clorox) and Lysol are examples of *disinfectants.* Disinfectants are used in radiology departments to clean equipment and to remove microorganisms from areas such as radiographic tables. *Antiseptics* are also used to stop the growth of microorganisms, but these are often applied to the skin, not to radiographic equipment. *Antifungal* medications can be administered systemically or topically to treat or prevent fungal infections. *Antibacterial* medications (*bacteriostatics*) also can be administered systemically or externally. Tetracycline is a systemic antibacterial medication.

98. **(C)** Kilovoltage (kV) and half-value layer (HVL) change both the quantity and the quality of the primary beam. The principal qualitative factor of the primary beam is kilovoltage, but an increase in kilovoltage will also affect an increase in the number (intensity) of x-ray photons produced at the target. HVL is defined as the amount of material necessary to decrease the intensity (quantity) of the beam to one-half of its original value, thereby effecting a change in both beam quality and quantity. The milliampere seconds value is adjusted to regulate the number (intensity) of x-ray photons produced at the target. X-ray beam quality is unaffected by changes in the milliampere seconds value. Distance/SID impacts x-ray beam intensity and spatial resolution, and has no effect on beam quality.

99. **(A)** The abdomen is divided anatomically into nine regions and four quadrants. The region designation usually is used for anatomic studies, whereas the quadrant designation is used most often to describe the location of a lesion, pain, tumor, or other abnormality. Some of the structures found in the left upper quadrant (LUQ) are the fundus of the stomach, the left kidney and suprarenal gland, and the splenic flexure.

100. **(D)** For negligent tort liability, four elements must be present—duty (what should have been done), breach (deviation from duty), injury sustained, and cause (as a result of breach). The assessment of duty is determined by the professional standard of care. Examples of negligent torts include patient injury as a result of a fall while unattended on an x-ray table, in a radiographic room, or on a stretcher without side rails or safety belt. Radiographing the wrong patient and radiographing the opposite limb are other examples of negligence. If patient injury results from

misperformance of a duty in the routine scope of practice of the radiographer, most courts will apply *res ipsa loquitur,* that is, "the thing speaks for itself." If the patient is obviously injured as a result of the radiographer's actions, it becomes the radiographer's burden to disprove negligence. In many instances, the hospital and/or radiologist will also be held responsible according to *respondeat superior,* or "the master speaks for the servant."

101. **(B)** To change nongrid to grid exposure, or to adjust exposure when changing from one grid ratio to another, recall the factor for each grid ratio:

No grid = 1 × original mAs
5:1 grid = 2 × original mAs
6:1 grid = 3 × original mAs
8:1 grid = 4 × original mAs
12:1 grid = 5 × original mAs
16:1 grid = 6 × original mAs

The grid conversion formula is

$$\frac{mAs_1}{mAs_2} = \frac{grid\ factor_1}{grid\ factor_2}$$

Substituting known quantities:

$$\frac{6}{x} = \frac{3}{5}$$
$$3x = 30$$

Thus, $x = 10$ mAs with a 12:1 grid.
Slightly different conversion factors are often recommended for digital equipment.

102. **(C)** Hypoglycemic reactions can be very severe and should be treated with an immediate dose of sugar in the form of juice or candy. Symptoms of hypoglycemia include fatigue, restlessness, irritability, and weakness. Diabetic patients who have not taken their insulin prior to a fasting examination should be given priority, and their examinations should be expedited as quickly as possible.

103. **(B)** The distal humerus articulates with the radius and ulna to form the elbow joint. The lateral aspect of the distal humerus presents a raised, smooth, rounded surface, the *capitulum,* which articulates with the superior surface of the radial head. The *trochlea* is on the medial aspect of the distal humerus and articulates with the semilunar notch of the ulna. Just proximal to the capitulum and trochlea are the *lateral* and *medial epicondyles;* the medial is more prominent and palpable (Fig. 6-24). The *olecranon fossa* is found on the *posterior* distal humerus and functions to accommodate the olecranon process with the elbow in extension. The *proximal* humerus also presents the greater and lesser tubercles on its anterior surface; between the tubercles is the bicipital, or intertubercular, groove.

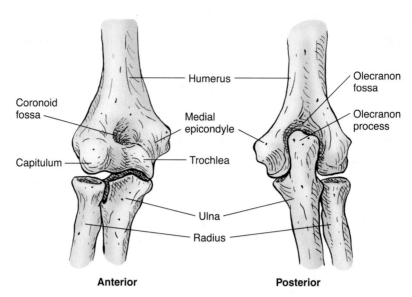

Coronoid fossa

Humerus

Medial epicondyle

Capitulum

Trochlea

Ulna

Radius

Olecranon fossa

Olecranon process

Anterior   **Posterior**

Figure 6-24

104. (B) The posterior oblique positions (LPO and RPO) are used to demonstrate the zygapophyseal articulations of L1–L4. When correctly positioned, the classic "Scotty dog" would be visualized. If the zygapophyseal articulations are not "open," that is, clearly visualized, and the pedicle is seen on the *posterior* aspect of the vertebral body, patient *rotation should be decreased.*

If the zygapophyseal articulations are not clearly visualized, and the pedicle is seen on the *anterior* aspect of the vertebral body, patient *rotation should be increased.*

105. (D) It is important to limit tabletop exposure during undertable fluoroscopy because the SSD is so much less than in overhead radiography; therefore, a much higher skin dose is delivered to the patient. For this reason, the tabletop exposure rate during fluoroscopy should not exceed *21 mGy$_a$/min/mA at 80 kV.* During high-level control fluoroscopy, the maximum permissible tabletop intensity is 200 mGy$_a$/min. To determine the exposure in this case, multiply *21 mGy$_a$ × 2 min × 3 mA = 126 mGy$_a$.*

106. (C) A *controlled area* is one that is occupied by radiation workers; the exposure rate in a controlled area must not exceed 1 mSv/week (100 mR/week). An *uncontrolled area* is one that is occupied by the general population; the exposure rate must not exceed 10 mR/week. Shielding requirements vary according to several factors, one of them being occupancy factor.

107. (D) Gonadal shielding should be used when the gonads lie within 5 cm of the collimated primary beam, when the patient has reasonable reproductive potential, and when clinical objectives permit. Because their reproductive organs lie outside the abdominal cavity, male patients are more easily and effectively shielded than are female patients, whose reproductive organs lie within the abdominal cavity. Therefore, radiographic examinations of the male abdomen and pelvic structures should include evidence of gonadal shielding.

108. (B) *Radiograph* shown in *Figure 6-11A* was performed PA, and *radiograph* shown in *Figure 6-11B* was performed AP, as evidenced by the bony pelvis anatomy. The PA projection (Fig. 6-11A) shows the ilia more foreshortened, giving the pelvis a "closed" appearance, whereas in the AP projection the ilia and bladder area appears more "open." There was an appropriate selection of technical factors, for the required anatomic structures are well visualized—renal shadows, psoas muscle, lumbar transverse processes, and inferior margin of the liver.

109. (B) An artifact associated with digital imaging and grids is *aliasing* or the *moiré* effect. If the direction of the lead strips and the grid lines per inch (i.e., grid frequency) matches the scan frequency of the scanner/reader, this artifact can occur. Aliasing (or moiré effect) appears as superimposed images slightly out of alignment, an image "wrapping" effect. This most commonly occurs in mobile radiography with stationary grids and can be a problem with DR flat-panel detectors.

110. (C) The radiograph shown in Figure 6-12 illustrates a plantodorsal projection of the calcaneus. The patient usually is positioned with the leg extended and the long axis of the plantar surface perpendicular to the tabletop/IR. The CR is directed 40° cephalad to the base of the third metatarsal. Structures that should be visualized include the sustentaculum tali, trochlear process, and calcaneal tuberosity.

111. (A) As radiation passes through tissue, different types of ionization processes can take place depending on the photon energy and the type of material being irradiated. In the *photoelectric effect,* a relatively low-energy photon uses all its energy to eject an inner-shell electron from the target atom, leaving a vacancy in that shell. An electron from the shell beyond drops down to fill the vacancy and in so doing emits a characteristic ray. This type of interaction contributes most to patient dose because all the x-ray photon energy is being transferred to tissue.

In *Compton scatter,* a high–energy-incident photon uses some of its energy to eject an outer-shell electron. In so doing, the incident photon is deflected with reduced energy but usually retains most of its original energy and exits the body as an energetic scattered photon. In Compton scatter, the scattered radiation will either contribute to image fog or pose a radiation hazard to personnel depending on its direction of exit. In *classic scatter,* a low-energy photon interacts with an atom but causes no ionization; the incident photon disappears in the atom and then immediately reappears and is released as a photon of identical energy but with changed direction. *Thompson scatter* is another name for classic scatter.

112. **(B)** The tibia is the larger and medial of the two long bones of the lower leg. Proximally, it presents the tibial *plateau* with its articular facets and *intercondylar* eminences/tubercles, medial and lateral *condyles,* and tibial tuberosity anteriorly. The body/shaft of the bone also features the anterior crest. Distally, the tibia presents the medial *malleolus* medially and fibular notch laterally.

113. **(D)** The thicker and denser the anatomic part being studied, the less bright will be the fluoroscopic image. Both milliamperage and kilovoltage affect the fluoroscopic image in a way similar to the way they affect the radiographic image. For optimal contrast, especially taking patient dose into consideration, higher kilovoltage and lower milliamperage generally are preferred.

114. **(B)** The absorption characteristics of the body tissues vary considerably from one body part to another. Some body parts, such as the chest, exhibit very different absorption characteristics of adjacent tissues. Some body tissues possess low-subject contrast, such as the abdomen. Adjacent tissues/organs of the abdomen have similar absorption characteristics. When differences in absorption characteristics are minimal, body tissues absorb radiation more uniformly.

High-kilovoltage (and low-milliampere seconds) factors can be used when adjacent tissues are very dissimilar, such as in the thorax. The high kilovoltage provides uniform penetration, decreasing the significant differential absorption of adjacent tissue structures. Compensating filtration is also used to "even out" tissue densities in uneven anatomic parts, such as the thoracic spine.

The photoelectric effect is the interaction between x-ray photons and matter that occurs at low kilovoltage levels—levels that tend to produce less part penetration and emphasize very different absorption characteristics.

115. **(A, D, and F)** Radiation exposure to personnel during fluoroscopic procedures is always lowest when staff is positioned at right angles to the center of the x-ray beam. The C-arm image intensifier should always be positioned above the patient, and the x-ray tube below the patient. In this way, personnel radiation exposure dose to the head and neck is reduced. Exposure dose is higher at the head and foot of the x-ray table, so personnel should always avoid those positions.

116. **(B)** The four types of body habitus describe differences in visceral shape, position, tone, and motility. One body type is *hypersthenic,* the very large individual with short, wide heart and lungs, high transverse stomach and gallbladder, and peripheral colon. The *sthenic* individual is the average, athletic, most predominant type. The *hyposthenic* patient is somewhat thinner and a little more frail, with organs positioned somewhat lower and medial. The *asthenic* type is smaller in the extreme, with a long thorax, a very long and medial, almost pelvic stomach and a low medial gallbladder. The asthenic colon is medial and redundant.

117–118. **(117, C; 118, D)** Diarthrotic joints, also described as synovial, are freely movable. The majority of human articulations are the diarthrotic/synovial type, and there are several types of diarthrotic articulations. The image shown in Figure 6-13 is a PA projection of the hand and wrist; an oblique projection of the thumb is obtained. The letter *T* is pointing out the first carpometacarpal joint, formed by the base of the first metacarpal and the trapezium. This is classified as a *sellar* or saddle joint. The sellar articulation permits flexion, extension, adduction, adduction, and circumduction (no rotation). The letter S is pointing out the second metacarpophalangeal joint, which is classified as *ellipsoid* or condyloid. Ellipsoid articulations permit flexion, extension, abduction, adduction, and circumduction (no axial movement). Another example of an ellipsoid articulation is the radiocarpal joint.

119. **(D)** The cervical intervertebral foramina lie 45° to the midsagittal plane (MSP) and 15°–20° to the transverse plane. When the *anterior* oblique position (i.e., LAO or RAO) is used, the CR is directed 15°–20° *caudad,* and the foramina disclosed are those closer to the IR. When the posterior oblique position (i.e., LPO or RPO) is used, the CR is directed 15°–20° cephalad, and the cervical intervertebral foramina demonstrated are those farther from the IR. There is, therefore, some magnification of the foramina (because of the OID) in the posterior oblique positions.

120. **(B)** As the size of the irradiated area increases, the quantity of tissue exposure increases. Dose area product (DAP) expresses the dose of radiation to a particular volume of tissue, thereby being a potentially better indicator of risk than dose values alone. DAP is expressed in terms of cGy-cm^2. An *increased* field size will *increase* the DAP even if the technical factors (dose) remain unchanged.

DAP can be monitored using a DAP meter in both radiographic and fluoroscopic procedures. The DAP meter is radiolucent and is mounted just below the radiographic collimator, measuring x-radiation before it reaches the part. Skin dose can be determined by dividing the skin area exposed by the DAP measurement. This value represents potential deterministic effect to that tissue.

121. (A) When the arm is placed in the AP position, the epicondyles are parallel to the plane of the cassette, and the shoulder is placed in external rotation. In this position, an AP projection of the humerus, elbow, and forearm can be obtained. For the lateral projection of the humerus, elbow, or forearm, the epicondyles must be perpendicular to the plane of the cassette.

122. (A) If the ionization chamber is centered more posteriorly, to a thinner and less-dense structure (spinous process), then the exposure received would be correct for that less-dense structure. The spinous processes would be well visualized, but the higher tissue density vertebral bodies and surrounding structures (pedicles and lamina) *would be underexposed.* Accurate selection of photocells and precise positioning are critical with the use of automatic exposure devices.

123. (A) *Septic shock* can result when the body is invaded by bacteria, infection, or some type of toxin; there are often accompanying signs of acute septicemia and hypotension. Septic shock can occur in individuals having weakened immune systems. Shock caused by an abnormally low volume of blood in the body is termed as *hypovolemic shock. Neurogenic shock* can be caused by some kind of trauma to the nervous system, that is, spinal cord injury or extreme psychological stress. *Cardiogenic shock* is related to the heart and caused by failure of the heart to pump adequate blood to the body's vital organs.

124. (A) The kidneys and ureters do not lie parallel to the horizontal in the AP position. In the RPO and LPO positions, the kidney that is *farther away/elevated* is placed *parallel* to the horizontal (IR). The kidney that is *closer* is placed *perpendicular* to the horizontal (IR). The *ureter* of the *downside* is removed from superimposition on the vertebrae and better visualized.

125. (B) Occupationally exposed individuals are required to use devices that will record and provide documentation of the radiation they receive over a given period of time, traditionally 1 month. The most commonly used personnel dosimeters are the OSL, the TLD, and the film badge. These devices must be worn *only* for documentation of occupational exposure. They must not be worn for any medical or dental x-rays one receives as a patient, and they are not used to measure naturally occurring background radiation. The occupational effective dose is assumed to be *10% of the monitor dose,* although it may be somewhat less than that.

126. (A) Primary radiation barriers are barriers that protect from the primary, or useful, x-ray beam. Secondary radiation barriers are those that protect from secondary or scattered radiation. Examples of primary barriers are the radiographic room walls and floors because the primary beam often can be directed toward them. Secondary radiation barriers include lead aprons, gloves, thyroid shields, the radiographic room ceiling, and the control booth. These will protect from exposure to scattered radiation only. Secondary radiation barriers will not protect from the useful beam.

127. (D) According to the inverse-square law of radiation, the intensity or exposure rate of radiation from its source is inversely proportional to the square of the distance. Thus, as distance from the source of radiation increases, exposure rate decreases. If the distance between the x-ray source and the image receptor is doubled, the image receptor will receive one-fourth of the original x-ray value.

128. (A) Muscle cells have a fairly low radiosensitivity, and nerve cells are the least radiosensitive in the body (in fetal life, however, nerve cells are highly radiosensitive). Lymphocytes, a type of white blood cell concerned with the immune system, have the greatest radiosensitivity of all body cells. Spermatids are also highly radiosensitive, although not to the same degree as lymphocytes.

129. (A) *Cathartics* are used to stimulate defecation (bowel movements). *Emetics,* such as ipecac, function to induce vomiting. *Diuretics* are used to promote urine elimination in individuals whose tissues are retaining excessive fluid. *Antitussives* are used to inhibit coughing.

130. (C) X-ray tube targets are constructed according to the *line-focus principle*—the focal spot is angled (usually 12°–17°) to the vertical. As the actual focal spot is projected downward, it is foreshortened; thus, the effective focal spot is smaller than the actual focal spot. As the focal spot is projected toward the cathode end of the x-ray beam, it becomes larger and approaches its actual size. Figure 6-25 illustrates the variation of the effective focal spot size along the longitudinal tube axis.

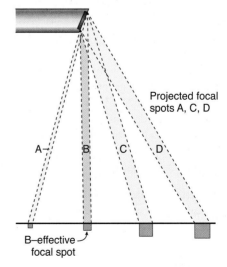

Figure 6-25

131. (D) Extravasation occurs when medication or contrast medium is injected into the tissues surrounding a vein rather than into the vein itself. It can happen when the patient's veins are particularly deep and/or small. If this happens, the needle should be removed, pressure applied to prevent formation of a hematoma, and then hot packs applied to relieve pain.

132. (D) Weight-bearing lateral projections of the foot are requested often to evaluate the longitudinal arch structure of the foot. The patient stands on a small platform. The x-ray cassette is placed between the feet, in a slot provided on the platform, with the top of the cassette against the medial aspect of the foot. The CR is directed to enter the lateral aspect of the foot perpendicular to the base of the fifth metatarsal and to exit the medial side of the foot.

133. (C) Figure 6-14 is an AP projection of the left hip. The leg is internally rotated, placing the femoral neck parallel to the IR. The labels indicate the following anatomic parts: A, sacroiliac joint; B, anterior inferior iliac spine; C, femoral head; D, greater trochanter; E, intertrochanteric crest; F, lesser trochanter; G, femoral neck; H, ischial tuberosity; I, obturator foramen; J, pubis; K, greater sciatic notch.

134. (C) Lead aprons are secondary radiation barriers and must contain at least 0.25-mm Pb equivalent, usually in the form of lead-impregnated vinyl (according to CFR 20). Many radiology departments routinely use lead aprons containing 0.5 mm Pb (the NCRP recommends 0.5-mm Pb equivalent minimum). These aprons are heavier, but they attenuate a higher percentage of scattered radiation.

135. (A) Droplet transmission occurs when an infected individual talks, coughs, or sneezes and droplets are placed in the air. The infectious droplets can be inhaled or otherwise accepted by an uninfected person. Examples of conditions spread by droplet transmission include influenza, most pneumonias, pertussis (whooping cough), pharyngitis, diphtheria, and mumps. Droplet precautions include providing the patient with a private room. The door may be left open because droplets usually do not spread more than 3 feet. A mask should be used when a procedure involves less than 3 feet proximity with the patient. Standard precautions are always used.

136. (B) *Stochastic* effects of radiation are nonthreshold and randomly occurring. Examples of stochastic effects include carcinogenesis and genetic effects. The chance of occurrence of stochastic effects is directly related to the radiation dose, that is, as radiation dose increases, there is a greater likelihood of genetic alterations or development of cancer. Tissue effects (formerly called deterministic or nonstochastic effects) are predictable threshold responses, that is, a certain quantity of radiation must be received before the effect will occur, and the greater the dose, the more severe is the effect. Tissue effects can be early (erythema, epilation, decreased WBC, and radiation sickness) or late (reduced fertility, cataracts, sterility, and fibrosis).

137. (E) It must be considered that every patient may be a carrier of MRSA (methicillin-resistant *Staphylococcus aureus*), which is readily colonized on the skin. Any disease spread by direct or close (indirect) contact, such as *MRSA, Clostridium difficile,* and some wounds, requires contact precautions. Contact-precaution procedures require a private patient room and the use of gloves and a gown for anyone coming in direct contact with the infected individual or the infected person's environment. Some facilities may require health care workers to wear a mask when caring for a patient with MRSA.

138. (D) The ability of x-ray photons to penetrate a body part has a great deal to do with the composition of that part (e.g., bone vs. soft tissue vs. air) and the presence of any pathologic condition. Pathologic conditions can alter the normal nature of the anatomic part. Some conditions, such as osteomalacia, fibrosarcoma, and paralytic ileus (obstruction), result in a decrease in body tissue density. When body tissue density decreases, x-rays will penetrate the tissues more readily, that is, there is more x-ray penetrability. In conditions such as ascites, where body tissue density increases as a result of the accumulation of fluid, x-rays will not readily penetrate the body tissues, that is, there is less x-ray penetrability.

139. (C) A number of milliamperage and exposure time settings can produce the same milliampere seconds value. Each of the following milliamperage and time combinations produces 10 mAs: 100 mA and 0.1 s, 200 mA and 0.05 s, 300 mA and 0.033 s (33 ms), and 400 mA and 0.025 s (25 ms). These milliamperage and exposure time combinations should produce identical receptor exposure. This is known as the *reciprocity law*. The radiographer can make good use of the reciprocity law when manipulating technical factors to decrease exposure time and decrease motion unsharpness.

140. (D) The pulmonary apices are often at least partially obscured by the clavicles. To visualize the entire lung apex and any suspicious areas, the clavicles must be "removed." This can be accomplished with the AP axial lordotic position. Through the arching of the patient's back and the cephalad angulation, the clavicles are projected upward and out of the pulmonary apices. Decubitus positions are used primarily to see air–fluid levels. Lateral and dorsal decubitus positions show fluid in the side that is down and air in the side that is up.

141. (D) A transthoracic projection is used to obtain a lateral projection of the upper half to two-thirds of the humerus when the arm cannot be abducted. The affected arm is placed next to the upright Bucky, the unaffected arm rests on the head, and the CR is directed horizontally through the thorax, exiting the upper humerus. Both superoinferior and inferosuperior projections of the shoulder require abduction of the arm.

142. **(C)** The radiographic subject, the patient, is composed of many different tissue types of varying densities (i.e., subject contrast), resulting in varying degrees of photon attenuation and absorption. This differential absorption contributes to the various shades of gray (i.e., scale of radiographic contrast) on the finished image. Normal tissue density may be significantly altered in the presence of pathology. For example, destructive bone disease can cause a dramatic decrease in tissue density. Abnormal accumulation of fluid (such as in ascites) will cause a significant increase in tissue density. Muscle atrophy or highly developed muscles similarly will decrease or increase tissue density.

143. **(B)** The heart superimposes a homogeneous tissue density over the sternum in the RAO position, thus providing clearer radiographic visualization of its bony structure. If the LAO position were used to project the sternum to the right of the thoracic vertebrae, the posterior ribs and pulmonary markings would cast confusing shadows over the sternum because of their differing densities. Prominent pulmonary markings can be obliterated using a "breathing technique," that is, using an exposure time long enough (with appropriately low milliamperage) to equal at least a few respirations.

144. **(D)** The posterior oblique positions (i.e., LPO and RPO) of the lumbar vertebrae demonstrate the zygapophyseal joints closer to the IR. The left zygapophyseal joints are demonstrated in the LPO position, whereas the right zygapophyseal joints are demonstrated in the RPO position. The lateral position is useful to demonstrate the intervertebral disk spaces, intervertebral foramina, and spinous processes.

145. **(B)** DF uses exposure, rather than continuous fluoroscopic exposure. DF photospot images, which are simply still-frame images, require less patient dose (unless more than necessary are taken), and offer postprocessing capability. DF also offers *road-mapping* capability—a technique useful in procedures involving guidewire/catheter placement. Another feature is the *last-image-hold* feature. During the fluoroscopic examination, the most recent fluoroscopic image can be stored on the monitor (last-image hold), thereby reducing the need for continuous x-ray exposure. This technique can offer significant reductions in the radiation exposure to the patient and personnel. The length of the procedure is an important consideration in patient dose; the longer the procedure, the *greater* the dose.

146. **(C)** A grid is a thin wafer placed between the patient and the IR to collect scattered radiation. It is made of alternating strips of lead and a radiolucent material such as plastic or aluminum. If the interspace material were also made of lead, little or no radiation would reach the IR, and no image would be formed.

147. **(D)** Whenever a radiation worker could receive 10% or more of the annual TEDE limit, that person must be provided with a radiation monitor. The annual TEDE limit for radiation workers is 50 mSv, but it is the responsibility of the radiographer to practice the ALARA principle, that is, to keep radiation dose as low as reasonably achievable.

148. **(B)** Beam restriction is used to determine the size of the x-ray field. This size should never be larger than the IR size. Because the size of the irradiated area can be made smaller, patient dose is reduced. Beam restriction reduces the production of scattered radiation that leads to fog and, therefore, improves contrast resolution. Spatial resolution is related to factors affecting recorded detail, not contrast resolution.

149. **(D)** An increase in technical factors will be required when imaging pathologic conditions that cause greater attenuation of the x-ray beam. The x-ray beam suffers more attenuation as the thickness and/or density of the tissues increases. Examples include conditions involving an increase in part size as a result of fluid accumulation (*edema*) following trauma, an accumulation of fluid in the abdomen (*ascites*), or an increase in bone size and density (*acromegaly*) as a result of an endocrine disorder. The radiographer needs a good working knowledge of pathologic conditions, their effect on the body, and the resulting modifications in technical factors required.

150. **(D)** In the AP projection of the lumbar spine, the disk spaces of L1–L4 are perpendicular to the IR and well visualized, but the L5–S1 disk space is angled 30°–35° cephalad to the perpendicular. If the CR is directed 30°–35° cephalad midway between the ASIS and the pubic symphysis, the L5–S1 interspace will be well demonstrated.

151. **(B)** All four medications are found routinely on a typical emergency cart. *Heparin* is used to decrease coagulation and often used in the cardiovascular imaging suite to inhibit coagulation on catheters. *Norepinephrine* functions to raise the blood pressure, whereas *nitroglycerin* functions as a vasodilator, relaxing the walls of blood vessels and increasing circulation. *Lidocaine* is used as a local anesthetic or antidysrhythmic.

152. **(B)** Focal spot blur, or geometric blur, is caused by photons emerging from a large focal spot. Because the projected focal spot is greatest at the cathode end of the x-ray tube, geometric blur is also greatest at the corresponding part (cathode end) of the radiograph. The projected focal spot size becomes progressively smaller toward the anode end of the x-ray tube.

153. **(B)** The CCD and CMOS are used to record the fluoroscopic image as it emerges from the output phosphor of

the image intensifier and is transmitted through the fiberoptic bundle. The CCD and CMOS replace the TV camera tube and are compact in size. CCDs produce no image vignetting as was experienced with TV camera tubes. CCDs provide better DQE, SNR, contrast, and resolution. CMOS is significantly less expensive, has higher speed, consumes much less power, but produces somewhat lesser image quality.

154. (A) The photoelectric effect and Compton scattering are the two predominant interactions between x-ray photons and matter in diagnostic radiology. In the photoelectric effect, the low–energy-incident photon is absorbed by the tissues being radiographed. In Compton scatter, the high–energy-incident photon uses only part of its energy to eject an outer-shell electron. It retains much of its original energy in the form of a scattered x-ray. Radiologic personnel can be exposed to that high-energy scattered radiation, especially in fluoroscopy and mobile radiography. Lead aprons are used to protect us from exposure to scattered radiation during these procedures.

155. (A) The bones of the foot include the 7 tarsal bones, 5 metatarsal bones, and 14 phalanges. The base of the fifth metatarsal has a prominent tuberosity (number 4), which is a common fracture site. There are two sesamoid bones (number 5) located within the flexor tendon just proximal to the first metatarsophalangeal joint. The calcaneus (os calcis), or heel bone, is the largest tarsal (numbers 6 and 7). It serves as attachment for the Achilles tendon posteriorly, articulates anteriorly with the cuboid bone (number 3), presents three articular surfaces superiorly for its articulation with the talus (number 1), and has a prominent shelf on its anteromedial edge called the *sustentaculum tali*. The inferior surface of the talus (astragalus) articulates with the superior calcaneus to form the three-faceted subtalar joint. The talus also articulates anteriorly with the navicular (number 2). Articulating anteriorly with the navicular are the three cuneiform bones—medial/first, intermediate/second, and lateral/third. The navicular articulates laterally with the cuboid.

156. (A) Location of the heels of the hands is of great importance during CPR. They should be placed about 1½ inches superior to the xiphoid tip. In this way, the heart will receive the compressions it requires without causing internal injuries. Rib fractures can depress and cause injury to the lung tissues within the rib cage.

157. (B) OID can affect receptor exposure when OID acts as an air gap. If a 6-inch air gap is introduced between the part and IR, much of the scattered radiation emitted from the part will not reach the IR, as shown in Figure 6-26. The OID thus is acting as a low-ratio grid and receptor exposure is therefore decreased.

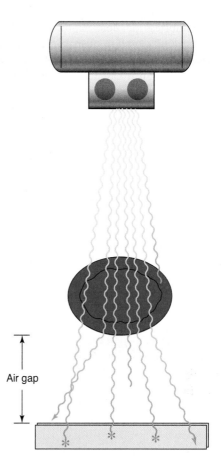

Air gap

Figure 6-26

158. (B) For an AP projection of the hip, two bony landmarks are used. The CR is directed perpendicular to a point located 2 inches medial to the ASIS at the level of the greater trochanter. A point midway between the iliac crest and the pubic symphysis is too superior and medial to coincide with the hip articulation.

159. (D) The intensity of radiation at a given distance from point source is inversely proportional to the square of the distance. If the distance from the point source is cut in half (from 4 m to 2 m), the dose received will be 4 times greater (12 mGy$_a$). If the distance from the point source is cut in half once again (from 2 m to 1 m), the dose received will again be 4 times greater (48 mGy$_a$). This can also be calculated by using the inverse-square law equation:

$$\frac{I_1}{I_2} = \frac{D_2^2}{D_1^2}$$

Substituting known factors:

$$\frac{3}{x} = \frac{1}{16}$$

$$x = 48 \text{ mGy}_a \text{ at 1 m}$$

160. (D) The shortest possible exposure time should be used to minimize motion unsharpness. Motion causes unsharpness that destroys detail. Careful and accurate patient instruction is essential for minimizing voluntary motion. Suspended respiration eliminates respiratory motion. Using the shortest possible exposure time is essential to decreasing involuntary motion. Immobilization can also be useful in eliminating motion unsharpness.

161. (A) Oral administration of barium sulfate is used to demonstrate the upper digestive system: esophagus, fundus, and body and pylorus of the stomach and barium progression through the small bowel/intestine. The small intestine is composed of the duodenum, jejunum, and *ileum.*

162. (D) DNA is the most radiosensitive molecule. It is also the most important molecule because it contains each cell's genetic information. With respect to deterministic effects, if a sufficient number of cells of the same type are damaged, that organ or tissue can be damaged or destroyed as a result of *cell death.* DNA damage can also cause stochastic effects by producing abnormal metabolic activity characteristic of *malignant* disease/tumors. Damage to germ cells can also result in stochastic/*genetic* effects.

163. (A) The image intensifier's input phosphor is 6–9 times larger than the output phosphor. It receives the remnant radiation emerging from the patient and converts it into a fluorescent light image. Very close to the input phosphor, separated only by a thin, transparent layer, is the photocathode. The photocathode is made of a photoemissive alloy, usually a cesium and antimony compound. The fluorescent light image strikes the photocathode and is converted to an electron image, which is focused by the electrostatic lenses to the small output phosphor.

164. (D) Adverse reactions to the intravascular administration of iodinated contrast medium are not uncommon, but although the risk of a life-threatening reaction is relatively rare, the radiographer must be alert to recognize and deal effectively with a serious reaction should it occur. Flushed appearance and nausea, occasionally vomiting, and a few hives characterize a minor reaction. Early symptoms of a possible anaphylactic reaction include constriction of the throat, possibly owing to laryngeal edema, dysphagia (difficulty in swallowing), and itching of the palms and soles. The radiographer must maintain the patient's airway, summon the radiologist, and call a "code."

165. (B) As OID increases, magnification increases. Viscera and structures within the body will be varying distances from the IR depending on their location within the body and the position used for the exposure. The size of a particular structure or image can be calculated using the following formula:

$$\frac{\text{Image size}}{\text{Object size}} = \frac{\text{SID}}{\text{SOD}\,(\text{SOD} = \text{SID} - \text{OID})}$$

Substituting known quantities:

$$\frac{9\,\text{cm}}{x\,\text{cm}} = \frac{105\,\text{cm}}{87\,\text{cm}}$$
$$105x = 783$$

Thus, $x = 7.45$ cm (approximate actual size). The relationship between SID, SOD, and OID is illustrated in Figure 6-27.

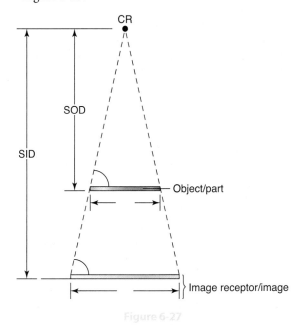

Figure 6-27

166. (B) *Anaphylaxis* is an acute reaction characterized by sudden onset of urticaria, respiratory distress, vascular collapse, or systemic shock; it sometimes leads to death. It is caused by ingestion or injection of a sensitizing agent such as a drug, vaccine, contrast agent, or food or by an insect bite. *Asthma* is characterized by difficulty in breathing, causing bronchospasm. It is often precipitated by stress, and although dyspnea is a symptom, oxygen is not administered. Asthmatics carry a nebulizer that contains a medication to relieve the bronchospasm, thereby relieving their breathing distress. Asthma and rhinitis are examples of allergic reactions.

167. (C) The x-ray tube's glass envelope and oil coolant are considered inherent (built-in) filtration. Thin sheets of aluminum are added to make a total of at least 2.5-mm Al equivalent filtration in stationary radiographic equipment operated above 70 kV. Stationary radiographic equipment using 50–70 kV require 1.5-mm Al equivalent filtration. The function of the filtration is to remove the low-energy photons that serve only to contribute to skin dose.

168. (A) The *autotransformer* (number 1) controls/selects the amount of voltage sent to the primary winding of the high-voltage transformer and operates on the principle of self-induction. The *step-up* (high-voltage) *transformer* (primary coil is number 2; secondary coil is number 3) operates on the principle of mutual induction. The step-up transformer functions to change low voltage to the high voltage necessary to produce x-ray photons. The x-ray tube is identified as number 7.

169. (C) In the simplified x-ray circuit shown, the *autotransformer* is labeled number 1, the primary coil of the *high-voltage transformer* is number 2, and the *secondary coil* is labeled number 3. The autotransformer selects the voltage that will be sent to the high-voltage transformer to be stepped up to the thousands of volts required for x-ray production. At the midpoint of the secondary coil is the *grounded milliamperage meter* (number 4). Because the milliamperage meter is in the control panel and is associated with high voltage, it must be grounded. The *rectification system,* which is used to change alternating current to unidirectional current, is indicated by the number 5. The rectification system is located between the secondary coil of the high-voltage transformer (number 3) and the x-ray tube (number 7).

170. (D) Disease processes can affect body tissue in terms of tissue density, effective atomic number, and thickness—these all affect the attenuation characteristics of the x-ray beam in the tissues. Bronchiectasis, pneumonia, and pneumonectomy are considered additive because they all involve an increase in tissue density. *Bronchiectasis* is a chronic dilatation of the bronchi with accumulation of fluid. *Pneumonia* is inflammation of the lung(s) with accumulation of fluid. Pneumonectomy is surgical removal of a lung; the absence of air will require additional beam intensity. Additional bony tissues and the pathologic presence of fluid are additive pathologic conditions and require an increase in technical factors. Destructive conditions such as osteoporosis, atrophy, emphysema, and bowel obstruction require a decrease in technical factors.

171. (A) The shorter the SID, the greater is the skin dose (ESE). This is why there are specific SSD restrictions in fluoroscopy. X-ray beam quality has a significant effect on patient skin dose. The use of high kilovoltage produces more high-energy penetrating photons, thereby decreasing skin dose. Filtration is used to remove the low-energy photons that contribute to skin dose from the primary beam. Although milliamperage regulates the number of x-ray photons produced, it does not affect photon quality.

172. (D) Breast tissue has very low subject contrast, but it is imperative to visualize microcalcifications and subtle tissue density differences. Fine detail is necessary to visualize any microcalcifications; therefore, a small focal spot tube is essential. High, short-scale contrast (and, therefore, low kilovoltage) is needed to accentuate minute differences in tissue density. A compression device serves to even out differences in tissue thickness (thicker at the chest wall, thinner at the nipple) and decrease OID and helps to decrease the production of scattered radiation.

173. (D) Some medications cannot be taken orally. They may be destroyed by the GI juices or may irritate the GI tract. Medications that are administered by any route other than orally are said to be given *parenterally.* This can include intravenous, intramuscular, topical, intrathecal, or subcutaneous modes of medication administration.

174. (A) The ARRT establishes principles of professional conduct to ensure the best services possible to patients entrusted to our care. These principles are detailed in the ARRT two-part *Standards of Ethics,* which includes the Code of Ethics and the Rules of Ethics. The 10-part *Code of Ethics* is aspirational; the 23 *Rules* of Ethics are enforceable and violation can result in professional sanction. The ARRT Ethics Committee provides peer review of cases (misdemeanor, felony, etc.) to ensure adherence to standards of professional behavior and possession of the moral character required to practice in the health care professions. If the violator's actions demonstrate that moral character is lacking, that individual can be sanctioned—that is, reprimanded, suspended, revoked, ineligible for certification, and so on, or other sanctions deemed appropriate by the Ethics Committee.

175. (D) The size (thickness) and pathology (nature) of the part has an impact on the *number* of x-ray photons transmitted through the part, thereby impacting *receptor exposure.* Body structures that are located some distance from the image receptor result in magnification of those structures, thereby impacting size *distortion* and *spatial resolution.*

176. (C) CCDs have been used to replace the television camera associated with image intensification. They are much more compact than a television camera and can efficiently capture the fluoroscopic image. In comparison to television cameras, CCDs provide better resolution and contrast and have a higher DQE (detective quantum efficiency) and SNR (signal-to-noise ratio). Efficiency of CMOS has improved greatly over the past decade. Advantages of CMOS over CCDs include significantly less cost, greater speed, and much more energy efficiency (less power consumption). The CCD still provides somewhat better image quality.

177–178. (177, B; 178, D) The image seen in Figure 6-17 is a unilateral frog-leg mediolateral projection of the right hip and proximal femur. The letter K identifies the femoral head and letter P is the acetabulum. The letter H identifies the femoral neck, letter A is the greater trochanter, letter F is the lesser trochanter, and letter J identifies the intertrochanteric line/crest. The letter S identifies the obturator foramen with its surrounding bony structures.

179. (A, B, and E) X-ray equipment operated above 70 kV requires total filtration of 2.5-mm aluminum equivalent. Filtration reduces patient's skin exposure by removing the low-energy, long-wavelength x-ray photons—thus increasing beam quality and "hardening" the x-ray beam. Low-energy photons that are absorbed by the filter contribute only to patient skin dose and have no impact on exit radiation or image formation.

180. (B) The effects of a quantity of radiation delivered to a body depend on several factors—the amount of radiation received, the size of the irradiated area, and how the radiation is delivered in time. If the radiation is delivered in portions over a period of time, it is said to be *fractionated* and has a less harmful effect than if the radiation were delivered all at once. With fractionation, cells have an opportunity to repair, so some recovery occurs between doses.

181. (D) Quality control refers to our equipment and its safe and accurate operation. Various components must be tested at specified intervals and test results must be within specified parameters. Any deviation from those parameters must be corrected. Examples of equipment components that are tested annually are the focal spot size, linearity, reproducibility, filtration, kilovoltage, and exposure time. Congruence is a term used to describe the relationship between the collimator light field and the actual x-ray field—they must be congruent (i.e., match) to within 2% of the SID. Radiographic equipment collimators should be inspected and verified as accurate semiannually, that is, twice a year. Kilovoltage settings can most effectively be tested using an electronic kilovoltage meter; to meet the required standards, the kilovoltage should be accurate to within ±4 kV. Reproducibility testing should specify that radiation output be consistent to within ±5%.

182. (A) Special consideration must be given to each patient according to his or her condition. Should an injured patient require assistance with dressing and undressing, it is important to remember that clothing should be *removed from* the *un*injured side first and *placed on* the *injured* side first. Elderly and very thin patients, and those who will be required to lie on the x-ray table for a lengthy period of time, benefit greatly from a foam pad placed under them—that is between them and the x-ray table.

183. (B) The internal rotation position places the humeral epicondyles perpendicular to the IR, the humerus in a true lateral position, and the lesser tubercle in profile. The external rotation position places the humeral epicondyles parallel to the IR, the humerus in a true AP position, and the greater tubercle in profile. The neutral position is used often for the evaluation of calcium deposits in the shoulder joint.

184. (A) *Assault* is the threat of touching or harming, with the apparent ability to carry out the threat. If a patient feels threatened by a health care provider either because of the provider's tone or pitch of voice or because of words that are threatening, an assault charge may be made. *Battery* refers to the unlawful laying of hands on a patient. Battery could be accused if a patient were moved about roughly or touched in a manner that is inappropriate or without the patient's consent. *False imprisonment* may be considered if a patient states that he or she no longer wishes to continue with a procedure and is ignored or if restraining devices are used improperly or used without a physician's order. *Invasion-of-privacy* issues arise when there has been a disclosure of confidential information.

185. (D) The stomach is normally angled with the fundus lying posteriorly and the body, pylorus, and duodenum inferior to the fundus and angling anteriorly. Therefore, when the patient ingests barium and lies AP recumbent, the heavy barium gravitates easily to the fundus and fills it. With the patient PA recumbent, barium gravitates inferiorly to the body, pylorus, and duodenum, displacing air into the fundus.

186. (C) Quality control refers to our equipment and its safe and accurate operation. Various components must be tested at specified intervals and test results must be within specified parameters. Any deviation from those parameters must be corrected. Examples of equipment components that are tested annually are the focal spot size, linearity, reproducibility, filtration, kilovoltage, and exposure time. Congruence is a term used to describe the relationship between the collimator light field and the actual x-ray field—they must be congruent (i.e., match) to within 2% of the SID. Radiographic equipment collimators should be inspected and verified as accurate semiannually, that is, twice a year. Kilovoltage settings can most effectively be tested using an electronic kilovoltage meter; to meet the required standards, the kilovoltage should be accurate to within ±4 kV. Reproducibility testing should specify that radiation output be consistent to within ±5%.

187. (B) Figure 6-18 illustrates a lateral thoracic spine. Motion from "breathing technique" has been used to blur out the superimposed pulmonary vascular markings and bony rib details to better demonstrate the bony structure of the thoracic spine. Because the shoulder area of the upper thoracic spine is so much thicker and denser than the lower thoracic area, use of the anode heel effect is also a valuable tool here. The thicker shoulder area is placed under the more intense cathode end of the x-ray beam, and the thinner anatomic part is placed under the anode end of the x-ray beam.

188. (D) All three pathologic conditions involve processes that render tissues more easily penetrated by the x-ray beam. *Pneumothorax* is a collection of air or gas in the pleural cavity. *Emphysema* is a chronic pulmonary disease characterized by an increase in the size of the air-containing terminal bronchioles. These two conditions add air to the tissues, making them more easily penetrated. *Multiple myeloma* is a condition characterized by infiltration and destruction of bone and marrow. Each of these conditions requires that factors be decreased from the normal to avoid overexposure.

189. **(C)** *Diuretics* are used to promote urine elimination in individuals whose tissues are retaining excessive fluid. They are used in treating hypertension, congestive heart failure, and edema. *Cathartics* are used to stimulate defecation (bowel movements); they are used as preparation for some x-ray examinations such as barium enemas. *Emetics* function to induce vomiting, and *antitussives* are used to inhibit coughing.

190. **(B)** Computed radiography (CR) image plates (IPs) have a protective function (for the PSP within) and can be used in the Bucky tray or directly under the anatomic part. They need not be light-tight because the PSP is not light sensitive. The IP has a thin lead-foil backing to absorb any backscatter. The PSP has a layer of europium-activated barium fluorohalide that functions as the image receptor. It can store the latent image for several hours; in about 8 h, the IP will lose approximately 25% of the information. It is strongly recommended to process PSP plates as soon as possible after the exposure.

191. **(D)** The greater the number of electrons making up the electron stream and bombarding the target, the greater is the number of x-ray photons produced. Although kilovoltage usually is associated with the energy of the x-ray photons because a greater number of more energetic electrons will produce more x-ray photons, an increase in kilovoltage will also increase the number of photons produced. Specifically, the quantity of radiation produced increases as the square of the kilovoltage. The material composition of the tube target also plays an important role in the number of x-ray photons produced. The higher the atomic number, the denser and more closely packed are the atoms making up the material, and therefore, the greater is the chance of an interaction between a high-speed electron and the target material.

192. **(B)** Radiographic rating charts enable the operator to determine the maximum safe milliamperage, exposure time, and kilovoltage for a particular exposure using a particular x-ray tube. An exposure that can be made using the large focal spot may not be safe when the small focal spot of the same x-ray tube is used. The total number of heat units an exposure generates also influences the amount of stress (in the form of heat) imparted to the anode. Single-phase heat units are determined by the product of milliamperage × time × kilovoltage. Three-phase and high-frequency heat units are determined from the product of milliamperage × time × kilovoltage × 1.4.

193. **(B)** A cross-sectional image of the abdomen is shown in Figure 6-19. The large, homogeneous structure on the right, labeled 14, is the *liver*. The gallbladder is often seen on the medial border of the liver but is not visualized here. The left kidney is labeled 5; the right kidney is seen clearly on the opposite side labeled 11. The vertebra is seen in the posterior center, and the psoas muscles are seen just posterior to the vertebra. Just anterior to the body of the vertebra is the circular *aorta,* labeled 7. The *inferior vena cava* (number 12) is seen to the left of the aorta. The circular structure just anterior to the inferior vena cava is the *portal vein* (number 13). Number 1 is the stomach, number 2 is the splenic/left colic flexure, number 3 is the pancreas, and number 4 is the spleen. Numbers 6 and 10 are portions of the left and right adrenal glands—not normally seen at this level. Number 8 is the celiac trunk; the common hepatic artery is seen branching to the right, and the splenic artery is seen branching to the left. Number 9 is a part of the diaphragmatic crura connecting the vertebrae and diaphragm.

194. **(B)** The control monitor that comes with the month's supply of dosimeters is used strictly as a standard for comparison with the personnel monitors used for the month. The control monitor should be stored in a radiation-free area, away from the radiographic rooms. When the control monitor has been processed, its exposure reading is compared with and subtracted from that of the monitors worn in radiation areas for that month. Exposure readings greater than that of the radiation-free monitor are typically reported in millirem units.

195. **(D)** According to the patient's bill of rights, the patient's verbal request supersedes any prior written consent. It is not appropriate to dismiss the patient without notifying the referring physician and the radiologist. The patient may very well need a particular radiographic examination to make a proper diagnosis or for preoperative planning, and the radiographer must inform the physician of the patient's decision immediately.

196. **(B)** The *input phosphor* of an image intensifier receives remnant radiation emerging from the patient and converts it to a fluorescent light image. Directly adjacent to the input phosphor is the *photocathode,* which is made of a photoemissive alloy (usually, a cesium and antimony compound). The fluorescent light image strikes the photocathode and is converted to an electron image. The electrons are carefully focused, to maintain image resolution, by the *electrostatic focusing lenses,* through the *accelerating anode* and to the *output phosphor* for conversion back to light.

197. (B) *Resolution* describes how closely fine details may be associated and still be recognized as separate details before seeming to blend into each other and appear as one. The degree of resolution transferred to the image receptor is a function of the resolving power of each of the system components and can be expressed in line pairs per millimeter (lp/mm), line-spread function (LSP), or modulation transfer function (MTF). Line pairs per millimeter can be measured using a resolution test pattern; a number of resolution test tools are available. LSP is measured using a 10-μ x-ray beam; MTF measures the amount of information lost between the object and the IR.

198–200. (198, B; 199, D; 200, C) The uppermost/first set of *collimator shutters* (5) closest to the x-ray tube port window function to reduce *off-focus radiation*. As high-speed electrons encounter the focal spot, as many as 25% of them can interact with other surfaces, for example, the glass envelope and the anode stem. This produces low-energy Brems photons that contribute to patient dose or are evidenced as exposed areas outside the collimated field. This off-focus radiation can be significantly reduced by the fixed diaphragm/uppermost collimator shutters (5) located just outside the x-ray tube's port window. The tube housing, whose function is to reduce leakage radiation, also assists with reducing off-focus radiation.

The x-ray tube Pyrex glass envelope is labeled number 6 and its port window is number 4. Numbers 1 and 2 represent the induction motor parts; number 1 is the stator, number 2 is the rotor. The induction motor functions to *rotate the anode*. Number 3 is the anode target which is made of *tungsten*.

SUBSPECIALTY LIST

Question Number and Subspecialty correspond to subcategories in each of the four ARRT examination specification sections

1. Image production/image acquisition and technical evaluation
2. Image production/image acquisition and technical evaluation
3. Procedures/extremities
4. Patient care
5. Image production/equipment operation and quality assurance
6. Procedures/head, spine and pelvis
7. Safety/radiation physics and radiobiology
8. Patient care
9. Procedures/thorax and abdomen
10. Safety/radiation physics and radiobiology
11. Procedures/thorax and abdomen
12. Safety/radiation physics and radiobiology
13. Image production/equipment operation and quality assurance
14. Procedures/extremities
15. Procedures/extremities
16. Procedures
17. Patient care
18. Safety/radiation protection
19. Procedures/thorax and abdomen
20. Image production/equipment operation and quality assurance
21. Safety/radiation protection
22. Patient care
23. Image production/image acquisition and technical evaluation
24. Procedures/thorax and abdomen
25. Procedures/head, spine and pelvis
26. Image production/image acquisition and technical evaluation
27. Safety/radiation protection
28. Procedures/thorax and abdomen
29. Image production/image acquisition and technical evaluation
30. Image production/equipment operation and quality assurance
31. Safety/radiation protection
32. Procedures/thorax and abdomen
33. Procedures/head, spine and pelvis
34. Image production/equipment operation and quality assurance
35. Procedures/thorax and abdomen
36. Patient care
37. Image production/equipment operation and quality assurance
38. Image production/image acquisition and technical evaluation
39. Procedures/extremities
40. Image production/equipment operation and quality assurance
41. Patient care
42. Safety/radiation protection
43. Patient care
44. Safety/radiation protection
45. Image production/image acquisition and technical evaluation
46. Procedures/extremities
47. Patient care
48. Image production/equipment operation and quality assurance
49. Image production/equipment operation and quality assurance
50. Procedures/extremities
51. Patient care
52. Safety/radiation protection
53. Safety/radiation protection
54. Procedures/extremities
55. Safety/radiation protection
56. Safety/radiation physics and radiobiology
57. Safety/radiation protection
58. Patient care
59. Patient care
60. Procedures/extremities
61. Safety/radiation protection
62. Patient care
63. Procedures/extremities
64. Safety/radiation physics and radiobiology
65. Procedures/thorax and abdomen
66. Safety/radiation physics and radiobiology
67. Procedures/head, spine and pelvis
68. Procedures/head, spine and pelvis
69. Procedures/extremities
70. Procedures/extremities
71. Procedures/thorax and abdomen
72. Image production/equipment operation and quality assurance

73. Patient care
74. Image production/equipment operation and quality assurance
75. Image production/image acquisition and technical evaluation
76. Image production/image acquisition and technical evaluation
77. Procedures/extremities
78. Procedures/head, spine and pelvis
79. Safety/radiation physics and radiobiology
80. Procedures/extremities
81. Safety/radiation protection
82. Image production/image acquisition and technical evaluation
83. Patient care
84. Safety/radiation physics and radiobiology
85. Patient care
86. Procedures/extremities
87. Procedures/extremities
88. Safety/radiation physics and radiobiology
89. Procedures/extremities
90. Patient care
91. Safety/radiation physics and radiobiology
92. Image production/equipment operation and quality assurance
93. Patient care
94. Safety/radiation protection
95. Procedures/extremities
96. Procedures/thorax and abdomen
97. Patient care
98. Image production/image acquisition and technical evaluation
99. Procedures/thorax and abdomen
100. Patient care
101. Image production/image acquisition and technical evaluation
102. Patient care
103. Procedures/extremities
104. Procedures/head, spine and pelvis
105. Safety/radiation protection
106. Safety/radiation protection
107. Safety/radiation protection
108. Procedures/thorax and abdomen
109. Image production/image acquisition and technical evaluation
110. Procedures/extremities
111. Safety/radiation physics and radiobiology
112. Procedures/extremities
113. Image production/equipment operation and quality assurance
114. Image production/image acquisition and technical evaluation
115. Safety/radiation protection
116. Procedures/thorax and abdomen
117. Procedures/extremities
118. Procedures/extremities
119. Procedures/head, spine and pelvis
120. Image production/image acquisition and technical evaluation
121. Procedures/extremities
122. Image production/image acquisition and technical evaluation
123. Patient care
124. Procedures/thorax and abdomen
125. Safety/radiation protection
126. Safety/radiation protection
127. Safety/radiation physics and radiobiology
128. Safety/radiation physics and radiobiology
129. Patient care
130. Image production/image acquisition and technical evaluation
131. Patient care
132. Procedures/extremities
133. Procedures/head, spine and pelvis
134. Safety/radiation protection
135. Patient care
136. Safety/radiation physics and radiobiology
137. Patient care
138. Image production/image acquisition and technical evaluation
139. Image production/image acquisition and technical evaluation
140. Procedures/thorax and abdomen
141. Procedures/extremities
142. Image production/image acquisition and technical evaluation
143. Procedures/thorax and abdomen
144. Procedures/head, spine and pelvis
145. Image production/equipment operation and quality assurance
146. Image production/image acquisition and technical evaluation
147. Safety/radiation protection
148. Safety/radiation protection
149. Image production/image acquisition and technical evaluation
150. Procedures/head, spine and pelvis
151. Patient care
152. Image production/equipment operation and quality assurance

153. Image production/equipment operation and quality assurance
154. Safety/radiation protection
155. Procedures/extremities
156. Patient care
157. Image production/image acquisition and technical evaluation
158. Procedures/head, spine and pelvis
159. Safety/radiation protection
160. Image production/image acquisition and technical evaluation
161. Procedures/thorax and abdomen
162. Safety/radiation physics and radiobiology
163. Image production/equipment operation and quality assurance
164. Patient care
165. Image production/equipment operation and quality assurance
166. Patient care
167. Safety/radiation protection
168. Safety/radiation physics and radiobiology
169. Safety/radiation physics and radiobiology
170. Image production/image acquisition and technical evaluation
171. Safety/radiation physics and radiobiology
172. Image production/image acquisition and technical evaluation
173. Patient care
174. Patient care
175. Image production/image acquisition and technical evaluation
176. Image production/equipment operation and quality assurance

177. Procedures/head, spine and pelvis
178. Procedures/head, spine and pelvis
179. Safety/radiation physics and radiobiology
180. Safety/radiation physics and radiobiology
181. Image production/equipment operation and quality assurance
182. Patient care
183. Procedures/extremities
184. Patient care
185. Procedures/thorax and abdomen
186. Image production/equipment operation and quality assurance
187. Procedures/head, spine and pelvis
188. Image production/image acquisition and technical evaluation
189. Patient care
190. Image production/equipment operation and quality assurance
191. Safety/radiation physics and radiobiology
192. Image production/equipment operation and quality assurance
193. Procedures/thorax and abdomen
194. Safety/radiation protection
195. Patient care
196. Image production/equipment operation and quality assurance
197. Image production/equipment operation and quality assurance
198. Safety/radiation physics and radiobiology
199. Safety/radiation physics and radiobiology
200. Safety/radiation physics and radiobiology

This chapter incorporates the Targeted Reading lists from Chapters 1 to 5.

Practice Test 2

QUESTIONS

DIRECTIONS: Each of the numbered items or incomplete statements in this section is followed by answers or by completions of the statement. Select the *one* letter answer or completion that is *best* in each case.

1. How are LET and biologic response (RBE) related?
- ❏ A. They are inversely related
- ❏ B. They are directly related
- ❏ C. They are related in a reciprocal fashion
- ❏ D. They are unrelated

2. A graphic representation of signal values representing various absorbing properties within the part being imaged is called a
- ❏ A. processing algorithm
- ❏ B. DICOM
- ❏ C. histogram
- ❏ D. window

3. The term *dysplasia* refers to
- ❏ A. difficulty speaking
- ❏ B. abnormal development of tissue
- ❏ C. malposition
- ❏ D. difficult or painful breathing

4. A positive contrast agent
1. absorbs x-ray photons
2. is composed of elements having high atomic number
3. is seen as a dark area on the image
- ❏ A. 1 only
- ❏ B. 1 and 2 only
- ❏ C. 2 and 3 only
- ❏ D. 1, 2, and 3

5. The quantity that is reflective of dose and the volume of tissue exposed is
- ❏ A. R in air
- ❏ B. absorbed dose
- ❏ C. dose area product
- ❏ D. entrance skin exposure

6. Proper body mechanics includes a wide base of support. The base of support is the portion of the body
- ❏ A. in contact with the floor or other horizontal surface
- ❏ B. in the midportion of the pelvis or lower abdomen
- ❏ C. passing through the center of gravity
- ❏ D. none of the above

7. The femorotibial articulation shown in Figure 7-1 could be better demonstrated by
- ❏ A. rotating the patient forward
- ❏ B. rotating the patient backward
- ❏ C. angling the central ray (CR) about 5° caudad
- ❏ D. angling the CR about 5° cephalad

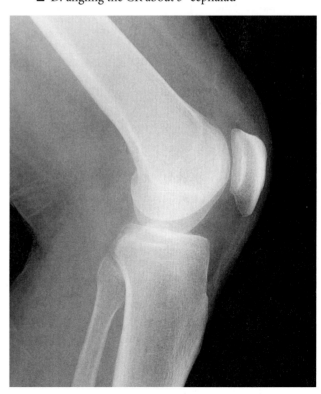

Figure 7-1. Used with permission of Stamford Hospital, Department of Radiology.

8. Which of the following types of adult tissue cells are considered radiosensitive?
   1. Brain cells
   2. Epithelial tissue
   3. Nerve cells
   4. Muscle cells
   5. Intestinal crypt cells
   6. Lymphocytes
       ❑ A. 1, 4, and 6
       ❑ B. 2, 5, and 6
       ❑ C. 1, 4, and 5
       ❑ D. 2, 3, and 4
       ❑ E. 3, 5, and 6

9. Geometric unsharpness will be *least obvious*
   1. at long SIDs
   2. with small focal spots
   3. at the anode end of the image
       ❑ A. 1 only
       ❑ B. 1 and 2 only
       ❑ C. 2 and 3 only
       ❑ D. 1, 2, and 3

10. Which of the dose–response curves shown in Figure 7-2 illustrate(s) a threshold dose?
    1. Curve number 1
    2. Curve number 2
    3. Curve number 3
        ❑ A. 1 only
        ❑ B. 2 only
        ❑ C. 1 and 3 only
        ❑ D. 2 and 3 only

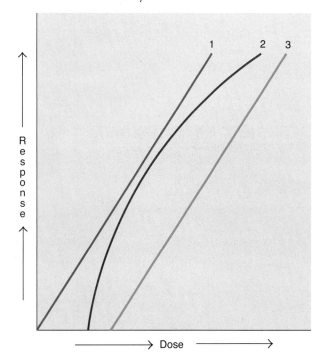

Figure 7-2

11. The carpal scaphoid can be demonstrated in which of the following projection(s) of the wrist?
    1. PA oblique
    2. PA with radial deviation
    3. PA with elbow elevated 20°
        ❑ A. 1 only
        ❑ B. 1 and 2 only
        ❑ C. 1 and 3 only
        ❑ D. 1, 2, and 3

12. Dorsal decubitus projections of the chest are used to evaluate small amounts of
    1. fluid in the posterior chest
    2. air in the posterior chest
    3. fluid in the anterior chest
        ❑ A. 1 only
        ❑ B. 1 and 2 only
        ❑ C. 2 and 3 only
        ❑ D. 1, 2, and 3

13. Which of the following is a functional study used to demonstrate the degree of AP motion present in the cervical spine?
    ❑ A. Moving mandible position
    ❑ B. AP open-mouth projection
    ❑ C. Laterals in flexion and extension
    ❑ D. AP right and left bending

14. Which of the following is/are evaluation criterion/criteria for a PA chest radiograph of the heart and lungs?
    1. Ten pairs of posterior ribs should be seen above the diaphragm
    2. The medial ends of the clavicles should be equidistant from the vertebral column
    3. The scapulae should be seen through the upper lung fields
        ❑ A. 1 only
        ❑ B. 1 and 2 only
        ❑ C. 2 and 3 only
        ❑ D. 1, 2, and 3

15. Select the correct statements regarding the structure indicated by the number 7 in Figure 7-3.
    1. It represents the glass envelope
    2. It absorbs scattered radiation
    3. It is lead-lined
    4. It decreases leakage radiation
    5. It represents the tube housing
    6. It "hardens" the x-ray beam
        ❑ A. 1, 2, and 3
        ❑ B. 2, 4, and 6
        ❑ C. 3, 4, and 5
        ❑ D. 3, 5, and 6
        ❑ E. 4, 5, and 6

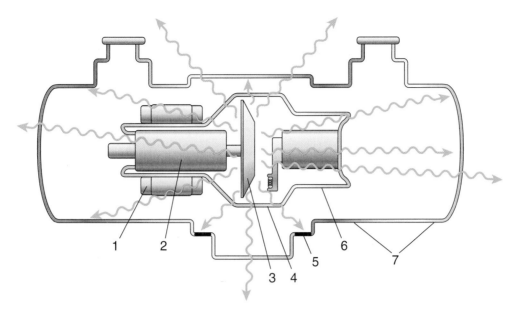

Figure 7-3

16. Which of the following is a fast-acting vasodilator used to lower blood pressure and relieve the pain of angina pectoris?
- ❏ A. Digitalis
- ❏ B. Dilantin
- ❏ C. Nitroglycerin
- ❏ D. Cimetidine (Tagamet)

17. Technical factors of 80 kV and 8 mAs are used for a particular nongrid exposure. What should be the new milliampere seconds value if an 8:1 grid is added?
- ❏ A. 16 mAs
- ❏ B. 24 mAs
- ❏ C. 32 mAs
- ❏ D. 40 mAs

18. Which of the following statements is/are *true* with regard to the two CT images seen in Figure 7-4?
1. Figure 7-4A illustrates more superior structures
2. The images are sagittal reconstructions
3. The examination was performed without artificial contrast
- ❏ A. 1 only
- ❏ B. 1 and 3 only
- ❏ C. 2 and 3 only
- ❏ D. 1, 2, and 3

19. The structure labeled number 7 in Figure 7-4B is the
- ❏ A. IVC
- ❏ B. aorta
- ❏ C. spleen
- ❏ D. left kidney

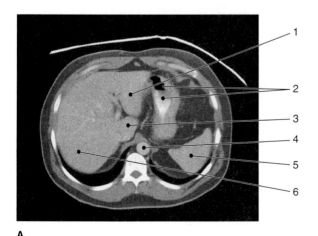
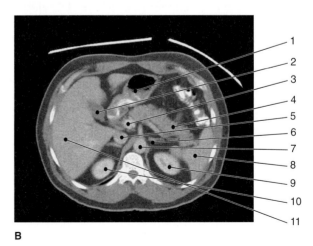

Figure 7-4. Used with permission of Stamford Hospital, Department of Radiology.

20. An illness of unknown or obscure cause is said to be
- ❏ A. systemic
- ❏ B. epidemic
- ❏ C. idiopathic
- ❏ D. pathogenic

21. The annual dose limit for occupationally exposed individuals is valid for
- ❏ A. alpha, beta, and x-radiations
- ❏ B. x- and gamma radiations only
- ❏ C. beta, x-, and gamma radiations
- ❏ D. all ionizing radiations

22. The sampling frequency in CR is expressed as
- ❏ A. pixel density
- ❏ B. the relationship between focal spot and matrix sizes
- ❏ C. light spread between the IP and the light guide of the scanner
- ❏ D. TFT array size

23. Features of digital fluoroscopy (DF) that contribute to patient dose reduction include
1. last-image hold
2. pulsed exposure
3. longer procedure times
- ❏ A. 1 only
- ❏ B. 1 and 2 only
- ❏ C. 2 and 3 only
- ❏ D. 1, 2, and 3

24. Which of the following is the approximate skin dose for 5 min of fluoroscopy performed at 1.5 mA?
- ❏ A. 31.5 mGy
- ❏ B. 105 mGy
- ❏ C. 157 mGy
- ❏ D. 210 mGy

25. To image suspected abdominal free air in an infant, which of the following projections of the abdomen will demonstrate the condition with the *lowest* patient dose?
- ❏ A. PA erect with grid
- ❏ B. Left lateral decubitus with grid
- ❏ C. Left lateral decubitus without grid
- ❏ D. Recumbent AP without grid

26. An AP oblique projection (lateral rotation) of the elbow will demonstrate the
1. olecranon process within the olecranon fossa
2. capitulum of the humerus
3. radial head free of superimposition
- ❏ A. 1 only
- ❏ B. 1 and 2 only
- ❏ C. 2 and 3 only
- ❏ D. 1, 2, and 3

27. Referring to Figure 7-5, which heart chamber pumps oxygenated blood into the aorta and to all body tissues?
- ❏ A. 2
- ❏ B. 6
- ❏ C. 4
- ❏ D. 5

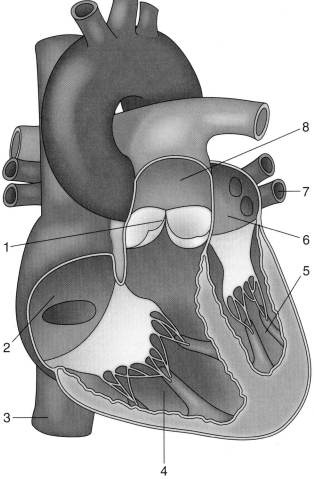

Figure 7-5

28. Which of the following contribute to x-ray beam attenuation and receptor exposure?
1. Tissue density
2. Pathology
3. Muscle development
- ❏ A. 1 and 2 only
- ❏ B. 1 and 3 only
- ❏ C. 2 and 3 only
- ❏ D. 1, 2, and 3

29. The risk of inoculation with HIV is considered high for which of the following routes of transmission?

1. Contaminated blood
2. Perinatal exposure
3. Accidental needlestick

   ❏ A. 1 only
   ❏ B. 1 and 2 only
   ❏ C. 2 and 3 only
   ❏ D. 1, 2, and 3

30. The active matrix array for indirect conversion systems uses

   ❏ A. amorphous silicon
   ❏ B. amorphous selenium
   ❏ C. detector elements
   ❏ D. TFT

31. The position illustrated in Figure 7-6 can be used successfully to demonstrate the

1. PA oblique sternum
2. left anterior ribs
3. barium-filled gastric fundus

   ❏ A. 1 only
   ❏ B. 1 and 2 only
   ❏ C. 2 and 3 only
   ❏ D. 1, 2, and 3

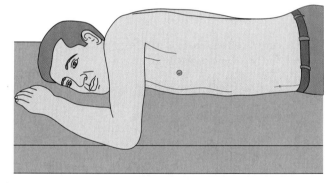

Figure 7-6

32. The AP axial projection of the pulmonary apices requires the CR to be directed

   ❏ A. 15° cephalad
   ❏ B. 15° caudad
   ❏ C. 30° cephalad
   ❏ D. 30° caudad

33. When electric signals are sampled for conversion to a digital image, what sampling frequency is required to maintain image resolution?

   ❏ A. At least half the number of pixels required to form the image must be sampled
   ❏ B. At least twice the number of pixels required to form the image must be sampled
   ❏ C. Raw images are sharp and do not require digital processing
   ❏ D. Sampling frequency must be half the frequency of the input signal

34. Which of the following image intensifier modes will result in the lowest patient dose?

   ❏ A. 25-inch mode
   ❏ B. 17-inch mode
   ❏ C. 12-inch mode
   ❏ D. Diameter does not affect patient dose

35. Abdominal viscera located in the retroperitoneum include the

1. kidneys
2. duodenum
3. ascending and descending colon

   ❏ A. 1 only
   ❏ B. 1 and 2 only
   ❏ C. 2 and 3 only
   ❏ D. 1, 2, and 3

36. The fact that x-ray intensity across the primary beam can vary as much as 45% describes the

   ❏ A. line-focus principle
   ❏ B. transformer law
   ❏ C. anode heel effect
   ❏ D. inverse-square law

37. Which of the x-ray circuit devices shown in Figure 7-7 requires alternating current for effective operation?

1. Number 1
2. Number 2
3. Number 7

   ❏ A. 1 only
   ❏ B. 1 and 2 only
   ❏ C. 2 and 3 only
   ❏ D. 1, 2, and 3

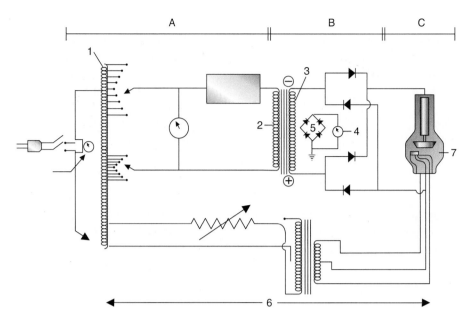

Figure 7-7

38. Referring to the simplified x-ray circuit shown in Figure 7-7, what is indicated by the number 6?
- ❏ A. Step-up transformer
- ❏ B. Autotransformer
- ❏ C. Filament circuit
- ❏ D. Rectification system

39. The infection streptococcal pharyngitis (strep throat) is caused by a
- ❏ A. virus
- ❏ B. fungus
- ❏ C. protozoon
- ❏ D. bacterium

40. The brightness level of the fluoroscopic image depends on
1. milliamperage
2. kilovoltage
3. patient thickness
- ❏ A. 1 only
- ❏ B. 1 and 2 only
- ❏ C. 1 and 3 only
- ❏ D. 1, 2, and 3

41. The advantages of high-frequency generators over earlier types of generators include
1. smaller size
2. nearly constant potential
3. lower patient dose
- ❏ A. 1 only
- ❏ B. 1 and 2 only
- ❏ C. 1 and 3 only
- ❏ D. 1, 2, and 3

42. Which of the following combinations would deliver the least amount of heat to the anode of a three-phase, 12-pulse x-ray unit?
- ❏ A. 400 mA, 0.12 s, 90 kV
- ❏ B. 300 mA, 0.5 s, 70 kV
- ❏ C. 500 mA, 0.033 s, 85 kV
- ❏ D. 700 mA, 0.06 s, 120 kV

43. A signed consent form is necessary prior to performing all the following procedures, *except*
- ❏ A. myelogram
- ❏ B. cardiac catheterization
- ❏ C. upper GI series
- ❏ D. interventional vascular procedure

44. The *best* projection to demonstrate the articular surfaces of the femoropatellar articulation is the
- ❏ A. AP knee
- ❏ B. PA knee
- ❏ C. tangential (sunrise) projection
- ❏ D. tunnel view

45. If the entrance dose for a particular radiograph is 25 mGy, the radiation exposure at 1 m from the patient will be approximately
- ❏ A. 250 mGy
- ❏ B. 2.5 mGy
- ❏ C. 0.25 mGy
- ❏ D. 0.025 mGy

46. In amorphous selenium flat-panel detectors, the term *amorphous* refers to a
- ❏ A. crystalline material having typical crystalline structure
- ❏ B. crystalline material lacking typical crystalline structure
- ❏ C. toxic crystalline material
- ❏ D. homogeneous crystalline material

47. It is recommended that a thermoluminescent dosimeter (TLD) or OSL be worn
- ❏ A. under the lead apron at waist level
- ❏ B. outside the lead apron at waist level
- ❏ C. under the lead apron at collar level
- ❏ D. outside the lead apron at collar level

48. Which of the filament conductors seen in Figure 7-8 carries high voltage?
1. Conductor number 1
2. Conductor number 2
3. Conductor number 3
- ❏ A. 1 only
- ❏ B. 2 only
- ❏ C. 3 only
- ❏ D. 1 and 2 only

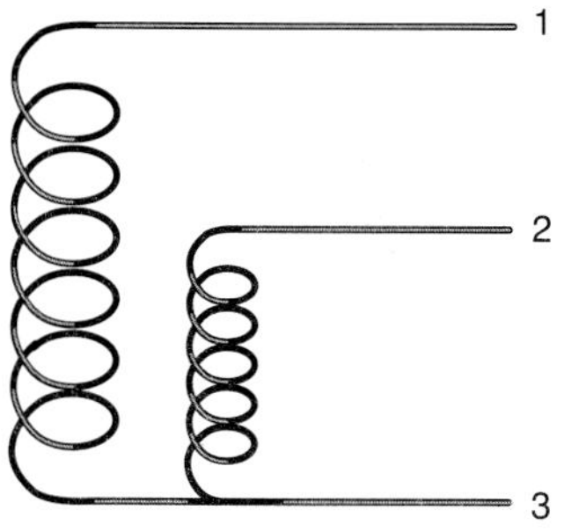

Figure 7-8

49. Which of the following procedures demonstrate renal function?
1. IVU
2. Excretory urography
3. Retrograde urography
- ❏ A. 1 only
- ❏ B. 1 and 2 only
- ❏ C. 2 and 3 only
- ❏ D. 1, 2, and 3

50. When the collimated field must extend past the edge of the body, allowing primary radiation to strike the tabletop, as in a lateral lumbar spine radiograph, what may be done to prevent excessive receptor exposure owing to undercutting?
- ❏ A. Reduce the milliampere seconds
- ❏ B. Reduce the kilovoltage
- ❏ C. Use a shorter SID
- ❏ D. Use lead rubber to absorb tabletop primary radiation

51. The sternoclavicular joints will be *best* demonstrated in which of the following positions?
- ❏ A. Apical lordotic
- ❏ B. Anterior oblique
- ❏ C. Lateral
- ❏ D. Weight-bearing

52. Typical patient demographic and examination information include(s)
1. type of examination
2. accession number
3. date and time of examination
- ❏ A. 1 only
- ❏ B. 1 and 2 only
- ❏ C. 2 and 3 only
- ❏ D. 1, 2, and 3

53. Which of the following is the *most frequent* site of hospital-acquired infection (HAI)?
- ❏ A. Urinary tract
- ❏ B. Blood
- ❏ C. Respiratory tract
- ❏ D. Digestive tract

54. Which of the following statements is/are *true* regarding the control dosimeter that accompanies each shipment of personnel radiation monitors?
1. It should be stored away from all radiation sources
2. It should be stored in the main work area
3. It should be used to replace an employee's lost monitor
- ❏ A. 1 only
- ❏ B. 2 only
- ❏ C. 1 and 3 only
- ❏ D. 2 and 3 only

55. Which of the following x-ray circuit devices operate(s) on the principle of mutual induction?
1. High-voltage transformer
2. Filament transformer
3. Autotransformer
- ❏ A. 1 only
- ❏ B. 1 and 2 only
- ❏ C. 1 and 3 only
- ❏ D. 1, 2, and 3

56. The two types of cells in the body are
- ❏ A. connective and nerve
- ❏ B. genetic and connective
- ❏ C. somatic and nerve
- ❏ D. somatic and genetic

57. If a radiograph were made of an average size knee using automatic exposure control (AEC) and all three photocells were selected, the resulting radiograph would demonstrate
- ❏ A. excessive receptor exposure
- ❏ B. insufficient receptor exposure
- ❏ C. poor detail
- ❏ D. adequate exposure

58. Which of the following involve(s) intentional misconduct?

1. Invasion of privacy
2. False imprisonment
3. Patient sustaining injury from a fall while left unattended
   - ❏ A. 1 only
   - ❏ B. 3 only
   - ❏ C. 1 and 2 only
   - ❏ D. 2 and 3 only

59. Which of the following terms/units is used to express the resolution of a diagnostic image?

- ❏ A. Line pairs per millimeter (lp/mm)
- ❏ B. Speed
- ❏ C. Latitude
- ❏ D. Kiloelectronvolts (keV)

60. Pathologic or abnormal conditions that would require an *increase* in technical factors include all of the following, *except*

- ❏ A. atelectasis
- ❏ B. pneumoperitoneum
- ❏ C. Paget disease
- ❏ D. congestive heart failure

61. In 1906, Bergonié and Tribondeau theorized that undifferentiated cells are highly radiosensitive. Which of the following is/are characteristic(s) of undifferentiated cells?

1. Young cells
2. Highly mitotic cells
3. Precursor cells
   - ❏ A. 1 only
   - ❏ B. 1 and 2 only
   - ❏ C. 1 and 3 only
   - ❏ D. 1, 2, and 3

62. The submentovertical (SMV) oblique axial projection of the zygomatic arches requires that the skull be rotated

- ❏ A. 15° toward the affected side
- ❏ B. 15° away from the affected side
- ❏ C. 45° toward the affected side
- ❏ D. 45° away from the affected side

63. Which of the following statements regarding Figure 7-9 are correct?

1. The patient is in an erect position
2. Duodenal mucosa is visualized
3. The image was made in the RAO position
4. The patient is in a recumbent position
5. The image is part of a lower GI examination
6. The image was made in the LPO position
   - ❏ A. 1, 3, and 5
   - ❏ B. 2, 4, and 6
   - ❏ C. 3, 4, and 5
   - ❏ D. 2, 5, and 6
   - ❏ E. 2, 3, and 4

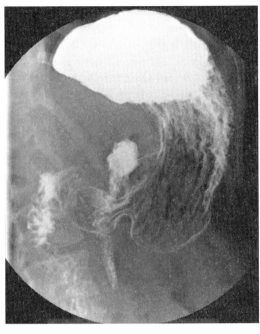

Figure 7-9. Used with permission of Stamford Hospital, Department of Radiology.

64. Image noise is likely to increase with an increase in

1. scattered radiation
2. quantum mottle
3. SNR
   - ❏ A. 1 only
   - ❏ B. 1 and 2 only
   - ❏ C. 2 and 3 only
   - ❏ D. 1, 2, and 3

65. The chest radiograph shown in Figure 7-10 demonstrates

- ❏ A. breathing motion
- ❏ B. aliasing artifact
- ❏ C. double exposure
- ❏ D. off-level grid cutoff

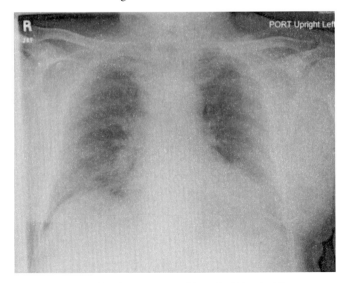

Figure 7-10. Used with permission of Stamford Hospital, Department of Radiology.

66. Which of the following functions to increase the milliamperage?
- ❏ A. Increasing the speed of anode rotation
- ❏ B. Increasing the transformer turns ratio
- ❏ C. Using three-phase rectification
- ❏ D. Increasing the heat of the filament

67. Which of the following is/are correct regarding care of protective leaded apparel?
1. Lead aprons should be fluoroscoped yearly to check for cracks
2. Lead gloves should be fluoroscoped yearly to check for cracks
3. Lead aprons should be hung on appropriate racks when not in use
- ❏ A. 1 only
- ❏ B. 1 and 2 only
- ❏ C. 1 and 3 only
- ❏ D. 1, 2, and 3

68. The ethical principle that refers to bringing about good, or benefiting others, is called
- ❏ A. fidelity
- ❏ B. veracity
- ❏ C. nonmaleficence
- ❏ D. beneficence

69. Which of the following is/are considered long-term somatic effect(s) of exposure to ionizing radiation?
1. Life span shortening
2. Carcinogenesis
3. Cataractogenesis
- ❏ A. 1 only
- ❏ B. 1 and 2 only
- ❏ C. 2 and 3 only
- ❏ D. 1, 2, and 3

70. Advantages of direct digital radiography (DR) over computed radiography (CR) include
1. DR is less expensive
2. DR has immediate readout
3. IPs are not needed for DR
- ❏ A. 1 only
- ❏ B. 1 and 2 only
- ❏ C. 2 and 3 only
- ❏ D. 1, 2, and 3

71. Desirable conditions for viewing digital images include
1. decreased ambient light
2. reduced monitor glare
3. well-lit area
- ❏ A. 1 only
- ❏ B. 1 and 2 only
- ❏ C. 2 and 3 only
- ❏ D. 1, 2, and 3

72. All of the following statements regarding the bony thorax are true, *except*
- ❏ A. the first seven pairs of ribs are called vertebrosternal, or true, ribs
- ❏ B. the only articulation between the thorax and the upper extremity is the sternoclavicular joint
- ❏ C. the gladiolus is the upper part of the sternum and is quadrilateral in shape
- ❏ D. the anterior ends of the ribs are about 4 inches below the level of the vertebral ends

73. Structure number 3 in Figure 7-11 is best demonstrated in which of the following positions?
- ❏ A. LPO
- ❏ B. RAO
- ❏ C. Lateral
- ❏ D. AP

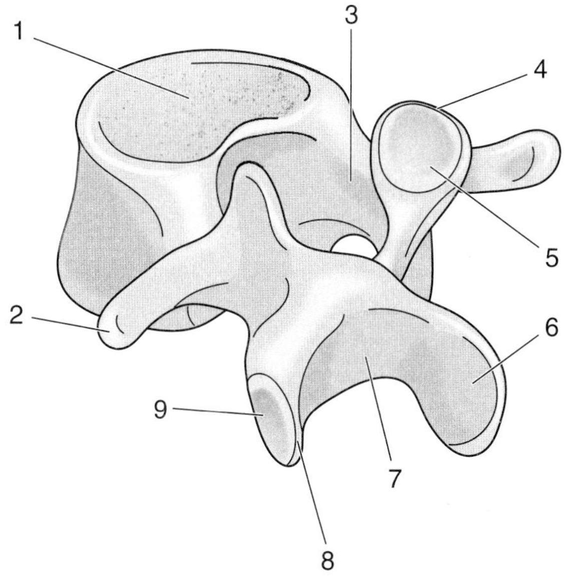

Figure 7-11

74. The late effects of radiation are considered to
1. have no threshold dose
2. be directly related to dose
3. occur within hours of exposure
- ❏ A. 1 only
- ❏ B. 1 and 2 only
- ❏ C. 2 and 3 only
- ❏ D. 1, 2, and 3

75. The lesser tubercle of the humerus will be visualized in profile in the
- ❏ A. AP shoulder external rotation radiograph
- ❏ B. AP shoulder internal rotation radiograph
- ❏ C. AP elbow radiograph
- ❏ D. lateral elbow radiograph

76. The radiation dose to a part depends on which of the following?

1. Type of tissue interaction(s)
2. Quantity of radiation
3. Biologic differences
   - ❏ A. 1 only
   - ❏ B. 1 and 2 only
   - ❏ C. 1 and 3 only
   - ❏ D. 1, 2, and 3

77. With the patient in an erect 45° LPO and the CR directed 2 inches medial and 2 inches inferior to the upper outer border of the left shoulder, which of the following will be visualized to best advantage?

- ❏ A. Coronoid process free of superimposition
- ❏ B. Coracoid process free of superimposition
- ❏ C. Glenoid cavity in profile
- ❏ D. Greater tubercle in profile

78. Which of the following groups of technical factors would deliver the *lowest* patient dose?

- ❏ A. 2.5 mAs, 100 kV
- ❏ B. 5 mAs, 90 kV
- ❏ C. 5 mAs, 70 kV
- ❏ D. 10 mAs, 80 kV

79. While measuring blood pressure, the first pulse that is heard, is recorded as the

- ❏ A. diastolic pressure
- ❏ B. systolic pressure
- ❏ C. venous pressure
- ❏ D. valvular pressure

80. Which of the following is/are valid evaluation criterion/criteria for a lateral projection of the forearm?

1. The radius and the ulna should be superimposed distally
2. The coronoid process and the radial head should be partially superimposed
3. The humeral epicondyles should be superimposed
   - ❏ A. 1 only
   - ❏ B. 1 and 2 only
   - ❏ C. 2 and 3 only
   - ❏ D. 1, 2, and 3

81. At what frequency must the radiographic equipment be checked for linearity and reproducibility?

- ❏ A. Annually
- ❏ B. Biannually
- ❏ C. Semiannually
- ❏ D. Quarterly

82. According to the line-focus principle, an anode having a small angle results in

1. improved resolution/sharpness
2. less focal spot blur
3. more pronounced heel effect
   - ❏ A. 1 and 2 only
   - ❏ B. 1 and 3 only
   - ❏ C. 2 and 3 only
   - ❏ D. 1, 2, and 3

83. Which of the following best describes the position shown in Figure 7-12?

- ❏ A. LPO
- ❏ B. RPO
- ❏ C. LAO
- ❏ D. RAO

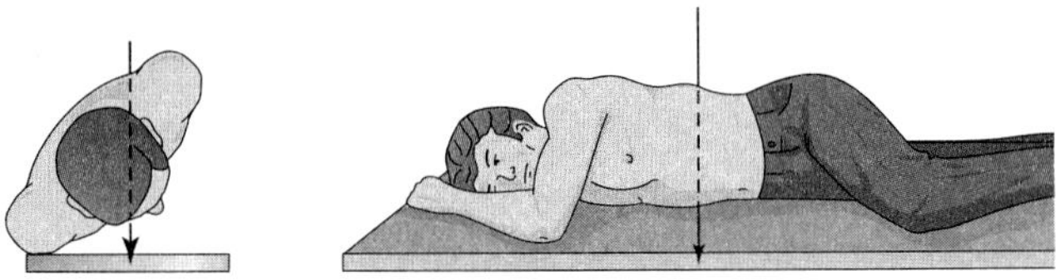

Figure 7-12

84. Which of the following expresses the *gonadal dose* that, if received by every member of the population, would be expected to produce the same total genetic effect on that population as the actual doses received by each of the individuals?

- ❏ A. Lethal dose
- ❏ B. Maximum permissible dose
- ❏ C. Somatically significant dose
- ❏ D. Genetically significant dose

85. A patient with an upper respiratory tract infection is transported to the radiology department for a chest examination. Who should be masked?

1. Technologist
2. Transporter
3. Patient
   - ❏ A. 1 only
   - ❏ B. 1 and 2 only
   - ❏ C. 3 only
   - ❏ D. 1, 2, and 3

86. The kilovoltage settings on radiographic equipment must be tested annually and must be accurate to within

- ❏ A. ±2 kV
- ❏ B. ±5 kV
- ❏ C. ±8 kV
- ❏ D. ±12 kV

87. The radiograph shown in Figure 7-13 exhibits a loss of receptor exposure as a result of

❏ A. x-ray tube angulation across grid lines
❏ B. exceeding the focusing distance
❏ C. incorrect grid placement
❏ D. insufficient SID

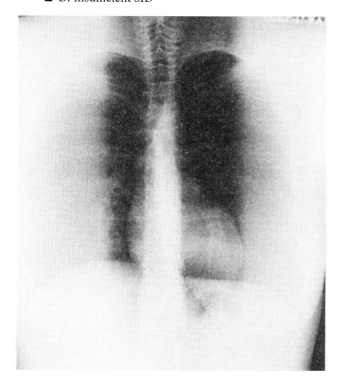

Figure 7-13. Used with permission of Stamford Hospital, Department of Radiology.

88. When examining a patient whose elbow is in partial flexion

❏ A. the AP projection requires two separate positions and exposures
❏ B. the AP projection is made through the partially flexed elbow, resting on the olecranon process, CR perpendicular to IR
❏ C. the AP projection is made through the partially flexed elbow, resting on the olecranon process, CR parallel to the humerus
❏ D. the AP projection is eliminated from the routine

89. Which of the following functions to protect the x-ray tube and the patient from overexposure in the event that the phototimer fails to terminate an exposure?

❏ A. Circuit breaker
❏ B. Fuse
❏ C. Backup timer
❏ D. Rheostat

90. To demonstrate the glenoid fossa in profile, the patient is positioned

❏ A. 45° oblique, affected side up
❏ B. 45° oblique, affected side down
❏ C. 25° oblique, affected side up
❏ D. 25° oblique, affected side down

91. Which of the following groups of technical factors will produce the *least* receptor exposure?

❏ A. 200 mA, 0.25 s, 70 kV, 12:1 grid
❏ B. 500 mA, 0.10 s, 90 kV, 8:1 grid
❏ C. 400 mA, 0.125 s, 80 kV, 12:1 grid
❏ D. 300 mA, 0.16 s, 70 kV, 8:1 grid

92. In which of the following procedures is quiet, shallow breathing recommended during the exposure to obliterate prominent pulmonary vascular markings?

1. RAO sternum
2. Lateral thoracic spine
3. AP scapula
❏ A. 1 only
❏ B. 1 and 2 only
❏ C. 2 and 3 only
❏ D. 1, 2, and 3

93. Which of the following statements is/are true regarding the lateral projection of the lumbar spine?

1. The MSP is parallel to the tabletop
2. The vertebral foramina are well visualized
3. The pedicles are well visualized
❏ A. 1 only
❏ B. 1 and 2 only
❏ C. 1 and 3 only
❏ D. 1, 2, and 3

94. An increase in the kilovoltage applied to the x-ray tube increases the

1. percentage of high-energy photons produced
2. exposure rate
3. patient absorption
❏ A. 1 only
❏ B. 1 and 2 only
❏ C. 2 and 3 only
❏ D. 1, 2, and 3

95. Which of the following is/are associated with magnification fluoroscopy?

1. Higher patient dose than nonmagnification fluoroscopy
2. Higher voltage to the focusing lenses
3. Image intensifier focal point closer to the input phosphor
❏ A. 1 only
❏ B. 1 and 2 only
❏ C. 2 and 3 only
❏ D. 1, 2, and 3

96. Correct positioning of the AP forearm includes which of the following element(s)?

1. Interepicondylar line parallel to the IR
2. Forearm extended and supinated
3. Epicondyles superimposed
❏ A. 1 only
❏ B. 1 and 2 only
❏ C. 2 and 3 only
❏ D. 1, 2, and 3

97. The structure indicated by the number 6 in Figure 7-14 is the

- ❏ A. cecum
- ❏ B. descending colon
- ❏ C. vermiform appendix
- ❏ D. terminal ileum

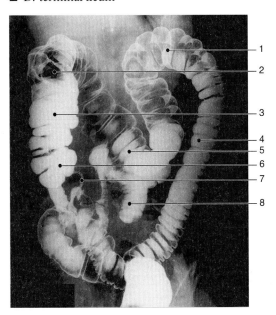

Figure 7-14. Used with permission of Stamford Hospital, Department of Radiology.

98. The structure indicated by the number 1 in Figure 7-14 is the

- ❏ A. left colic flexure
- ❏ B. right colic flexure
- ❏ C. transverse colon
- ❏ D. sigmoid colon

99. Which of the following exposures would most likely deliver the greatest dose to the thyroid?

- ❏ A. AP skull
- ❏ B. PA skull
- ❏ C. PA esophagus
- ❏ D. PA chest

100. Which of the following conditions require(s) a decrease in technical factors?

1. Emphysema
2. Osteomalacia
3. Atelectasis
   - ❏ A. 1 only
   - ❏ B. 1 and 2 only
   - ❏ C. 2 and 3 only
   - ❏ D. 1, 2, and 3

101. If 0.5 Gy was delivered during a 6-min fluoroscopic examination, what was the dose rate?

- ❏ A. 0.3 mGy/min
- ❏ B. 3.0 mGy/min
- ❏ C. 8.33 mGy/min
- ❏ D. 83.3 mGy/min

102. Characteristic(s) of a 16:1 grid include which of the following?

1. It absorbs more useful radiation than an 8:1 grid
2. It has more centering latitude than an 8:1 grid
3. It is used with higher kilovoltage exposures than an 8:1 grid
   - ❏ A. 1 only
   - ❏ B. 1 and 3 only
   - ❏ C. 2 and 3 only
   - ❏ D. 1, 2, and 3

103. An exposure was made at 40-inch SID using 5 mAs and 105 kV, using an 8:1 grid. Another image of the same part is made using a 12:1 grid and 90 kV. Which of the following exposure times will be *most appropriate,* using 400 mA, to maintain the original receptor exposure?

- ❏ A. 0.01 s
- ❏ B. 0.03 s
- ❏ C. 0.1 s
- ❏ D. 0.3 s

104. All of the following statements regarding three-phase current are true, *except*

- ❏ A. three-phase current is constant-potential direct current
- ❏ B. three-phase equipment produces more x-rays per milliampere second than single-phase equipment
- ❏ C. three-phase equipment produces higher average-energy x-rays than single-phase equipment
- ❏ D. the three-phase waveform has less ripple than the single-phase waveform

105. The pyloric canal and duodenal bulb are *best* demonstrated during an upper GI series in which of the following positions?

- ❏ A. RAO
- ❏ B. Left lateral
- ❏ C. Recumbent PA
- ❏ D. Recumbent AP

106. The decision as to whether to deliver ionic or nonionic contrast medium should include a preliminary patient history including, but not limited to

1. patient age
2. history of respiratory disease
3. history of cardiac disease
   - ❏ A. 1 and 2
   - ❏ B. 1 and 3
   - ❏ C. 2 and 3
   - ❏ D. 1, 2, and 3

107. A satisfactory radiograph was made without a grid using a 72-inch SID and 8 mAs. If the distance is changed to 40 inches and a 12:1 ratio grid is added, what should be the new milliampere seconds value?

- ❏ A. 9.5 mAs
- ❏ B. 12 mAs
- ❏ C. 21 mAs
- ❏ D. 26 mAs

108. Which of the following statements regarding SNR is most accurate?
- ❏ A. SNR increases as mAs increases
- ❏ B. Low SNR is desirable
- ❏ C. Low SNR improves resolution
- ❏ D. SNR increases as kV decreases

109. The dose from all types of ionizing radiation and its associated risk to human tissues is defined as
- ❏ A. effective dose (EfD)
- ❏ B. equivalent dose (EqD)
- ❏ C. doubling dose
- ❏ D. weighting exposure

110. The regular measurement and evaluation of radiographic equipment components and their performance is most accurately termed as
- ❏ A. postprocessing
- ❏ B. quality assurance
- ❏ C. quality control
- ❏ D. quality congruence

111. The radiograph in Figure 7-15 could be improved in which of the following ways?
- ❏ A. The MSP should be 45° to the plane of the IR
- ❏ B. The MSP should be 90° to the plane of the IR
- ❏ C. The chin should be elevated slightly
- ❏ D. The head should be flexed slightly

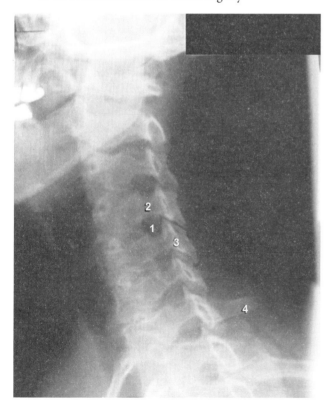

Figure 7-15

112. What is the anatomic structure indicated by the number 3 in the radiograph in Figure 7-15?
- ❏ A. Spinous process
- ❏ B. Transverse process
- ❏ C. Pedicle
- ❏ D. Intervertebral foramen

113. With the patient positioned as shown in Figure 7-16, how should the CR be directed to *best* demonstrate the intercondyloid fossa?
- ❏ A. Perpendicular to the popliteal depression
- ❏ B. 40° caudad to the popliteal depression
- ❏ C. Perpendicular to the long axis of the femur
- ❏ D. 40° cephalad to the popliteal depression

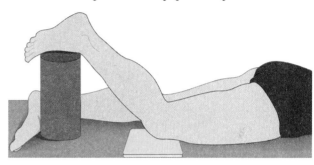

Figure 7-16

114. What feature is used to display RIS information about current patients?
- ❏ A. HIS
- ❏ B. Modality work list
- ❏ C. PACS
- ❏ D. DICOM

115. The most common cause of x-ray tube failure is
- ❏ A. a cracked anode
- ❏ B. a pitted anode
- ❏ C. vaporized tungsten on glass envelope
- ❏ D. insufficient heat production

116. A patient who has been recumbent for some time and gets up quickly may suffer from light-headedness or feel faint. This is called
- ❏ A. dyspnea
- ❏ B. orthopnea
- ❏ C. hypertension
- ❏ D. orthostatic hypotension

117. If a quantity of radiation is delivered to a body over a short period of time, its effect
- ❏ A. will be greater than if it were delivered over a long period of time
- ❏ B. depends solely on the distance factor
- ❏ C. has no relation to how it is delivered in time
- ❏ D. depends solely on the radiation quantity

118. Which of the labeled bones in Figure 7-17 identifies the tarsal cuboid?

❏ A. Number 2
❏ B. Number 3
❏ C. Number 6
❏ D. Number 7

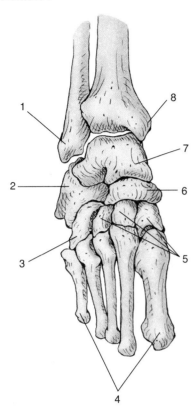

Figure 7-17

119. What does the number 1 in Figure 7-17 identify?

❏ A. Medial malleolus
❏ B. Lateral malleolus
❏ C. Medial cuneiform
❏ D. Talus

120. Select the three correct completions: Scattered radiation exposure to head and neck regions of personnel during C-arm fluoroscopic procedures can be reduced by placing

❏ A. the fluoroscopy tube over the patient
❏ B. staff at the foot of the x-ray table
❏ C. staff at right angles to the center of the x-ray beam
❏ D. the fluoroscopy tube under the patient
❏ E. the image intensifier over the patient
❏ F. staff at the head of the x-ray table

121. Brightness and contrast resolution in digital imaging can be influenced by

1. window level (WL)
2. window width (WW)
3. lookup table (LUT)

❏ A. 1 only
❏ B. 1 and 2 only
❏ C. 2 and 3 only
❏ D. 1, 2, and 3

122. Sterile technique is required when contrast agents are administered

❏ A. through a nasogastric tube
❏ B. intrathecally
❏ C. rectally
❏ D. orally

123. Which of the following groups of digital system technical factors would be *most appropriate* for a sthenic adult abdomen, using an iodinated contrast agent?

❏ A. 6 mAs, 75 kV
❏ B. 3 mAs, 85 kV
❏ C. 1.5 mAs, 75 kV
❏ D. 6 mAs, 95 kV
❏ E. 1.5 mAs, 105 kV

124. Which of the four baselines illustrated in Figure 7-18 should be used for a lateral projection of facial bones?

❏ A. Baseline 1
❏ B. Baseline 2
❏ C. Baseline 3
❏ D. Baseline 4

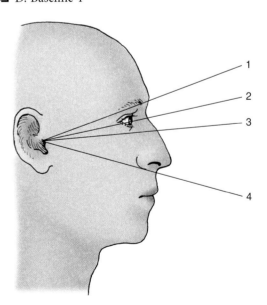

Figure 7-18

125. Which of the following statements is/are true regarding the radiograph shown in Figure 7-19?
1. The part is rotated
2. Pneumothorax is present
3. Adequate inspiration is demonstrated
   - ❏ A. 1 only
   - ❏ B. 2 only
   - ❏ C. 1 and 2 only
   - ❏ D. 1, 2, and 3

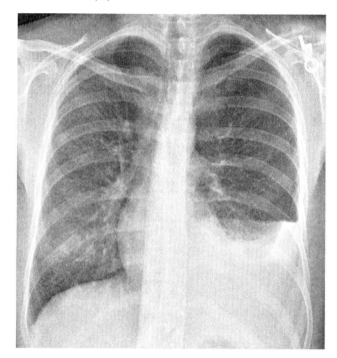

Figure 7-19

126. Which of the following is/are used to control the production of scattered radiation?
1. Collimators
2. Optimal kV
3. Use of grids
   - ❏ A. 1 only
   - ❏ B. 1 and 2 only
   - ❏ C. 2 and 3 only
   - ❏ D. 1, 2, and 3

127. Which of the following is/are included in whole-body dose equivalents?
1. Gonads
2. Lens
3. Extremities
   - ❏ A. 1 only
   - ❏ B. 1 and 2 only
   - ❏ C. 2 and 3 only
   - ❏ D. 1, 2, and 3

128. The AP oblique projection of the ilium requires that the
   - ❏ A. unaffected side be elevated 40°
   - ❏ B. affected side be elevated 40°
   - ❏ C. unaffected side be elevated 25°
   - ❏ D. affected side be elevated 20°

129. To eject a K-shell electron from a tungsten atom, the incoming electron must have energy of *at least*
   - ❏ A. 60 keV
   - ❏ B. 70 keV
   - ❏ C. 80 keV
   - ❏ D. 90 keV

130. What is the name of the plane indicated by the number 1 in Figure 7-20?
   - ❏ A. Midcoronal plane
   - ❏ B. Midsagittal plane
   - ❏ C. Transverse plane
   - ❏ D. Horizontal plane

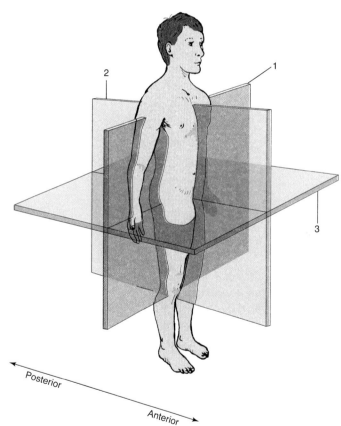

Figure 7-20

131. Which of the following is the most likely site for a lumbar puncture?
❏ A. S1–S2
❏ B. L3–L4
❏ C. L1–L2
❏ D. C6–C7

132. Which of the following is/are characteristic(s) of anemia?
1. Decreased number of circulating red blood cells
2. Decreased hemoglobin
3. Hematuria
❏ A. 1 only
❏ B. 1 and 2 only
❏ C. 1 and 3 only
❏ D. 1, 2, and 3

133. Differences between body habitus types are likely to affect all of the following, *except*
❏ A. the size and shape of an organ
❏ B. the position of an organ
❏ C. the position of the diaphragm
❏ D. the degree of bone porosity

134. The effective energy of an x-ray beam is increased by increasing the
1. added filtration
2. kilovoltage
3. milliamperage
❏ A. 1 only
❏ B. 2 only
❏ C. 1 and 2 only
❏ D. 1, 2, and 3

135. Which of the illustrations in Figure 7-21 most closely portrays the hypersthenic body type?
❏ A. Illustration number 1
❏ B. Illustration number 2
❏ C. Illustration number 3
❏ D. Illustration number 4

136. The reduction in x-ray photon intensity as the photon passes through a material is termed
❏ A. anode heel effect
❏ B. grid cutoff
❏ C. attenuation
❏ D. divergence

137. Which of the following positions can be used to effectively demonstrate the left colic flexure during radiographic examination of the large bowel?
1. RAO
2. LAO
3. RPO
❏ A. 1 only
❏ B. 1 and 2 only
❏ C. 1 and 3 only
❏ D. 2 and 3 only

138. Which of the following is recommended for a cervical spine having recent trauma or known fracture?
❏ A. Erect AP and lateral
❏ B. Recumbent AP and open mouth
❏ C. Flexion and extension laterals
❏ D. Dorsal decubitus lateral

139. Maslow's hierarchy of basic human needs includes which of the following?
1. Self-esteem
2. Love and belongingness
3. Death with dignity
❏ A. 1 only
❏ B. 1 and 2 only
❏ C. 2 and 3 only
❏ D. 1, 2, and 3

140. A radiograph exposed using a 12:1 ratio grid may exhibit a loss of receptor exposure at its lateral edges because the
❏ A. SID was too great
❏ B. grid failed to move during the exposure
❏ C. x-ray tube was angled in the direction of the lead strips
❏ D. CR was off-center

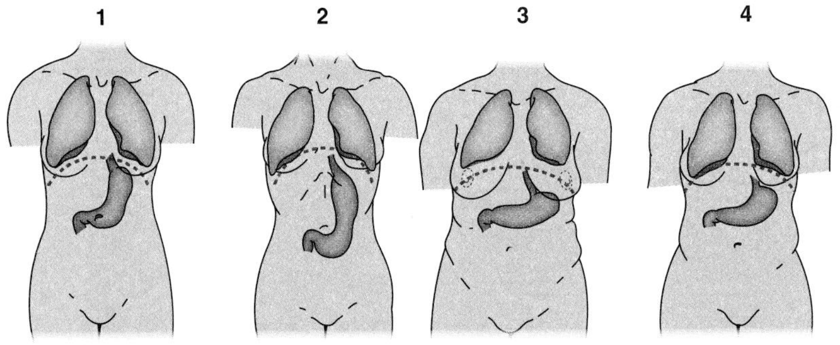

Figure 7-21. Reproduced with permission from Saia DA. *LANGE Radiography Review Flashcards.* New York: McGraw Hill, 2015.

141. Which of the following technical changes is *most likely* to permit the greatest reduction in patient dose?
- ❏ A. Increasing the mAs by half and decreasing the kV by 15%
- ❏ B. Increasing kilovoltage by 15% and cutting the milliampere seconds value in half
- ❏ C. Changing collimation from 10 × 12 to 14 × 17
- ❏ D. Changing from an 8:1 grid technique to nongrid

142. The trapezium is identified in Figure 7-22 as
- ❏ A. number 3
- ❏ B. number 4
- ❏ C. number 5
- ❏ D. number 6

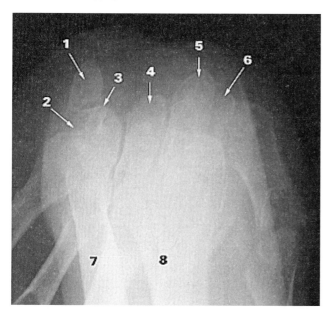

Figure 7-22

143. The major difference between excretory and retrograde urography is that
- ❏ A. they each require a different type of contrast agent
- ❏ B. intravenous studies require more images
- ❏ C. retrograde studies do not demonstrate function
- ❏ D. more contrast medium–induced adverse reactions occur in retrograde studies

144. In myelography, the contrast medium generally is injected into the
- ❏ A. cisterna magna
- ❏ B. individual intervertebral disks
- ❏ C. subarachnoid space between the first and second vertebrae
- ❏ D. subarachnoid space between the third and fourth lumbar vertebrae

145. Body substances and fluids that are considered infectious or potentially infectious include
1. feces
2. breast milk
3. wound drainage
- ❏ A. 1 only
- ❏ B. 1 and 2 only
- ❏ C. 2 and 3 only
- ❏ D. 1, 2, and 3

146. Which of the following is/are demonstrated in the lateral projection of the cervical spine?
1. Intervertebral joints
2. Zygapophyseal joints
3. Intervertebral foramina
- ❏ A. 1 only
- ❏ B. 1 and 2 only
- ❏ C. 2 and 3 only
- ❏ D. 1, 2, and 3

147. Contaminated needles are disposed of in special containers in which of the following ways?
- ❏ A. Recap the needle, remove syringe, dispose of
- ❏ B. Do not recap needle, remove from syringe, dispose of
- ❏ C. Recap the needle, dispose of entire syringe
- ❏ D. Do not recap needle, dispose of entire syringe

148. Acceptable method(s) of minimizing motion unsharpness is/are
1. suspended respiration
2. short exposure time
3. patient instruction
- ❏ A. 1 only
- ❏ B. 1 and 2 only
- ❏ C. 1 and 3 only
- ❏ D. 1, 2, and 3

149. Which acronym is used to help rescuers remember the correct CPR step sequence?
- ❏ A. BLS
- ❏ B. ACB
- ❏ C. CAB
- ❏ D. SLB

150. Which of the following would be the safest interval of time for a fertile woman to undergo abdominal radiography without significant concern for irradiating a recently fertilized ovum?
- ❏ A. The first 10 days following the cessation of menstruation
- ❏ B. The first 10 days following the onset of menstruation
- ❏ C. The 10 days preceding the onset of menstruation
- ❏ D. About 14 days before menstruation

151. What is the anatomic structure indicated by number 1 in the radiograph shown in Figure 7-23?

❑ A. Mandibular angle
❑ B. Coronoid process
❑ C. Zygomatic arch
❑ D. Maxillary sinus

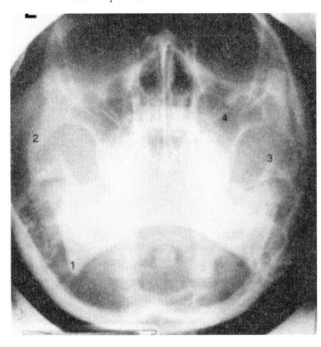

Figure 7-23

152. What is the anatomic structure indicated by number 3 in the radiograph in Figure 7-23?

❑ A. Mandibular angle
❑ B. Coronoid process
❑ C. Zygomatic arch
❑ D. Maxillary sinus

153. Esophageal varices are best demonstrated in which of the following positions?

❑ A. Erect
❑ B. Recumbent
❑ C. Fowler
❑ D. Sims

154. Heat production at the anode increases when using

1. high mAs factors
2. a small focal spot
3. high kV factors
4. low-ratio grids
   ❑ A. 1, 2, and 4
   ❑ B. 1 and 2 only
   ❑ C. 2 and 3 only
   ❑ D. 1, 2, and 3

155. With which of the following does the lateral extremity of the clavicle articulate?

❑ A. Manubrium
❑ B. Coracoid process
❑ C. Coronoid process
❑ D. Acromion process

156. With the patient supine, the left side of the pelvis elevated 25°, and the CR entering 1 inch medial to the left anterosuperior iliac spine (ASIS), which of the following is demonstrated?

❑ A. Left sacroiliac joint
❑ B. Left ilium
❑ C. Right sacroiliac joint
❑ D. Right ilium

157. Double-focus x-ray tubes have two

1. focal spots
2. filaments
3. anodes
   ❑ A. 1 only
   ❑ B. 1 and 2 only
   ❑ C. 1 and 3 only
   ❑ D. 2 and 3 only

158. What is the anatomic structure indicated by number 6 in the radiograph shown in Figure 7-24?

❑ A. Superior articular process
❑ B. Pars interarticularis
❑ C. Transverse process
❑ D. Lamina

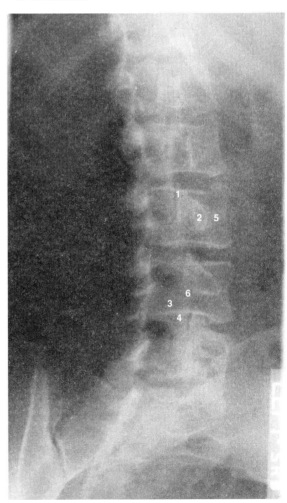

Figure 7-24. Used with permission of Stamford Hospital, Department of Radiology.

159. What is the anatomic structure indicated by number 3 in the radiograph in Figure 7-24?
- ❏ A. Superior articular process
- ❏ B. Pars interarticularis
- ❏ C. Transverse process
- ❏ D. Lamina

160. The drug diphenhydramine is classified as a/an
- ❏ A. diuretic
- ❏ B. antipyretic
- ❏ C. antihistamine
- ❏ D. emetic

161. Which of the following cell types is the *least* radiosensitive?
- ❏ A. Myelocytes
- ❏ B. Myocytes
- ❏ C. Megakaryocytes
- ❏ D. Erythroblasts

162. Which of the following is/are essential to high-quality mammographic examinations?
1. Small focal spot x-ray tube
2. Short-scale contrast
3. Use of a compression device
- ❏ A. 1 only
- ❏ B. 1 and 2 only
- ❏ C. 1 and 3 only
- ❏ D. 1, 2, and 3

163. The degree of difference between remnant beam signals is termed
- ❏ A. window level
- ❏ B. window width
- ❏ C. subject contrast
- ❏ D. receptor contrast

164. What is the anatomic structure indicated by the number 10 in Figure 7-25?
- ❏ A. Coracoid process
- ❏ B. Ulnar styloid process
- ❏ C. Radial styloid process
- ❏ D. Radial notch

165. Which of the following correctly identifies the head of the ulna in the illustration in Figure 7-25?
- ❏ A. Number 3
- ❏ B. Number 4
- ❏ C. Number 5
- ❏ D. Number 9

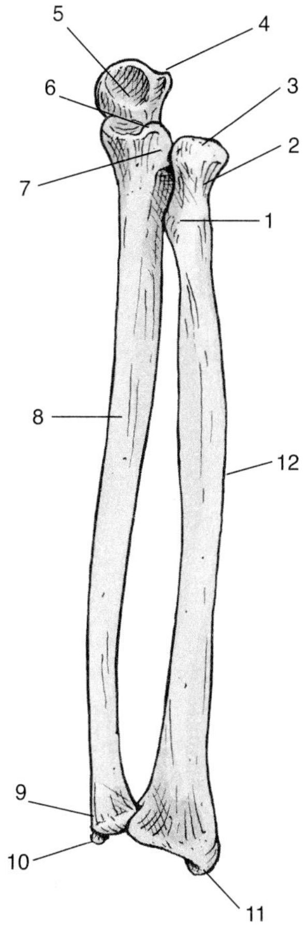

Figure 7-25

166. Which of the following waveforms has the lowest percentage voltage ripple?
- ❏ A. Single-phase
- ❏ B. Three-phase, six-pulse
- ❏ C. Three-phase, 12-pulse
- ❏ D. High-frequency

167. What percentage of x-ray attenuation does a 0.5-mm lead equivalent apron at 75 kV provide?
- ❏ A. 51%
- ❏ B. 66%
- ❏ C. 75%
- ❏ D. 88%

168. Which of the following drugs may be used to prolong blood clotting time?
1. Heparin
2. Diphenhydramine
3. Lidocaine
- ❏ A. 1 only
- ❏ B. 1 and 2 only
- ❏ C. 1 and 3 only
- ❏ D. 1, 2, and 3

169. Which of the following procedures may be used to better demonstrate the interphalangeal joints of the toes?

1. Angle the CR 15° caudad
2. Angle the CR 15° cephalad
3. Place a sponge wedge under the foot with the toes elevated 15°
   ❏ A. 1 only
   ❏ B. 1 and 2 only
   ❏ C. 1 and 3 only
   ❏ D. 2 and 3 only

170. The *most commonly used* method of low-flow oxygen delivery is the

❏ A. oxygen mask
❏ B. nasal cannula
❏ C. respirator
❏ D. oxyhood

171. The femoral neck can be located

❏ A. parallel to the femoral shaft
❏ B. perpendicular to the femoral shaft
❏ C. perpendicular to a line drawn from the ASIS to the pubic symphysis
❏ D. perpendicular to a line from the iliac crest to the pubic symphysis

172. The vessels seen as numbers 1 and 2 in Figure 7-26 function to convey

❏ A. oxygenated blood to the lungs
❏ B. deoxygenated blood to the lungs
❏ C. oxygenated blood to the left atrium
❏ D. deoxygenated blood to the right atrium

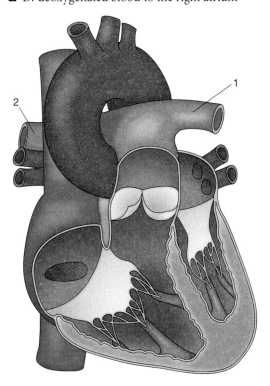

Figure 7-26

173. Improper support of a patient's fractured lower leg (tibia/fibula) while performing radiography could result in

1. movement of fracture fragments
2. tearing of soft tissue, nerves, and blood vessels
3. initiation of muscle spasm
   ❏ A. 1 and 2 only
   ❏ B. 1 and 3 only
   ❏ C. 2 and 3 only
   ❏ D. 1, 2, and 3

174. Personnel radiation monitor reports must include which of the following information?

1. Dose equivalents for report period
2. Dosimeter type
3. Radiation quality
   ❏ A. 1 only
   ❏ B. 1 and 2 only
   ❏ C. 2 and 3 only
   ❏ D. 1, 2, and 3

175. The intertrochanteric crest is located on the

❏ A. proximal posterior femur
❏ B. proximal anterior femur
❏ C. distal posterior femur
❏ D. distal anterior femur

176. The ethical principle that aspires to, above all, do no harm describes

❏ A. fidelity
❏ B. veracity
❏ C. nonmaleficence
❏ D. beneficence

177. A radiographer would be in violation of the American Registry of Radiologic Technologists (ARRT) *Code of Ethics for the Profession of Radiologic Technology* for all of the following, *except*

❏ A. failing to wear a lead apron when performing mobile radiography
❏ B. failing to participate in continuing education
❏ C. communicating information regarding suspected child abuse to the referring physician
❏ D. refusing to participate in new and innovative technical procedures

178. Hospitals and other health care providers must ensure patient confidentiality in compliance with which of the following legislation?

❏ A. MQSA
❏ B. MRSA
❏ C. HIPAA
❏ D. HIPPA

179. Another name for Hirschsprung disease, the most common cause of lower GI obstruction in neonates, is

- ❏ A. intussusception
- ❏ B. volvulus
- ❏ C. congenital megacolon
- ❏ D. pyloric stenosis

180. An exposure was made using 300 mA and 50 ms. If the exposure time is changed to 22 ms, which of the following milliamperage selections would *most* closely approximate the original receptor exposure?

- ❏ A. 300 mA
- ❏ B. 400 mA
- ❏ C. 600 mA
- ❏ D. 700 mA

181. A technique chart should include which of the following information?

1. Recommended SID
2. Grid ratio
3. CR angulation
  - ❏ A. 1 only
  - ❏ B. 1 and 2 only
  - ❏ C. 1 and 3 only
  - ❏ D. 1, 2, and 3

182. What is the established fetal dose-limit guideline for pregnant radiographers during the entire gestation period?

- ❏ A. 1 mSv
- ❏ B. 5 mSv
- ❏ C. 50 mSv
- ❏ D. 100 mSv

183. The acquired immune deficiency syndrome (AIDS) virus may be transmitted

1. by sharing contaminated needles
2. from mother to child during birth
3. by intimate contact with body fluids
  - ❏ A. 1 only
  - ❏ B. 1 and 2 only
  - ❏ C. 1 and 3 only
  - ❏ D. 1, 2, and 3

184. Which type of personnel radiation monitor is an ionization chamber that uses Bluetooth technology to relate its data mobile device or any computer with Internet access and USB connection?

- ❏ A. Pocket dosimeter
- ❏ B. Direct ion storage dosimeter
- ❏ C. Optically stimulated luminescence dosimeter
- ❏ D. Thermoluminescent dosimeter

185. Which of the following are considered *most* radiosensitive?

- ❏ A. Lymphocytes
- ❏ B. Ova
- ❏ C. Neurons
- ❏ D. Myocytes

186. The National Council on Radiation Protection and Measurements (NCRP) recommends an annual occupational effective (stochastic) dose equivalent limit of

- ❏ A. 50 mSv
- ❏ B. 100 mSv
- ❏ C. 25 mSv
- ❏ D. 200 mSv

187. Which of the following is/are associated with magnification fluoroscopy?

1. Increased mA
2. Smaller portion of the input phosphor is used
3. Image intensifier focal point moves closer to the output phosphor
  - ❏ A. 1 only
  - ❏ B. 1 and 2 only
  - ❏ C. 2 and 3 only
  - ❏ D. 1, 2, and 3

188. Alignment of x-ray tube, part, and IR are essential to avoid

1. distortion
2. magnification
3. image noise
4. foreshortening
5. elongation
  - ❏ A. 1, 3, and 4
  - ❏ B. 1, 4, and 5
  - ❏ C. 1, 2, and 5
  - ❏ D. 2, 4, and 5
  - ❏ E. 2, 3, and 4

189. Linear energy transfer (LET) may be *best* described as

- ❏ A. the amount of energy delivered per distance traveled in tissue
- ❏ B. the unit of absorbed dose
- ❏ C. radiation equivalent man
- ❏ D. radiation absorbed dose

190. Which of the following anomalies is/are possible if an exposure dose of 400 mGy (40 rad) were delivered to a pregnant uterus in the 3rd week of pregnancy?

1. Skeletal anomaly
2. Organ anomaly
3. Neurologic anomaly
  - ❏ A. 1 only
  - ❏ B. 2 only
  - ❏ C. 2 and 3 only
  - ❏ D. 1, 2, and 3

191. When interviewing a patient, what is it that the health care professional can observe?

❑ A. Symptoms
❑ B. History
❑ C. Objective signs
❑ D. Subjective signs

192. Which of the following can function to double the receptor exposure?

1. Double the mAs
2. Increase kV by 15%
3. Increase SID by 8 inches
    ❑ A. 1 only
    ❑ B. 1 and 2 only
    ❑ C. 2 and 3 only
    ❑ D. 1 and 3 only

193. Which of the following is/are characteristics of a patient with pulmonary emphysema?

1. Hyperventilation
2. Increased AP diameter of the chest
3. Shoulder girdle elevation
    ❑ A. 1 only
    ❑ B. 1 and 2 only
    ❑ C. 2 and 3 only
    ❑ D. 1, 2, and 3

194. The primary function of filtration is to reduce

❑ A. patient skin dose
❑ B. operator dose
❑ C. image noise
❑ D. scattered radiation

195. Which of the following statements is/are *true* regarding the PA axial projection of the paranasal sinuses?

1. The CR is directed caudally to the orbitomeatal line (OML)
2. The petrous pyramids are projected into the lower third of the orbits
3. The frontal sinuses are visualized
    ❑ A. 1 only
    ❑ B. 1 and 2 only
    ❑ C. 2 and 3 only
    ❑ D. 1, 2, and 3

196. Spatial resolution is directly related to

1. SID
2. tube current
3. focal spot size
    ❑ A. 1 only
    ❑ B. 1 and 2 only
    ❑ C. 2 and 3 only
    ❑ D. 1, 2, and 3

197. The Centers for Disease Control and Prevention (CDC) suggests that health care workers protect themselves and their patients from blood and body fluid contamination by using

❑ A. strict isolation precautions
❑ B. standard precautions
❑ C. respiratory precautions
❑ D. sterilization

198. X-ray tube life may be extended by

1. using high-milliampere seconds, low-kilovoltage technical factors
2. avoiding lengthy anode rotation
3. avoiding exposures to a cold anode
    ❑ A. 1 only
    ❑ B. 1 and 2 only
    ❑ C. 2 and 3 only
    ❑ D. 1, 2, and 3

199. Which of the following is *most likely* to occur as a result of using a 30-inch SID with a 14 × 17 inches IR to image a fairly homogeneous structure?

❑ A. Production of quantum mottle
❑ B. Noticeable receptor exposure variation between opposite ends of the IR
❑ C. Production of scatter radiation fog
❑ D. Excessively short-scale contrast

200. Which of the following radiographic examinations require(s) the patient to be NPO 8–10 h prior to examination for proper patient preparation?

1. Abdominal survey
2. Upper GI series
3. BE
    ❑ A. 1 and 2 only
    ❑ B. 1 and 3 only
    ❑ C. 2 and 3 only
    ❑ D. 1, 2, and 3

ANSWERS AND EXPLANATIONS

1. **(B)** LET expresses the rate at which photon or particulate energy is transferred to (absorbed by) biologic material (through ionization processes); it depends on the type of radiation and absorber characteristics. *Relative biologic effectiveness* (RBE) describes the degree of response or amount of biologic change that one can expect of the irradiated material. As the amount of transferred energy (LET) increases (from interactions occurring between radiation and biologic material), the amount of biologic effect/damage also will increase, that is, the two are directly related.

2. **(C)** A *histogram* is a graph usually having several peaks and valleys representing the pixel values/absorbing properties of the various tissues, and so on, that make up the imaged part. These various attenuators include things such as bone, muscle, air, contrast agents, foreign bodies, and pathology. The various pixel values, then, represent image contrast. If the histogram has a rather flat "tail," this represents underexposed areas at the periphery of the image, which can skew the overall histogram analysis. The radiographer selects the particular processing algorithm on the computer/control panel that corresponds to the anatomic part and projection being performed. DICOM (Digital Imaging and Communications in Medicine) refers to the standard for communication between PACS and HIS/RIS systems. *Windowing* refers to the radiographer's postprocessing adjustment of contrast and brightness (at the workstation).

3. **(B)** *Dysplasia* refers to abnormal development of tissue—often demonstrated radiographically in skeletal imaging. Difficulty in speaking is termed *dysphasia*. *Malposition* refers to an anatomic structure located in a place other than the norm, for example, situs inversus. Difficult or painful breathing is termed *dyspnea*.

4. **(B)** Contrast media having high atomic number are called *radiopaque* because x-ray photons have difficulty penetrating these dense materials. Radiopaque contrast agents appear white on the x-ray image because many x-ray photons have been absorbed by these materials (e.g., barium and iodine). These are referred to *positive* contrast agents—composed of dense (i.e., *high atomic number*) material through which x-rays will not pass easily. *Radiolucent* (negative) contrast agents appear black on the finished image because x-ray photons pass through easily. An example of a radiolucent contrast agent is air.

5. **(C)** Dose area product (DAP) expresses the radiation dose leaving the x-ray tube *times* the area of the x-ray field. DAP meters measure the *product* of in-air radiation and the area of the x-ray field. There is heightened awareness of radiation skin dose these days, particularly in interventional fluoroscopic procedures. It is recommended that maximum radiation skin dose is better estimated using a DAP meter. This is generally thought to provide more useful information in potential high-dose procedures then simply recording the fluoroscopic time. The DAP meter is a type of ionization chamber that is placed just beyond the x-ray collimators and must capture the entire x-ray field to provide an accurate reading. DAP is sometimes called KAP (kerma air product).

6. **(A)** Proper body mechanics includes a wide base of support. The *base of support* is the portion of the body that is in contact with the floor or some other horizontal plane. The *center of gravity* is the midpoint of the pelvis or lower abdomen, depending on body build. The *line of gravity* is the abstract line passing vertically through the center of gravity. Proper body mechanics can help to prevent painful back injuries by making proficient use of the muscles in the arms and legs.

7. **(D)** The knee is formed by the proximal tibia, the patella, and the distal femur, which articulate to form the femorotibial and femoropatellar joints. The distal posterior femur presents two large *medial* and *lateral condyles* separated by the deep intercondyloid fossa. Because the medial femoral condyle is further from the IR, it is magnified and will obscure the femorotibial joint space, as seen in Figure 7-1. If the CR is angled about 5° cephalad, the medial femoral condyle will be projected superiorly and superimposed on the lateral femoral condyle, thus opening the joint space. The patient should lie on the affected side with the patella perpendicular to the tabletop and the knee flexed 20°–30°. Rotating the part forward or backward will affect visualization of the *femoropatellar* joint.

8. **(B)** Because muscle, brain, and nerve tissues perform specific functions and are formed of highly differentiated cells that do not divide, they are relatively insensitive to ionizing radiation exposure. *Epithelial* cells cover the outer surface of the body; they also line body cavities and tubes and passageways leading to the exterior. They contain very little intercellular substance and are devoid of blood vessels. Because epithelial cells constantly regenerate through mitosis, they are very *radiosensitive*. *Lymphocytes* are important in the production of antibodies, have a life span of only about 24 h, and are the most radiosensitive type of blood cell. *Intestinal crypt cells* are immature stem cells and highly radiosensitive.

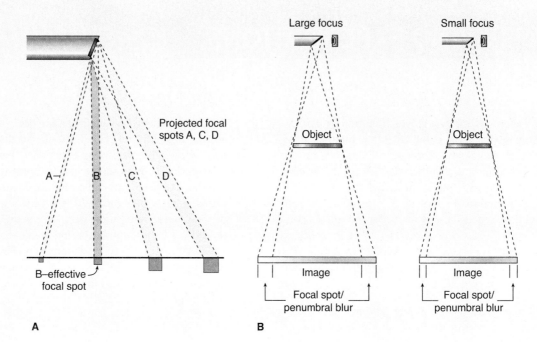

Figure 7-27

9. **(D)** The x-ray tube anode is designed according to the line-focus principle, that is, with the focal track beveled (Fig. 7-27). This allows a larger actual focal spot to project a smaller effective focal spot, resulting in improved detail/sharpness with less blur (less geometric unsharpness) as seen in 7-27A. However, because of the target angle, penumbral blur varies along the longitudinal tube axis, being greater at the cathode end of the image and less at the anode end of the image as seen in 7-27B. Therefore, better detail/sharpness will be appreciated using small focal spots at the anode end of the x-ray beam and at longer SIDs.

10. **(D)** Three dose–response (dose–effect) curves are illustrated in Figure 7-2, representing the body's response to ionizing radiation exposure. *Dose* is indicated by the horizontal axis (increasing to the right); *response* is indicated by the vertical axis (increasing upward). Two of the curves (numbers 1 and 3) are *linear*, that is, *response is directly related to dose*. Curve 2 is not a straight line and is, therefore, *nonlinear*. Curves 2 and 3 show that a particular dose (*threshold quantity*) of radiation is required before any effect will occur; therefore, curve 2 is *nonlinear threshold*, and curve 3 is *linear threshold*. Curve 1, however, shows that any dose of radiation (theoretically, even a single x-ray photon, i.e., there is no threshold) can result in a particular biologic effect; therefore, it is *linear nonthreshold*.

11. **(A)** The scaphoid can be difficult to image because its curved shape lends itself to foreshortening and self-superimposition. The lateral carpals, especially the scaphoid, are well demonstrated in the PA oblique projection. The *ulnar* deviation maneuver helps to overcome the scaphoid's self-superimposition. The scaphoid may also be demonstrated with less foreshortening with the

wrist PA and elevated 20°. The CR is directed perpendicular to the carpal scaphoid.

The medial carpals, especially the pisiform, are well demonstrated in the AP oblique projection with the radial deviation maneuver.

12. **(A)** The *dorsal decubitus* position is obtained with the patient supine and the x-ray beam directed horizontally. The finished image looks similar to a lateral projection of the chest. However, small amounts of fluid will gravitate to the posterior chest, and small amounts of air will rise to the anterior chest. The *ventral decubitus* position is obtained with the patient prone and the x-ray beam directed horizontally. The finished image can demonstrate small amounts of fluid anteriorly and small amounts of air posteriorly.

13. **(C)** The degree of anterior and posterior motion is occasionally diminished with a whiplash-type injury. Anterior (forward, flexion) and posterior (backward, extension) motion is evaluated in the lateral position with the patient assuming flexion and extension as best as he or she can. Left and right bending images of the thoracic and lumbar vertebrae are obtained frequently when evaluating scoliosis. The AP open-mouth projection is used to evaluate the first two cervical vertebrae. The moving mandible AP projection is used to demonstrate the entire cervical spine while blurring out the superimposed mandible.

14. **(B)** Sufficient inspiration is demonstrated by the visualization of 10 pairs of posterior ribs projected above the diaphragm. Rotation of the chest is detected by asymmetry in the distance between the medial ends of the clavicles and the vertebral column. The scapulae should be free of superimposition with the lung fields; this is

accomplished by rolling the shoulders forward while positioning for the PA projection.

15. (C) The number 7 (Fig. 7-3) points out the *lead-lined x-ray tube housing.* The glass enclosed x-ray tube (number 6) is within the lead-lined housing. When high-speed electrons strike surfaces other than the tungsten target (number 3), x-rays are produced and emitted in all directions (isotropically). X-ray tubes have a lead-lined metal protective housing (number 7) to absorb much of this "*leakage radiation.*" Leakage radiation must not exceed 1 mGy$_a$/h at a distance of 1 m from the tube housing. Because the production of x-rays requires the use of high voltage, the tube housing also serves to protect from electric shock. The production of x-rays involves the production of large quantities of heat, which can be damaging to the x-ray tube. Therefore, an oil coolant surrounds the x-ray tube to further insulate it and to absorb heat from the x-ray tube structures.

The tube housing is unrelated to scatter or hardening of the x-ray beam.

16. (C) *Angina pectoris* is a spasmodic chest pain that is frequently caused by oxygen deficiency in the myocardium. The pain often radiates down the left arm and up to the left jaw. Angina pectoris attacks frequently are associated with exertion or emotional stress in individuals with coronary artery disease. Pain may be relieved with a vasodilator, such as *nitroglycerin* given sublingually or transdermally. *Digitalis* is used to treat congestive heart failure. *Dilantin* is used in the control of seizure disorders, and *cimetidine* (Tagamet) is used to treat duodenal ulcers.

17. (C) To change nongrid to grid exposure, or to adjust exposure when changing from one grid ratio to another, remember the factor for each grid ratio:

No grid = 1 × original mAs
5:1 grid = 2 × original mAs
6:1 grid = 3 × original mAs
8:1 grid = 4 × original mAs
10:1, 12:1 grid = 5 × original mAs
16:1 grid = 6 × original mAs

Therefore, to change from nongrid exposure to an 8:1 grid, multiply the original milliampere seconds value by a factor of 4. Thus, a new setting of 32 mAs is required. Slightly different conversion factors are often recommended for digital equipment.

18. (A) The images shown in Figure 7-4 are *axial* CT images of the abdomen *with contrast.* In Figure 7-4A, the liver (number 1, left lobe; number 6, right lobe; number 3, caudate lobe), barium-filled stomach (number 2), spleen (number 5), and aorta (number 4) are seen. More *inferior* structures, such as the inferior vena cava (number 5) and kidneys (number 9 and number 10) are seen in Figure 7-4B.

19. (B) Figure 7-4B is an axial CT section of the abdomen with contrast. Structures demonstrated include the barium-filled stomach (number 1), the gallbladder (number 2), duodenum (number 3), pancreas (number 4), IVC (number 5), left adrenal gland (number 6), aorta (number 7), spleen (number 8), left kidney (number 9), right kidney (number 10), and liver (number 11).

20. (C) *Idiopathic* refers to a disease of unknown or unclear cause. The term *systemic* refers to or concerns a (body) system. An *epidemic* describes a disease that swiftly affects a large number of people in a particular geographic region. Anything that is or can be disease-producing is termed *pathogenic.*

21. (C) The occupational dose limit is valid for beta, x-, and gamma radiations. Because alpha radiation is rapidly ionizing, so traditional personnel monitors will not record alpha radiation. Because alpha particles are capable of penetrating only a few centimeters of air, they are practically harmless as an external source.

22. (A) Sampling frequency used in CR is expressed as *pixels per millimeter* or *pixel density.* Mobile spot size impacts spatial resolution but has no impact on pixel density or sampling frequency. Light spread between the IP and scanner light guide refers to CR but does not impact sampling frequency. TFT arrays are not part of CR systems; TFT arrays are found in direct and indirect digital detector systems.

23. (B) DF uses exposure, rather than continuous fluoroscopic exposure. DF photospot images, which are simply still-frame images, need no chemical processing, require less patient dose (unless more than necessary are taken), and offer postprocessing capability. DF also offers *road-mapping* capability—a technique useful in procedures involving guidewire/catheter placement. Another feature is the *last-image-hold* feature. During the fluoroscopic examination, the most recent fluoroscopic image can be stored on the monitor (last-image hold), thereby reducing the need for continuous x-ray exposure. This technique can offer significant reductions in the radiation exposure to the patient and personnel. The length of the procedure is an important consideration in patient dose; the longer the procedure, the *greater* the dose.

24. (C) Fluoroscopic skin dose is greater than radiographic skin dose because the x-ray source is much closer to the patient. The generally accepted rule is that the skin receives 21 mGy$_a$/min/mA. Therefore, 21 mGy for 5 min at 1.5 mA equals 21 × 5 × 1.5 = 157.5 mGy approximate skin dose.

25. (C) *Air–fluid levels* are demonstrated in the erect or decubitus position. Grid radiography requires about a 3–4 times greater dose than nongrid radiography. A left lateral decubitus projection without a grid, then, would demonstrate fluid levels with a considerably smaller dose to the infant. A recumbent AP projection would not demonstrate air–fluid levels.

26. (C) The radial head and neck are projected free of superimposition in the AP oblique projection (*lateral* rotation) of the elbow. The humeral capitulum is also well demonstrated in this external oblique position. The AP oblique projection (*medial* rotation) of the elbow superimposes the radial head and neck on the proximal ulna. It demonstrates the olecranon process within the olecranon fossa, and it projects the coronoid process free of superimposition.

27. (D) Figure 7-5 illustrates the component parts of cardiopulmonary circulation. Deoxygenated blood enters the RA (2) from the superior and inferior (3) venae cavae. Blood flows from RA through the right atrioventricular/tricuspid valve into the RV (4). RV contraction opens the pulmonary semilunar valve (1) and blood flows into the pulmonary artery (8) to the lungs and undergoes oxygenation. Newly oxygenated blood enters LA (6) via four pulmonary veins (7).

Oxygenated blood flows from the LA through left atrioventricular/mitral valve into the LV (5). *LV contraction opens the aortic semilunar valve and blood flows into the ascending aorta.* The aorta and its branches distribute oxygenated blood to all body tissues. CO_2 is collected by the venous system, and deoxygenated blood is returned via the superior and inferior (3) venae cavae to the RA (2).

28. (D) The radiographic subject (the patient) is composed of many different tissue types of varying densities, resulting in varying degrees of photon attenuation and absorption. This *differential absorption* contributes to the variation in x-ray intensity reaching the image receptor. Normal tissue density may be significantly altered in the presence of pathology. Destructive bone disease can cause a dramatic decrease in tissue density. Abnormal accumulation of fluid (as in ascites) will cause a significant increase in tissue density. Muscle atrophy or highly developed muscles will similarly decrease or increase tissue density.

29. (B) The overall chance that a person will become infected with HIV is high through sexual contact, fluids containing infected blood, contaminated needles or blood, from mother to fetus via the placenta, and through breast milk. The most common occupational exposure is via the HIV infected needlestick but, according to the CDC, the probability of infection is only 0.3%.

30. (A) DR uses solid-state detector plates (FPDs) as the x-ray IR to intercept the x-ray beam.

Indirect-capture systems are FPDs that use TFTs or CCDs. Both indirect-capture systems involve *scintillation*. Scintillators include cesium iodide (CsI), gadolinium oxysulfide (Gd_2O_2S), and *amorphous silicon* (a-Si).

The scintillator captures x-ray photons and emits light. That light is then recorded via CCD *or* TFT. *Direct*-capture systems use *amorphous selenium* (a-Se) and TFTs. Amorphous selenium, a semiconductor, is the x-ray photon detector. Upon x-ray exposure, x-ray energy is converted to an electrical signal in a single layer of material, such as the semiconductor a-Se. Electric voltage is applied to both surfaces of the a-Se, electron hole pairs are created, and charges are read by TFT arrays located on the surfaces. The electrical signal is transferred directly to the ADC.

Systems *without* a scintillation/light conversion step have a *higher* DQE, with the exception of the new complementary metal oxide semiconductor (*CMOS*) capture systems. In general, amorphous selenium TFTs used in direct-capture systems have the highest DQE.

DR affords the additional advantage of immediate display.

31. (B) The RAO position is shown in Figure 7-6. The RAO position is often used to superimpose the sternum onto the heart shadow, providing uniform receptor exposure throughout the sternum. This position is also used to see axillary portions of left anterior ribs; in the anterior oblique positions, the affected side is away from the IR. The RAO position can also be used to demonstrate the barium-filled pylorus and duodenum, and the esophagus can be projected between the vertebrae and heart in this position. The degree of obliquity depends on the patient's body habitus—greater obliquity is required for thinner chests. Barium-filled gastric fundus would be demonstrated in either the AP recumbent or LPO position.

32. (A) It is occasionally necessary to view the lung apices free of superimposition with the clavicles. This objective can be achieved in an AP axial projection. The patient is positioned AP erect with the CR directed 15°–20° cephalad, entering the manubrium. An AP axial projection can also be obtained with the patient in the lordotic position. If sufficient lordosis can be assumed, the CR is directed perpendicular to the IR.

33. (B) The polyenergetic x-ray beam is captured very efficiently by the digital receptors. However, the range of x-ray photons is so large that *raw images* are unclear and require digital processing to be of diagnostic quality. X-ray photons are converted to electrical signals, which are then available for processing and postprocessing. Digital processing permits visualization of an infinite number of tissue densities captured by the digital detector. According to the Nyquist theorem, when the electric signals are sampled for conversion to a digital image, the sampling frequency must be more than twice the frequency of the input signal to best duplicate that original signal. At least twice the number of pixels required to form the image must be sampled, or resolution will be compromised.

34. **(A)** When a change to a larger diameter mode is made, the voltage on the electrostatic focusing lenses is decreased, and the result is a less *magnified but brighter* image. The milliamperage will be automatically decreased to compensate for the increase in brightness, resulting in *lower* patient dose in the *larger* diameter modes.

35. **(D)** Structures located behind the parietal peritoneum are called *retroperitoneal.* Retroperitoneal structures include the kidneys, adrenal glands, pancreas, duodenum, ascending and descending colon, portions of the aorta, and the inferior vena cava.

36. **(C)** A beveled focal track extends around the periphery of the anode disk; when a small angle is used, the beveled edge allows for a smaller effective focal spot and better detail. The disadvantage, however, is that photons are noticeably absorbed by the "heel" of the anode, resulting in a smaller percentage of x-ray photons at the anode end of the x-ray beam and a concentration of x-ray photons at the cathode end of the beam. This is known as the *anode heel effect* and can cause a primary beam variation of up to 45%. The anode heel effect becomes more pronounced as the SID decreases, as IR size increases, and as target angle decreases.

37–38. **(37, B; 38, C)** The *autotransformer* (number 1) controls/selects the amount of voltage sent to the primary winding of the high-voltage transformer and operates on the principle of self-induction. The *step-up* (high-voltage) *transformer* (primary coil is number 2; secondary coil is number 3) operates on the principle of mutual induction. The step-up transformer functions to change low voltage to the high voltage necessary to produce x-ray photons. All the x-ray circuit transformers—the autotransformer, the step-up/high-voltage transformer, and the step-down/filament transformer—require AC for their operation. The step-down/filament transformer is located in filament circuit (6). The x-ray tube is identified as number 7. The x-ray tube requires unidirectional current for efficient operation; AC coming from the high-voltage transformer is changed to unidirectional current by the circuit rectifiers (5).

39. **(D)** Streptococcal pharyngitis (strep throat) is caused by bacteria. To know this, you have to remember that bacteria are classified according to their morphology (i.e., size and shape). The three classifications are spirals, rods (bacilli), and spheres (cocci). Viruses, unlike bacteria, cannot live outside a human cell. Viruses attach themselves to a host cell and invade the cell with their genetic information. Various fungal infections may grow on the skin (cutaneously), or they may enter the skin. Fungal infections that enter the circulatory or lymphatic system can be deadly. Protozoa are one-celled organisms classified by their motility. Ameboids move by locomotion, flagella use their protein tail, cilia possess numerous short protein tails, and sporozoans actually are not mobile.

40. **(D)** The thicker and denser the anatomic part being studied, the less bright will be the fluoroscopic image. Both milliamperage and kilovoltage affect the fluoroscopic image in a way similar to the way they affect the radiographic image. For optimal contrast, especially taking into consideration the patient dose, higher kilovoltage, and lower milliamperage generally are preferred.

41. **(D)** High-frequency generators first appeared in mobile x-ray units and were then adopted by mammography and CT equipment. Nowadays, more and more radiographic equipment use high-frequency generators. Their compact size makes them popular, and the fact that they produce nearly constant potential voltage helps to improve image quality and decrease patient dose (fewer low-energy photons to contribute to skin dose).

42. **(C)** Radiographic rating charts enable the operator to determine the maximum safe milliamperage, exposure time, and kilovoltage for a particular exposure using a particular x-ray tube. An exposure that can be made using the large focal spot may not be safe when the small focal spot of the same x-ray tube is used. The total number of heat units an exposure generates also influences the amount of stress (in the form of heat) imparted to the anode. Single-phase heat units are determined by the product of milliamperage × time × kilovoltage. *Three-phase and high-frequency* heat units are determined from the product of milliamperage × time × kilovoltage × 1.4. In the examples given then, group (A) produces 6048 HU, group (B) produces 14,700 HU, group (C) produces 1983 HU, and group (D) produces 7056 HU. Therefore, group (C) technical factors will deliver the *least amount of heat* to the anode.

43. **(C)** A signed consent form (informed consent) is not necessary prior to performing an upper GI series. Informed consent is necessary before performing any procedure that is considered invasive or that carries considerable risk. A myelogram, a cardiac catheterization, and an interventional vascular procedure are all invasive procedures, and all carry some degree of risk. A physician should explain to the patient what those risks are as well as the risk of not having the procedure. In addition, the patient should be made aware of alternative procedures and the risks associated with the alternatives. Only after the patient has been made aware and all questions have been answered appropriately should the informed consent be signed. A radiographer is not responsible for obtaining informed consent. However, in some institutions, it may be departmental procedure for the radiographer to check the chart and see whether there is a signed consent form in place.

44. **(C)** The tangential (sunrise) projection is used to demonstrate the articular surfaces of the femur and patella. It is also used to demonstrate vertical fractures of the patella. The AP, PA, and oblique projections of the knee are used primarily to evaluate the joint space and articulating structures. The tunnel view is used to demonstrate the intercondyloid fossa.

45. **(D)** During radiography and fluoroscopy, radiation scatters from the patient in all directions. In fact, the patient is the single most important scattering object in both radiographic and fluoroscopic procedures. The approximate intensity (quantity) of scattered radiation at 1 m from the patient is 0.1% of the entrance dose. Therefore, if the entrance dose for this exposure is 25 mGy, the intensity of radiation at 1 m from the patient is 0.1% of that, or 0.025 mGy ($0.001 \times 25 = 0.025$).

46. **(B)** Flat-panel detectors used in DR are often made of an amorphous selenium (a-Se)–coated thin film transistor (TFT) array. They function to convert the x-ray energy (emerging from the radiographed part) into an electrical signal. The TFT capacitors send the electrical signal to the analog-to-digital converter (ADC) to be changed to a digital signal. *Amorphous selenium* refers to a crystalline material (selenium) that lacks its crystalline structure. Amorphous selenium or silicon is used to produce the direct-conversion flat-panel detectors used in DR.

47. **(D)** Most of the occupational exposure received by radiographers is received during fluoroscopy and mobile radiography, and the use of lead aprons is required during both these procedures. The position of the personnel monitor relative to the lead apron, therefore, becomes important. It is recommended that the badge be worn outside the lead apron at collar level. In this position, the badge will record the maximum possible exposure received by the radiographer and will provide a realistic estimate of thyroid and lens exposure.

48. **(C)** The basic components of the x-ray tube are the *anode* (positive electrode) and *cathode* assembly (negative electrode), enclosed within an evacuated (vacuum) *glass envelope.*

The x-ray tube glass enclosure is made of glass that is heat resistant to maintain the necessary vacuum for the production of x-rays. The cathode assembly consists of one or more *filaments,* their supporting wires, and a *nickel focusing cup.* The filament is a fine (approximately 0.2 mm diameter) 1- to 2-cm coil of tungsten wire that, when heated to incandescence by approximately 4 amps of current, boils off/releases outer-shell tungsten electrons. This event is called *thermionic emission.* Most x-ray tubes actually have two or more filaments and are called *double-focus tubes.* The typical x-ray tube has two filaments, one small and one large (Fig. 7-8), to direct electrons to either the small or large anode focal spot. Each filament is closely embraced by a negatively charged focusing cup that serves to direct the electrons toward the anode. The two filaments are arranged in a three-wire/conductor system. A low-voltage conductor carries low voltage to heat the selected (large or small) filament.

The third conductor is common to both filaments and carries the high voltage.

49. **(B)** Retrograde urography is not considered a functional study of the urinary system. IVU, and excretory/descending urography are all considered functional urinary tract studies because the contrast medium is introduced intravenously and excreted by the kidneys. Retrograde urography involves introduction of contrast medium into the kidneys via catheter, thereby demonstrating their *structure* but not their *function.*

50. **(D)** When the primary beam is restricted to an area near the periphery of the body, sometimes part of the illuminated area overhangs the edge of the body. If the exposure is then made, scattered radiation from the tabletop (where there is no absorber) will undercut the part, causing excessive receptor exposure. If, however, a *lead rubber mat* is placed on the overhanging illuminated area, most of this scatter will be absorbed. This is frequently helpful in lateral lumbar spine and AP shoulder radiographs.

51. **(B)** The (diarthrotic) sternoclavicular joints are formed by the medial (sternal) extremities of the clavicles and the clavicular notches of the manubrium (of the sternum). They can be demonstrated in the LAO and RAO positions. The LAO position demonstrates the left sternoclavicular joint, whereas the RAO position demonstrates the joint on the right. The patient is obliqued about 15° with the side of interest adjacent to the IR.

52. **(D)** Patient demographic and examination information originates from the hospital/facility HIS, where it is obtained when the patient is initially registered. That information is available or retrievable when the patient is scheduled, or arrives, for imaging services. *Typical patient information includes name, DOB or age, sex, ID number, accession number, examination being performed, date and time of examination.*

Additional information may be available on the examination requisition; more information is usually entered by the technologist at the time of the examination.

A feature that is useful in sorting examinations and decreasing (but not eliminating) errors is the modality work list (MWL). The MWL "brings up" existing RIS information, that is, the examinations scheduled for each imaging area—for example, x-ray, CT, MRI, mammography, and ultrasound. The technologist selects the correct patient, which includes that patient's particular demographics, from the particular MWL.

It is essential that the technologist is attentive to detail and accuracy when entering patient information; errors in patient demographics entry, and entry duplication, must be avoided.

53. **(A)** HAIs are also called *nosocomial.* Despite the efforts of infectious disease departments, HAIs continue to be a problem in hospitals these days. This is at least partly because of there being a greater number of older, more vulnerable patients and an increase in the number of invasive procedures performed these days (i.e., needles and catheters). The most frequent site of HAI is the urinary tract, followed by wounds, the respiratory tract, and blood.

54. **(A)** The control badge is an important part of the monitoring system. It should be stored somewhere away from radiation sources. At the end of the monitoring period, when the badges are returned to the dosimetry service, the exposure to the control badge (which should be zero) is compared with the exposure received by the rest of the personnel monitors. If the control badge is stored near radiation or used to replace someone's lost badge, there is no standard for comparison for the rest of the group of monitors.

55. **(B)** In mutual induction, two coils are in close proximity, and a current is supplied to one of the coils. As the magnetic field associated with every electric current expands and "grows up" around the first coil, it interacts with and "cuts" the turns of the second coil. This interaction, motion between magnetic field and coil (conductor), induces an electromotive force (emf) in the second coil. This is *mutual induction,* the production of a current in a neighboring circuit. Transformers, such as the high-voltage transformer and the filament (step-down) transformer, operate on the principle of mutual induction. The autotransformer operates on the principle of self-induction. Both the transformer and the autotransformer require the use of alternating current.

56. **(D)** The human body is composed of approximately 80% water; the remaining 20% is a combination of substances, such as proteins, carbohydrates, and lipids. The smallest functional unit of the body is the *cell;* the structure/content of which often determines its function. Cells form tissues and organs that also have functional characteristics. The two basic types of cells are *somatic* and *genetic.* Somatic cells are all the body's cells (bone, muscle, nerve, etc.) except those concerned with reproduction—those cells are termed genetic.

DNA is located in the nucleus of each cell, packaged into thread-like structures called *chromosomes.* Each chromosome is made up of DNA tightly coiled many times around proteins called histones that support its structure. Passed from parents to offspring, DNA contains the specific instructions that make each individual unique.

Chromosomes are visible, under microscope, in the cell's nucleus only when the cell is dividing (*mitosis*). Most of what researchers know about chromosomes has been learned by observing chromosomes during mitotic activity. Division of *somatic* cells is *mitosis,* whereas (reduction) division of *genetic* cells is *meiosis.*

Every chromosome has a constricted portion called its *centromere,* which divides the chromosome into two sections, or "arms." The chromosome's short arm is called its "p arm." The chromosome's long arm is called its "q arm." The location of the centromere on each chromosome is often used to assist description of the location of specific genes.

57. **(B)** Proper functioning of the AEC device depends on accurate positioning by the radiographer. The correct photocell(s) must be selected, and the anatomic part of interest must completely cover the photocell(s) to achieve the desired receptor exposure. If a photocell is left uncovered, scattered radiation from the part being examined will cause premature termination of exposure and an underexposed radiograph.

58. **(C)** Invasion of privacy—that is, public discussion of privileged and confidential information—is intentional misconduct. False imprisonment, such as unnecessarily restraining a patient, is also intentional misconduct. However, if a radiographer left a weak patient standing while leaving the room to check images or get supplies and the patient fell and sustained an injury that would be considered unintentional misconduct or negligence.

59. **(A)** *Resolution* describes how closely fine details may be associated and still be recognized as separate details before seeming to blend into each other and appear "as one." The degree of resolution transferred to the IR is a function of the resolving power of each of the system components and can be expressed in line pairs per millimeter (lp/mm). It can be measured using a resolution test pattern; a variety of resolution test tools are available. The star pattern generally is used for focal spot size evaluation. Resolution can also be expressed in terms of line-spread function (LSP) or modulation transfer function (MTF). LSP is measured using a 10-μm x-ray beam; MTF measures the amount of information lost between the object and the IR.

60. **(B)** Pathologic processes and abnormal conditions that alter tissue composition or thickness can have a significant effect on receptor exposure. The radiographer must be aware of these variants and processes to make an appropriate and accurate adjustment of technical factors.

Examples of *additive* pathologic conditions:

- Ascites
- Rheumatoid arthritis
- Paget disease
- Pneumonia
- Atelectasis
- Congestive heart failure
- Edematous tissue

Examples of *destructive/subtractive* pathologic conditions:

- Osteoporosis
- Osteomalacia
- Pneumoperitoneum
- Emphysema
- Degenerative arthritis
- Atrophic and necrotic conditions

61. (D) Cells that are termed *undifferentiated* are immature or young. They have no specific function and/or structure. They are usually precursor cells; their most important function is to divide. Mitosis is the most radiosensitive part of the cell cycle.

62. (A) The oblique axial projection is valuable when the zygomatic arches cannot be demonstrated bilaterally with the submentovertical projection because they are not prominent enough or because of a depressed fracture. The patient still may be positioned as for an SMV projection, but the head is obliqued 15° toward the side being examined. This serves to move the zygomatic arch away from superimposed structures and provides a slightly oblique axial projection of the arch (Fig. 7-28). This position is very useful in cases of depressed fracture of the zygomatic arch.

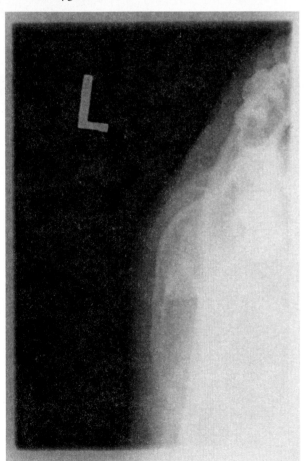

Figure 7-28

63. (B) The image shown in Figure 7-9 is part of an upper GI examination. Barium sulfate has been taken by mouth; the stomach and the first portion of the small intestine are visualized. The fundus is filled with barium, which indicates that the patient is recumbent; the proximal portion of the stomach is posterior while the body and pylorus lie more anteriorly. The vertebra indicates that the patient is in an oblique position. The fundus has barium, so this must be an LPO position. The mucosal folds of the duodenum are well visualized. If this position has been performed erect, barium fluid levels would be seen within the stomach.

64. (B) *Noise* is a term used to describe any undesirable fluctuations in the brightness of an image. Common types of image noise are fog from scattered radiation and quantum mottle/noise, which often results from insufficient x-ray intensity (milliampere seconds). SNR refers to signal-to-noise ratio. The signal is the x-ray photons. The higher the SNR, the less image noise.

65. (B) The image shown in Figure 7-10 illustrates *aliasing artifact,* or Moiré effect. Aliasing, or Moiré, has the appearance of somewhat wavy linear lines and can occur in computed radiography when using *stationary grids.* If the grid's lead strip pattern (i.e., frequency) matches the scanning (sampling) pattern of the scanner/reader, the resulting interference can cause aliasing (also called Moiré) artifact. When sampling frequencies are decreased, aliasing/Moiré is less evident. As sampling frequencies increase, aliasing/Moiré is more obvious.

66. (D) The thoriated tungsten filament of the cathode assembly is heated by its own filament circuit. This circuit provides current and voltage to heat the filament to incandescence, at which time it undergoes thermionic emission (the liberation of valence electrons from filament atoms). The greater the number of electrons flowing between the cathode and the anode, the greater is the tube current (milliamperage). *Rectification* (single- or three-phase) is the process of changing alternating current to unidirectional current. A greater number of secondary transformers turn functions to increase voltage and decrease current.

67. (D) Proper care of leaded protective apparel is required to ensure its continued usefulness. If lead aprons and gloves are folded, cracks will develop, and this will decrease their effectiveness. Both items should be fluoroscoped annually to check for the formation of cracks.

68. (D) Fidelity, veracity, nonmaleficence, and beneficence are all ethical principles. *Nonmaleficence* is the principle that refers to the prevention of harm. *Beneficence* is the ethical principle that refers to bringing about good or benefiting others. *Fidelity* refers to faithfulness and *veracity* refers to truthfulness.

69. (D) Follow-up studies have been done on individuals receiving accidental exposure to radiation (e.g., medical personnel, uranium miners, and children irradiated in vivo). Pioneer radiation workers developed leukemia and other cancers, their vision was clouded by the formation of cataracts, and their lives were shorter than those of their colleagues. With sophisticated equipment and knowledge of radiation protection these days, none of these situations should occur.

70. (C) CR is less expensive primarily because it is compatible with existing equipment. DR requires existing equipment to be modified or new equipment purchased. Because there is an image plate (IP), CR can be conveniently used for mobile studies; mobile units often come equipped for DR as well. After image processing, the IP is erased and reused. DR offers the advantage of immediate visualization of the x-ray image; in CR, there is a short delay.

71. (B) Digital images are best viewed in areas with low-lighting levels that will avoid undesirable monitor screen glare. Digital images usually have a black "mask" covering the white unexposed areas, further reducing objectionable ambient light and glare. If the radiographer views images in a brightly lit area, the image can appear excessively dark. The same image, when reviewed by the radiologist, might look most adequate. As light level increases, the pupils of the eye contract and admit less light, causing images to appear dark. It is an effect similar to walking from a sunny day into a dark theater.

72. (C) The sternum has three parts: the uppermost portion is the *manubrium* (and is quadrilateral in shape), the midportion is the *body* or *gladiolus,* and the distal portion is the *ensiform* or *xiphoid process.* The sternum supports the clavicles superiorly and provides attachment for the ribs laterally. The first seven pairs of ribs are true, or *vertebrosternal,* ribs because they attach directly to the sternum. The ribs angle obliquely anteriorly and inferiorly so that their anterior portions are 3–5 inches inferior to their posterior attachment. The *sternoclavicular joints* afford the only bony attachment between the thorax and the upper extremity.

73. (C) Figure 7-11 illustrates a lumbar vertebra. The structure labeled number 3 is the pedicle. Lumbar pedicles, and the intervertebral foramina which they help to form, are best demonstrated in the lateral projection. Number 1 is the vertebral body, number 2 is a transverse process, number 4 is the superior articular process, number 5 is its facet, number 6 is the spinous process, number 7 is the lamina, number 8 is the inferior articular process, and number 9 is its facet.

74. (B) Exposure to high doses of radiation results in *early* effects. Examples of early effects are blood changes and erythema. If the exposed individual survives, then *late,* or long-term, effects must be considered. Individuals who receive small amounts of low-level radiation (e.g., those who are occupationally exposed) are concerned with the late effects of radiation exposure—effects that can occur many years after the initial exposure. *Late* effects of radiation exposure, such as carcinogenesis, are considered to be related to the linear nonthreshold dose–response curve—that is, there is *no safe dose;* theoretically, even one x-ray photon can induce a later response.

75. (B) The greater and lesser tubercles are prominences on the proximal humerus, separated by the bicipital groove. The AP projection of the humerus in external rotation demonstrates the greater tubercle in profile (Fig. 7-29A). With the arm placed in internal rotation, the humerus is placed in a true lateral position, and the lesser tubercle is demonstrated (Fig. 7-29B).

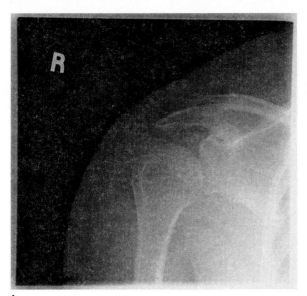 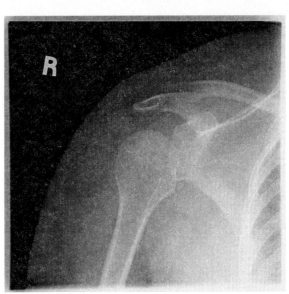

A   B

Figure 7-29

76. (D) Photoelectric interaction in tissue involves complete absorption of the incident photon, whereas Compton interactions involve only partial transfer of energy. The larger the quantity of radiation and the greater the number of photoelectric interactions, the greater is the patient dose. Radiation dose to more radiosensitive tissues, such as gonadal tissue or blood-forming organs, is more harmful than the same dose to muscle tissue.

77. (C) The AP oblique projection (LPO, RPO position/ Grashey method) is used to demonstrate the glenoid fossa in profile. The position is most comfortably performed in the erect position. The body is rotated 35°–45° toward the affected side. The CR is directed 2 inches medial and 2 inches inferior to the upper outer border of the shoulder. The glenohumeral joint space is open and the glenoid cavity is demonstrated in profile.

78. (A) Because patient dose is regulated by the quantity of x-ray photons delivered to the patient, the milliampere seconds value regulates patient dose. Highly energetic x-ray photons (high kilovoltage) are more likely to penetrate the patient rather than be absorbed by biologic tissue. Consequently, the use of high-kilovoltage and low-milliampere seconds technical factors is preferred in an effort to reduce patient dose.

79. (B) With the blood pressure cuff wrapped snugly around the patient's brachial artery and the pump inflated to approximately 180 mm Hg, the valve is opened only slightly to release pressure very slowly. With the stethoscope over the brachial artery, listen for the pulse while watching the mercury column (gauge). Note the point at which the first pulse is heard as the systolic pressure. As the valve is opened further, the sound is louder; the point at which it suddenly becomes softer is recorded as the diastolic pressure.

80. (D) To accurately position a lateral forearm, the elbow must form a 90° angle with the humeral epicondyles superimposed. The radius and ulna are superimposed distally. Proximally, the coronoid process and radial head are partially superimposed. Failure of the elbow to form a 90° angle or the hand to be lateral results in a less than satisfactory lateral projection of the forearm.

81. (A) Quality control refers to our equipment and its safe and accurate operation. Various components must be tested at specified intervals and test results must be within specified parameters. Any deviation from those parameters must be corrected. Examples of equipment components that are tested annually are the focal spot size, linearity, reproducibility, filtration, kilovoltage, and exposure time. Reproducibility specifies that radiation output must be consistent to within ±5%. Linearity tests x-ray output with increasing milliampere seconds; mGy$_a$/ mAs should be accurate to within 10%. Kilovoltage settings can most effectively be tested using an electronic kilovoltage meter; to meet the required standards, the

kilovoltage should be accurate to within ±4 kV. Congruence is a term used to describe the relationship between the collimator light field and the actual x-ray field—they must be congruent to within 2% of the SID. Radiographic equipment collimators should be inspected and verified as accurate semiannually.

82. (A) The line-focus principle states that the effective focal spot is smaller than the actual focal spot. The line-focus principle also illustrates that as the target angle decreases, the effective focal spot decreases (providing improved resolution/sharpness). When anode angles are made smaller, the *actual* focal spot size can be larger (permitting greater heat load capacity) while still maintaining a small *effective* focal spot size. It must be remembered, however, that a steep (small) target angle increases the anode heel effect, and part coverage may be compromised.

83. (D) The patient is seen to be in a recumbent oblique position in Figure 7-12. When the anterior surface is closer to the IR, the position is described as an *anterior oblique* position. Because the right side is closer to the IR, it is a *right anterior oblique* position. When the posterior surface is closer to the IR, the position is described as posterior oblique position.

84. (D) The *genetically significant dose* (GSD) illustrates that large exposures to a few people are cause for little concern when diluted by the total population. On the contrary, we all share the burden of the radiation that is received by the total population, and especially as the use of medical radiation increases, each individual's share of the total exposure increases.

85. (C) A patient with a respiratory disease can transmit infectious organisms via airborne contamination (if the patient sneezes or coughs). Therefore, patients with upper respiratory tract infection should be transported wearing a mask to prevent the possibility of airborne contamination. It is not necessary for the radiographer to be masked.

86. (B) Quality control refers to our equipment and its safe and accurate operation. Various components must be tested at specified intervals and test results must be within specified parameters. Any deviation from those parameters must be corrected. Examples of equipment components that are tested annually are the focal spot size, linearity, reproducibility, filtration, kilovoltage, and exposure time. Kilovoltage settings can most effectively be tested using photodiodes or ion chambers; to meet required standards, the kilovoltage should be accurate to within ±5 kV of the kilovoltage selected on the control panel. If the kilovoltage is outside of that range, the generator must be recalibrated.

Congruence is a term used to describe the relationship between the collimator light field and the actual x-ray field—they must be congruent (i.e., match) to within 2% of the SID. Collimators should be inspected and verified as accurate semiannually, that is, twice a year. Reproducibility testing should specify that radiation output be consistent to within ±5%.

87. **(C)** If the x-ray tube is angled significantly *across the lead strips* of a focused grid, there is uniform loss of receptor exposure (grid cutoff). Insufficient or excessive *distance* with focused grids causes loss of receptor exposure (grid cutoff) along the periphery of the image. Figure 7-13 demonstrates grid cutoff everywhere except along a central vertical strip of the image. This receptor exposure loss is due to the focused grid's being placed *upside down*. Thus, the middle vertical lead strips allow x-rays to pass, but because the lead strips angle laterally, they are directly opposite to the direction of the x-ray photons (rather than parallel to them), and severe grid cutoff (loss of exposure to the IR) results.

88. **(A)** When a patient's elbow needs to be examined in partial flexion, the lateral projection offers little difficulty, but the AP projection requires special attention. If the AP projection is made with a perpendicular CR and the olecranon process resting on the tabletop, the articulating surfaces are obscured. With the elbow in partial flexion, *two exposures are necessary* to achieve an AP projection of the elbow joint articular surfaces. One is made with the forearm parallel to the IR (humerus elevated), which demonstrates the proximal forearm. The other is made with the humerus parallel to the IR (forearm elevated), which demonstrates the distal humerus. In both cases, the CR is perpendicular if the degree of flexion is not too great or angled slightly into the joint space with greater degrees of flexion.

89. **(C)** A phototimer is one type of automatic exposure device. When it is installed in an x-ray unit, it is calibrated to produce radiographic densities as required by the radiologist. Once the part being radiographed has been exposed to produce the proper receptor exposure, the phototimer automatically terminates the exposure. *The manual timer should be used as a backup timer should the phototimer fail to terminate the exposure, thus protecting the patient from overexposure and the x-ray tube from excessive heat load.* The backup timer should be set to 150% (1.5 times) longer than the anticipated exposure time; 600 mAs not be exceeded. Circuit breakers and fuses are circuit devices used to protect circuit elements from overload. In case of current surge, the circuit will be broken, thus preventing equipment damage. A rheostat is a type of variable resistor.

90. **(B)** When viewing the glenoid fossa from the anterior, it is seen to angle posteriorly and approximately 45°. To view it in profile, then, it must be placed so that its surface is perpendicular to the IR. The patient is positioned in a 45° oblique, affected-side-down position, which places the glenoid fossa approximately perpendicular to

the IR. The arm is abducted slightly, the elbow is flexed, and the hand and forearm are placed over the abdomen. The CR is directed perpendicular to the glenohumeral joint.

91. **(A)** The milliampere seconds values are almost identical. Of the remaining factors, kilovoltage and grid ratio both affect receptor exposure. Decreased kilovoltage (choices A and D) decreases penetration and therefore the number of photons reaching the IR. High-ratio grids (choices A and C) also limit the number of photons reaching the IR thereby decreasing receptor exposure. Therefore, (A) is the best answer, having *both* low kilovoltage *and* high-ratio grid.

92. **(D)** Pulmonary vascular markings often are prominent in the elderly and in smokers. Quiet, shallow breathing may be used during a long exposure (with a compensating low milliamperage) to blur them out. Oblique sternum, AP scapula, and lateral thoracic spine projections are examinations in which this technique is useful.

93. **(C)** With the patient in the lateral position, the MSP is parallel to the x-ray tabletop. Because the *inter*vertebral foramina, which are formed by the pedicles, are 90° to the MSP, they are well demonstrated in the lateral projection. The intervertebral joints (i.e., disk spaces) are also well demonstrated. The spinal cord passes through the vertebral foramina, which would not be visualized in conventional radiography of the lumbar spine.

94. **(B)** As the kilovoltage is increased, a greater number of electrons are driven across to the anode with greater force. Therefore, as energy conversion takes place at the anode, *more* high-energy photons are produced. However, because they are *higher energy* photons, there will be less patient absorption.

95. **(D)** The input phosphor of image intensifiers is usually made of cesium iodide. For each x-ray photon absorbed by cesium iodide, approximately 5000 light photons are emitted. As the light photons strike a photoemissive *photocathode,* a number of electrons are released from the photocathode and focused toward the output side of the image tube by voltage applied to the negatively charged *electrostatic focusing lenses.* The electrons are then accelerated through the neck of the tube where they strike the small (0.5–1 inch) *output phosphor* (zinc cadmium sulfide) that is mounted on a flat glass support. The entire assembly is enclosed within a 2- to 4-mm-thick vacuum glass envelope. Remember that the image on the output phosphor is *minified, brighter,* and *inverted* (electron focusing causes image inversion).

Input phosphor diameters of 5–12 inches are available. Although smaller diameter input phosphors improve resolution, they do not permit a large FOV, that is, viewing of large patient areas.

Dual- and triple-field image intensifiers are available that permit *magnified* viewing of fluoroscopic images. To achieve magnification, the *voltage* to the focusing lenses is increased and a *smaller* portion of the input phosphor is used, thereby resulting in a smaller FOV. Because minification gain is now decreased, the image is not as bright. The milliamperage is automatically increased to compensate for the loss in brightness when the image intensifier is switched to magnification mode. Entrance skin exposure (ESE) can increase dramatically as the FOV decreases (i.e., as magnification increases).

As FOV decreases, *magnification* of the output phosphor image increases, there is less *noise* because increased milliamperage provides a greater number of x-ray photons, and *contrast* and *resolution* improve. The *focal point* in the magnification mode is *further away from* the output phosphor (as a result of increased voltage applied to the focusing lenses) and therefore the output image is magnified.

96. **(B)** The *AP projection* of the forearm requires that the elbow be extended and the hand supinated. The interepicondylar line must be parallel to the IR, to avoid overlap of the radius and ulna. The shoulder and elbow should be on the same plane. Superimposition of the epicondyles is a requirement of the *lateral* forearm projection.

97-98. **(97, A; 98, A)** The image shown in Figure 7-14 is a double-contrast BE, oblique position. Because the left colic/splenic flexure (number 1) is "open," this is either an RPO or LAO position. The right colic/hepatic flexure (number 2), ascending colon (number 3), the descending colon (number 4), and transverse colon (number 5) are demonstrated. Barium has refluxed from the cecum (number 6) into the terminal ileum (number 8). Number 7 is the vermiform process/appendix.

99. **(A)** Remember that the x-ray beam is polyenergetic/ heterogeneous—made up of many energies of x-ray photons. The use of aluminum filtration to decrease the number of low-energy photons entering the body does not solve the problem completely. Remaining low-energy photons will be absorbed by the tissue structures closest to the entering x-ray beam. If the patient is positioned for an AP projection, anterior structures will receive a higher (entry) dose than posterior structures, that is, the exit dose is less. If the patient is positioned for a PA projection, posterior structures will receive the higher entry dose. Abdomen imaging performed in the PA projection, whenever possible, will reduce exposure to the gonads. Skull and cervical spine projections performed PA will reduce exposure to the lens of the eye and to the thyroid.

A PA chest radiograph delivers about 0.01 mGy to the thyroid; a PA skull radiograph, about 0.08 mGy; and a PA esophagram, about 0.09 mGy. An AP skull radiograph delivers about 0.92 mGy to the thyroid. As can be seen from these examples, giving some thought to projection/ position selection can decrease critical organ dose significantly.

100. **(B)** *Subcutaneous emphysema* is a pathologic distension of tissues with air; *pulmonary emphysema* is a chronic disease characterized by overdistension of the alveoli with air. *Osteomalacia* is a softening of bone so that it becomes flexible, brittle, and deformed. All three of these conditions involve a decrease in tissue density and, therefore, require a decrease in technical factors. *Atelectasis* is a collapsed or airless lung; it requires an increase in technical factors.

101. **(D)** If 0.5 Gy was delivered during a 6-min fluoroscopic examination, the dose rate is determined by dividing the dose (0.5 Gy) by the length of the exam (6 min). Therefore, the dose rate is 0.8333 Gy/min, which is equal to 83.33 mGy/min.

102. **(B)** High-kilovoltage exposures produce large amounts of scattered radiation, and high-ratio grids are used often with high-kilovoltage techniques in an effort to absorb more of this scattered radiation. However, as more scattered radiation is absorbed, more primary radiation is absorbed as well. This accounts for the increase in milliampere seconds required when changing from an 8:1 to a 16:1 grid. In addition, precise centering and positioning become more critical; a small degree of inaccuracy is more likely to cause grid cutoff in a high-ratio grid.

103. **(B)** The use of high kilovoltage with a fairly low-ratio grid will be ineffective in ridding the remnant beam of scattered radiation. To reduce the amount of scattered radiation reaching the image receptor in this example, it has been decided to decrease the kilovoltage by 15%, thus making it necessary to increase the milliampere seconds from 5 to 10 mAs. Because an increase in the grid ratio to 12:1 is also desired, another change in milliampere seconds will be required (remember, 10 mAs is now the *old* mAs):

$$\frac{10\,(\text{old mAs})}{x\,(\text{new mAs})} = \frac{4\,(8{:}1\text{ grid factor})}{5\,(12{:}1\text{ grid factor})}$$

$$4x = 50$$

Thus, $x = 12.5$ mAs at 90 kV. Now, determine the *exposure time* required with 400 mA to produce 12.5 mAs:

$$400x = 12.5$$

$$x = 0.03\text{ s exposure}$$

Slightly different conversion factors are often recommended for digital equipment.

104. **(A)** Three-phase current is obtained from three individual alternating currents superimposed on, but out of step with, one another by 120°. The result is an *almost* constant-potential current, with only a very small voltage ripple (4%–13%), producing more x-rays per milliampere second, and at a higher average energy, than single-phase equipment.

105. (A) The RAO position affords a good view of the pyloric canal and duodenal bulb. It is also a good position for the barium-filled esophagus, projecting it between the vertebrae and the heart. The left lateral projection of the stomach demonstrates the left retrogastric space, the recumbent PA projection is used as a general survey of the gastric surfaces, and the recumbent AP projection with slight left oblique affords a double contrast of the pylorus and duodenum.

106. (D) All the choices listed in the question should be part of a preliminary patient history before deciding to inject ionic or nonionic contrast media. As patients age, their general health decreases and are, therefore, more likely to suffer from adverse reactions. Patients with a history of respiratory disease, such as asthma or emphysema and COPD, are more likely to have a reaction and to suffer greater distress in the event of a reaction. Patients with cardiac disease run an increased risk of changes in heart rate and myocardial infarction. Patients also should be screened for decreased renal or hepatic function, sickle cell disease, diabetes, and pregnancy.

107. (B) According to the inverse-square law of radiation, as the distance between the radiation source and the IR decreases, the exposure rate increases. Therefore, a decrease in technical factors is first indicated to compensate for the distance change. The following formula (exposure-maintenance formula) is used to determine new milliampere seconds values when changing distance:

$$\frac{mAs_1}{mAs_2} = \frac{D_1^2}{D_2^2}$$

Substituting known values:

$$\frac{8}{x} = \frac{5184}{1600}$$
$$5184x = 12{,}800$$

Thus, x = 2.47 mAs at 40-inch SID. To then compensate for adding a 12:1 grid, you must multiply the 2.47 mAs by a factor of 5. Thus, 12 mAs are required to produce a receptor exposure similar to the original image. The following are the factors used for milliampere seconds conversion from nongrid to grid:

No grid = 1 × original mAs
5:1 = grid 2 × original mAs
6:1 = grid 3 × original mAs
8:1 = grid 4 × original mAs
12:1 = grid 5 × original mAs
16:1 = grid 6 × original mAs

Slightly different conversion factors are often recommended for digital equipment.

108. (A) That portion of the x-ray beam striking the IR and representing image anatomy is called the *signal*. Some of the initial x-ray beam is absorbed via photoelectric interaction; some is scattered via Compton scatter (creating *noise*). Signal-to-noise ratio (SNR) is an important factor in all of medical imaging. Noise impairs image resolution; a high SNR is desirable (more signal, less noise). Generally speaking, SNR increases as milliampere seconds value increases; however, this is at the expense of patient dose. It is the responsibility of the radiographer to select technical factors and techniques that will provide a quality diagnostic image while keeping the ALARA concept in mind and minimizing patient dose.

109. (A) The term *effective dose* (EfD) refers to the dose from radiation sources internal and/or external to the body and is expressed in units of Sievert or rem. The factors used to determine effective dose (*EfD*) are as follows:

EfD = radiation weighting factor (W_r) × tissue weighting factor (W_t) × absorbed dose (D)

The term *equivalent dose* (EqD) refers to the product of the absorbed dose (Gy/rad) and its radiation weighting factor (W_r). Equivalent dose does not include the tissue weighting factor (W_t). Doubling dose is that amount of ionizing radiation that would cause twice/double the number of normally occurring mutations.

110. (C) Quality control refers to our equipment and its safe and accurate operation. Various components must be tested at specified intervals and test results must be within specified parameters. Any deviation from those parameters must be corrected. Examples of equipment components that are tested annually are the focal spot size, linearity, reproducibility, collimation, filtration, kilovoltage, and exposure time. Quality assurance is associated with patients and staff and their interactions and relationships. Congruence is a term used to describe the relationship between the collimator light field and the actual x-ray field—they must be congruent (i.e., match) to within 2% of the SID. Postprocessing refers to the windowing or other manipulation of a digital image.

111. (C) An oblique projection of the cervical spine is shown in Figure 7-15. The first two cervical vertebrae are poorly visualized because of superimposition with the mandible; the chin should be elevated to correct this problem. Otherwise, the positioning is satisfactory, with good demonstration of the remainder of the cervical intervertebral foramina. The patient has been accurately rotated 45°, and a 15°–20° tube angle was used.

112. (B) An oblique projection of the cervical spine is shown in Figure 7-15. The patient has been accurately positioned RAO with the MSP 45° to the IR and the CR angled 15°–20° caudad, but the chin should be elevated to avoid superimposition on the first two cervical vertebrae. This position offers excellent delineation of the intervertebral foramina (number 1) formed by the adjacent vertebral notches of pedicles (number 2). This projection gives an "on end" view of the transverse processes (number 3). A portion of the spinous processes (number 4) may be seen, especially in the lower cervical vertebrae.

113. **(B)** To demonstrate the intercondyloid fossa, the CR must be directed perpendicular to the long axis of the tibia (Fig. 7-30). Because the knee is flexed so that the tibia forms a 40° angle with the IR, the CR must be directed 40° caudad to place the CR perpendicular to the long axis of the tibia. Directing the CR to the popliteal depression aligns the CR parallel with the knee joint space.

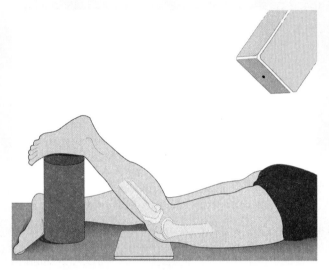

Figure 7-30

114. **(B)** Patient demographic and examination information originates from the hospital/facility HIS, where it is obtained when the patient is initially registered. That information is available or retrievable when the patient is scheduled, or arrives, for imaging services. Typical patient information includes name, DOB or age, sex, ID number, accession number, examination being performed, date and time of examination. Additional information may be available on the examination requisition; more information is usually entered by the technologist at the time of the examination.

A feature that is useful in sorting examinations and decreasing (but not eliminating) errors is the *modality work list* (MWL). The MWL "brings up" existing RIS information, that is, the examinations scheduled for each imaging area—for example, x-ray, CT, MRI, mammography, and ultrasound. The technologist selects the correct patient, which includes that patient's particular demographics, from the particular MWL. It is essential that the technologist is attentive to detail and accuracy when entering patient information; errors in patient demographics entry, and entry duplication, must be avoided.

PACS is used by health care facilities to economically store, archive, exchange, and transmit digital images from multiple imaging modalities.

RIS and HIS can be integrated with PACS for electronic health information storage. The purpose of HIS is to manage health care information and documents electronically, and to ensure data security and availability. RIS is a system for tracking radiological and imaging procedures. RIS is used for patient registration and scheduling, radiology workflow management, reporting and printout, manipulation and distribution and tracking of patient data, and billing. RIS complements HIS and is critical to competent workflow to radiologic facilities.

115. **(C)** Excessive heat production is a major problem in x-ray production. Of the energy required to produce x-rays, 0.2% is transformed to x-rays, and 99.8% is transformed to heat. The copper anode stem and the oil surrounding the x-ray tube help to move heat away from the face of the anode. Excessive heat can cause pitting of the anode (resulting in decreased output) or actual cracking of the anode, or damage to the rotor bearings (resulting in tube failure). As the cathode filament is heated for exposure after exposure, some of its tungsten is vaporized and deposited on the inner surface of the glass envelope near the tube window. After a time, this can cause electric arcing and tube failure. This is the most common cause of tube failure because it can occur even with normal use.

116. **(D)** A patient who has been recumbent for some period of time and gets up quickly may suffer from light-headedness or feel faint. This is called *orthostatic hypotension*. It is best to have patients sit up and dangle their feet from the table for a moment while being supported and then assist them off the table. Patients also will feel better emotionally if they are not rushed or treated like they are on an assembly line. Always assist patients on and off of the radiographic table. Even healthy, young outpatients can injure themselves. Patients with dyspnea (difficulty breathing) or orthopnea (difficulty breathing when recumbent) are unable to lie supine. *Dyspnea* and *orthopnea* refer to difficulty breathing; this may be due to a heart condition, asthma, strenuous exercise, or excessive anxiety. *Hypertension* refers to the condition of elevated blood pressure.

117. **(A)** The effects of a quantity of radiation delivered to a body depend on several factors—the amount of radiation received, the size of the irradiated area, and how the radiation is delivered in time. If the radiation is delivered in portions over a period of time, it is said to be *fractionated* and has a *less harmful* effect than if the radiation were delivered all at once. With fractionation, cells have an opportunity to repair, and so some recovery occurs between doses.

118–119. **(118, B; 119, B)** An anterior view of the foot and ankle bones is shown in Figure 7-17. The ankle joint is formed by the articulation of the tibia, fibula, and talus (number 7). The tibial (medial) malleolus is labeled 8; the fibular (lateral) malleolus is labeled 1. The talus articulates with the calcaneus (number 2) inferiorly and with the navicular (number 6) anteriorly. The cuboid (number 3) is seen anterior to the calcaneus, and the three cuneiforms (number 5) are anterior to the navicular.

120. (C, D, and E) Radiation exposure to personnel during fluoroscopic procedures is always lowest when staff is positioned at right angles to the center of the x-ray beam. The C-arm image intensifier should always be positioned above the patient, and the x-ray tube below the patient. In this way, personnel radiation exposure dose to the head and neck is reduced. Exposure dose is higher at the head and foot of the x-ray table, so personnel should always avoid those positions.

121. (D) The radiographer selects a *processing algorithm* by selecting the anatomic part and particular projection on the computer/control panel. The CR unit then matches that information with a particular *lookup table* (LUT)—a characteristic curve that best matches the anatomic part being imaged. The observer is able to review the image and, if desired, change its appearance (through "windowing"); doing so changes the LUT. Histogram analysis and use of the appropriate *LUT* together function to produce predictable image quality in CR. In addition, the radiographer can manipulate, that is, change and enhance, the digital image displayed on the display monitor through *postprocessing.* One way to alter image contrast and/or brightness is through *windowing.* The term *windowing* refers to some change made to window width and/or window level, that is, a change in the LUT. Change in window width affects change in the number of gray shades, that is, *image contrast.* Change in window *level* affects change in the image *brightness.* Therefore, windowing and other postprocessing mechanisms permit the radiographer to affect changes in the image and produce "special effects," such as *contrast enhancement, edge enhancement,* and *image stitching.*

122. (B) Sterile technique is required for administration of contrast media by the intravenous and intrathecal (intraspinal) methods. Aseptic technique is used for administration of contrast media by the oral and rectal routes as well as through the nasogastric tube.

123. (B) Lower kilovoltage (about 75–80 kV) was used in analog imaging to enhance the photoelectric effect and, in turn, to better visualize the iodinated contrast-filled structures. In analog imaging, high kilovoltage produced scattered radiation that could obliterate the effect of the contrast agent. In digital imaging, higher kilovoltage can be used because digital processing corrects for scattered radiation. Use of higher kilovoltage also helps reduce the patient dose.

124. (C) The infraorbitomeatal line (IOML) is an imaginary line extending from the infraorbital margin to the external auditory meatus and is represented by number 3 in Figure 7-18. The IOML is used for most lateral skull projections, including lateral projections of facial bones. The skull is positioned so that the MSP is parallel to the IR, the interpupillary line is perpendicular to the IR, and the IOML is parallel to the long (transverse) axis of the IR. Number 1 is the glabellomeatal line, number 2 is the OML (orbitomeatal line), and number 4 is the acanthomeatal line. These baselines are used to obtain accurate positioning in skull radiography.

125. (D) *Pneumothorax,* the presence of air in the pleural cavity, is seen (as well as a large pleural effusion) in Figure 7-19. A large pneumothorax is usually accompanied by a partial or complete collapse of the lung (atelectasis). Radiographic indications of atelectasis include elevation of the hemidiaphragm of the affected side and an increase in tissue density of the collapsed lung. Thoracentesis is the procedure required to remove significant amounts of air, blood, or other fluids in the pleural cavity. *Rotation* of the chest is illustrated by unequal distances between the medial aspect of the clavicles and the vertebral column. Adequate *inspiration* is indicated by visualization of 10 posterior ribs seen above the diaphragm.

126. (B) As kilovoltage is increased, x-ray photons begin to interact with atoms of tissue via the Compton-scattered interaction. Scattered x-ray photons result, which serve only to add unwanted, undiagnostic densities (scattered radiation fog) to the radiologic image. (Although Compton scatter reduces patient dose compared with photoelectric interactions, it can pose a significant radiation hazard to personnel during fluoroscopic procedures.) Therefore, the use of *optimal kilovoltage* is recommended to reduce the production of scattered radiation. Scattered radiation is also a function of the size and content of the irradiated field. The greater the volume and atomic number of the tissue, the greater is the production of scattered radiation. Although there is little that can be done about the atomic number of the structure to be radiographed, every effort can be made to keep the field size restricted to the essential area of interest in an effort to decrease production of scattered radiation. Grids have no effect on the production of scattered radiation, but they are very effective in removing scattered radiation from the beam before it strikes the IR.

127. (B) Whole-body dose is calculated to include all the especially radiosensitive organs. The *gonads,* the *lens* of the eye, and the *blood-forming organs* are particularly radiosensitive. The annual dose limit to the less sensitive skin, hands, and feet (extremities) is 500 mSv/year.

128. (A) *Pelvis* is the Latin word for *basin,* so-named for its shape. The curved ilia are foreshortened in the direct AP projection. The AP *oblique* projection is used to place the affected ilium parallel to the IR. The *unaffected side is elevated 40°* to place the ilium parallel to the IR. The sagittal plane passing through the affected hip is centered to the grid and the IR is centered at the level of the ASIS.

129. (B) X-ray photons are produced in two ways as high-speed electrons interact with target tungsten atoms. First, if the high-speed electron is attracted by the nucleus of a tungsten atom and changes its course, as the electron is "braked," energy is given up in the form of an x-ray photon. This is called *Bremsstrahlung* (braking) *radiation,* and it is responsible for most of the x-ray photons produced at the conventional tungsten target. Second, a high-speed electron having energy of at least 70 keV may eject a tungsten K-shell electron, leaving a vacancy in the shell. An electron from the next energy level, the L shell, drops down to fill the vacancy, emitting the difference in energy as a K-characteristic ray. Characteristic radiation makes up only about 15% of the primary beam.

130. (A) The midcoronal plane (number 1; Fig. 17-20) divides the body into anterior and posterior halves. A coronal plane is any plane parallel to the midcoronal plane. The midsagittal plane (number 2) divides the body into left and right halves. A sagittal plane is any plane parallel to the midsagittal plane. A transverse or horizontal plane (number 3) is perpendicular to the midsagittal plane and midcoronal plane, dividing the body into superior and inferior portions.

131. (B) The spinal cord is a column of nervous tissue about 17 inches (44 cm) in length. It is somewhat flattened anteroposteriorly and extends from the medulla oblongata of the brain to the level of L2 within the spinal canal. Because the adult spinal cord ends at the level of L2, a lumbar puncture usually is performed below that level—generally, at the level of L3–L4. A lumbar puncture may be performed for the removal of spinal fluid for diagnostic purposes or for the injection of medications.

132. (B) *Anemia* is a blood condition typically characterized by a decreased number of circulating red blood cells and decreased hemoglobin; it has many causes. Adequate hemoglobin is required to provide oxygen to the body. Anemia is treated according to its cause. *Hematuria* is the term used to describe blood in the urine and is unrelated to anemia.

133. (D) The four types of body habitus are (from upper extreme to lower extreme) hypersthenic, sthenic, hyposthenic, and asthenic. The gallbladder and stomach are higher and more lateral and the large bowel more peripheral in the hypersthenic individual. The diaphragm is in a higher position in the hypersthenic individual. Recognition of a patient's body habitus and its characteristics is an important part of accurate radiography. Bone porosity generally is unrelated to body habitus.

134. (C) As filtration is added to the x-ray beam, the lower energy photons are removed, and the overall energy or wavelength of the beam is greater. As kilovoltage is increased, more high-energy photons are produced, and again, the overall or average energy of the beam is greater. *An increase in milliamperage serves to increase the number of photons produced at the target but is unrelated to their energy.*

135. (C) The four types of body habitus, from largest to most slight, are *hypersthenic, sthenic, hyposthenic,* and *asthenic.* In Figure 7-21, number 1 is hyposthenic, number 2 is asthenic, number 3 is hypersthenic, and number 4 is sthenic. The characteristics and the prevalence of each habitus type are listed in the following text. The term *body habitus* refers to the body's physical appearance. Variations in body habitus have a significant effect on the shape, location, and position of thoracic and abdominal organs, and can affect their function and motility. Illustrations 1–4 show how greatly the position of the diaphragm, lungs, and stomach can differ among the various body habitus.

Body Habitus: Types, Characteristics, and Prevalence

Hypersthenic and asthenic characterize the *extremes* in body types:

Hypersthenic (5%)
- Body—large and heavy
- Bony framework—thick, short, and wide
- Lungs and heart—high
- Stomach—transverse
- Colon/large bowel—peripheral
- Gallbladder—high and lateral

Asthenic (10%)
- Body—slender and light
- Bony framework—delicate
- Thorax—long and narrow
- Stomach—very low and long (fishhook)
- Colon/large bowel—low, medial, and redundant
- Gallbladder—low and medial

Sthenic and hyposthenic types characterize the *more average* body types:

Sthenic (50%)
- Build—average and athletic
- Similar to hypersthenic, but modified by elongation of abdomen and thorax

Hyposthenic (35%)
- Somewhat slighter, less robust
- Similar to asthenic, but stomach, intestines, and gallbladder situated higher in abdomen

136. (C) The reduction in x-ray beam intensity that results from scattering (Compton) and absorption (photoelectric) processes is termed *attenuation.* The anode heel effect is related to the variation in x-ray beam intensity as it emerges in a divergent cone-shaped fashion from the x-ray tube, with greater intensity being at the cathode end of the beam. Grid cutoff is absorption of the useful remnant beam as a result of misalignment or miscentering with the grid.

137. **(D)** The hepatic (right colic) and splenic (left colic) flexures are not generally well demonstrated in the AP and PA projections. To "open" the flexures, oblique projections are required. The left anterior oblique (LAO, left PA oblique) and right posterior oblique (RPO, right PA oblique) positions are used to demonstrate the splenic flexure. The hepatic flexure is usually well demonstrated in the RAO and LPO positions.

138. **(D)** The radiographer must check with the physician before any movement of the cervical spine in patients having had recent injury or known fracture or subluxation. Movement of the traumatized cervical spine could cause further injury. Cervical collar must not be removed unless done so/authorized by the physician. A *horizontal beam lateral,* performed in the *dorsal decubitus position,* is the first image obtained when suspecting cervical trauma, fracture, subluxation, and others.

139. **(B)** Psychologist Abraham Maslow described a hierarchy, or pyramid, of needs with primary (physiologic) needs at the base and secondary (nonphysiologic) needs at higher levels. Maslow postulated that as the most basic survival needs are met, new needs emerge. At the bottom of the hierarchy are physiologic needs such as food, water, air, rest, and so on. One step up in the hierarchy is safety and security. Next is love and belongingness, followed by self-esteem and the esteem of others. Last is self-actualization, which is a kind of spiritual growth, satisfaction from life achievement, the feeling of leaving one's mark.

140. **(A)** If the SID is above or below the recommended focusing distance, the primary beam at the lateral edges will not coincide with the angled lead strips. Consequently, there will be absorption of the primary beam, termed *grid cutoff.* If the grid failed to move during the exposure, there would be grid lines throughout. CR angulation in the direction of the lead strips is appropriate and will not cause grid cutoff. If the CR were off-center, there would be uniform loss of receptor exposure.

Grids are valuable tools for reducing the quantity of scattered radiation reaching the IR. Their disadvantages are twofold. They require a significant increase in patient dose, and they require precise positioning and centering, which can be problematic especially in mobile imaging. However, *virtual grids* are very useful in helping to overcome these problems. Figure 7-31A and B illustrates the usefulness of virtual grids. Figure 7-31A is an abdomen radiograph obtained without using a grid; Figure 7-31B is the same abdomen obtained using a virtual grid. We see that image contrast is improved and patient dose is 50% lower than that required with a physical grid.

141. **(D)** Converting from an 8:1 grid to nongrid requires about a fourfold decrease in milliampere seconds. Increasing the kilovoltage by 15% and cutting the milliampere seconds in half would reduce patient dose by half. Increasing milliampere seconds will always increase exposure dose. Therefore, the largest decrease will occur with removal of a grid.

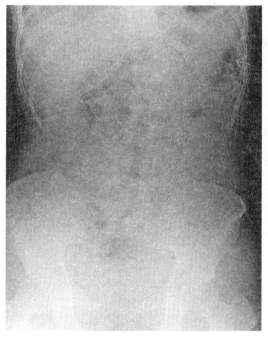

A

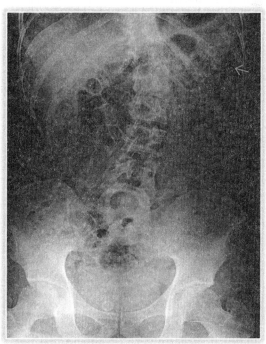

B

Figure 7-31. **A** and **B:** Used with permission of FUJIFILM Medical Systems USA, Inc.

142. **(D)** An inferosuperior projection (carpal canal/tunnel position) is seen in Figure 7-22. The pisiform is seen as number 1, the triquetrum as number 2, the hook of the hamate as number 3, the capitate as number 4, the scaphoid as number 5, the trapezium as number 6, the ulna as number 7, and the radius as number 8.

143. **(C)** Retrograde urography requires ureteral catheterization so that a contrast medium can be introduced directly into the pelvicalyceal system. This procedure provides excellent opacification and structural information but does not demonstrate the function of these structures. Intravenous studies, such as the IVU, demonstrate function.

144. **(D)** Generally, contrast medium is injected into the subarachnoid space between the third and fourth lumbar vertebrae. Because the spinal cord ends at the level of the first or second lumbar vertebra, this is considered to be a relatively safe injection site. The cisterna magna can be used, but the risk of contrast medium entering the ventricles and causing side effects increases. Diskography requires injection of contrast medium into the individual intervertebral disks.

145. **(D)** Body substance precaution procedures identify various body fluids as infectious or potentially infectious. These body substances include pleural, pericardial, peritoneal, and amniotic fluids; synovial fluid; cerebrospinal fluid (CSF); breast milk; and vaginal secretions, as well as nasal secretions, tears, saliva, sputum, feces, urine, and wound drainage.

146. **(B)** Intervertebral joints are well visualized in the lateral projection of all the vertebral groups. Cervical articular facets (forming zygapophyseal joints) are 90° to the MSP and, therefore, are well demonstrated in the lateral projection. The cervical intervertebral foramina lie 45° to the MSP (and 15°–20° to a transverse plane) and, therefore, are demonstrated in the oblique position.

147. **(D)** Most needlesticks occur while attempting to recap a needle. Several diseases, including hepatitis and human immunodeficiency virus (HIV) infection, can be transmitted via a needlestick. Therefore, do not attempt to recap a needle, but rather dispose of the entire syringe with needle attached in the special container that is available.

148. **(D)** Motion causes unsharpness that destroys detail. Careful and accurate patient instruction is essential for minimizing voluntary motion. Suspended respiration eliminates respiratory motion. Using the shortest possible exposure time is essential to decrease involuntary motion. Immobilization can also be very useful in eliminating motion unsharpness.

149. **(C)** The sudden cessation of productive ventilation and circulation is called cardiopulmonary arrest. The radiographer should be trained in basic life support (BLS) for health care providers. The American Heart Association (AHA) uses the acronym CAB, representing *c*irculation, *a*irway, *b*reathing to help individuals remember CPR step sequence. AHA says that the life of an adult who suddenly collapses can be saved using hands-only CPR. AHA states that compressions should be fast and forceful. Chest compressions should begin soon. Compressions should be about 100/min and the chest should be compressed at least 2 inches in each compression. Airway should be established using the head-tilt, chin-lift movement. If the victim is not breathing normally, the professional rescuer should begin mouth-to-mouth breathing. One cycle is considered to be 30 chest compressions followed by two rescue breaths.

150. **(B)** The most hazardous time for abdominal irradiation is in the earliest stages of pregnancy, when many women are unaware that they are pregnant. For this reason, *it is recommended that elective radiologic procedures be performed within the first 10 days following the onset of the menses.* It is during this time that the danger of irradiating a recently fertilized ovum is most unlikely. About 14 days before the onset of menses is when the ovarian follicle ruptures and liberates an ovum.

151–152. **(151, A; 152, B)** A parietoacanthal projection (Waters position) of the skull is shown in Figure 7-23. The chin is elevated sufficiently to project the petrous ridges below the *maxillary sinuses* (number 4). Note that the foramen rotundum is seen near the upper margin of the maxillary sinuses. Other paranasal sinus groups are not well visualized in this position, although a modification with the mouth open may be taken to demonstrate the sphenoidal sinuses. This is also the single best projection to demonstrate the facial bones. The *zygomatic arch* (number 2) is well demonstrated; the mandible, its *angle* (number 1), and the *coronoid process* (number 3) are also well demonstrated. The odontoid process is seen projected through the foramen magnum. The *mastoid* air cells are seen adjacent to the mandibular angle as multiple small, air-filled, bony spaces.

153. **(B)** Esophageal varices are best demonstrated when there is increased venous pressure and when blood is flowing against gravity. Therefore, to demonstrate the twisted, dilated condition of venous varicosities, esophagrams must be performed in the recumbent position. In the erect position, the veins appear smoother and normal. The Fowler position describes a position in which the patient's head is higher than the feet, and the Sims position is preferred for insertion of the enema tip.

154. **(B)** Excessive heat production is a major problem in x-ray production. Of the energy required to produce x-rays, 0.2% is transformed to x-rays, and 99.8% is transformed to heat. The copper anode stem and the oil surrounding the x-ray tube help to move heat away from the face of the anode. Heat production is increased with the use of *high*-milliampere seconds technical factors far

more than with high-kilovoltage factors and can be particularly harmful when using a *small focal spot.* Excessive heat can cause pitting of the anode (resulting in decreased output) or actual cracking of the anode or damage to the rotor bearings (resulting in tube failure). As the cathode filament is heated for exposure after exposure, some of its tungsten is vaporized and deposited on the inner surface of the glass envelope near the tube window. After a time, this can cause electric arcing and tube failure. This is the most common cause of tube failure because it can occur even with normal use. Grid ratio is unrelated to heat production at the anode.

155. **(D)** The S-shaped clavicle (collar bone) is usually the last bone to completely ossify, at about age 21, and is one of the most commonly fractured bones in young people. Its medial end articulates with the sternum to form the sternoclavicular joint; the clavicle articulates laterally with the scapula's acromion process, forming the acromioclavicular joint. Superior dislocation of the acromioclavicular joint is a common athletic injury.

156. **(A)** The sacroiliac joints angle posteriorly and medially 25° to the MSP. Therefore, to demonstrate them with an AP oblique projection, the affected side must be elevated 25°. This places the joint space perpendicular to the IR and parallel to the CR. When the PA oblique projection is used, the unaffected side will be elevated 25°.

157. **(B)** A double-focus tube has two focal spot sizes available. These focal spots actually are two available paths on the focal track. There are also two filaments. When the small focal spot is selected, the small filament is heated, and electrons are driven across to the smaller portion of the focal track. When the large focal spot is selected, the large filament is heated, and electrons are driven across to the larger portion of the focal track.

158-159. **(158, B; 159, D)** An LAO position of the lumbar spine is shown in Figure 7-24. The patient is positioned so that the lumbar spine is 45° to the IR. The zygapophyseal joints (those closest to the IR) are well demonstrated in this position. The typical Scottie dog image is depicted. The "ear" (number 1) of the Scottie is the superior articular process, and the "front leg" (number 4) is the inferior articular process. The Scottie's "eye" (number 2) is the pedicle, its "body" (number 3) is the lamina, its "nose" (number 5) is the transverse process, and its "neck" (number 6) is the pars interarticularis.

160. **(C)** An antihistamine is used to relieve allergic effects. Benadryl (*diphenhydramine hydrochloride*) is an example of an antihistamine that is often on hand in radiology departments in the event of a minor reaction to contrast media. An antipyretic is used to reduce fever. Tylenol (*acetaminophen*) is an example of an antipyretic. Ipecac is a medication used to induce vomiting and is classified as an *emetic.* This is easy to remember if you think of what an emesis basin is for. A *diuretic* is a medication that stimulates the *production of urine.* Lasix (furosemide) is an example of a diuretic.

161. **(B)** Bergonié and Tribondeau theorized in 1906 that all precursor cells are particularly radiosensitive (e.g., stem cells found in bone marrow). There are several types of stem cells in bone marrow, and the different types differ in degree of radiosensitivity. Of these, red blood cell precursors, or *erythroblasts,* are the most radiosensitive. White blood cell precursors, or *myelocytes,* follow. Platelet precursor cells, or *megakaryocytes,* are even less radiosensitive. *Myocytes* are mature muscle cells and are fairly radioresistant.

162. **(D)** Breast tissue has very low-subject contrast, but it is imperative to visualize microcalcifications and subtle density differences. Fine detail is necessary to visualize any microcalcifications; therefore, a small focal spot tube is essential. Short-scale (high) contrast (and, therefore, low kilovoltage) is needed to accentuate any differences in tissue density. A compression device serves to even out differences in tissue thickness (thicker at the chest wall, thinner at the nipple) and decrease OID and helps to decrease the production of scattered radiation.

163. **(C)** The absorption characteristics of body tissues can vary considerably from one body part to another. Adjacent tissues of some body parts, such as the chest, exhibit quite different absorption characteristics. Conversely, adjacent abdominal tissues have very similar absorption characteristics. The emerging remnant beam signals (photons) mirror those differences; this describes *subject contrast.*

164-165. **(164, B; 165, D)** An anterior view of the forearm is shown in Figure 7-25. The proximal anterior surface of the ulna (number 8) presents a rather large pointed process at the anterior margin of the semilunar (trochlear) notch (number 5) called the *coronoid process* (number 6). The olecranon process is identified as number 4, and the radial notch of the ulna is number 7. Distally, the ulnar head is number 9, and its styloid process is labeled 10. The radius (number 12) is the lateral bone of the forearm. The radial head is number 3, the radial neck is number 2, and the radial tuberosity is number 1. Distally, the radial styloid process is labeled 11.

166. **(D)** Single-phase current has a 100% voltage drop between peak voltages. Three-phase current decreases this voltage drop considerably. Three-phase, six-pulse current has about a 13% voltage drop between peak voltages, and three-phase, 12-pulse current has only about a 4% drop between peak voltages. However, high-frequency current is almost constant potential, having less than 1% voltage ripple.

167. **(D)** Lead aprons are worn by occupationally exposed individuals during fluoroscopic and mobile x-ray procedures. Lead aprons are available with various lead

equivalents; 0.5- and 1.0-mm lead equivalents are the most common. The 1.0-mm lead equivalent apron will provide close to 100% protection at most kilovoltage levels, but it is used rarely because it weighs anywhere from 12 to 24 pounds. A 0.25-mm lead equivalent apron will attenuate about 97% of a 50-kV x-ray beam, 66% of a 75-kV beam, and 51% of a 100-kV beam. A 0.5-mm lead equivalent apron will attenuate about 99.9% of a 50-kV beam, 88% of a 75-kV beam, and 75% of a 100-kV beam.

168. (A) *Heparin* is produced by the body (especially in the liver) and functions to prevent intravascular clotting. Heparin is also produced artificially and used to treat thromboembolic disorders. Lidocaine and Benadryl are drugs that are usually available on crash carts for emergency use. *Lidocaine* is used to treat ventricular arrhythmias, and *Benadryl* is used to treat allergic reactions and acute anaphylaxis.

169. (D) Because the toes curve naturally downward, the interphalangeal joints are not well demonstrated in the AP (dorsoplantar) projection. To "open" the interphalangeal joints, the CR should be directed 15° cephalad. Another method is to place a 15° foam sponge wedge under the foot, elevating the toes 15° from the IR; the CR then would be directed perpendicularly.

170. (B) The most commonly used method of low-flow oxygen delivery is the nasal cannula. It can be used to deliver oxygen at rates from 1 to 4 mL/min at concentrations of 24%–36%. The nasal cannula also provides increased patient freedom to eat and talk, which a mask does not. Masks are used for higher flow concentrations of oxygen, over 5 mL/min; depending on the type of mask, they can deliver anywhere from 35% to 60% oxygen. Respirators and ventilators are high-flow delivery mechanisms that are used for patients who are in severe respiratory distress or are unable to breathe on their own. Oxyhoods or tents generally are used for pediatric patients who may not tolerate a mask or cannula. The amount of oxygen delivered is somewhat unpredictable, especially if the opening is accessed frequently. Oxygen delivery may be between 20% and 100%.

171. (C) The landmarks that can be used in radiography of the bony pelvis are the iliac crest, the ASIS, the pubic symphysis, the greater trochanter, the ischial tuberosity, and the tip of the coccyx. With the patient in the anatomic position, the femoral neck is located 2½ inches distal on a line drawn perpendicular to the midpoint of a line drawn between the ASIS and the pubic symphysis. It is recommended to rotate the legs inward about 15°, whenever possible, to place the femoral neck parallel to the IR.

172. (B) Numbers 1 and 2 indicate the right and left pulmonary arteries in Figure 7-26. The pulmonary arteries carry deoxygenated blood from the right ventricle to the lungs for oxygenation. That describes pulmonary

circulation. *Systemic circulation* refers to oxygenated blood flowing from the left atrium, through the mitral/bicuspid valve, through the aortic semilunar valve into the left ventricle, through the aorta and all the arterial branches, to tissue capillaries, then the return of deoxygenated blood to the heart through veins and ultimately to the superior and inferior venae cavae into the right atrium.

173. (D) Improper support of a patient's fractured lower leg (tibia/fibula) while performing radiography could result in movement of the fracture fragments, which can cause tearing of the soft tissue, nerves, and blood vessels. In addition, lack of support may cause muscle spasm, which can make closed reduction of some fractures difficult.

174. (D) According to state and federal law, personnel radiation monitor reports must be retained as legal documents. Information that must be included in these documents includes the user's personal data, that is, name, birth date, sex, identification number (usually Social Security Number), type of monitor (e.g., film badge, TLD, or OSL dosimeter), radiation quality, dose equivalent (i.e., deep, eye, and shallow) for that exposure period (usually 1 month), the quarterly accumulated dose equivalent (i.e., deep, eye, and shallow), year-to-date dose equivalent (i.e., deep, eye, and shallow), lifetime dose equivalent (i.e., deep, eye, and shallow), number of monitors received year to date, and inception date (month and year) of the dosimeter.

175. (A) The femur is the longest and strongest bone in the body. The femoral shaft is bowed slightly anteriorly and presents a long, narrow ridge posteriorly called the *linea aspera*. The proximal femur consists of a head that is received by the pelvic acetabulum. The femoral neck, which joins the head and shaft, normally angles upward about 120° and forward (in anteversion) about 15°. The greater and lesser trochanters are large processes on the posterior proximal femur. The intertrochanteric crest runs obliquely between the trochanters posteriorly; the intertrochanteric line parallels the intertrochanteric crest on the anterior femoral surface. The intercondyloid fossa, a deep notch found on the distal posterior femur between the large femoral condyles and the popliteal surface, is a smooth surface just superior to the intercondyloid fossa.

176. (C) Fidelity, veracity, nonmaleficence, and beneficence are all ethical principles. *Nonmaleficence* is the principle that refers to the prevention of harm. *Beneficence* is the ethical principle that refers to bringing about good or benefiting others. *Fidelity* refers to faithfulness, and *veracity* refers to truthfulness.

177. (C) A radiographer who fails to wear a lead apron when performing portable radiography is in direct violation of the ARRT *Code of Ethics for the Profession of Radiologic Technology*. Although this may seem to some to be a personal decision, the fact is that our profession demands that we protect not only others but also ourselves from unnecessary radiation exposure. Participating in continuing education is every radiographer's duty, and not only is in keeping with the ARRT *Code of Ethics* but also is mandatory for renewal of ARRT certification these days. Under normal circumstances, patient confidentiality is of the utmost importance, and radiographers always must respect a patient's right to privacy. There are special circumstances, however, where a radiographer is negligent if he or she does not communicate confidential information to the proper individuals. These cases include suspected cases of child abuse and any instance where the welfare of an individual or community is at risk. The professional radiographer is encouraged to investigate new and innovative techniques. As technology continues to grow, we must grow with it. There are often new and better ways to perform procedures, especially as equipment changes occur.

178. (C) Hospital information systems must ensure confidentiality in compliance with Health Insurance Portability and Accountability Act of 1996 (HIPAA) regulations. Most institutions now have computerized, paperless systems that accomplish the same information transmittal; these systems must ensure confidentiality in compliance with HIPAA regulations. The health care professional generally has access to the computerized system only via personal password, thus helping to ensure confidentiality of patient information. All medical records and other individually identifiable health information, whether electronic, on paper, or oral, are covered by HIPAA legislation and by subsequent Department of Health and Human Services (HHS) rules that took effect in April, 2001.

179. (C) Hirschsprung disease, or congenital megacolon, is caused by the absence of some or all of the bowel ganglion cells—usually in the rectosigmoid area but occasionally more extensively. Hirschsprung disease is the most common cause of lower GI obstruction in neonates and is treated surgically by excision of the affected area followed by reanastomosis with the normal, healthy bowel. Hirschsprung disease is diagnosed by BE or, in mild cares, by rectal biopsy. Intussusception is "telescoping" of the bowel, causing (mechanical) obstruction. Volvulus is twisting of the bowel on itself causing (mechanical) obstruction. Pyloric stenosis is a condition of the upper GI tract.

180. (D) Because 50 ms is equal to 0.050 s, and mA × time = mAs, the original milliampere seconds value was 15 mAs. Now, it is only necessary to determine what milliamperage must be used with 22 ms to provide the same 15 mAs (and thus the same receptor exposure). Because mA × time = mAs,

$$0.022x = 15$$
$$x = 682 \ (700 \text{ mA})$$

181. (B) *Technique charts* are technical factor guides that help technologists produce radiographs with consistent receptor exposure and contrast. They suggest a group of technical factors to be used for a particular projection of a stated part, at a particular SID with a particular grid ratio, and focal spot size. *Technique charts do not take into account the nature of the part* (disease and atrophy).

182. (B) The pregnant radiographer poses a special radiation protection consideration because the safety of the unborn individual must be considered. It must be remembered that the developing fetus is particularly sensitive to radiation exposure. Established guidelines state that the occupational radiation exposure to the fetus must not exceed 5 mSv (500 mrem) during the entire gestation period.

183. (D) Epidemiologic studies indicate that AIDS can be transmitted only by intimate contact with body fluids of an infected individual. This can occur through the sharing of contaminated needles, through sexual contact, and from mother to baby at childbirth (perinatal). AIDS can also be transmitted by transfusion of contaminated blood.

184. (B) The newest type of personnel monitoring device is the direct ion storage dosimeter (DIS); it is a digital ionization dosimeter. The DIS eliminates the need to collect and send dosimeters for monthly or quarterly processing. The user wears the DIS, which looks like a small flash drive, in the same way as other monitors such as an OSL (optically stimulated luminescence) dosimeter. The DIS has a gas-filled ionization chamber within and uses Bluetooth technology to relate its raw data via mobile device or any computer with Internet access and a USB connection. Occupational exposure can be read, and reread, at any time without loss of information.

The pocket dosimeter, or pocket ionization chamber, resembles a penlight and has a thimble ionization chamber within. Ions are counted and radiation quantity is registered in milliroentgens (mR). The use of the pocket dosimeter is indicated when working with high exposures or large quantities of radiation for short periods of time, so that an immediate reading is available to the user. The pocket dosimeter is sensitive and accurate but has limited application in diagnostic radiography.

185. (A) Mature white blood cells (*lymphocytes*) are considered the most radiosensitive cells. *Ova* (female germ cells) are very radiosensitive, but not to the same degree as lymphocytes. *Myocytes* (muscle cells) and especially *neurons* (nerve cells) are actually radioresistant.

186. (A) A 1984 review of radiation exposure data revealed that the average annual dose equivalent for monitored radiation workers was approximately 2.3 mSv (0.23 rem). The fact that this is approximately one-tenth the recommended limit indicates that the limit is adequate for radiation protection purposes. Therefore, the NCRP reiterates its 1971 recommended annual limit of 50 mSv (5 rem).

187. (B) The input phosphor of image intensifiers is usually made of cesium iodide. For each x-ray photon absorbed by cesium iodide, approximately 5000 light photons are emitted. As the light photons strike a photoemissive *photocathode,* a number of electrons are released from the photocathode and focused toward the output side of the image tube by voltage applied to the negatively charged *electrostatic focusing lenses.* The electrons are then accelerated through the neck of the tube where they strike the small (0.5–1 inch) *output phosphor* that is mounted on a flat glass support. The entire assembly is enclosed within a 2- to 4-mm-thick vacuum glass envelope. Remember that the image on the output phosphor is *minified, brighter,* and *inverted* (electron focusing causes image inversion).

Input phosphor diameters of 5–12 inches are available. Although smaller diameter input phosphors improve resolution, they do not permit a large FOV, that is, viewing of large patient areas.

Dual- and triple-field image intensifiers are available that permit *magnified* viewing of fluoroscopic images. To achieve magnification, the *voltage* to the focusing lenses is increased and a *smaller* portion of the input phosphor is used, thereby resulting in a smaller FOV. Because minification gain is now decreased, the image is not as bright. The milliamperage is automatically increased to compensate for the loss in brightness when the image intensifier is switched to magnification mode. Entrance skin exposure (ESE) can increase dramatically as the FOV decreases (i.e., as magnification increases).

As FOV decreases, *magnification* of the output phosphor image increases, there is less *noise* because increased milliamperage provides a greater number of x-ray photons, and *contrast* and *resolution* improve. The focal point in the magnification mode is *further away from* the output phosphor (as a result of increased voltage applied to the focusing lenses) and therefore the output image is magnified.

188. (B) There are two types of distortion: size and shape. Size distortion is magnification and is caused by excessive OID or insufficient SID. Shape distortion is impacted by tube, parts, and IR alignment. The two types of shape distortion are elongation and foreshortening. X-ray tube angulation can create elongation, whereas angulation of the part with respect to the IR causes foreshortening. Both can cause significant misrepresentation of the actual part as seen in Figure 7-32.

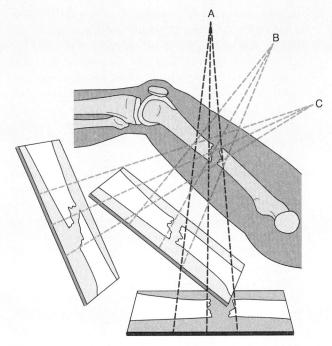

Figure 7-32

189. (A) The velocity and charge of particulate radiation determine the amount of energy transferred (and, therefore, the number of ionizations) to the tissue traversed. A greater LET (number of ionizations) is delivered by particles with a slower velocity and greater charge. The greater the LET and the number of ionizations, the greater is the biologic effect. The unit of absorbed dose is the Gy_t. The unit of effective dose is the Sievert.

190. (B) Irradiation during *pregnancy,* especially in early pregnancy, must be avoided. The fetus is particularly radiosensitive during the first trimester, during much of which time pregnancy may not even be suspected. High-risk examinations include pelvis, hip, femur, lumbar spine, cystograms and urograms, and upper and lower gastrointestinal (GI) series. During the first trimester, specifically the 2nd to 10th weeks of pregnancy (i.e., during major organogenesis), if the radiation dose is sufficient, fetal anomalies can be produced. *Skeletal and/or organ anomalies* can appear if irradiation occurs in the early part of this time period, and *neurologic anomalies* can be formed in the latter part; *mental retardation* and childhood *malignant diseases,* such as cancers or leukemia, and retarded growth/development also can result from irradiation during the first trimester. Fetal irradiation during the second and third trimesters is not likely to produce anomalies but rather, with sufficient dose, some type of childhood malignant disease. Fetal irradiation during the first 2 weeks of gestation can result in *embryonic resorption* or *spontaneous abortion.* It must be emphasized, however, that the likelihood of producing fetal anomalies at doses less than 200 mGy (20 rad) is exceedingly small and that most general diagnostic examinations are likely to deliver fetal doses of less than 10–20 mGy (1–2 rad).

191. (C) Interviewing skills and the collection of valuable, objective, and subjective patient data (clinical history) are an important function of the health care professional. Objective data are those that are discernible to the senses of the interviewer—objective signs that can be heard, seen, or felt. Subjective data are those that can be discerned only by the patient—pain, emotions, and so on. Chief complaint is the principal medical problem as stated by the patient.

192. (B) Milliampere seconds is directly proportional to receptor exposure. Doubling the milliampere seconds will double the receptor exposure. When milliampere seconds cannot be adjusted, increasing the kilovoltage by 15% will produce approximately the same results. An increase in SID would decrease receptor exposure.

193. (C) Emphysema is a chronic obstructive pulmonary disease (COPD) characterized by pathologic distension of the pulmonary alveoli with (destructive) changes in their walls, resulting in a loss of elasticity. Emphysema is seen occasionally following asthma or tuberculosis, but it is caused most frequently by cigarette smoking. Because the emphysematous patient's greatest difficulty is exhalation, it becomes a conscious, forced effort. Breathing is shallow and rapid. Forced and ineffective breathing results in expansion of the AP diameter of the chest and elevated shoulder girdle in established emphysema. Hyperventilation results from too frequent deep breaths in the anxious or tense individual. This results in a feeling of dizziness and tingling of the extremities.

194. (A) It is our ethical responsibility to minimize radiation dose to patients. X-rays produced at the target make up a heterogeneous primary beam. There are many "soft" (low-energy) photons that, if not removed, would contribute only to greater patient dose. They are too weak to penetrate the patient and expose the IR. These soft x-rays penetrate only a small thickness of tissue before being absorbed.

195. (C) Paranasal sinuses must be examined in the upright position to demonstrate any air/fluid levels. The CR must be parallel to the floor so that any air/fluid levels do not get obliterated with a tube angle technique. The PA axial (Caldwell) projection of the paranasal sinuses is used to demonstrate the frontal and ethmoidal sinuses. A small radiolucent sponge is placed between the forehead and upright Bucky and head adjusted so that the OML forms an angle of 15° with the horizontal CR. The CR is directed to exit the nasion. This projection demonstrates the petrous pyramids in the lower third of the orbits, thus permitting optimal visualization of the frontal and ethmoidal sinuses.

196. (A) As SID increases, so does spatial resolution/recorded detail because magnification is decreased. Therefore, SID is directly related to spatial resolution. As focal spot size increases, spatial resolution decreases because more penumbral blur is produced. Focal spot size is thus inversely related to spatial resolution/radiographic sharpness. Tube current affects receptor exposure and is unrelated to special resolution.

197. (B) Standard blood and body fluid precautions serve to protect health care workers and patients from the spread of diseases, such as AIDS and AIDS-related complex. Although the precautions are indicated for *all* patients, special care must be emphasized when working with patients whose infectious status is unknown (e.g., the emergency trauma patient). Gloves must be worn if the radiographer may come in contact with blood or body fluids. A gown should be worn if the clothing may become contaminated. Blood spills should be cleaned with a solution of 1 part bleach to 10 parts water.

198. (C) X-ray tube life may be extended by using technical factors that produce a minimum of heat (a lower milliampere seconds and higher kilovoltage combination) whenever possible. When the rotor is activated, the filament current is increased to produce the required electron source (thermionic emission). Prolonged rotor time, then, can lead to shortened filament life owing to early vaporization. Large exposures to a cold anode will heat the anode surface, and the temperature difference between surface and interior can cause cracking of the anode. This can be avoided by proper warming of the anode prior to use, thereby allowing sufficient dispersion of heat through the anode.

199. (B) Because x-ray photons are produced at the tungsten target, they more readily diverge toward the cathode end of the x-ray tube. As they try to diverge toward the anode, they interact with, and are absorbed by, the anode "heel." Consequently, there is a greater intensity of x-ray photons at the cathode end of the x-ray beam. This phenomenon is known as the *anode heel effect*. Because shorter SIDs and larger IR sizes require greater divergence of the x-ray beam to provide coverage, the anode heel effect will be accentuated.

200. (C) There is no preparation required for an abdominal survey. For an upper GI series and a lower GI series (BE), the patient should be NPO, or have nothing by mouth, for 8–10 h prior to the examination. In addition, a low-residue diet may be imposed, fluid intake may be increased, and cleansing enemas and laxatives may be prescribed to rid the colon of fecal matter.

SUBSPECIALTY LIST

Question Number and Subspecialty correspond to subcategories in each of the four ARRT examination specification sections

1. Safety/radiation physics and radiobiology
2. Image production/equipment operation and quality assurance
3. Patient care
4. Image production/image acquisition and technical evaluation
5. Safety/radiation physics and radiobiology
6. Patient care
7. Procedures/extremities
8. Safety/radiation physics and radiobiology
9. Image production/image acquisition and technical evaluation
10. Safety/radiation physics and radiobiology
11. Procedures/extremities
12. Procedures/thorax and abdomen
13. Procedures/head, spine and pelvis
14. Procedures/thorax and abdomen
15. Image production/equipment operation and quality assurance
16. Patient care
17. Image production/image acquisition and technical evaluation
18. Procedures/thorax and abdomen
19. Procedures/thorax and abdomen
20. Patient care
21. Safety/radiation protection
22. Image production/image acquisition and technical evaluation
23. Image production/equipment operation and quality assurance
24. Safety/radiation protection
25. Procedures/thorax and abdomen
26. Procedures/extremities
27. Procedures/thorax and abdomen
28. Image production/image acquisition and technical evaluation
29. Patient care
30. Image production/equipment operation and quality assurance
31. Procedures/thorax and abdomen
32. Procedures/thorax and abdomen
33. Image production/image acquisition and technical evaluation
34. Image production/equipment operation and quality assurance
35. Procedures/thorax and abdomen
36. Image production/equipment operation and quality assurance
37. Image production/equipment operation and quality assurance
38. Image production/equipment operation and quality assurance
39. Patient care
40. Image production/equipment operation and quality assurance
41. Image production/equipment operation and quality assurance
42. Image production/equipment operation and quality assurance
43. Patient care
44. Procedures/extremities
45. Safety/radiation physics and radiobiology
46. Image production/equipment operation and quality assurance
47. Safety/radiation protection
48. Image production/equipment operation and quality assurance
49. Procedures/thorax and abdomen
50. Image production/image acquisition and technical evaluation
51. Procedures/thorax and abdomen
52. Patient care
53. Patient care
54. Safety/radiation protection
55. Image production/equipment operation and quality assurance
56. Image production/equipment operation and quality assurance
57. Image production/equipment operation and quality assurance
58. Patient care
59. Image production/image acquisition and technical evaluation
60. Image production/image acquisition and technical evaluation
61. Safety/radiation physics and radiobiology
62. Procedures/head, spine and pelvis
63. Procedures/thorax and abdomen
64. Image production/image acquisition and technical evaluation

65. Image production/image acquisition and technical evaluation
66. Image production/image acquisition and technical evaluation
67. Safety/radiation protection
68. Patient care
69. Safety/radiation physics and radiobiology
70. Image production/equipment operation and quality assurance
71. Image production/equipment operation and quality assurance
72. Procedures/thorax and abdomen
73. Procedures/head, spine and pelvis
74. Safety/radiation physics and radiobiology
75. Procedures/extremities
76. Safety/radiation physics and radiobiology
77. Procedures/extremities
78. Safety/radiation protection
79. Patient care
80. Procedures/extremities
81. Image production/equipment operation and quality assurance
82. Image production/image acquisition and technical evaluation
83. Procedures/thorax and abdomen
84. Safety/radiation protection
85. Patient care
86. Image production/equipment operation and quality assurance
87. Image production/image acquisition and technical evaluation
88. Procedures/extremities
89. Safety/radiation protection
90. Procedures/extremities
91. Image production/image acquisition and technical evaluation
92. Procedures/thorax and abdomen
93. Procedures/head, spine and pelvis
94. Safety/radiation protection
95. Image production/equipment operation and quality assurance
96. Procedures/extremities
97. Procedures/thorax and abdomen
98. Procedures/thorax and abdomen
99. Safety/radiation protection
100. Image production/image acquisition and technical evaluation
101. Safety/radiation protection
102. Image production/image acquisition and technical evaluation
103. Image production/image acquisition and technical evaluation

104. Image production/equipment operation and quality assurance
105. Procedures/thorax and abdomen
106. Patient care
107. Image production/image acquisition and technical evaluation
108. Image production/equipment operation and quality assurance
109. Safety/radiation physics and radiobiology
110. Image production/equipment operation and quality assurance
111. Procedures/head, spine and pelvis
112. Procedures/head, spine and pelvis
113. Procedures/extremities
114. Patient care
115. Image production/equipment operation and quality assurance
116. Patient care
117. Safety/radiation physics and radiobiology
118. Procedures/extremities
119. Procedures/extremities
120. Safety/radiation protection
121. Image production/image acquisition and technical evaluation
122. Patient care
123. Procedures/thorax and abdomen
124. Procedures/head, spine and pelvis
125. Procedures/thorax and abdomen
126. Image production/image acquisition and technical evaluation
127. Safety/radiation protection
128. Procedures/head, spine and pelvis
129. Safety/radiation physics and radiobiology
130. Procedures/thorax and abdomen
131. Procedures/head, spine and pelvis
132. Patient care
133. Procedures/thorax and abdomen
134. Safety/radiation physics and radiobiology
135. Procedures/thorax and abdomen
136. Safety/radiation physics and radiobiology
137. Procedures/thorax and abdomen
138. Procedures/head, spine and pelvis
139. Patient care
140. Image production/image acquisition and technical evaluation
141. Safety/radiation protection
142. Procedures/extremities
143. Procedures/thorax and abdomen
144. Procedures/head, spine and pelvis
145. Patient care
146. Procedures/head, spine and pelvis

147. Patient care
148. Procedures/thorax and abdomen
149. Patient care
150. Safety/radiation protection
151. Procedures/head, spine and pelvis
152. Procedures/head, spine and pelvis
153. Procedures/thorax and abdomen
154. Image production/equipment operation and quality assurance
155. Procedures/extremities
156. Procedures/head, spine and pelvis
157. Image production/equipment operation and quality assurance
158. Procedures/head, spine and pelvis
159. Procedures/head, spine and pelvis
160. Patient care
161. Safety/radiation physics and radiobiology
162. Procedures/thorax and abdomen
163. Image production/equipment operation and quality assurance
164. Procedures/extremities
165. Procedures/extremities
166. Image production/equipment operation and quality assurance
167. Safety/radiation protection
168. Patient care
169. Procedures/extremities
170. Patient care
171. Procedures/head, spine and pelvis
172. Procedures/thorax and abdomen
173. Patient care
174. Safety/radiation protection
175. Procedures/extremities
176. Patient care
177. Patient care
178. Patient care
179. Patient care
180. Image production/image acquisition and technical evaluation
181. Image production/image acquisition and technical evaluation
182. Safety/radiation protection
183. Patient care
184. Safety/radiation protection
185. Safety/radiation physics and radiobiology
186. Safety/radiation protection
187. Image production/equipment operation and quality assurance
188. Image production/image acquisition and technical evaluation
189. Safety/radiation physics and radiobiology
190. Safety/radiation physics and radiobiology
191. Patient care
192. Image production/image acquisition and technical evaluation
193. Patient care
194. Safety/radiation protection
195. Procedures/head, spine and pelvis
196. Image production/image acquisition and technical evaluation
197. Patient care
198. Image production/equipment operation and quality assurance
199. Image production/image acquisition and technical evaluation
200. Procedures/thorax and abdomen

TARGETED READING

This chapter incorporates the Targeted Reading lists from Chapters 1 to 5.

INDEX

INDEX

Note: Page number followed by *f* indicates figure only.

A

Abdomen, 90
    AP supine projection, 62, 96
    cross-sectional image of, 274, 275*f*, 297
    CT images, 305, 305*f*, 327
    CT section of, 305*f*, 327
    dorsal decubitus position, 65, 100
    lateral projection, 96
    left lateral decubitus without grid, 306, 327
    quadrants, 63, 99, 265, 287
Abdominal cavity, free air in, 63, 98
Abdominal irradiation, 342
Abdominal viscera, 307
Abduction, 89
Abscess, 285
Absorption, 138, 201
Acetabulum, 96
    dome of, 47, 83
    RPO position (Judet method) of, 39, 75
Acid-fast bacillus (AFB), 31
Acquired immunodeficiency syndrome (AIDS), 13, 31, 323, 345
Acromegaly, 270, 292
Acromioclavicular (AC) joint, 69, 69*f*, 104
    radiographic examination of, 54, 90
    separation, 59, 94
Acromion process, 256, 257*f*, 264, 277, 286
Acute radiation syndrome, 114, 124, 135, 148
    early symptoms of, 126, 151
Adduction, 62, 89, 96
Advance health care directive, 13, 30, 32
AEC. *See* Automatic exposure control (AEC)
Airborne precautions, 5, 11, 20, 24, 29
    negative-pressure room in, 6, 21
Air–fluid levels, 327
Air kerma, 122, 129, 142, 145, 155
Alcohol-based hand antiseptic sanitizers, 18
Algorithm, 167, 167*f*, 189
Algorithms (computer programs), 264, 286
Aliasing, 244, 249, 266, 288
Aliasing artifact, 167, 189, 332
Allergens, 30
Allergy, 12, 30
Aluminum filters, 119, 123, 142, 146
Aluminum oxide crystals, 122, 145
American Heart Association (AHA), 342
American Registry of Radiologic Technologists (ARRT), 322, 344
Amorphous selenium, 235
Amphiarthrodial joints, 98
Amphiarthrotic joints, 86
Ampoule, 16
Analgesic, effects of, 260, 281
Analog-to-digital converter (ADC), 173, 195, 246
Anaphylactic reaction, contrast agents, 23
Anaphylactic shock, 19
Anaphylaxis, 259, 272, 280, 294

Anatomically programmed radiography (APR), 170, 191
Anatomic compression, during imaging, 116, 138
Anemia, 318, 340
Aneurysms, 12, 29
Angina pectoris, 7, 9, 23, 26, 305, 327
Angulation, 76
Ankle
    AP projection of, 59, 94
    AP stress studies of, 62, 97
    lateral projection of, 55, 91
    medial oblique projection of, 261, 282
Ankle mortise, 39, 74
    15° medial oblique projection, 56, 92
    talofibular articulation, 39, 74, 74*f*
    talotibial articulation, 39, 74, 74*f*
Annual occupational whole-body dose-equivalent limit, 119, 121, 141, 144, 155
    for extremities, 130, 133, 157, 160
    for lens of eye, 131, 157, 158
    for students, 133, 157, 160
Anode, 241
    angle, 227, 244
    cold, excessive heat to, 219, 234
    cooling chart, 227, 227*f*, 244
    focal track, 225, 241
    hazardous technical factors for, 256, 277
    heat hazard to, 218, 234
    heel effect, 173, 183*f*, 194, 201, 203–204, 225, 241, 274, 274*f*, 296, 329, 347
    loss of rotation and melt on focal track, 220, 235
    rotating, 222, 222*f*, 238, 241
    rotor-bearing damage, 219, 234
    stem, 228, 228*f*, 245
Anoxic condition, 283
Anterior inferior iliac spine, 269, 269*f*, 291
Antidote, 30
Antipyretic, in fever, 14, 32
Antisepsis, 11, 28
Antiseptics, 28, 287
Antitussives, 18, 290
Anxiety, reduction of, prior to examination, 4, 18
Aperture diaphragms, 220, 236
Apical pulse, 27
Apophysis, 84, 90, 104
Appendicitis, 106
Apposition, 41, 76
AP recumbent position, 64, 99
ARRT Code of Ethics, 15, 273, 295
ARRT Code of Ethics for the Profession of Radiologic Technology, 344
ARRT Rules of Ethics, 1, 15
Arthrodesis, 283
Arthrography
    knee, 66, 101
    shoulder, 67, 101, 102*f*
Artifacts, 199
Ascites, 269, 270, 291, 292
Asphyxia, 95

Aspiration, 60, 95
Assault, 21, 273, 296
Asthenic patient, 52, 87, 289
Asthma, 280, 294
Asystole, 95
Atelectasis, 15, 74, 76, 95, 101, 261, 282, 336
Atlantoaxial articulation and odontoid process, 44, 44*f*, 80
Atlantoaxial joint, 46, 82–83
Atlas, 71, 106
Atrial septal defect, 25, 90
Attenuation, 117, 139, 179, 201, 256, 276–277, 340
Aura, 24
Autoclaving, 19. *See also* Sterilization
Automated language lines, 28
Automatic brightness control (ABC), 138, 155, 242
Automatic exposure control (AEC), 170, 192, 226, 228, 240, 243, 245, 263, 284, 309, 331
    backup timer functions, 219, 235
    essential function of, 224, 240
    exposure termination, 229, 246
    minimum response time of, 227, 244
    parallel-plate ionization chamber, 243
Automatic exposure control devices, 121, 144, 168, 190, 331
    backup timer in, 168, 190
Automatic exposure rate control (AERC), 219, 234, 247
Automatic implantable cardioverter defibrillators (AICDs), 26
Autonomy, 24
Autotransformer, 224, 241, 272, 272*f*, 295, 308, 329
Avulsion fracture, 44, 80

B

Background (environmental) radiation, sources of, 114, 135
Back strain, reducing of, 5, 20
Bacteria classification, 329
Bacteriocidals, 28
Bacteriostatics, 28
Barium enema (BE), 6, 8, 21, 25, 257, 278
Barium-filled stomach, lateral projections of, 58, 93, 93*f*
Barium sulfate
    contrast examination, 10, 27
    oral administration of, 271, 294
    suspension, 99
        contraindications to, 64, 99
Basic life support (BLS), 342
Battery, 6, 21, 296
Battery-powered mobile units, 226, 243
Beam restriction, 196, 270, 292
    advantages of, 130, 156
Beam restrictors, 125, 150, 220, 236
Beam signals, 168, 321, 343
Beam splitter, 221, 237–238
Becquerel, 155